I0056081

Drug Conception, Design and Manufacturing

Drug Conception, Design and Manufacturing

Edited by **Brendon Krauss**

SYRAWOOD
PUBLISHING HOUSE

New York

Published by Syrawood Publishing House,
750 Third Avenue, 9th Floor,
New York, NY 10017, USA
www.syrawoodpublishinghouse.com

Drug Conception, Design and Manufacturing
Edited by Brendon Krauss

© 2016 Syrawood Publishing House

International Standard Book Number: 978-1-68286-201-8 (Hardback)

This book contains information obtained from authentic and highly regarded sources. Copyright for all individual chapters remain with the respective authors as indicated. All chapters are published with permission under the Creative Commons Attribution License or equivalent. A wide variety of references are listed. Permission and sources are indicated; for detailed attributions, please refer to the permissions page and list of contributors. Reasonable efforts have been made to publish reliable data and information, but the authors, editors and publisher cannot assume any responsibility for the validity of all materials or the consequences of their use.

The publisher's policy is to use permanent paper from mills that operate a sustainable forestry policy. Furthermore, the publisher ensures that the text paper and cover boards used have met acceptable environmental accreditation standards.

Trademark Notice: Registered trademark of products or corporate names are used only for explanation and identification without intent to infringe.

Printed in the United States of America.

Contents

Preface   IX

Chapter 1   **Investigation on *in vitro* dissolution rate enhancement of indomethacin by using a novel carrier sucrose fatty acid ester**   1
Songa Ambedkar Sunil, Meka Venkata Srikanth, Nali Sreenivasa Rao, Vengaladasu Raju and Kolapalli Venkata Ramana Murthy

Chapter 2   **Development and characterization of chitosan-polycarbophil interpolyelectrolyte complex-based 5-fluorouracil formulations for buccal, vaginal and rectal application**   11
Mohamed S Pendekal and Pramod K Tegginamat

Chapter 3   **Effects of tight *versus* non tight control of metabolic acidosis on early renal function after kidney transplantation**   22
Farhad Etezadi, Pejman Pourfakhr, Mojtaba Mojtahedzade, Atabak Najafi, Reza Shariat Moharari, Kourosh Karimi Yarandi and Mohammad Reza Khajavi

Chapter 4   **Evaluation of the antinociceptive and anti-inflammatory effects of essential oil of *Nepeta pogonosperma* Jamzad et Assadi in rats**   28
Taskina Ali, Mohammad Javan, Ali Sonboli and Saeed Semnanian

Chapter 5   **Natural gums as sustained release carriers: development of gastroretentive drug delivery system of ziprasidone HCl**   36
Rajamma AJ, Yogesha HN and Sateesha SB

Chapter 6   **Cost-effectiveness of adding-on new antiepileptic drugs to conventional regimens in controlling intractable seizures in children**   45
Zahra Gharibnaseri, Abbas Kebriaeezadeh, Shekoufeh Nikfar, Gholamreza Zamani and Akbar Abdollahiasl

Chapter 7   **Large scale screening of commonly used Iranian traditional medicinal plants against urease activity**   51
Farzaneh Nabati, Faraz Mojab, Mehran Habibi-Rezaei, Kowsar Bagherzadeh, Massoud Amanlou and Behnam Yousefi

Chapter 8   **Inhibition of HIV and HSV infection by vaginal lactobacilli *in vitro* and *in vivo***   60
Rezvan Zabihollahi, Elahe Motevaseli, Seyed Mehdi Sadat, Ali Reza Azizi-Saraji, Sogol Asaadi-Dalaie and Mohammad Hossein Modarressi

Chapter 9   **Genistein abrogates G2 arrest induced by curcumin in p53 deficient T47D cells**   67
Puji Astuti, Esti D Utami, Arsa W Nugrahani and Sismindari Sudjadi

Chapter 10   *In vitro* α-glucosidase inhibitory activity of phenolic constituents from aerial
parts of *Polygonum hyrcanicum*   74
Fahimeh Moradi-Afrapoli, Behavar Asghari, Soodabeh Saeidnia, Yusef Ajani,
Mobina Mirjani, Maryam Malmir, Reza Dolatabadi Bazaz, Abbas Hadjiakhoondi,
Peyman Salehi, Mattias Hamburger and Narguess Yassa

Chapter 11   **GC-MS analysis of insecticidal essential oil of flowering aerial parts of**
***Saussurea nivea* Turcz**   80
Sha Sha Chu, Guo Hua Jiang and Zhi Long Liu

Chapter 12   **Neuroprotective properties of *Melissa officinalis* after hypoxic-ischemic injury**
both *in vitro* and *in vivo*   85
Mohammad Bayat, Abolfazl Azami Tameh, Mohammad Hossein Ghahremani,
Mohammad Akbari, Shahram Ejtemaei Mehr, Mahnaz Khanavi and
Gholamreza Hassanzadeh

Chapter 13   **Preparation and evaluation of inhalable itraconazole chitosan based polymeric**
micelles   95
Esmaeil Moazeni, Kambiz Gilani, Abdolhossein Rouholamini Najafabadi,
Mohamad Reza Rouini, Nasir Mohajel, Mohsen Amini and
Mohammad Ali Barghi

Chapter 14   **Structural relationships and vasorelaxant activity of monoterpenes**   104
Tamires Cardoso Lima, Marcelo Mendonça Mota, José Maria Barbosa-Filho,
Márcio Roberto Viana Dos Santos and Damião Pergentino De Sousa

Chapter 15   **Terpenes From the Root of *Salvia hypoleuca* Benth**   108
Soodabeh Saeidnia, Mitra Ghamarinia, Ahmad R Gohari *and Alireza Shakeri

Chapter 16   **Formulation and evaluation of microsphere based oro dispersible tablets of**
itopride hcl   114
Sanjay Shah, Sarika Madan and SS Agrawal

Chapter 17   **Anticancer activity of *Pupalia lappacea* on chronic myeloid leukemia K562 cells**   126
Alvala Ravi, Mallika Alvala, Venkatesh Sama, Arunasree M Kalle,
Vamshi K Irlapati and B Madhava Reddy

Chapter 18   **Modified Gadonanotubes as a promising novel MRI contrasting agent**   136
Rouzbeh Jahanbakhsh, Fatemeh Atyabi, Saeed Shanehsazzadeh, Zahra Sobhani,
Mohsen Adeli and Rassoul Dinarvand

Chapter 19   **Design and characterization of diclofenac diethylamine transdermal patch**
using silicone and acrylic adhesives combination   145
Dandigi M Panchaxari, Sowjanya Pampana, Tapas Pal, Bhavana Devabhaktuni
and Anil Kumar Aravapalli

Chapter 20   **Metformin loaded non-ionic surfactant vesicles: optimization of formulation,**
effect of process variables and characterization   159
Anchal Sankhyan and Pravin K Pawar

Chapter 21   **Design and evaluation of Lumefantrine – Oleic acid self nanoemulsifying ionic**
complex for enhanced dissolution   167
Ketan Patel, Vidur Sarma and Pradeep Vavia

Chapter 22   **Isolation and characterization of exopolysaccharide with immunomodulatory activity from fermentation broth of *Morchella conica***   **177**
Chao-an Su, Xiao-yan Xu, De-yun Liu, Ming Wu, Fan-qing Zeng, Meng-yao Zeng, Wei Wei, Nan Jiang and Xia Luo

Chapter 23   **Biological activity and microscopic characterization of *Lythrum salicaria* L**   **183**
Azadeh Manayi, Mahnaz Khanavi, Soodabeh Saiednia, Ebrahim Azizi, Mohammad Reza Mahmoodpour, Fatemeh Vafi, Maryam Malmir, Farideh Siavashi and Abbas Hadjiakhoondi

Chapter 24   **A cytotoxic hydroperoxy sterol from the brown alga, *Nizamuddinia zanardinii***   **190**
Maryam Hamzeloo Moghadam, Jamileh Firouzi, Soodabeh Saeidnia, Homa Hajimehdipoor, Shahla Jamili, Abdolhossein Rustaiyan and Ahmad R Gohari

Chapter 25   **Anti-inflammatory effects of apo-9′-fucoxanthinone from the brown alga, *Sargassum muticum***   **194**
Eun-Jin Yang, Young Min Ham, Wook Jae Lee, Nam Ho Lee and Chang-Gu Hyun

Chapter 26   **Statistical optimization of a novel excipient (CMEC) based gastro retentive floating tablets of propranolol HCl and it's *in vivo* buoyancy characterization in healthy human volunteers**   **201**
Venkata Srikanth Meka, Sreenivasa Rao Nali, Ambedkar Sunil Songa, Janaki Ram Battu and Venkata Ramana Murthy Kolapalli

Chapter 27   **A system dynamics model for national drug policy**   **213**
Akbar Abdollahiasl, Abbas Kebriaeezadeh, Rassoul Dinarvand, Mohammad Abdollahi, Abdol Majid Cheraghali, Mona Jaberidoost and Shekoufeh Nikfar

Permissions

List of Contributors

Preface

The process of drug design and manufacturing has undergone a lot of change with time owing to scientific and technological advances. This book contains some path-breaking studies conducted across the world in the field of drug design and manufacturing. Topics such as formulation, conception, classification, assessment, clinical investigation of drugs, etc. have been covered within this book. It compiles contributions made by eminent scientists and researchers. It would be very useful for graduate and post graduate students pursuing pharmacology or associated fields of study.

This book has been the outcome of endless efforts put in by authors and researchers on various issues and topics within the field. The book is a comprehensive collection of significant researches that are addressed in a variety of chapters. It will surely enhance the knowledge of the field among readers across the globe.

It gives us an immense pleasure to thank our researchers and authors for their efforts to submit their piece of writing before the deadlines. Finally in the end, I would like to thank my family and colleagues who have been a great source of inspiration and support.

Editor

Investigation on *in vitro* dissolution rate enhancement of indomethacin by using a novel carrier sucrose fatty acid ester

Songa Ambedkar Sunil*, Meka Venkata Srikanth, Nali Sreenivasa Rao, Vengaladasu Raju and Kolapalli Venkata Ramana Murthy

Abstract

Background and the purpose of the study: The purpose of the present investigation was to characterize and evaluate solid dispersions (SD) of indomethacin by using a novel carrier sucrose fatty acid ester (SFE 1815) to increase its in vitro drug release and further formulating as a tablet.

Methods: Indomethacin loaded SD were prepared by solvent evaporation and melt granulation technique using SFE 1815 as carrier in 1:0.25, 1:0.5 1:0.75 and 1:1 ratios of drug and carrier. Prepared SD and tablets were subjected to in vitro dissolution studies in 900 mL of pH 7.2 phosphate buffer using apparatus I at 100 rpm. The promising SD were further formulated as tablets using suitable diluent (DCL 21, Avicel PH 102 and pregelatinised starch) to attain the drug release similar to that of SD.. The obtained dissolution data was subjected to kinetic study by fitting the data into various model independent models like zero order, first order, Higuchi, Hixon-Crowell and Peppas equations. Drug and excipient compatibility studies were confirmed by fourier transform infrared spectroscopy, X-ray diffraction, differential scanning calorimetry and scanning electron microscopy.

Results: The in vitro dissolution data exhibited superior release from formulation S_6 with 1:0.5 drug and carrier ratio using solvent evaporation technique than other SDs prepared at different ratio using solvent evaporation and melt granulation technique. The in vitro drug release was also superior to that of the physical mixtures prepared at same ratio and also superior to SD prepared using common carriers like polyvinyl pyrollidone and PEG 4000 by solvent evaporation technique. Tablets (T_8) prepared with DCL21 as diluent exhibited superior release than the other tablets. The tablet formulation (T_8) followed first order release with Non-Fickian release.

Conclusion: SFE 1815 a novel third generation carrier can be used for the preparation of SD for the enhancement of *in vitro* drug release of indomethacin an insoluble drug belonging to BCS class II.

Keywords: Solid dispersions, Indomethacin, Sucrose Fatty Acid Ester, Dissolution rate

Introduction

The therapeutic efficacy of a drug product intended to be administered by the oral route depends upon its absorption in the gastro-intestinal tract to end with bioavailability. It is well established that dissolution is recurrently the rate-limiting step in the gastrointestinal absorption of a drug from a solid dosage form which belongs to BCS class II (low soluble and high permeable). The drug release from poorly soluble drugs has been shown to be unpredictable and still remains a problem to the pharmaceutical industry [1]. Several methods that have been employed to improve the solubility of poorly water soluble drugs include increasing the particle surface area available for dissolution by milling [2], improving the wettability with surfactants or doped crystals [3], decreasing crystallinity by preparing a solid dispersion [4], use of inclusion compounds such as cyclodextrin derivatives [5], use of polymorphic forms or solvated compounds [6] and use of salt forms. There are several advantages and disadvantages for the above given methods. Solid dispersions (SD) represent an ideal pharmaceutical technique for increasing the dissolution, absorption and

* Correspondence: sunilsonga@gmail.com
A.U. College of Pharmaceutical Sciences, Andhra University, Visakhapatnam, 530003 India

therapeutic efficacy of drugs with poor aqueous solubility. The term "solid dispersion" refers to the dispersion of one or more active ingredients in an inert carrier or matrix in the solid state prepared by melting, solvent, or melting solvent methods [7] which has been used by various researchers who have reported encouraging results with different drugs [8]. The method of preparation and the type of the carrier used are important in influencing the properties of such solid dispersions [9]. Among the carriers used in the formation of solid dispersions, polyethylene glycol and polyvinyl pyrrolidone are the most commonly used. The first generation (urea) and second generation (PEG, polyvinyl pyrrolidone, HPMC, hydroxylpropyl cellulose, starch derivatives, cyclodextrins) of carriers have many disadvantages when compared to the use of third generation carriers (poloxamer, gelucire, sucrose fatty acid esters) which are non-ionic and led to development of superior solid dispersions.

Sucrose fatty acid esters (SFE) are nonionic surface active agents which are mono-, di-, and tri-esters of sucrose with fatty acids, manufactured from purified sugar or hydrogenated edible tallow or edible vegetable oils. These consist of sucrose residues as the hydrophilic group or polar head and fatty acid residues as the lipophilic group or non-polar head with a unique emulsification property that tolerates any temperature variation [10,11]. SFE are currently regulated by the U.S. Food and Drug Administration (FDA) as food additives under chapter 21, section 172.859 of the Federal Code of Regulations (CFR). However, studies of SFE in the area of commonly used tablet formulations are limited and emphasize using specific types of SFE for particular approaches. These are non-toxic and biodegradable, as they can be enzymatically hydrolyzed to sucrose and fatty acids prior to intestinal absorption or excreted in faeces, depending on the degree of esterfication with a wide range of HLB values 1 – 16 [12,13].

The present investigation was focused on exploring sucrose fatty acid ester as a drug carrier to increase the drug solubility and the dissolution rate of indomethacin by formation of solid dispersions using various methods. The dissolution characteristics and physicochemical modification of the indomethacin-SFE solid dispersions were investigated by in vitro dissolution test, FTIR, XRD, SEM and thermal analysis (DSC). These solid dispersions were formulated into tablets after optimizing with suitable diluent used in the study and were evaluated for physicochemical characterization.

Experimental
Materials
Indomethacin was a gift sample from Macleods pharmaceuticals Ltd. India. Sucrose fatty acid ester 1815 was obtained from Mitsubishi-Kagaku Foods Corporation,

Japan. Avicel PH 102 was obtained from FMC Biopolymer. DCL 21 was purchased from Zeel Pharmaceuticals, India. All other chemicals were of reagent grade and used as received.

Methods
Composition of solid dispersions
Solid dispersions contained of 1:0.25, 1:0.5, 1:0.75 and 1:1 of indomethacin and SFE 1815 prepared by melt granulation and solvent evaporation methods. Physical mixtures were prepared only for the promising ratio for comparision. Table 1 lists the solid dispersions prepared along with the method employed for preparation, composition and codes.

Preparation of solid dispersions
Melt granulation method
Accurately weighed amounts of carrier were placed in an aluminum pan on a hot plate and melted, with constant stirring, at a temperature of about 50 °C. An accurately weighed amount of indomethacin was incorporated into the melted carrier with stirring to ensure homogeneity. The mixture was heated until a clear homogeneous melt was obtained. The pan was then removed from the hot plate and allowed to cool at room temperature and the obtained damp mass is passed through sieve no #40. The granules obtained were transferred to a polybag and stored in desiccator for further studies.

Solvent evaporation method
Accurately weighed amounts of indomethacin and carrier (SFE 1815) were dissolved in minimum quantities of methanol in a china dish. The solution was stirred till slurry was formed. The solvent was evaporated under reduced pressure at 40 °C, and the resulting residue was dried under vacuum for 3 h, stored in a desiccator at

Table 1 Composition of different SD using SFE 1815

Code name	Method	Polymer	Ratio (Drug: polymer)
S_1	Melt Granulation	SFE 1815	1:0.25
S_2			1:0.5
S_3			1:0.75
S_4			1:1
S_5	Solvent Evaporation	SFE 1815	1:0.25
S_6			1:0.5
S_7			1:0.75
S_8			1:1
S_9	Physical Mixing	SFE 1815	1:0.5
S_{10}	Solvent Evaporation	PVP	1:0.5
S_{11}	Solvent Evaporation	PEG 4000	1:0.5

least overnight, ground in a mortar, and passed through mesh no #40.

Physical mixtures
Physical mixtures were obtained by pulverizing accurately weighed amounts of drug and polymer in a glass mortar and carefully mixed until a homogeneous mixture was obtained. Drug and carrier ratio of 1:0.5 were prepared and subsequently stored at room temperature in desiccator.

Preparation of tablets
SD powder, diluents, disintegrant and binder were weighed as per formulae given in Table 2, these were then passed through sieve no # 40, transferred to a poly bag and blended for 5 min. To this homogeneous blend, magnesium stearate presifted through # 60 was added and blended for 2 min. The resulting blend was compressed on Cadmach 16 station compression machine under a common compression force of 2-3 Kg/cm^2, using 6 mm, round, flat faced punches.

In vitro dissolution studies
Powder equivalent to indomethacin 25 mg for SD and tablets were introduced into dissolution medium. The dissolution medium is 900 mL of phosphate buffer pH 7.2, rotational speed of the basket was set at 100 rpm at 37 ± 0.5 °C. Aliquots (5 ml each) were withdrawn at predetermined time intervals by means of a syringe fitted with a 0.45 μm pre-filter and immediately replaced with 5 mL of fresh medium maintained at 37 ± 0.5 °C. The samples were analyzed for indomethacin using U.V. double beam Elico SL 210 model at 318 nm. For comparison, dissolution studies of pure indomethacin and INDOCAP marketed capsules along with PM and SD prepared with polyvinyl pyrollidone (PVP) and PEG 4000 at drug and polymer ratio of 1:0.5 employing solvent evaporation technique were also performed. All the dissolution experiments were carried out in triplicate. Comparison of dissolution profiles was done to quantify the difference in rate and extent of drug release as

influenced by the formulation and process variables in order to find out the mode of drug release and their kinetics.

Release kinetics
As a model-dependent approach, the dissolution data was fitted to five popular release models such as zero-order, first-order, Higuchi [14], Hixon-Crowel [15] and Korsmeyer -peppas equations. The order of drug release from matrix systems was described by using zero order kinetics or first orders kinetics. The mechanism of drug release from matrix systems was studied by using Higuchi and Hixon-Crowel equation. Model with the highest coefficient correlation (r) was judged to be a more appropriate model for the dissolution data.

According to Korsmeyer-Peppas equation, the release exponent n value is used to characterize different release mechanisms. If the n value is 0.5, the release mechanism follows Fickian diffusion. If n value is >0.45 or <0.89, the mechanism follows non-Fickian (anomalous) diffusion and when n = 0.89 it will be non-Fickian case II and if n > 0.89 it will be non-Fickian super case II transport [16]. The equations for different models are represented in Table 3.

Fourier transform infrared spectroscopy
FTIR spectra can be used to detect drug excipient interactions by following the shift in vibrational or stretching bands of key functional groups. FTIR spectra were obtained by using Alpha FTIR spectrophotometer (Bruker Optik GmbH, Germany). All the spectra were analyzed using OPUS 6.5 software. Samples were prepared by KBr pellet method, which had been prepared by gently mixing 1 mg of the sample with 200 mg of KBr. The spectra were scanned over a wave number range of 4000 - 500 cm^{-1}.

X-ray diffraction
The physical state of indomethacin in different samples was evaluated with X-ray powder diffraction. XRD is a powerful tool in detecting crystallinity. The X-ray

Table 2 Formulae of tablets

Formulation	T_1	T_2	T_3	T_4	T_5	T_6	T_7	T_8	T_9
Indo + SD	37.5	37.5	37.5	37.5	37.5	37.5	37.5	37.5	37.5
Pregelatinised Starch	25	55	75						
Avicel PH 102				25	55	75			
DCL 21							25	55	75
Crocarmellose Sodium	3	3	3	3	3	3	3	3	3
PVP K 30	3	3	3	3	3	3	3	3	3
Magnesium Stearate	1.5	1.5	1.5	1.5	1.5	1.5	1.5	1.5	1.5

Table 3 Mathematical models for comparison of dissolution profiles

Model	Equation
Zero-order	$Q_t = Q_0 + K_0$
First-order	$\ln Q_t = \ln Q_0 - K_1 t$
Higuchi	$Q_t = K_H \sqrt{t}$
Hixon-Crowell	$Q_r^{1/3} - Q_t^{1/3} = K_s t$
Korsmeyer-Peppas	$Q_t / Q_\infty = K_k t^n$

Q_t: amount of drug released in time t, Q_0: initial amount of drug in the Tablet, Q_r: remaining amount of the drug in tablet, Q_∞: fraction of drug released at time t, K_0, K_1, K_H, K_s, K_K – Rate order constants.

diffraction patterns were recorded on X-Ray diffractometer (PW 1729, Philips, Netherlands). XRD patterns were recorded using monochromatic Cu Kα radiation with Nitrogen filter at a voltage of 40 keV and a current of 40 mA. The sample was analyzed over 2θ range of 5-30° and the data was processed with Diffrac Plus V1.01 software.

Differential scanning calorimetry

DSC is a frequently used thermo analytical technique that generates data on melting endotherms and glass transitions. DSC was performed utilizing Mettler DSC 821 (Mettler-Toledo, Switzerland). Samples of 3-4 mg were encapsulated and hermetically sealed in flat bottomed aluminum pan with crimped on lid. Samples were allowed to equilibrate for 1 min and then heated in a nitrogen atmosphere over a temperature range from 25 °C to 240 °C with a heating rate of 5 °C/min. An empty aluminum pan is served as reference. Nitrogen was used as a purge gas, at the flow rate of 20 mL/min for all the studies. Reproducibility was checked by running the sample in triplicate. Thermograms were obtained by the STAR^e SW 9.10 software and reported.

Scanning electron microscopy

SEM has been employed to study the morphology of the samples. The samples were mounted on the SEM sample stab, using a double sided sticking tape and coated with gold (200 A°) under reduced pressure (0.001 torr) for 5 min using an ion sputtering device (Jeol JFC-1100 E, Japan). The gold coated samples were observed under the SEM (JEOL JSM-840A, Japan) and photomicrographs of suitable magnifications were obtained with the aid of a software system (LINK^{ISIS}, Oxford, UK).

Results and discussion
In vitro dissolution studies
Solid dispersions

Gradual increase in drug release of the prepared SD was observed with increase in concentration of the polymer up to an extent, further increase in concentration did not increase the drug release. Maximum drug release was obtained at the end of 30 min for S_6 by solvent evaporation technique using SFE 1815 polymer in 1:0.5 drug and polymer ratio. Whereas using the same polymer but employing melt granulation technique gave less drug release. The enhanced drug releases from SD prepared with solvent evaporation technique in this study are in co-relation with the previous study conducted by Patel et al. on SD prepared using PEG 6000 and PVP using solvent evaporation and melting methods [17]. Only 35.10%, 63.90%, 68.78% and 73.54% drug release was observed form pure drug, S_9 (PM), SD using PVP (S_{10}) and PEG 4000 (S_{11}) respectively in 30 min, whereas

99.77% drug was released from S_6 which is shown in Figure 1. Earlier workers also tried out to enhance the dissolution of indomethacin by SD technique, El-Badry et al. prepared SD using PEG4000 and Gelucire 50/13 using hot melting method, results have shown that more amount of carrier was required and also 90 min was required for complete release of drug [18]. The capability to enhance or increase the drug release and bioavailability of the insoluble drug by SFE 1815 depends upon the common factors like excellent wettability, which could be observed clearly from the solid dispersion since it rapidly left the surface and was dispersed in the bulk of the dissolution medium which markedly increased indomethacin solubility and also specific features like (i) HLB value – higher the HLB value greater is the ability to enhance (ii) length of fatty acid chain - shorter fatty acid increases the release more than the longer fatty acids [19] (iii) number of carbon atoms in the fatty acid chain [19] (v) proportion of monoesters –higher the proportion of monoesters higher is the hydrophilicity of the surfactant [12,20,21]. The main reason for better drug release of SD using SFE 1815 is the HLB value which is 15 and the number of monoesters (70%) in the ester composition of the carrier. The comparative dissolution profiles of S_6 with SD prepared with other carriers, PM prepared with same ratio as S_6, pure drug and marketed capsule are given in Figure 2.

It is well known from the literature and practical knowledge that the SD are unstable as such, but stable when formulated as a tablet dosage form. The best SD (S_6) prepared by solvent evaporation technique in 1:0.5 of drug: SFE1815 ratio was selected for the development of tablets, which gave a superior and enhanced release profile than SD prepared by melt granulation using same carrier, SD prepared by common carriers by solvent evaporation technique and PM.

Tablets were developed using different diluents (pregelatinised starch, Avicel PH102 and DLC 21) in different concentrations (25%, 55% and 75%). More than 99% of the drug was released from all the formulations. T_8 formulation with 55% w/w of DCL21 gave maximum drug release in 30 min. The initial lag in drug release when compared with SD was due to the disintegration time required for the tablet and the profiles are shown in Figure 3.

Even though pregelatinised starch is more soluble than Avicel PH102 the percent of drug released from the tablets was less when compared to Avicel PH102. The possible reason for that release could be the swelling nature of pregelatinsed starch [22]. As the concentration of the pregelatinized starch was increased, the percent of drug release decreased, which is one of the reason for its use in the development of sustained release tablets [23]. Tablets prepared with DCL 21 as diluent gave better

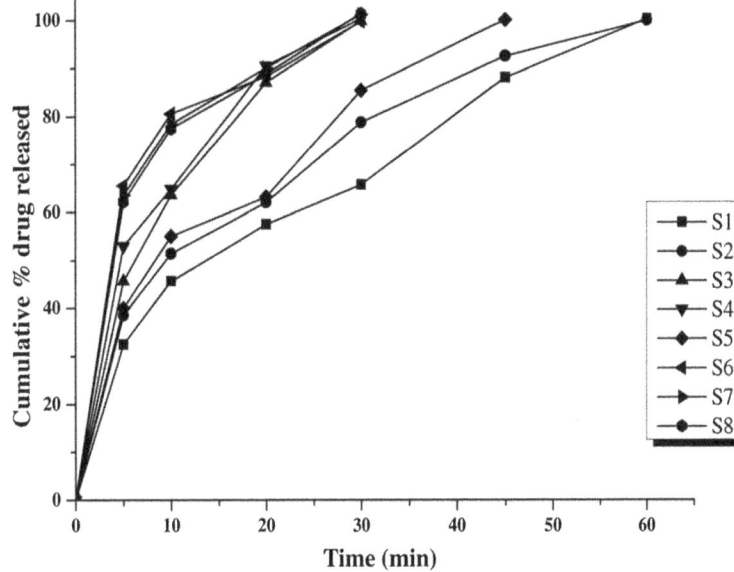

Figure 1 Dissolution profiles of solid dispersions with SFE 1815 as carrier, S_1–S_4 (melt granulation), S_5–S_8 (solvent evaporation).

release than those prepared with Avicel PH 102 due to the more hydrophilic nature and solubility of DCL 21.

Release kinetics

The drug release of indomethacin from the formulations T_2 and T_3 followed zero order kinetics which was indicated by higher 'r' values of zero order release model. T_1, T_4, T_5, T_6, T_7, T_8, and T_9 followed first order release model which was indicated by the higher 'r' value.

The relative contributions of drug diffusion and erosion to drug release were further confirmed by subjecting the dissolution data to Higuchi model and Hixon Crowell model. It was found that T_2 and T_3 followed zero order kinetics with Non-Fickian diffusion mechanism. T_1, T_4, T_5, T_7, T_8 and T_9 followed first order with Non-Fickian diffusion mechanism. T_6 formulation followed first order release with erosion mechanism as the 'r' value obtained is greater for Hixon Crowell mechanism.

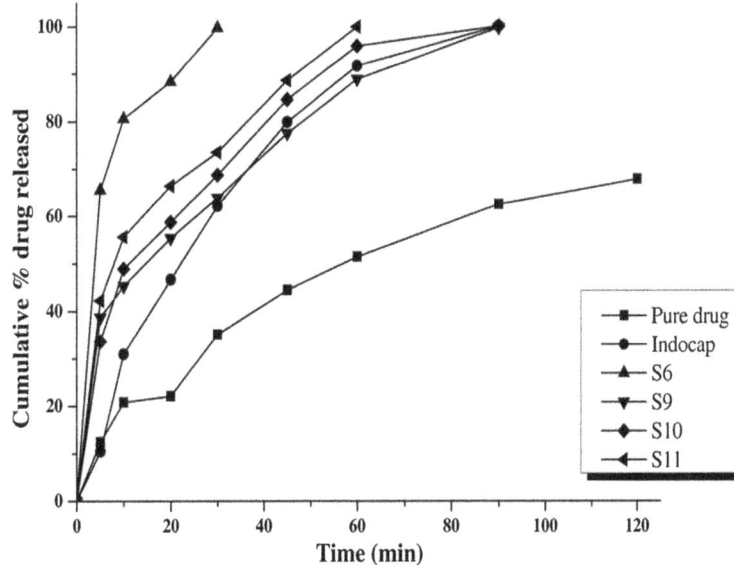

Figure 2 Comparative dissolution profiles of solid dispersions S_6 (SFE 1815), S_9 (physical mixtures), S_{10} (PVP), S_{11} (PEG 4000) along with pure drug and marketed capsule (Indocap).

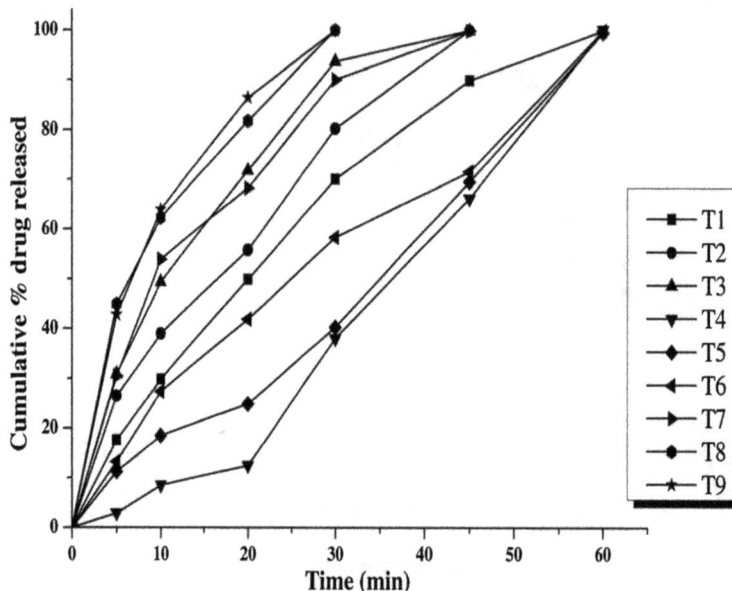

Figure 3 Dissolution profiles of tablets prepared with different diluents A) T_{1-3} (pregelatinised starch), T_{4-6} (Avicel PH102) and T_{7-9} (DCL 21).

The promising tablet formulation T_8 followed first order release with Non-Fickian diffusion mechanism. Results of various order plots for the tablets are shown in Table 4.

Fourier transform infrared spectroscopy

Pure indomethacin spectra showed characteristic peaks at 3020 cm^{-1} (aromatic C-H stretching), 2965 cm^{-1} (C-H stretching vibrations), 1761 cm^{-1} (C = O stretching vibrations), 1261 cm^{-1} (asymmetric aromatic O-C stretching), 1086 cm^{-1} (symmetric aromatic O-H stretching).

SD (S_6) and tablet formulation (T_8) also exhibited the characteristic peaks of indomethacin with no additional peaks observed in the spectra, indicating retention of chemical identity of indomethacin as shown in Figure 4. However, intensity of peaks corresponding to the drug was reduced or broadened in the SD and tablet formulations, possibly due to the mixing with the surfactant and addition of other excipients. The FTIR spectra data confirmed that SFE 1815 did not alter the performance characteristics indicating their compatibility of the drug.

X-ray diffraction

The X-ray diffractograms of pure drug indomethacin and promising formulations are shown in Figure 5. The diffractogram of indomethacin showed characteristic sharp intensity diffraction peaks at 2θ values of 11.51°, 12.76°, 16.62°, 19.54°, 21.84°, 22.78°, 26.64°, 27.47° and 29.35°, which reflected the crystalline nature of drug. Both the formulations (S_6 and T_8), showed diffraction peaks at respective 2θ values of pure indomethacin although their relative intensities were reduced or there was slight shift in their peaks, suggesting reduced degree of crystallinity of drug in these formulations.

Differential scanning calorimetry

The DSC thermogram of pure indomethacin exhibited a sharp endothermic peak at 164 °C corresponding to its melting point, indicating its crystalline nature. SFE 1815 showed endothermic melting peak at 54.2 °C. There is a shift in the melting peak of indomethacin in SD (S_6) and tablet (T_8) to 158.2 °C and 158.4 °C respectively as indicated in Figure 6. The shift observed in the melting peak of indomethacin in the formulations may be due to physical interaction between the drug and excipient. Compared to pure drug the melting peak was broadened to some extent in the formulations which may be due to changes in its crystalline form.

Table 4 Kinetic models of core tablets

Model	Zero Order		First order		Higuchi	Hixon-Crowel	Pepas	
Batch	R	K_0	r	K	r	r	r	n
T_1	0.990	1.56	0.998	0.028	0.979	0.928	0.995	0.771
T_2	0.991	1.587	0.958	0.024	0.931	0.915	0.979	0.858
T_3	0.982	1.687	0.944	0.023	0.893	0.888	0.986	0.881
T_4	0.977	1.66	0.984	0.049	0.990	0.985	0.997	0.719
T_5	0.979	2.10	0.983	0.051	0.992	0.968	0.996	0.610
T_6	0.938	2.13	0.976	0.087	0.993	0.997	0.991	0.552
T_7	0.937	2.07	0.982	0.072	0.994	0.993	0.984	0.532
T_8	0.935	2.97	0.992	0.083	0.998	0.973	0.999	0.560
T_9	0.934	3.05	0.999	0.099	0.998	0.990	0.995	0.573

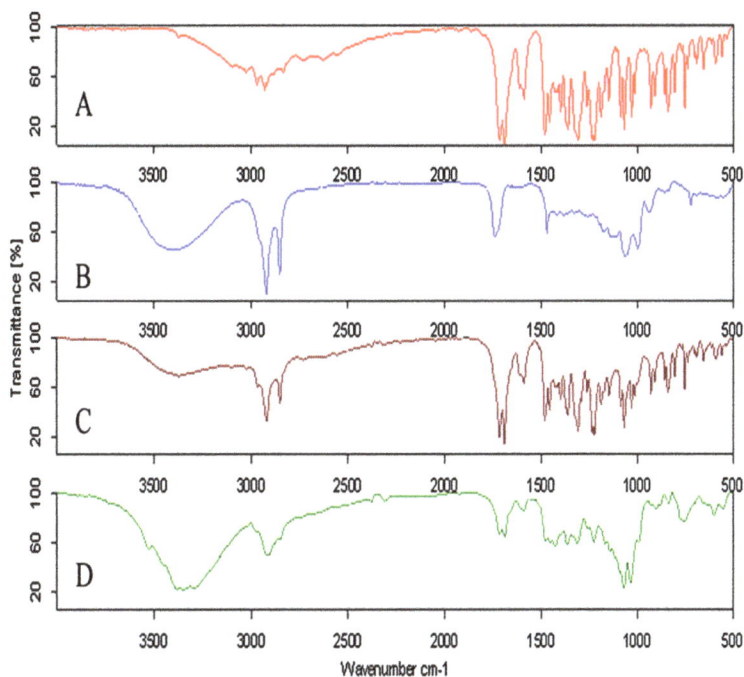

Figure 4 FTIR spectra of A) indomethacin, B) SFE 1815, C) S_6 and D) T_8.

Scanning electron microscopy

Figure 7, demonstrates the surface morphology of pure indomethacin as crystalline in nature. Surface morphology of S_6 and T_8 indicated that the individual surface properties of drug were changed during the compression process and surfactant might have been adsorbed on to the drug during the preparation of SD. The appearance of the solid dispersion was homogenous, with partial loss of drug crystallinity and reduction in particle size, which may be reason for faster dissolution of the drug and which was further confirmed by DSC and XRD studies.

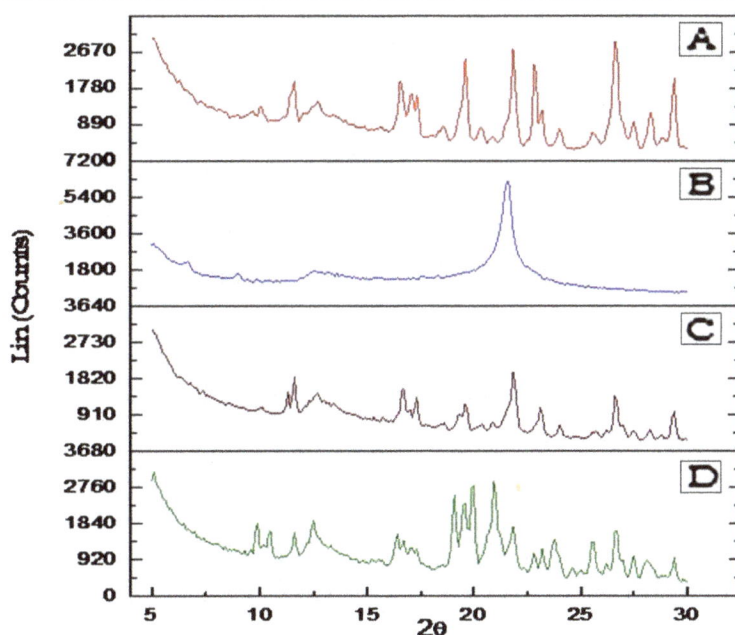

Figure 5 X-ray diffractograms of A) Indomethacin, B) SFE 1815 C) S_6 and D) T_8.

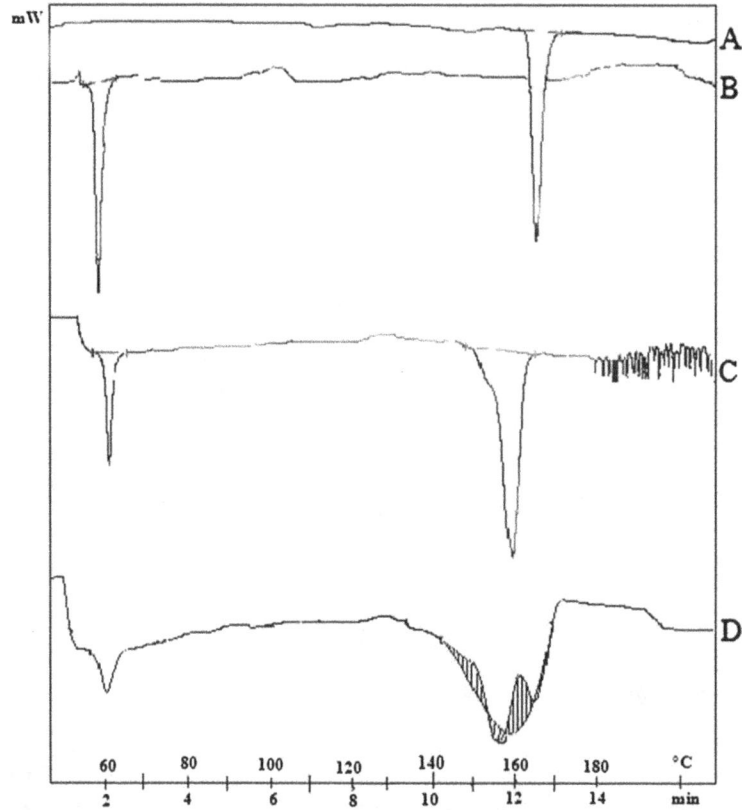

Figure 6 DSC chromatographs of A) Indomethacin B) SFE 1815 C) S_6 D) T_8.

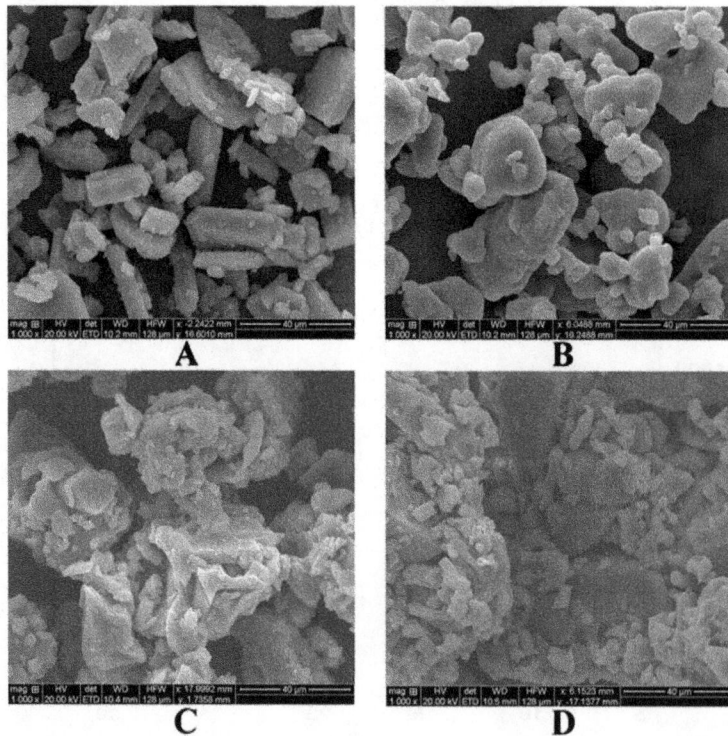

Figure 7 SEM photographs of A) Indomethacin, B) SFE1815 C) S_6 D) T_8.

Conclusion

This study clearly shows that SD of indomethacin with SFE 1815 employing solvent evaporation technique improves their dissolution rates. Solvent evaporation techniques used in the present study requires very few quantity of organic solvent and absence of specialized equipment. Mechanisms involved are solubilisation and improved wetting of the drug [24] in the SFE 1815 rich micro-environment formed at the surface of drug crystals after dissolution of the polymer [25]. Solid dispersions formulated with SFE 1815 improved the dissolution rate compared with physical mixtures and SD formulated using PVP and PEG 4000 at the same concentrations. As SFE 1815 belongs to third generation by virtue of their efficiency to increase the surface area and wide range of HLB, these are more efficient than other commonly used carriers to increase the solubility and dissolution. There are no reports to date on the usage of SFE 1815 as carriers. The crystallinity of the drugs was reduced in all solid dispersions which were evident from the XRD graphs and decreased intensity of the peaks from DSC thermograms. The same enhanced release was observed from the SD formulated as tablet dosage form with DCL21 as diluent.

Competing interests

The author(s) declare that they have no competing interests.

Acknowledgement

The author S. A. Sunil is thankful to UGC (University Grants Commission, India) for awarding senior research fellowship for carrying out this research. One of the authors S. A. Sunil is thankful to B. Janaki Ram, M. Chaithanya Krishna and G. Sirisha for providing valuable information to carry out this research work.

Author details

A.U. College of Pharmaceutical Sciences, Andhra University, Visakhapatnam, 530003 India.

Authors' contributions

SAS: The main author involved in the literature survey, compilation, acquisition of data, planning design and carrying out the research work, interpretation of data along with review of intellectual content and drafting of the final manuscript titled "Investigation on *in vitro* dissolution rate enhancement of indomethacin by using a novel carrier sucrose fatty acid ester". MVS: Co- research scholar who was involved in design of experimental formulas, carrying out the bench work for formulation of the solid dispersions and carrying out the dissolution studies. NSR: Co-research scholar involved in the analytical method development and interpretation of the FTIR studies. VR: Senior research scholar involved in the study, procurement of the novel third generation carrier sucrose fatty acid ester along with the softwares required for interpretation and drawing of dissolution profiles. KVRM: Research guide, who gave valuable suggestions in the design of experimental formulas, interpretation of the dissolution data along with the carrier role in the enhancement, critical review of the manuscript for intellectual content, vital and crucial review and approval of the final manuscript to be published. He also granted me permission to carry out research activities along with use of the equipment in the laboratory. All the above authors read and approved the final manuscript.

References

1. Ghebremeskel AN, Vemavarapu C, Lodayam M: Use of surfactants as plasticizers in preparing solid dispersions of poorly soluble API: Selection of polymer-surfactant combinations using solubility parameters and testing the processability. *Int J Pharm* 2007, 328:119–129.
2. Habib FS, Attia MA: Effect of particle size on the dissolution rate of monophenylbutazone solid dispersion in presence of certain additives. *Drug Dev Ind Pharm* 1985, 11:2009–2019.
3. Chow AHL, Hsia CK, Gordon JD, Young JWM, Vargha-Butler EI: Assessment of wettability and its relationship to the intrinsic dissolution rate of doped phenytoin crystals. *Int J Pharm* 1995, 126:21–28.
4. Flego C, Lovrecich M, Rubessa F: Dissolution rate of griseofulvin from solid dispersion with poly(vinylmethylether: maleic anhydride). *Drug Dev Ind Pharm* 1988, 14:1185–1202.
5. Pitha J: Amorphous water-soluble derivatives of cyclodextrins: nontoxic dissolution enhancing excipients. *J Pharm Sci* 1985, 74:987–990.
6. Sekiguchi K, Kanke M, Tsuda Y, Ishida K, Tsuda T: Dissolution behavior of solid drugs. III. Determination of the transition temperature between the hydrate and anhydrous forms of phenobarbital by measuring their dissolution rates. *Chem Pharm Bull* 1973, 21:1592–1600.
7. Chiou WL, Riegelman S: Pharmaceutical applications of solid dispersion systems. *J Pharm Sci* 1971, 60:1281–1302.
8. Sheu MT, Yeh CM, Sokoloski TD: Characterization and dissolution of fenofibrate solid dispersion systems. *Int J Pharm* 1994, 103:137–146.
9. Otsuka M, Onone M, Matsuda Y: Hygroscopic stability and dissolution properties of spray-dried solid dispersion of furosemide with Eudragit. *J Pharm Sci* 1996, 82:32–38.
10. Garti N, Clement V, Leser M, Aserin A, Fanun M: Sucrose ester microemulsions. *J Mol Liq* 1999, 80:253–96.
11. Muller AS, Gagnaire J, Queneau Y, Karaoglanian M, Maitre JP, Bouchu A: Winsor behaviour of sucrose fatty acid esters: choice of the cosurfactant and effect of the surfactant composition. *Colloids Surf A: Physicochem Eng Aspects* 2002, 203:55–66.
12. Shigeoka T, Izawa O, Kitazawa K, Yamauchi F: Studies on the metabolic fate of sucrose esters in rats. *Food Chem Toxicol* 1984, 22:409–14.
13. Noker PE, Lin TH, Hill DL, Shigeoka T: Metabolism of 14C-labelled sucrose esters of stearic acid in rats. *Food Chem Toxicol* 1997, 35:589–95.
14. Higuchi T: Mechanism of sustained-action medication. Theoretical analysis of rate of release of solid drugs dispersed in solid matrices. *J Pharm Sci* 1963, 52:1145–1149.
15. Hixson AW, Crowell JH: Dependence of reaction velocity upon surface and agitation. I. Theoretical considerations. *Ind Eng Chem* 1931, 23:923–931.
16. Peppas NA: Analysis of fickian and non-fickian drug release from polymers. *Pharm Acta Helv* 1985, 60:110–111.
17. Rakesh PP, Dhaval JP, Dipen BB, Jayvadan KP: Physicochemical characterization and dissolution study of solid dispersions of furosemide with polyethylene glycol 6000 and polyvinylpyrollidone K30. *Dissolution technologies* 2008, 15:17–25.
18. Mahmoud E, Gihan F, Mohamed F: Improvement of solubility and dissolution rate of indomethacin by solid dispersions n Gelucire 50/13 and PEG4000. *Saudi Pharmaceutical Journal* 2009, 17:217–225.
19. Zelko R, Orban A, Suvegh K: Tracking of the physical ageing of amorphous pharmaceutical polymeric excipients by positron annihilation spectroscopy. *J Pharm Biomed Anal* 2006, 40:249–254.
20. Husband FA, Samey DB, Barnard MJ, Wilde PJ: Comparison of foaming and interfacial properties of pure sucrose monolaurates, dilaurate and commercial preparations. *Food Hydrocolloids* 1998, 12:237–44.
21. Tual A, Bourles E, Barey P, Houdoux A, Desprairies M, Courthaudon JL: Effect of surfactant sucrose ester on physical properties of dairy whipped emulsions in relation to those of O/W interfacial layers. *J Colloid Interf Sci* 2006, 295:495–503.
22. Levina M, Ali R, Rajabi S: The Influence of excipients on drug release from hydroxypropyl methylcellulose matrices. *J Pharm Sci* 2004, 93:2746–2754.
23. Suvakanta D, Murthy PN, Lilakanta N, Chowdhury P: Kinetic modeling on drug release from controlled drug delivery systems. *Acta Poloniae Pharmaceutica drug research* 2010, 67:217–223.

24. Ahuja N, Katare OP, Singh B: **Studies on dissolution enhancement and mathematical modelling of drug release of a poorly water-soluble drug using water soluble carriers.** *Eur J Pharm Biopharm* 2007, **65:**26–38.
25. Craig DQM: **The mechanism of drug release from solid dispersion in water-soluble polymers.** *Int J Pharm* 2002, **231:**131–144.

Development and characterization of chitosan-polycarbophil interpolyelectrolyte complex-based 5-fluorouracil formulations for buccal, vaginal and rectal application

Mohamed S Pendekal* and Pramod K Tegginamat

Abstract

Background of the study: The present investigation was designed with the intention to formulate versatile 5-fluorouracil (5-FU) matrix tablet that fulfills the therapeutic needs that are lacking in current cancer treatment and aimed at minimizing toxic effect, enhancing efficacy and increasing patient compliance. The manuscript presents the critical issues of 5-FU associate with cancer and surpasses issues by engineering novel 5-FU matrix tablets utilizing chitosan- polycarbophil interpolyelectrolyte complex (IPEC).

Methods: Precipitation method is employed for preparation of chitosan and polycarbophil interpolyelectrolyte complex (IPEC) followed by characterization with Fourier transform infrared spectroscopy (FT-IR), Differential Scanning calorimeter (DSC) and X-ray Diffraction (XRD). 5-FU tablets were prepared by direct compression using IPEC. Six formulations were prepared with IPEC alone and in combination with chitosan, polycarbophil and Sodium deoxycholate. The formulations were tested for drug content, hardness, friability, weight variation, thickness, swelling studies, *in vitro* drug release (buccal, vaginal and rectal pH), *ex vivo* permeation studies, mucoadhesive strength and *in vivo* studies.

Results: FT-IR studies represent the change in spectra for the IPEC than single polymers.DSC study represents the different thermo gram for chitosan, polycarbophil and IPEC whereas in X-ray diffraction, crystal size alteration was observed. Formulations containing IPEC showed pH independent controlled 5-FU without an initial burst release effect in buccal, vaginal and rectal pH. Furthermore, F4 formulations showed controlled release 5-FU with highest bioadhesive property and satisfactory residence in both buccal and vaginal cavity of rabbit. 3% of SDC in formulation F6 exhibited maximum permeation of 5-FU.

Conclusion: The suitable combination of IPEC, chitosan and polycarbophil demonstrated potential candidate for controlled release of 5-FU in buccal, vaginal and rectal pH with optimum swelling approaching zero order release.

Keywords: Chitosan, Polycarbophil, Interpolyelectrolyte complex, pH independent drug release

Introduction

Extensive research has been made for the delivery of active drugs through buccal, vaginal and rectal cavity. The mucosa offers excellent opportunities to deliver active drugs both locally and systemically [1]. Over the last decade considerable progress in research towards the development of buccal, vaginal and rectal drug delivery for various diseases have been made.

Cancer is a disease involving all organs, races, ages and sex of the humans. Among all types of cancer, Oropharyngeal cancer, colorectal cancer contributes to world most burden and cervical cancer accounts for little extent. Oropharyngeal cancer develops in the part of the throat just behind the mouth called the oropharynx. Oropharynx includes the base of the tongue, soft palate, tonsils, tonsillar pillars and back wall of the throat [2].

* Correspondence: mohamedsaif.xlnc@gmail.com
Department of Pharmaceutics, JSS College of Pharmacy, JSS University, SS Nagar, Mysore-15, Karnataka, India

Cervical cancer involving the cervix that is narrow and lower part of uterus. About 90% of Oropharyngeal and cervical cancers are squamous cells carcinoma that begins in the epithelial lining in mouth and vagina. Whereas in colorectal cancer columnar cells are affected. Surgery, radiation therapy and chemotherapy are the most common therapies for treating cancer.

In chemotherapy, most of the anticancer drugs are parenterally administered attributable to poor oral bio-availability; this can be due to either poor absorption or significant first pass metabolism. However, limitation of parental are need to be sterile, time consuming, pain on administration and as also studies reported, approximately 90% of cancer patients prefer oral administration than intravenous administration [3,4].

5-FU is the drug of choice in oropharyngeal caner, colorectal cancer, stomach cancer and cervical cancer [5]. Chemically, 5-FU is a dipodic acid and highly polar in nature with pka values of 8.0 and 13.0 [6,7]. After oral administration, 5-FU is poorly absorbed with erratic variation in bioavailability ranging between 0 to 80%. 5-FU after parenteral administration it is rapidly eliminated with apparent terminal half life of approximately 8-20 min [8,9]. On intravenous administration 5-FU produces severe systemic toxic effects including gastrointestinal, hematological, neural, cardiac and dermatological origin [10]. These problems make 5-FU suitable candidate for Transbuccal/vaginal and rectal delivery.

Polymeric drug delivery systems are mainly designed for the efficient delivery of active drug. Among various polymeric drug delivery systems, interpolyelectrolyte complexes are most new, efficient form of polymeric carriers for novel drug delivery systems [11-14]. Chitosan polycarbophil IPEC has established its potential in drug delivery and have been most efficient form of IPEC compared to other complexes [15-17].

Most publications on 5-FU focused only on single drug delivery system like buccal gels, cervical patches, colorectal drug delivery. Hardly any articles reported on permeation studies and histological effects of 5-FU. Literature review revealed that there is no single drug delivery system available that can be given either through buccal, vaginal or rectal route. The prime goal has to design 5-FU multipurpose tablets with greater efficacy, potency, adoptability to need, minimal toxic effects and better patient compliance than the established marketed product.

Materials and methods
Materials
5-FU obtained from Strides Arcolab Ltd., Bangalore, India. Chitosan (Marine chemical, Cochin, India, Deacetylation degree: 85%, Viscosity: <200 mpa.s, Moisture content: <10%, Ash content: <1%, Insoluble: <1%, pH: 3-

6, Particle size: 80-100 mesh). Polycarbophil (Noveon AA-1)(Arihantt Trading Co., Mumbai, India, nature: pH:2.5-3, Ash content: 0.009 ppm, Density: (bulk) 0.19-0.24 g/cm^3. Equilibrium moisture content: 8-10%, pka: 6.0 ± 0.5, Glass transition temp: 100-105°C, Moisture content: 2.0% max, Specific gravity: 1.41).

Sodium deoxycholate, microcrystalline cellulose and Talc were from Zydus Cadila, India. All other chemicals and reagents used were of analytical grade.

Methods
Preparation of chitosan- polycarbophil complex (IPEC)
3% w/v Chitosan aqueous acetic acid solution and 3% w/v of polycarbophil acetic acid solution were mixed. The chitosan solution was added slowly to the polycarbophil solution under homogenization over a period of 20 min (5000 rpm) and the mixture was then stirred for a period of 1 hr at a speed of 1200 rpm with a mechanical stirrer. The formed gel was separated under vacuum pump and washed several times with a 2% v/v acetic acid solution to remove any non complexed polymeric material. The gel was dried in hot air oven and the dried complex was ground with a grinder. The powder was passed through a 200 μm sieve and used for further study.

Fourier transform infrared (FT-IR) spectroscopy study
The infrared absorption spectra of Chitosan, polycarbophil and IPEC were analyzed using a FT-IR spectrophotometer (8400S, Shimadzu, Japan). The pellets were prepared by pressing the sample with potassium bromide.

Differential scanning calorimetric (DSC)
Thermal analysis was carried out using a differential scanning calorimeter (DSC 50, Shimadzu Scientific Instruments, Japan) for Chitosan, polycarbophil and IPEC. The samples were placed in an aluminum-sealed pan and preheated to 200°C. The sample was cooled to room temperature and then reheated from 40 to 400°C at a scanning rate of 10°C/min.

Powder X-Ray diffraction
Powder x-ray diffraction patterns on Chitosan, Polycarbophil and IPEC were obtained by using an x-ray Diffractometer (Miniflex II Desktop X-ray Diffractometer, Rigaku Corporation, Tokyo, Japan). The samples were scanned from 6° to 40° (2θ) with an increment of 0.02° and measurement time of 10 s/increment.

Preparation of mucoadhesive matrix tablet
Mucoadhesive tablets were fabricated by direct compression method as shown Table 1. The accurate quantity of 5-FU and excipients were weighed. They were passed through sieve and thoroughly mixed using mortar and

Table 1 Formulation chart

Ingredients	F1	F2	F3	F4	F5	F6
5-flurouracil	20	20	20	20	20	20
IPEC	60	80	100	80	80	80
Chitosan	——	——	——	20	20	20
Polycarbophil	——	——	——	20	20	20
Sodium deoxycholate	——	——	——	—	3	4.5
Microcrystalline cellulose	65	45	25	5	2	0.5
Talc	5	5	5	5	5	5

Weight in mg.
Total weight of tablet is 150 mg.

Pestle. The blend was lubricated and then compressed into compacts by direct compression method using 8-mm flat-faced punches in KBr press (Techno search, Mumbai, India) at 1 ton pressure with a dwell time of 1 s.

Swelling studies

The swelling index of the prepared mucoadhesive 5-FU tablets was determined by weighing five tablets and recording their weights before placing them separately in weighed beakers. The total weight was recorded ($W1$). Four milliliters of phosphate buffer pH 6.8 (similarly with simulated vaginal fluid pH 4.2 and pH 7.4) was added to each beaker and then placed in an incubator at $37 \pm 0.5°C$. At time intervals of 2, 4, 6 and 8 h excess water was carefully removed, and the swollen tablets were weighed ($W2$). The experiment was repeated three times, and the average $W1$ and $W2$ were reported.

The swelling index was determined from the formula.

$$SI = (W2 - W1)/W1 \, X \, 100$$

In vitro release of matrix tablets

The drug release rate from buccal compacts was studied using the orbital shaking incubator using (Remi CIS 24, India) 30 mL of phosphate buffer pH 6.8. The temperature was maintained at $37 \pm 0.5°C$ and 50 rpm (rotation per min). For every one hour of time interval 3 mL sample was withdrawn, filtered through a Millipore filter of 0.45 μm pore size and assayed spectrophotometrically at 266 nm. Immediately after each sample withdrawal, a similar volume of phosphate buffer pH 6.8 was added to the dissolution medium.

The drug release rates from vaginal tablets were studied in 500 ml of simulated vaginal fluid pH 4.2 in type II dissolution apparatus. The temperature was maintained at $37 \pm 0.5°C$ and 50 rpm. For every one hour of time interval 10 mL sample was withdrawn, filtered through a Millipore filter of 0.45 μm pore size and assayed spectrophotometrically at 265 nm. Immediately after each sample withdrawal, a similar volume of simulated vaginal fluid was added to the dissolution medium.

In-vitro drug release for rectal tablets was performed using the dissolution apparatus I; 500 mL phosphate buffer (pH 7.4) maintained at $37 \pm 0.5°C$ was used as a dissolution medium. Basket was rotated at 50 rpm. 10 mL aliquots was taken at periodic time intervals and replaced by equal volume of phosphate buffer. The solution was suitably diluted and the absorbance was taken at 267 nm using UV visible Spectrophotometer.

Bioadhesive strength

Bioadhesive strength of the compacts was measure using modified physical balance as recently discussed [18]. *In vitro* bioadhesion studies were carried out using sheep buccal mucosa and modified two-armed balance. The phosphate buffer pH 6.8 was used as the moistening fluid. A glass stopper was suspended by a fixed length of thread on one side of the balance and was counter balanced with the weights on the other side. Fresh sheep buccal mucosa was collected from the slaughter house. It was scrapped off from the connective tissues and a thin layer of buccal mucosa was separated which was stored in tries buffer until used for the bioadhesion study. A circular piece of sheep buccal mucosa was cut and fixed to the tissue holder and was immersed in phosphate buffer pH 6.8 and the temperature was maintained at $37° \pm 1°C$. Then the tablet was fixed to a glass stopper with the help of cyanoacrylate adhesive and it was placed on the buccal mucosa by using a preload of 50gm and kept it aside for 3 min to facilitate adhesion bonding. After preloading time, the preload was removed and the weights were added on the other side of the balance until tablet detaches from the sheep buccal mucosa. The weight required to detach tablet from buccal mucosa was noted.

Ex vivo permeation study

Permeation study was carried out for the optimized formulation using Franz diffusion cell. The tablet was placed in the donor compartment on the sheep mucosa. The mucosal layer is on donor compartment. The receptor compartment was filled with phosphate buffer pH 6.8. The temperature was maintained at $37 \pm 0.5°C$ and 50 rpm. The amount of 5-FU permeated through sheep mucosa was determined by withdrawing 3 ml of aliquots from the receptor compartment using a syringe and immediately replacing the same volume of solution.

In vivo x-ray studies

The *in vivo* X-ray studies were approved by the Institutional Animal Ethical Committee of JSS College of Pharmacy (Mysore, Karnataka, India). The study was performed on healthy female rabbit, weighing between

1-1.5 kg. F4 formulation was modified by adding 20 mg of X-ray grade barium sulfate (20 mg of 5-FU was replaced). The prepared tablet was placed in buccal mucosa of healthy rabbit. During the study, the rabbit was not allowed to eat or drink. The rabbit was exposed to x-ray examinations and photographs were taken at 1st and 8th hr after administration of the tablet. Similarly procedure was followed for vaginal and rectal delivery.

Kinetic analysis

Drug release from simple swellable systems may be described by the power law expression and is defined by the following equation

$$M_t / M_\infty = Kt^n$$

Where M_t is the amount of drug released at time t, M_∞ is the overall amount of drug released, K_1 is the release constant; n is the release or diffusion exponent and M_t / M_∞ is the cumulative drug concentration released at time t (or fractional drug release).

The release exponent (n) value was used for interpretation of the release mechanism from the compacts. The dissolution data were modeled by using PCP disso v2.01 (Bharathi Vidhyapeeth, Deemed University, Pune, Maharashtra, India).

Statistical analysis

Statistical analyses of all data were undertaken using Graph Pad prism version 5.0 (Graph pad software Inc, San Diego, California, USA).

Results and discussion

In our previous paper, studies on Carbopol® 71 G and Noveon AA-1(polycarbophil) polymers and the influence of formulation expedients were evaluated in our laboratory on buccal bioadhesive tablet of Fluconazole [19]. Later, it was also shown in our laboratory that the interpolymer complex between Chitosan and Carbopol® 71 G as a suitable polymer for the development of novel drug delivery of miconazole for candidiasis [20].

In the light of vast previous experience and literature on Carbopol® 71 G and polycarbophil, we identified that polycarbophil, Carbopol and chitosan polymers are well suitable for particular pH. In contrast, chitosan-polycarbophil interpolyelectrolyte complex showed high potential as matrix former and used as new class of polymer carriers for creating novel drug delivery system [21]. Therefore based on the extensive review and previous experience on above cited polymers, chitosan-polycarbophil interpolyelectrolyte complex are taken into present investigation.

Characterization of IPEC

The interaction between chitosan and polycarbophil has been studied by several investigators [22,23]. The studies indicated that IPEC could be formed by the electrostatic interaction between the COO^- group of polycarbophil and NH_3^+ group of chitosan. The protonation of chitosan and dissociation of polycarbophil solution was successfully accomplished by solution of chitosan and polycarbophil in acetic acid solution. Subsequently, chitosan – polycarbophil interpolymer complex were prepared from these solutions. Figure 1 shows the superimposed IR spectra of Chitosan, polycarbophil and IPEC in 1000-2000 cm^{-1} and 1400-1800 cm^{-1}.

The degree of deacetylation of Chitosan is 85%, the amine group of 2-aminoglucose unit and the carbonyl group of 2-aminoglucose unit of chitosan showed absorption bands at 1589 and 1656 cm^{-1}, respectively [24]. Polycarbophil exhibits a broad band at 1713 cm^{-1} assigned to $C = O$ stretching (hydrogen-bonded). The weak band at 1415 cm^{-1} is due to the symmetric stretching of carboxylate anion (COO^-), bands 1230 and 1160 cm^{-1} are attributed to the C-O stretching [25,26]. In IR spectra, spectra of the physical mixture of two polymers or immiscible polymers will be the sum of the spectra of the individual compounds, whereas polymers after electrostatic interaction, there will be changes in the IR spectra such as Wave number shifts, band broadening and new absorption bands that are evidence of the polymers miscibility [27]. In IR spectra of Chitosan-polycarbophil IPEC, a new and strong band is observed at 1561 cm^{-1}. This band can be assigned due to the overlapping of asymmetric COO^- stretching vibration of polycarbophil and the NH_3^+ asymmetric bending vibration of chitosan which is agreement with literature to be located between 1550–1610 cm^{-1} [28]. In addition, another band at approximately 1402 cm^{-1} is a further evidence of the interaction because it is attributed to the symmetric COO^- stretching vibration [29].

Figure 2 shows the DSC thermo grams of chitosan, polycarbophil and IPEC. The DSC thermo grams of pure chitosan, exhibits one broad endothermic peak at 110°C associated to the evaporation of bound water, a glass transition at 240°C and an exothermic peak at about 320°C attributable to the polymer degradation. This includes saccharide rings dehydration, depolymerization and decomposition of deacetylated and acetylated chitosan units [30,31]. These peaks are agreement with other reported studies [32,33]. Polycarbophil thermo gram exhibits two endothermic peaks at 91°C and ~245°C. The first endothermic peak is short and narrow peak assigned to the evaporation of water from hydrophilic groups in the polymers and the second one corresponds to a thermal degradation through intermolecular anhydride formation and water elimination [34,35]. The

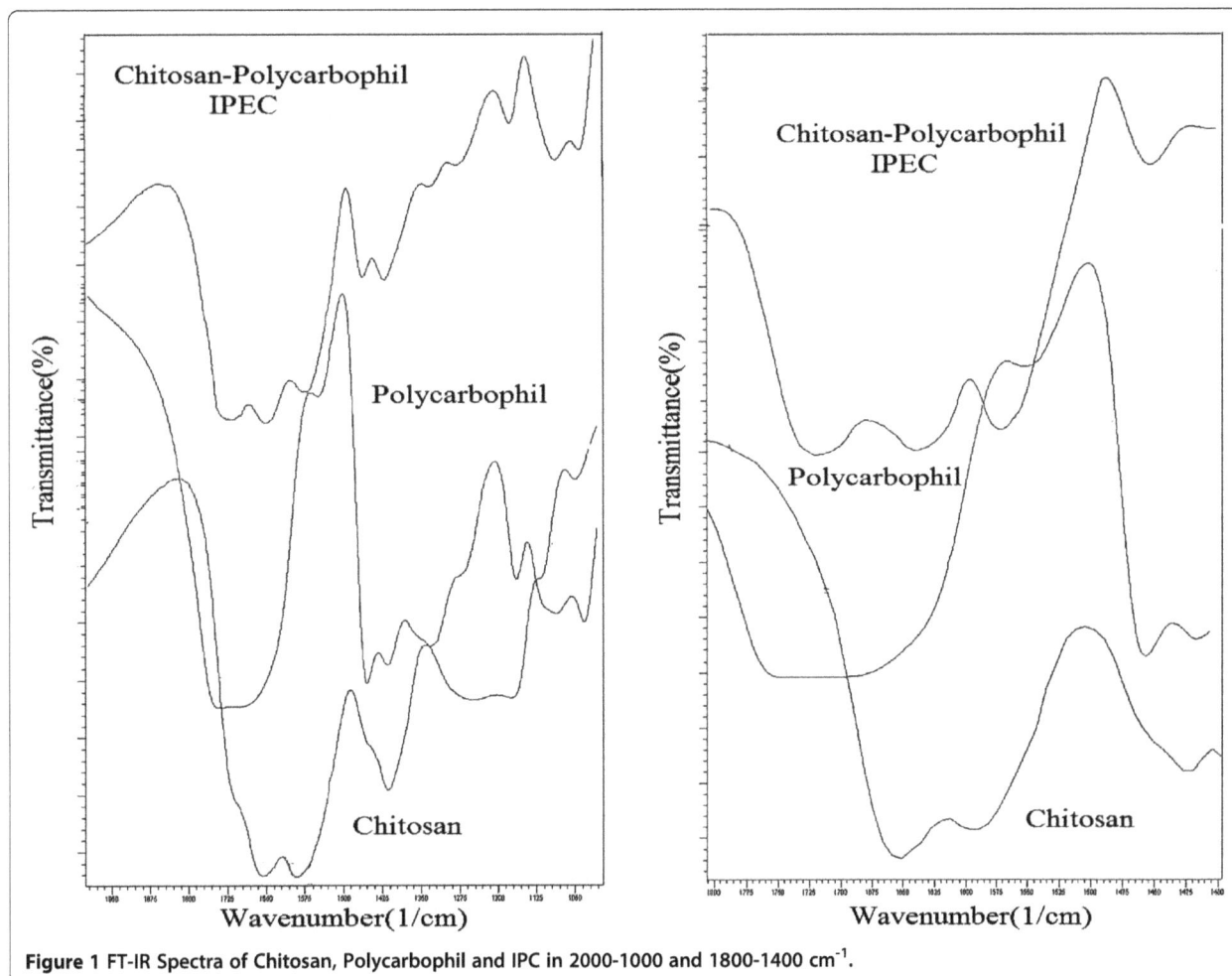

Figure 1 FT-IR Spectra of Chitosan, Polycarbophil and IPC in 2000-1000 and 1800-1400 cm^{-1}.

chitosan-polycarbophil IPEC thermo gram exhibit four endothermic peaks. The first one and second is associated with the vaporization of water situated at ~53°C and ~100°C in the chitosan polycarbophil IPEC. The second endothermic peak is probably related with the cleavage of the electrostatic interactions between the oppositely charged polymers, since it is not observed for the pure compounds. The appearance of new broad endotherm at 250°C is indicative of a compound with distinctive thermal behavior properties.

The X-ray diffraction of Chitosan, polycarbophil and IPEC were shown in Figure 3. The powder x-ray diffraction pattern of chitosan powder showed two prominent diffraction peaks at 10.6° (2θ) and 19.64° (2θ). A shoulder peak appears at 21.74° and also minor peak appears at 26.62°. The two prominent crystalline peaks at 10.6° and 19.64° are typical fingerprint for chitosan which were related to the hydrated and anhydrous crystals respectively [36]. Polycarbophil showed peaks at 18.88°, whereas IPEC showed peak at 19.92°. The typical peaks of chitosan disappeared and the IPEC showed an amorphous morphology after completing. The integration of polycarbophil into chitosan disrupted the crystalline structure of chitosan, hindering the formation of hydrogen bonding between amino groups and hydroxyl groups.

Characterization of matrix tablets
Pharmaceutical properties
The results of pharmaceutical properties are summarized in Table 2. The matrix tablets showed a diameter of 8 mm with negligible variation and therefore not included in the table. All the formulations showed satisfactory values within the limits of conventional oral tablets stated in the *Indian Pharmacopoeia* [37].

Swelling studies
F3 formulation containing higher concentration of IPEC showed pronouncedly higher swelling capabilities in vaginal, buccal and rectal pH compare to F1 and F2 formulation (lesser concentration of IPEC). The swelling for F3 formulation in vaginal, buccal and rectal pH was found to 802%, 798%, and 797% respectively. Further,

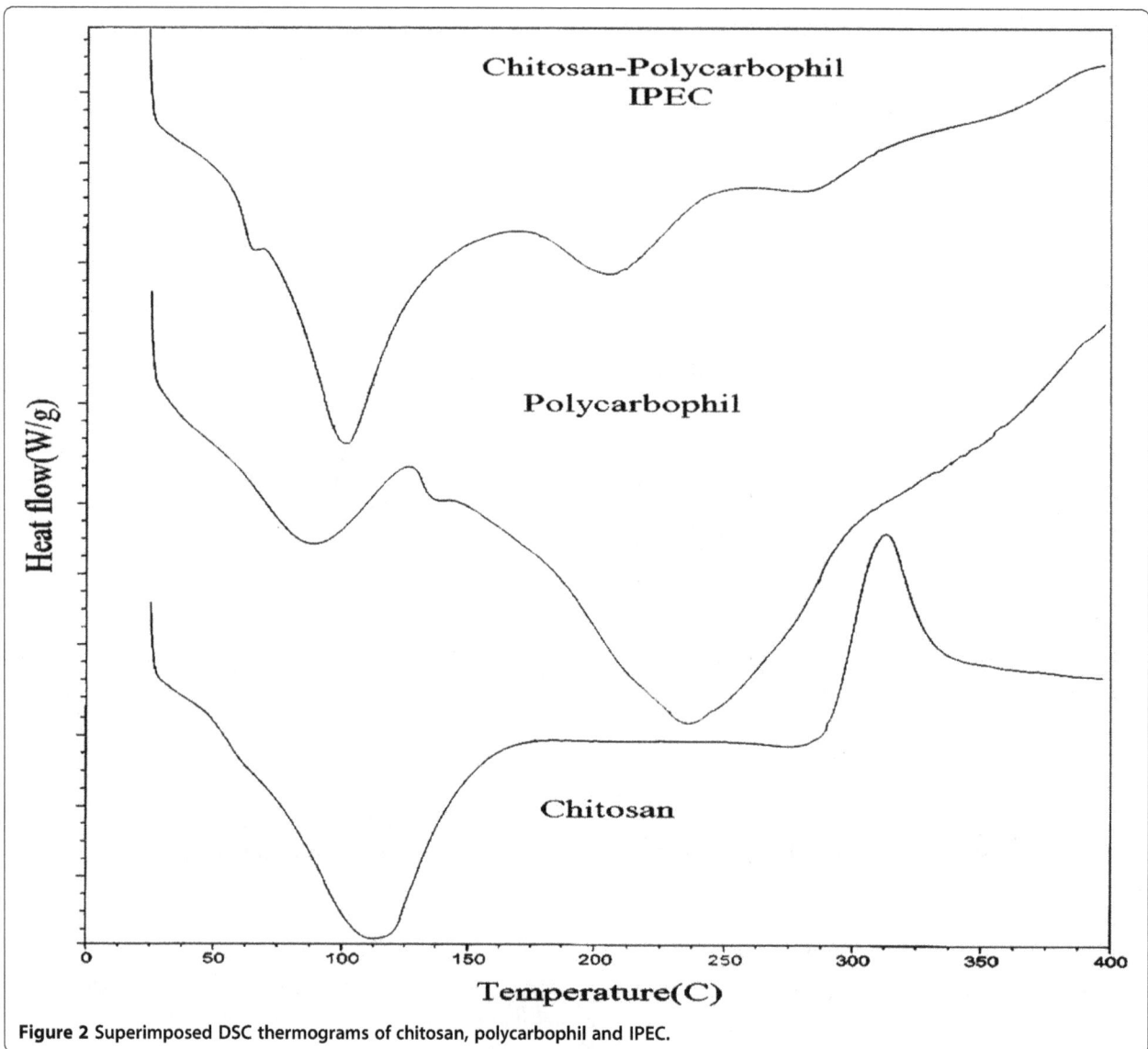

Figure 2 Superimposed DSC thermograms of chitosan, polycarbophil and IPEC.

the addition of chitosan and polycarbophil for F4 formulation in vaginal pH 4.2 reduces the swelling to 445%. Nearly same degree of swelling was observed for F5 and F6 as that of the formulation F4. The addition of sodium deoxycholate doesn't significantly alter the swelling in F5 and F6. The comparison of degree of swelling of all formulations in vaginal pH 4.2 was shown in Figure 4a. In pH 6.8, F2 formulation showed 785% of swelling i.e. lesser than F3 formulation. The F4 formulation found to be having 495% of least swelling; this may be explained due to dissociation of carboxylic group of polycarbophil in buccal pH 6.8. Swelling profiles of formulations in pH 6.8 was shown in Figure 4b. In pH 7.4, F4 formulation exhibited swelling of 481% that is as nearly similar in pH 4.2 and pH 6.8. Nearly same degree of swelling was observed for F5 and F6 as that of the formulation F4.

Swelling profiles of formulations in pH 7.4 was shown in Figure 4c.

These findings indicate the presence of IPEC alone in matrix tablet exhibit slow uniform pH independent swelling degree and also the presence of chitosan and polycarbophil in IPEC matrix tablets alters the swelling degree. Therefore the mechanism of drug release from IPEC matrix tablets was affected by the presence of chitosan and polycarbophil.

Bioadhesion studies

The mucoadhesive strength for all the formulations was shown in Figure 5. F1 formulation containing only IPEC shows least detachment force this may be explained due to the lacking of free functional groups which probably involved in the adhesion of the mucosa. F2 formulation

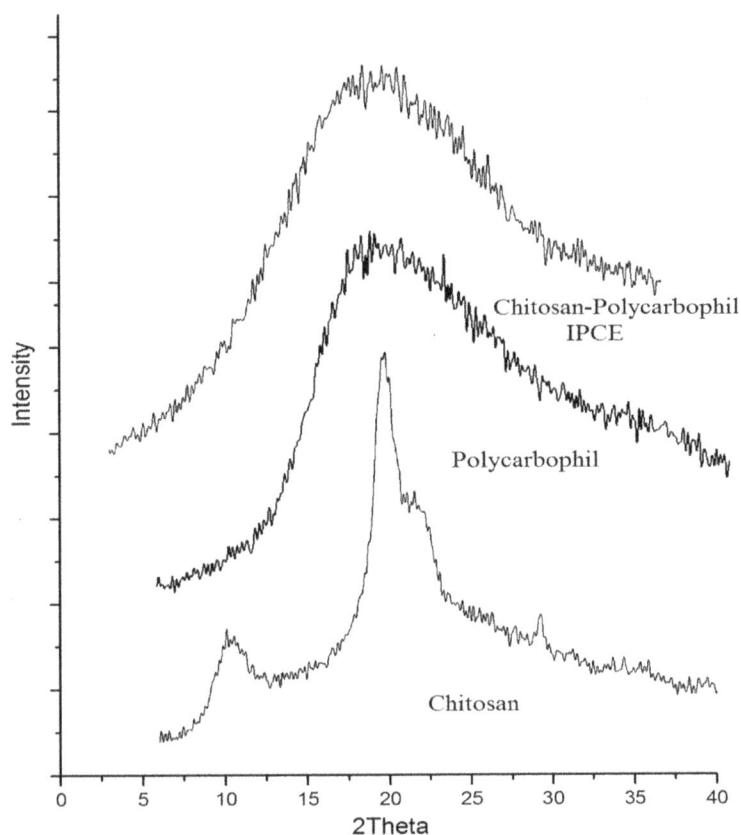

Figure 3 Superimposed XRD spectra of Chitosan, polycarbophil and IPEC.

having higher concentration of IPEC still exhibited least detachment force, even further increase in IPEC concentration in F3 formulation doesn't alters the detachment force. F4 formulation shows highest detachment force, this may be due to availability of free functional groups. F5 & F6 formulation containing sodium deoxycholate doesn't have any impact on the detachment force.

These findings indicate the presence of IPEC alone doesn't exhibit sufficient bioadhesion hence the presence of other polymers is necessary for development of bioadhesive matrix tablets. Therefore suitable combination of polymers along with IPEC is selected for producing sufficient bioadhesion without altering properties of IPEC.

In vitro drug release studies

In vitro drug release study of formulations in pH 4.2, 6.8 and 7.4 was shown in Figure 6a, b and c respectively. Initially 5-FU matrix tablets were made from IPEC and their *in vitro* drug release investigated and exhibited controlled release properties without any initial burst effect in buccal, vaginal and rectal pH .F1 & F2 formulations exhibited controlled drug release in buccal, vaginal and rectal pH with zero-order drug release. But F3 formulation, retarded drug release up to 70% in buccal, vaginal and rectal pH. Higher increase in concentration of IPEC forms gel layer around tablets that retards the drug release up to 70%. In spite of excellent

Table 2 Pharmaceutical properties

Formulation code	Thickness (mm)	Hardness (N)	Friability (%)	Weight (mg)	Drug content (%)
F1	2.03 ± 0.01	71 ± 3	0.08	149.4 ± 0.43	99.90 ± 0.09
F2	2.01 ± 0.05	72 ± 2	0.09	149.2 ± 1.00	99.91 ± 0.08
F3	2.03 ± 0.01	72 ± 3	0.06	150.0 ± 0.57	99.92 ± 0.05
F4	2.03 ± 0.02	73 ± 1	0.05	150.1 ± 1.00	99.94 ± 0.08
F5	2.01 ± 0.02	73 ± 3	0.03	149.2 ± 0.52	99.95 ± 0.05
F6	2.02 ± 0.02	73 ± 2	0.04	149.2 ± 0.44	99.92 ± 0.05

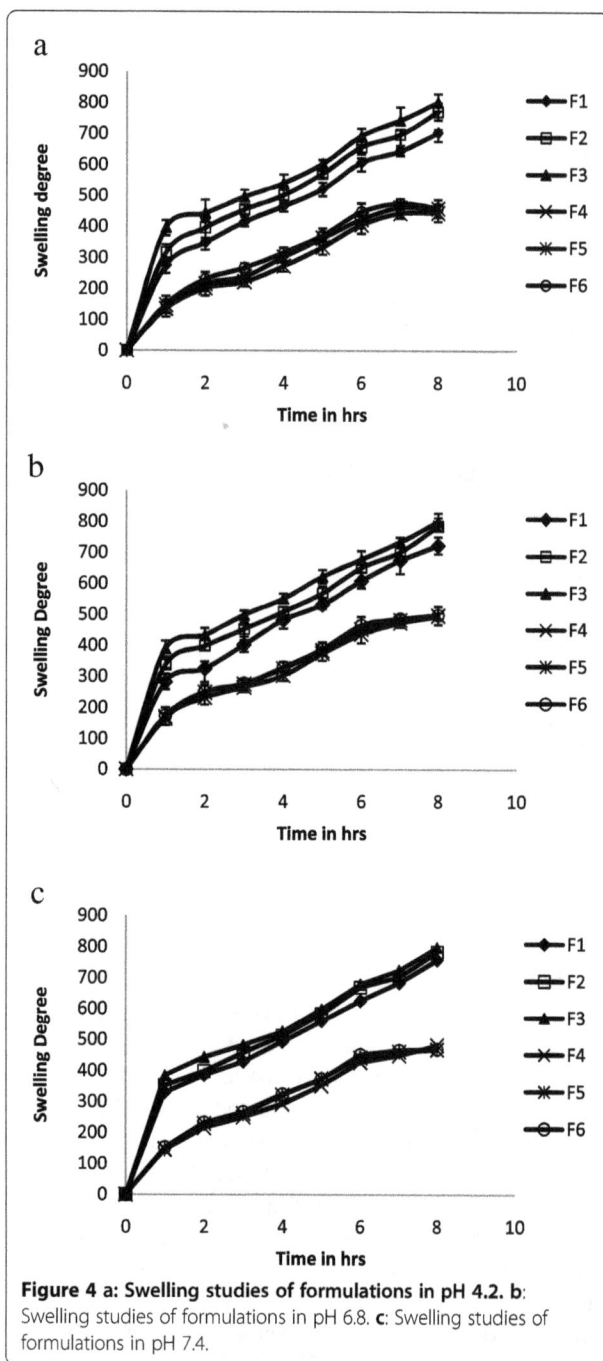

Figure 4 a: Swelling studies of formulations in pH 4.2. b: Swelling studies of formulations in pH 6.8. c: Swelling studies of formulations in pH 7.4.

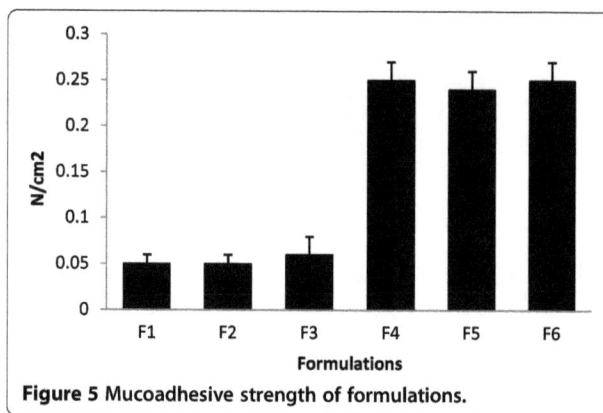

Figure 5 Mucoadhesive strength of formulations.

controlled 5-FU release up to 8 hr in buccal, vaginal and rectal pH, formulations containing IPEC (F1, F2 & F3) fails to attain sufficient mucoadhesive strength (mentioned in mucoadhesive studies). The study represents that alone IPEC can sustain the drug release but doesn't produces mucoadhesion. Hence, addition of chitosan and polycarbophil for IPEC formulation exhibited drug release up to 90% in 8 h in buccal, vaginal and rectal pH. This may be due to undissociation of carboxylic group of polycarbophil in pH 4.2, thereby neutralizing the gel

forming ability of chitosan. In buccal pH 6.8, the polycarbophil has the ability to swell and retard the drug release that is due to dissociation of carboxylic group. This property of polycarbophil is neutralized by chitosan that possesses gel forming property only in acidic pH. Similarly in rectal pH 7.4 the properties of polycarbophil and chitosan don't altered, hence similar drug profile was seen as in buccal and vaginal pH. F5 & F6 formulation containing SDC exhibited similar drug release profile as F4 formulation (Data not mentioned).

F4 formulation was subjected for kinetic study and the Correlation coefficients for F4 formulation in vaginal, buccal and rectal pH were found to 0.9964, 0.9957 and 0.9966 respectively. According to drug release exponent value (n), it is clear that F4 formulation approached zero-order drug release in vaginal, buccal and rectal pH (n value is 0.9). Thus the drug release is predicted as function of swelling for F4 formulation.

To confirm the similarity of F4 formulation dissolution profiles in buccal, vaginal and rectal pH, the similarity factor (f2) was used and was found above 80. Since the f2 values were higher than 50, these results confirmed that the drug release profiles were almost similar for F4 formulation for both buccal, vaginal pH and rectal pH.

Ex vivo permeation studies

5-FU permeation from formulations F5 and F6 across sheep mucosa over a period of 8 h is shown in Figure 7. The maximum permeation of 5-FU from F5 was 97% at 8 h compared with 63% from F6. Regression of the linear portions of the two plots gave Slopes and intercepts from which the permeation flux (slope divided by mucosal surface area) of F5 and F6 were calculated to be 8.5866 and 5.1333 $mg/cm^2/h$, respectively. While permeation coefficients were found be 2.1466 and 1.2833 cm/h for F5 and F6 formulations, respectively.

In formulation F5 addition of SDC 2% increased the cumulative percentage of drug permeated to 63%. This may be due to SDC extracted only mucosal lipid from the intercellular spaces. Thus, this enhances the diffusivity of

a

b

c

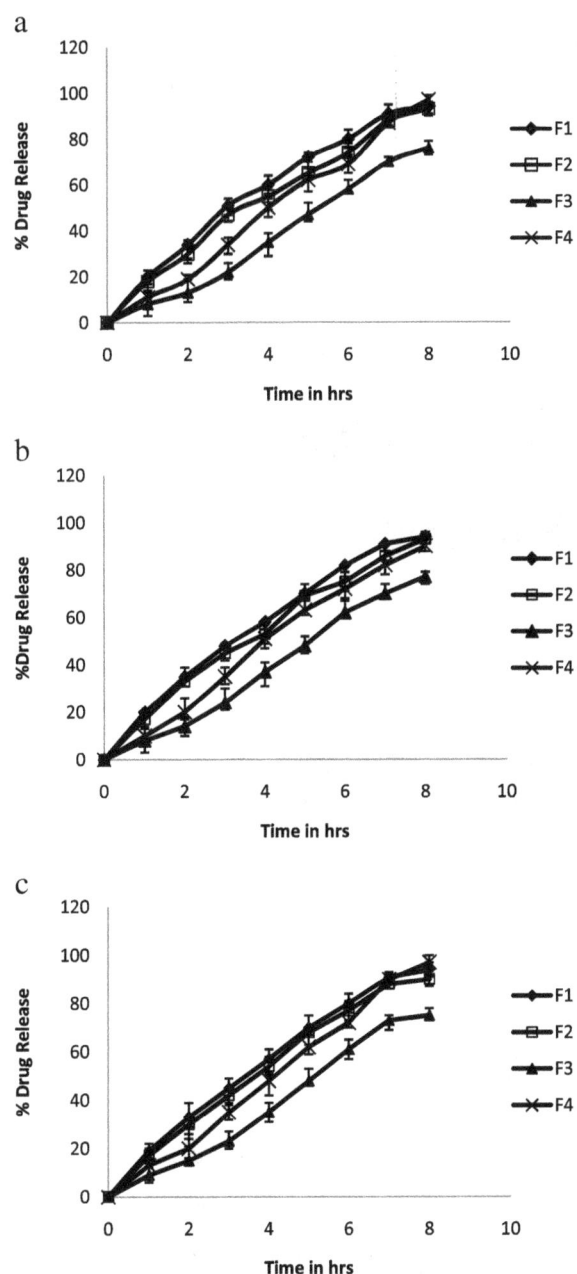

Figure 6 a: Dissolution profile of formulations F1-F4 in pH 4.2.
b: Dissolution profile of formulations F1-F4 in pH 6.8. **c**: Dissolution profile of formulations F1-F4 in pH 7.4.

Figure 7 Ex vivo permeation studies of F5 & F6 formulation.

uncoiling and extension of the protein helices, which leads to opening of the polar pathways for diffusion [39]. All these effects might contribute to enhancing the permeation of the drug.

In vivo X-ray studies

After administration of the optimized formulation (F4), developed by using barium sulfate, the duration of the tablet in the buccal, vaginal and rectal cavity was monitored by radiograms (Figure 8). The tablet adheres to the buccal, vaginal and rectal mucosa. The buccal tablet swells and retained till 8 h with little reduction in tablet size, as the tablet swells certain part of the tablet was swallowed by rabbit thereby the tablet size reduces. Whereas the tablet in vaginal cavity swells in 1 h and little reduction of size at 8 h. In rectal cavity tablet remained in cavity till 8 h.

Conclusion

All formulations studied showed good pharmaceutical properties. However, in consideration of swelling, drug release and mucoadhesion, some important differences have been highlighted. Formulation F3 containing only IPEC exhibited almost similar swelling in vaginal, buccal and rectal pH. Other two formulations F1 & F2 also containing lesser amount of IPEC produced less swelling than F3 formulation. The addition of polymer blends (chitosan and polycarbophil) to F3 formulation showed optimum swelling. These formulations, in fact, in addition to good swelling, lack sufficient mucoadhesion. F4 formulation demonstrated high mucoadhesive property. Further, the addition of SDC doesn't produce impact on mucoadhesion.

On the basis of these properties, it is clear that IPEC alone doesn't produce desired response hence, addition of polymeric blends is essential for developing the drug delivery system. The *in vitro* drug release study of F3 formulation demonstrated potential excipient for control

the 5-FU via the par cellular or polar route. Further increase in concentration of SDC (F6),i.e., 3%, increased the drug permeation up to 97% thus SDC in 3% extract lipids from the cell membranes, along with the extraction of mucosal lipid from the intercellular spaces by the formation of micelles. This resulted in enhancing passive diffusivity of the 5-FU via transcellular (crossing the cell membranes and entering the cell) and par cellular routes [38]. It was mentioned that SDC can also cause the

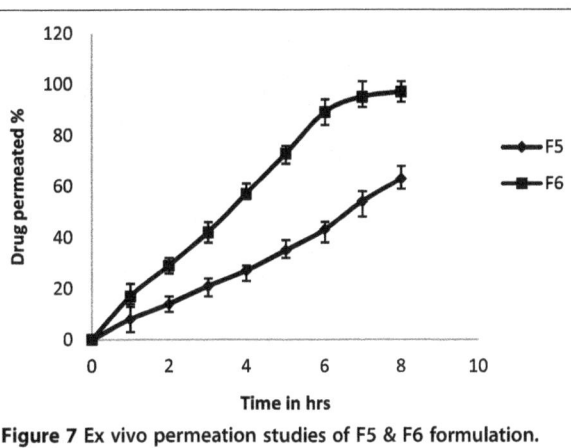

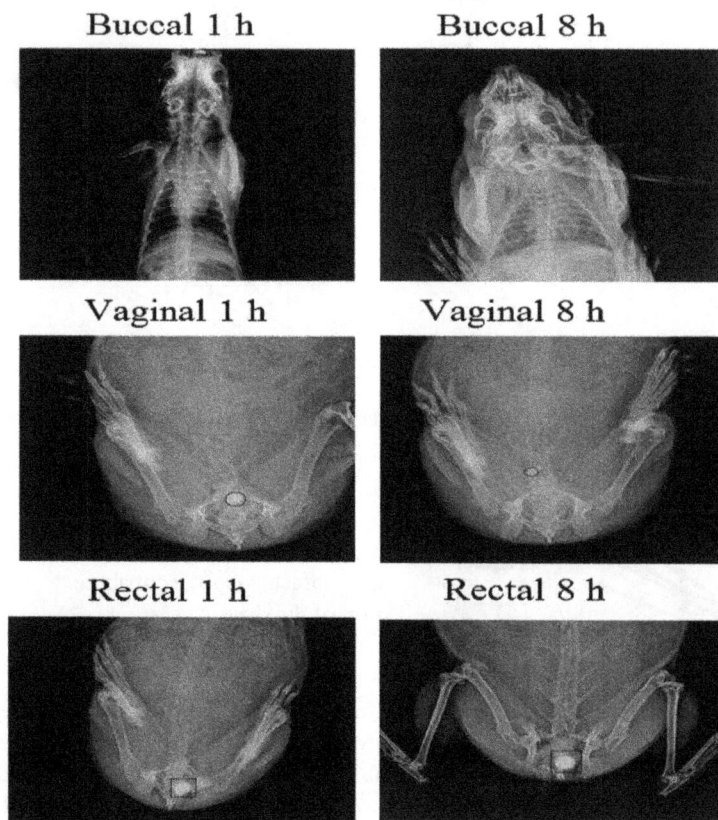

Figure 8 X-ray radiographic images of buccal and vaginal cavity at 1 and 8 h after ingestion of BaSO₄-loaded optimized F4 matrix tablet.

release and also possesses pH independent drug release. The matrix system with suitable combination of IPEC with polymeric blends (chitosan and polycarbophil) in F4 formulation able to produce desired drug release, bioadhesion, swelling and satisfactory *in vivo* residence. The desired bioadhesion can be achieved only with the addition of chitosan and polycarbophil; hence suitable combination played key role in the bioadhesion and subsequently maintains the pH independent drug release without initial burst release pattern. The addition of 3% Sodium deoxycholate to the F4 formulation demonstrated necessary 5-FU permeation.

Competing interests
Both authors declared that they have no competing interests.

Authors' contributions
MSP carried out preparation and characterization of chitosan-polycarbophil complex, involved in formulation of tablets, carried out physicochemical properties, swelling studies, bioadhesion studies, kinetic studies and statistical analysis. PKT carried out *in vitro* drug release studies, *in vivo* studies and has been involved in drafting the manuscript. Both authors read and approved the final manuscript.

Acknowledgment
The authors wish to thank the JSS University, Mysore, India for providing the facilities to complete this work.

References
1. DeVries ME, Bodde E, Coos J, Junginger HE: **Development in buccal drug delivey.** *Crit Rev ther Drug Carrier syst* 1991, **8**(3):271–303.
2. Dhiman MK, Dhiman A, Sawant KK: **Transbuccal delivery of 5-flurouracil: permeation enhancement and pharmacokinetic study.** *AAPS PharmaSciTech* 2009, **10**(1):258–265.
3. Rathbone MJ, Drummond BK, Tucker IG: **The oral cavity as a site for systemic drug delivery.** *Adv drug del rev* 1994, **13**:1–22.
4. Liu G, Franssen E, Fitch MI, Warner E: **Patient preferences for oral versus intravenous palliative chemotherapy.** *J Clin Oncol* 1997, **15**:110–115.
5. Calavresi P, Chabner BA: **The pharmacological basis of therapeutics.** In *Goodman and Gilmans*. 9th edition. Edited by Hardman JG, Limbird LE, Perry BM, Raymond WR. New Delhi: McGraw-Hill; 1996:125–1232.
6. Rudy BC, Senkowski BZ: **Flurouracil: Analytical profiles of drug substances.** In *Volume 2*. Edited by Klaus F. New York: Academic press; 1973:221–244.
7. Williams AC, Barry BW: **Terpenes and the lipid-protein partitioning theory of the skin penetration enhancement.** *Pharm res* 1991, **8**:17–24.
8. Dollery C: *Therapeutic drugs*. London: Churchill Livingstone Edinbugh; 1999.
9. Singh BN, Singh RB, Singh J: **Effects of ionization and penetration enhancers on the Transdermal delivery of 5-flurouracil through excised human stratum corneum.** *Int J pharm* 2005, **298**(1):98–107.
10. Diasio RB, Harris BE: *Clinical Pharmacokinetics* 1989, **16**:215.
11. Peppas NA, Khare AR: **Preparation, structure and diffusion behavior of hydrogels in controlled release.** *Adv Drug Deliv Rev* 1993, **11**:1–35.
12. Berger J, Reist M, Mayer JM, Felt O, Peppas NA, Gurny R: **Structure and interactions in covalently and ionically crosslinked chitosan hydrogels for biomedical applications.** *Eur J Pharm Biophar* 2004, **57**:19–34.

13. Nam K, Watanabe J, Ishihara K: **The characteristics of spontaneously forming physically cross-linked hydrogels composed of two water soluble phospholipids polymers for oral drug delivery carrier I: Hydrogel dissolution and insulin release under neutral pH condition.** *Eur J Pharm Sci* 2004, **23**:251–270.

14. Moustanfine RI, Kabonova TV, Kemonova VA, Van den Mooter G: **Characteristics of interpolyelectrolyte complexes of Eudragit E100 with Eudragit L100.** *J control rel* 2005, **103**:191–198.

15. Lu Z, Chen W, Hamman JH: **Chitosan-polycarbophil complexes in swellable matrix systems for controlled drug release.** *Curr drug deliv* 2007, **4**:257–63.

16. Lu Z, Chen W, Olivier EI, Hamman JH: **Matrix polymeric excipients: comparing a novel interpolyelectrolyte complex with hydroxypropylmethylcellulose.** *Drug Delivery* 2008, **15**:87–96.

17. Lu Z, Chen W, Hamman JH, Ni J, Zhai X: **Chitosan-polycarbophil interpolyelectrolyte complex as an excipient for bioadhesive matrix systems to control macromolecular drug delivery.** *Pharm Dev Tech* 2008, **13**:37–47.

18. Deshmukh VN, Jadhav JK, Sakarkar DM: **Formulation and *in vitro* evaluation of theophylline anhydrous bioadhesive tablets.** *Asian J Pharm* 2009, **3**:54–58.

19. Mohamed SP, Muzzammil S, Pramod TMP: **Preparation of Fluconazole buccal tablet and influence of formulation expedients on its properties.** *Acta Pharmaceutica Sinica* 2011, **46**(4):460–465.

20. Pendekal MS, Tegginamat PK: **A novel bucco-vaginal controlled release drug delivery system of miconazole nitrate for candidiasis-design and evaluation.** *Lat Am J Pharm* 2012, **31**(3):461–8.

21. Zhilei L, Weiyang C, Hamman JH: **Chitosan-polycarbophil interpolyelectrolyte complex as a matrix former for controlled release of poorly water-soluble drugs I: *in vitro* evaluation.** *Drug Dev Ind Phar* 2010, **36**(5):539–546.

22. Claudia LS, Jorge CP, Amilcar R, Alberto Pais ACC, Joao Sousa JS: **Films based on chitosan polyelectrolyte complexes for skin drug delivery: Development and characterization.** *J MemSci* 2008, **320**:268–279.

23. Siracha T, Nuttanan S, Wichan K, Desmond BW, Ampol M: **Fabrication of chitosan–polyacrylic acid complexes as polymeric osmogents for swellable micro/nanoporous osmotic pumps.** *Drug Dev Ind Phar* 2011, **37**(8):926–933.

24. Tien LCM, Lacroix MPI, Szabo PI, Mateescu MA: ***N*-acylated chitosan: hydrophobic matrices for controlled drug release.** *J Control Rel* 2003, **93**:1–13.

25. Dong J, Ozaki Y, Nakashima K: **Infrared, Raman, and near-infrared spectroscopic evidence for the coexistence of various hydrogen-bond forms in poly(acrylic acid).** *Macromolecules* 1997, **30**:1111.

26. Brandenburg K, Seydel U: *Fourier Transform Infrared Spectroscopy of Cell Surface Polysacharides.* New York: Wiley-Liss; 1996.

27. Stuart B: *Infrared Spectroscopy: Fundamentals and Applications.* West Sussex, England: John Wiley & Sons Ltd.; 2004.

28. Coates J: *Interpretation of Infrared Spectra.* Chichester: A Practical Approach. John Wiley & Sons Ltd.; 2000.

29. Brown CD, Kreilgaard L, Nakakura M, Caram-Lelham N, Pettit DK, Gombotz WR, Hoffman AS: **Release of PEGylated granulocyte-macrophage colonystimulating factor from chitosan/glycerol films.** *J Control Rel* 2001, **72**:35.

30. Mathew S, Brahmakumar M, Abraham TE: **Microstructural imaging and characterization of the mechanical, chemical, thermal, and swelling properties of starch-chitosan blend films.** *Biopolymers* 2006, **82**:176.

31. Sarmento B, Ribeiro A, Veiga F, Ferreira D: **Development and characterization of new insulin containing polysaccharide nanoparticles.** *Colloids Surf B Biointerfaces* 2006, **53**:193.

32. Neto CGT, Giacometti JA, Job AE, Ferreira FC, Fonseca JLC, Pereira MR: **Thermal analysis of chitosan based networks.** *Carbohyd Polym* 2005, **62**:97–103.

33. Sankalia MG, Mashru RC, Sankalia JM, Sutariya VB: **Reversed chitosan-alginate polyelectrolyte complex for stability improvement of alpha-amylase: optimization and physicochemical characterization.** *Eur J Pharm Biopharm* 2007, **65**:215.

34. Fan XD, Hsieh YL, Krochta JM, Kurth MJ: **Study on molecular interaction behavior and thermal and mechanical properties of polyacrylic acid and lactose blends.** *J Appl Polym Sci* 1921, **2001**:82.

35. Huang Y, Lu J, Xiao C: **Thermal and mechanical properties of cationic guar gum/poly(acrylic acid) hydrogel membranes.** *Polym Deg Stab* 2007, **92**:1072.

36. Wan Y, Creber KAM, Peppley B, Bui VT: **Synthesis, characterization and ionic conductive properties of phosphorylated chitosan membranes.** *Macromol Chem Physiol* 2003, **204**:850–858.

37. Indian pharmacopeia: *The Indian pharmacopeia commission.* India: Ghaziabad; 2007.

38. Hoogstraate AJ, Wertz PW, Squier CA, Bos Van Geest A, Abraham W, Garrison MD, Verhoef JC, Junginger HE, Bodde HE: **Effects of the penetration enhancer glycodeoxycholate on the lipid integrity in porcine buccal epithelium *in vitro*.** *Eur J Pharm Sci* 1997, **5**:189–98.

39. Gandhi R, Robinson J: **Mechanisms of penetration enhancement for transbuccal delivery of salicylic acid.** *Int J Pharm* 1992, **85**:129–40.

Effects of tight *versus* non tight control of metabolic acidosis on early renal function after kidney transplantation

Farhad Etezadi, Pejman Pourfakhr, Mojtaba Mojtahedzade, Atabak Najafi, Reza Shariat Moharari, Kourosh Karimi Yarandi and Mohammad Reza Khajavi[*]

Abstract

Background: Recently, several studies have been conducted to determine the optimal strategy for intra-operative fluid replacement therapy in renal transplantation surgery. Since infusion of sodium bicarbonate as a buffer seems to be safer than other buffer compounds (lactate, gluconate, acetate)that indirectly convert into it within the liver, We hypothesized tight control of metabolic acidosis by infusion of sodium bicarbonate may improve early post-operative renal function in renal transplant recipients.

Methods: 120 patients were randomly divided into two equal groups. In group A, bicarbonate was infused intra-operatively according to Base Excess (BE) measurements to achieve the normal values of BE (−5 to +5 mEq/L). In group B, infusion of bicarbonate was allowed only in case of severe metabolic acidosis (BE $\leq$ −15 mEq/L or bicarbonate $\leq$ 10 mEq/L or PH $\leq$ 7.15). Minute ventilation was adjusted to keep $PaCO_2$ within the normal range. Primary end-point was sampling of serum creatinine level in first, second, third and seventh post-operative days for statistical comparison between groups. Secondary objectives were comparison of cumulative urine volumes in the first 24 h of post-operative period and serum BUN levels which were obtained in first, second, third and seventh post-operative days.

Results: In group A, all of consecutive serum creatinine levels were significantly lower in comparison with group B. With regard to secondary outcomes, no significant difference between groups was observed.

Conclusion: Intra-operative tight control of metabolic acidosis by infusion of Sodium Bicarbonate in renal transplant recipients may improve early post-operative renal function.

Keywords: Acid–base disorder, Renal transplantation, Chronic renal failure, Sodium bicarbonate

Background

Kidney transplantation is a cardinal method and the most cost-effective treatment modality used for the patients with chronic renal failure (CRF) [1].

Experiments in animals show that premedication with Sodium Bicarbonate, before the development of ischemic damage in renal tubules, may have renoprotective effects [2,3]. It is obvious that transplanted kidney is under the risk of ischemic insult (warm and cold ischemic period).Furthermore, Infusion of sodium bicarbonate solution (8.4%), which is hyperosmolar, can shift intracellular water into interstitial and intra-vascular spaces leading to intravascular volume expansion and induces osmotic diuresis [4-6]. Meanwhile, the alkalization of the urine might increase the solubility of acidic materials accumulated in CRF patients and enhance their excretion through urine [7]. The main concern with bicarbonate infusion is CO2 retention in the body. In other words, every 100 mEq of bicarbonate can produce 2.24 l of CO_2 in the body. This amount equals to an average adult CO2 production during 10 min of normal activity [8]. The extra load of CO_2 can be exhaled by increasing pulmonary minute ventilation which could be easily achieved during general anesthesia.

* Correspondence: khajavim@tums.ac.ir
Sina Hospital, Tehran University of Medical Sciences, Hassan Abad sq, Tehran, Iran

During recent years, several studies have been conducted to determine the optimal strategy for intra-operative fluid replacement therapy in renal transplantation surgery [9-11]. Three types of crystalloids have been examined for this purpose.1- Normal saline which is the preferred IV fluids for administration during kidney transplant surgery [12]. Infusion of large-volume of NS during renal transplantation can lead to hyperchloremic acidosis. 2- Lactated Ringer's solution which contains lactate anion, and can be transformed into bicarbonate in the liver; its infusion prevents aggravation of metabolic acidosis and so, produces less hyperkalemia in comparison with normal saline solution. 3- Plasmalyte solution contains acetate and gluconate which can be converted to bicarbonate in the liver. It is obvious that a normal functional liver with adequate hepatic blood flow is a prerequisite for this buffer effect attributed to the aforementioned balanced salt solutions. On the other hand, it has been already shown that anesthetic agents might reduce the hepatic blood flow [13].

Additionally, lactate may be pro-inflammatory by itself [14]. Also, lactated Ringer's solution has been reported to induce hypercoagulable state [10,15].

With regard to the above-mentioned facts and relatively safe profile of Sodium bicarbonate, and lack of a clinical trial in literature which deals with acid–base balance during a renal transplant surgery we designed this study based on the following hypothesis: The adjustment of metabolic acidosis with infusion of Sodium bicarbonate, even before the implantation of the kidney may reduce the work-load of ischemic donor's kidney and as a result, may improve the early outcome of the transplanted kidney.

Methods

After receiving the approval of the ethics committee of Research Deputy of our University, a written informed consent was obtained from all eligible patients who were candidate for living-donor renal transplantation. After study registration at IRCT website as: "IRCT138902163829N2",this prospective study was conducted on 120 patients with American Society of Anesthesiologists (ASA) class 3 and 4 who underwent renal transplantation from August 2010 to August 2011 in urology and transplantation operating room of Sina Hospital in which about 8-12 kidney transplantations are being done monthly. The randomization was performed by using a computer generated table of random numbers. The inclusion criteria are patients of any age who are candidate for elective kidney transplantation. The exclusion criteria were severe congestive heart failure (EF $\leq$ 35%), recent use of acetazolamide (during the past 24 h), detection of serum potassium level higher than 6 mEq/L and lower than 2.9 mEq/L, and serum sodium

level higher than 155 mEq/L. Occurrence of severe hypotension (SBP $\leq$ 90 mmHg) indicates either more rapid fluid replacement than the protocol of the study or need for catecholamine infusion due to uncontrolled surgical bleeding. Therefore, it was another exclusion criterion of this study.

Patients, anesthesiologists and other anesthesia team members, who were responsible for postoperative evaluation of primary and secondary outcomes, were blinded to intra-operative interventions. All recipients had been undergoing hemodialysis the day before surgery. Standard monitoring according to the recommendations of ASA was used. For all patients radial arterial cannula was inserted before the induction of anesthesia in order to monitor blood pressure and obtain blood samples. Central venous catheter was inserted in the right internal jugular vein after induction of anesthesia for infusion of crystalloids and Sodium Bicarbonate and central venous pressure (CVP) monitoring in the patients.

General anesthesia was induced with a combination of IV midazolam (0.05 mg/kg), fentanyl (2 µg /kg) and sodium thiopental (4 mg/kg). Anesthesia was maintained using isoflurane in an air/oxygen mixture and the bolus injection of fentanyl (2 µg/kg) every hour; muscle relaxation was achieved by use of IV injection of atracurium (0.2 mg/kg every 20 min).

Intra-operative fluid replacement therapy was performed according to the following protocol: Every patient received 20-25 ml/kg/h of only NS titrated continuously during the anesthesia, while CVP was kept between10-15 cm H2O. All eligible patients were randomized into two groups, each of them consisting of 60 cases; the intervention group of patients (group A) was scheduled to receive sodium bicarbonate infusion (8.4%) for tight control of metabolic acidosis according to Base Excess (BE) measurements, which were determined by an arterial blood gas analyzer (Gem primer 3000, Instrumentation laboratory, USA) from the commencement of anesthesia. The first arterial blood sample was obtained *via* arterial cannula just after induction of anesthesia and then, every 30 min up to the end of operation.

In the case of BE lower than–5 mEq/L, the clinician was permitted to start sodium bicarbonate infusion to keep the BE values in normal range (between +5 mEq/L to–5 mEq/L) [8,16,17]. Accordingly, if the BE value was below–5 mEq/L, the total deficit of bicarbonate was calculated with respect to the volume of distribution of sodium bicarbonate (30% of body weight), and half of the total deficit was infused through the central venous catheter during 15 min in the group A [8].

In the control group (group B), the infusion of sodium bicarbonate was allowed only in case of severe metabolic acidosis (BE $\leq$–15 mEq/L or serum bicarbonate level $\leq$ 10 mEq/L or PH $\leq$ 7.15).

Blood products were administered, when clinically indicated based on ASA recommendations. Every unpredicted complication occurring during anesthesia was treated by the clinician caring for the patients.

The patients were ventilated on continuous mandatory ventilation (CMV) mode according to this initial setting: RR = 10, TV = 10 cc /kg, I/E ratio = 1/2.

The ventilator setting (RR or TV) was adjusted every 30 min (after observing ABG result) by the clinician responsible for patients' care to keep the $PaCO_2$ between 35 to 40 mmHg. Perioperative immunosuppressive therapies were administered to all patients according to our institutional protocol:

1. Mycophenolate mofetil (Cell Cept): 1-2 g
2. Cyclosporine (Neoral): 6.5-7 mg/kg
3. Prednisolone: 2 mg/kg

All of the transplantation surgeries were performed by the same surgical team including an urologist and a vascular surgeon. All of the donors received 0.25gr/kg of mannitol infusion just before procurement of the left kidney *via* an open approach. The donor kidneys were flushed with lactated Ringer's solution before being transferred to the operating room. Afterwards, the kidneys were implanted in the right or left retroperitoneal space of the recipients. All the recipients received 5,000 units of heparin intravenously (three minutes before performing the clamp). All patients received 5 mg/kg of furosemide just after declamping of the implanted kidney as a routine intervention. The mean arterial pressure (MAP) of the patients was recorded just before and 15 min after the injection of furosemide. Postoperative IV fluid therapy was the same for all of the patients as the following protocol: Urine output was replaced (one milliliter for one milliliter) with an IV infusion of dextrose 5%/0.45% Na Cl plus 20 mEq/L of Sodium Bicarbonate.

Our primary endpoint was to evaluate the effects of metabolic acidosis tight control while maintaining the normal intraoperative $PaCO_2$ on the postoperative early renal function through four consecutive sampling of the serum creatinine levels, which were measured on first, second, third and seventh postoperative days. As the secondary objective, the effect of intraoperative bicarbonate infusion on the urine volume and serum BUN level in the early postoperative period was evaluated. Serum BUN concentration levels were measured in the first, second, third, and seventh days of the postoperative period. Cumulative urine volumes in the recovery room and during the first six and twenty four hours after the surgery were recorded as well.

Statistical analysis

Data are presented as means ± SD for continuous variables and as percentages for categorical variables. A sample size of 60 in each group was calculated to have at least 80% power to detect the expected difference between treatment protocols with respect to the primary goal. A 0.7 mg/dl difference in the mean serum creatinine level was noted to be significant. All data were tested for normality using method of Kolmogorov-Smirnov. Sphericity assumption was checked by Mauchly test before comparisons. Different variants of multiple measurements were separately analyzed using GLM repeated measurement analysis. A p value less than 5% was considered significant. All the laboratory measurements were analyzed at the central laboratory of Sina University Hospital.

Results

One hundred twenty patients were randomized into two equal groups. Demographic characteristics and preoperative variables were comparable in the two groups (Table 1). In the intra-operative period, three patients in group A were excluded from the study because of severe surgical bleeding and life threatening hypotension. This event occurred for two of the patients in the group B. The follow up could not be indicated in three other patients of group A because of two biopsy proven acute rejections and one Doppler sonography proven graft thrombosis. Meanwhile, three cases of graft thrombosis and one case of acute rejection were also observed in group B. At last, data from fifty four patients in each

Table 1 Comparison of demographic and preoperative variables of both groups

Variable		Group A Mean ± SD	Group B Mean ± SD
Sex	Male	36 (66%)	33 (61%)
	Female	18 (34%)	21 (39%)
Age (yrs.)		42 ± 15	44 ± 15
Weight (kg)		65.6 ± 13.2	66.3 ± 20.6
Dialysis before surgery (h)		23 ± 4	23 ± 3
Baseline Hgb (g/dl)		11.9 ± 3.1	10.1 ± 1.9
Baseline Albumin (mg/dl)		3.9 ± 0.3	4.1 ± 0.2
Baseline MAP in operating room (mmHg)		110 ± 14	114 ± 13
Baseline PH		7.35 ± 0.04	7.34 ± 0.07
Baseline BE (mEq/L)		−4.4 ± 0.2	−4.6 ± 0.3
Baseline PaCO2 (mmHg)		35 ± 1.5	34 ± 1.6
Baseline Cr (mg/dl)		5.1 ± 1.3	5.1 ± 1.2
Baseline BUN (mg/dl)		90.0 ± 32.4	92.1 ± 33.1

[Data are reported as mean ± SD] Hgb = hemoglobin, BP = blood pressure, mEq/L = milli equivalent per litre, MAP = mean arterial pressure, BE = base excess, Cr = creatinine, Pa CO2 = arterial pressure of CO2 gas, BUN = blood urea nitrogen.

group were gathered and underwent statistical analysis. Flowchart of the study progress is depicted in Figure 1.

All patients received similar volumes of NS as fluid replacement therapy during the surgery (5.54 ± O.51 vs.5.70 ± 0.67 lit) and no patient received colloid or blood products throughout the transplantation. No significant difference exists regarding to the duration of surgery between the groups. Mean amount of bicarbonate infused during the surgery was 87.4 ± 50.7 mEqin group A. Since, mean change of BE during the surgery was –6 ± 2.7 mEq/Lin group B, there was no indication for sodium bicarbonate infusion in this group. Duration of warm and cold ischemia and the mean amount of bleeding were similar among the groups. Mean of PH values at the end of surgery was 7.39 ± 0.05in group A and it was 7.20 ± 0.03in the group B while, the mean of multiple PH measurements throughout the operation was 7.38 ± 0.04 in group A and it was 7.21 ± 0.05 in group B. In addition, mean of BE at the end of surgery in the group A was –1.6 ± 1.3 and it was –10.6 ± 2.9in the group B. MAP of the patients decreased 15 min after furosemide injection in both groups, but this decline was temporary and self-limited (Table 2).

We observed significantly lower serum creatinine level in the group A in comparison with the group B throughout the days of follow up (p = 0.001) (Table 3).

The cumulative urine volumes gathered in the first 24 h of our study in both groups were not significantly different (p = 0.075) (Table 3).

Serum BUN levels were measured four times throughout the study and in all of them, lower BUN levels were observed in the group A, but the difference was not statistically significant(p = 0.74) (Table 3).

Table 2 Comparison of intra-operative variables between groups

Variable	Group A	Group B
	Mean ± SD	Mean ± SD
Time of surgery (min)	222 ± 30	227 ± 31
Amount of sodium bicarbonate infused (mEq)	87 ± 50	0
Extent of BE change during operation (mEq/L)	–	–6 ± 2.7
Amount of NS infused during surgery (lit)	5.5 ± 0.5	5.7 ± 0.6
Time of cold ischemia (min)	3.9 ± 2	4.01 ± 2
Time of warm ischemia (min)	18.3 ± 1.9	18.1 ± 2.1
Blood loss (ml)	294.2 ± 112.8	291.1 ± 103.9
MAP of patients before furosemide injection	138 ± 24	119 ± 32
MAP of patients 15 min after furosemide injection	122 ± 15	109 ± 18
Mean of multiple PH values throughout operation	7.38 ± 0.04	7.21 ± 0.05
Mean of PH value at the end of surgery	7.39 ± 0.05	7.20 ± 0.03
BE at the end of surgery(mEq/L)	–1.6 ± 1.3	–10.6 ± 2.9

[Data are reported as mean ± SD] BE = base excess, NS = normal saline, MAP = mean arterial pressure, mEq/L = milli equivalent per litre.

Discussion

According to meticulous literature search, this study is the first one which evaluates effects of intra-operative metabolic acidosis tight control on early renal function after a kidney transplantation surgery.

The development of hyperchloremic metabolic acidosis during intra-operative period is a well-recognized complication attributed to infusion of large volumes of

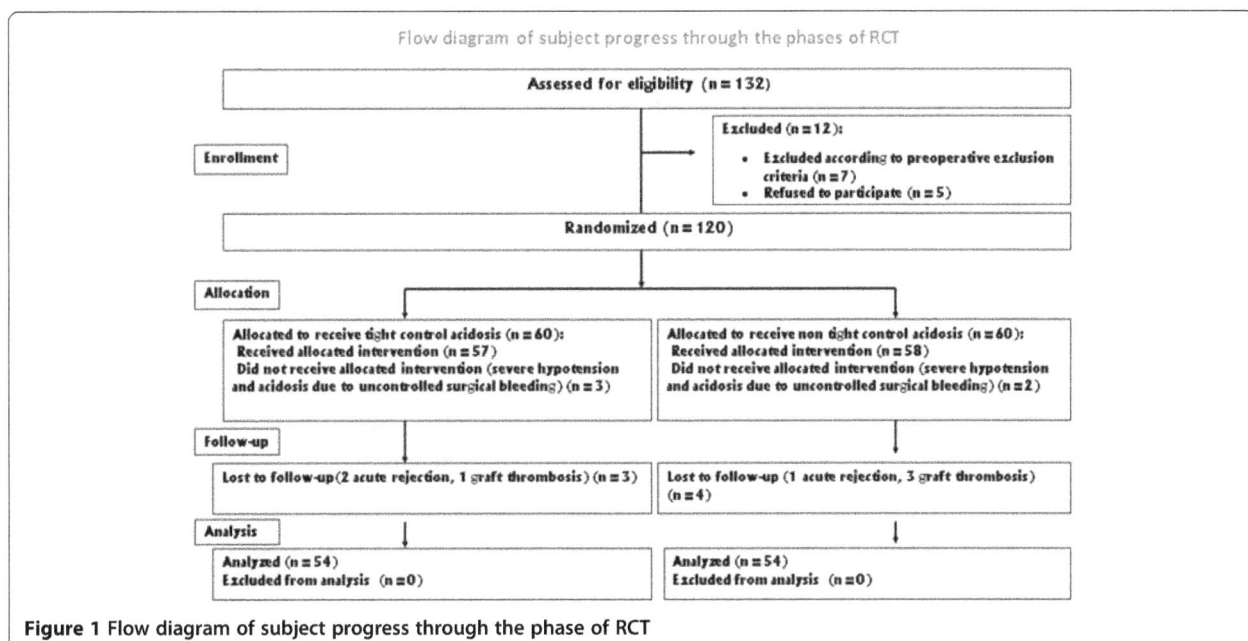

Figure 1 Flow diagram of subject progress through the phase of RCT

Table 3 Comparison of primary and secondary outcomes between groups

Measurements	Group A	Group B	P Value
	Mean ± SD	Mean ± SD	
Urine volume in Recovery (ml)	812 ± 492	377 ± 384	P = 0.075
Total Urine volume in 6 h (ml)	3696 ± 2401	1578 ± 1422	
Total Urine volume in 24 h (ml)	11279 ± 3937	9960 ± 5718	
Cr (mg/dl) 1st day	3.2 ± 0.8	3.5 ± 1.3	P = 0.001
Cr (mg/dl) 2nd day	1.7 ± 0.6	2.7 ± 1.2	
Cr (mg/dl) 3rd day	1.5 ± 0.5	2.5 ± 0.9	
Cr (mg/dl) 7th day	1.4 ± 0.3	2.2 ± 0.8	
BUN(mg/dl) 1st day	67.6 ± 21	79.2 ± 40	P = 0.74
BUN(mg/dl) 2nd day	56.4 ± 24.8	76.2 ± 48.7	
BUN(mg/dl) 3rd day	55.51 ± 30.3	81.11 ± 51.9	

[Data are reported as mean ± SD] Cr = creatinine, BUN = blood urea nitrogen.

NS solution [18,19]. It is worthwhile to mention that other types of anions (sulfate, phosphate, formate, etc.) have usually accumulated in CRF patients, but crystalloid replacement therapy doesn't change their plasma levels except some dilution that may ensue, and also they have a minor role in acid–base balance in comparison to such an abundant and strong anion like chloride. On the other hand, infusion of large volumes of crystalloids is a crucial strategy during a renal transplantation surgery [20]. Therefore, occurrence of hyperchloremic acidosis is unavoidable in these cases. With respect to normal range of serum chloride level (102-106 mEq/L) and the mean amount of NS solution infused (Table 2), every patient in this study received approximately 250 mEq extra load of chloride, which distributes throughout the extracellular fluid compartment [8]. Accordingly, after final equilibrium, serum chloride level is anticipated to raise about 10 mEq/L .According to Stewart-Fencl approach, 10 mEq/L of chloride excess results in 10 mEq/L decrease in Strong Ion Difference (SID) [16,17]. Consequently, such a decline in SID, reduces 10 mEq/L of the BE value measured by the ABG analyzer [16,17,21]. On the other hand, infusion of about 5l of NS during the surgery leads to 25% dilution of serum albumin concentration which is the main part of serum "A total"(an independent variable which includes sum of negative charges of weak anions such as phosphate and albumin). Hence, about +3 mEq/L increment in BE value takes place [16,17].

Thus, an acidifying force of about-10 mEq/L (hyperchloremia) faces an alkalinizing force of about +3 mEq/L (hypoalbuminemia).The final effect would be about-7 mEq/L of acidifying force. It must be mentioned that there are a few papers in the current literature which deal with the issue of optimal crystalloid therapy in a renal transplant surgery [9-11,22-26].

The effects of large-volume infusion of NS versus lactated Ringer's solution were compared by O'Malley et al. in renal transplant patients [9].They stated that lactated Ringer's solution may be as safe as NS. They incidentally found (through an intra-group analysis in NS group) a significantly higher urine volume and lower serum creatinine level in eight patients who were treated with bicarbonate to adjust metabolic acidosis. Accordingly, they suggested that metabolic acidosis was the probable reason of such a negative impact on renal functions in those patients who were not treated for acidosis. As they stated in their article, they did not define an algorithm for treatment of metabolic acidosis. So, to avoid the mentioned shortcoming, we designed a definite algorithm for treatment of metabolic acidosis in those who underwent a large volume infusion of NS. Surprisingly, our results support their findings regarding to beneficial effects of the metabolic acidosis control on a renal function. Several investigators have already suggested that hyperchloremia by itself may be the cause of such a detrimental effect on a renal function [22-24]. It must be pointed out that we normalized metabolic acidosis without enhancing excretion of extra load of chloride ion. Despite it, better early renal function tests were achieved. This finding may reveal that acidosis on its own, and not the chloride ion excess by itself is the cause of harmful effects on a renal function.

Hadimioglu et al. observed significantly larger urine output in NS group in comparison with lactated Ringer's and Plasmalyte solution groups in spite of significantly progressive rise of serum chloride level observed in the NS group [11]. However, they didn't find any significant difference between groups in terms of the renal function tests after the surgery. Their findings may support our concept that hyperchloremia on its own may be an innocent factor. Recently, Modi MP et al. through a letter to the editor stated that lactated Ringer's solution is as safe as NS in a renal transplant surgery [25]. Othman et al. have a different view point; they investigated on rapidity of fluid replacement therapy instead of the type of fluid which is used. They suggested that maintaining a given CVP in the renal transplant patients as a target by adjusting NS infusion rate, is superior to constant continuous infusion of NS in terms of an early postoperative renal function [26]. Another point that must be clarified is a probable negative impact of vasodilation and resulting hypotension induced by Lasix on the renal perfusion. Our results show a little reduction in MAP of both groups which seems clinically unimportant. The reason may be that vessels have been already dilated by anesthetic drugs in patients under general anesthesia, so minimal vasodilation is anticipated in these patients. In addition, equal amount of Lasix is injected to both groups, thus, it could not be regarded as a confounding factor in this study.

Our study may be subject to a number of limitations. 1-Only living donor transplantations were enrolled in this study. Thus, our results are merely applicable to this group of patients. 2- The other criticism is that a traditional marker (consecutive serum creatinine levels) was used as an indicator of an early renal function [27]. Because of logistical reasons, we could not use novel biomarkers of kidney injury like β2 Microglobulin, α- GluthationeS-transferase, etc. for this purpose. Although, the superiority of novel biomarkers over traditional ones is still unproven, use of novel biomarkers especially those which are specific for evaluation of ischemic renal insult may be advantageous in the transplanted kidney that is under such a risk.

Conclusion

Intraoperative metabolic acidosis tight control by using Sodium bicarbonate infusion, while keeping $PaCO_2$ level in normal range, may be an advantageous strategy to enhance the early postoperative kidney function in a renal transplant surgery.

Competing interest
The authors declare that they have no competing interests.

Authors' contributions
FE: Reviewing the literature, designing the study method, preparing the manuscript and final revision. PP: Conducting the study and gathering the data, preparing data for analysis. MM: Contributing to design the study method and interpreting the study results. AN: Participating in literature review and designing the study method. RSM: Conducting the study, participating in the analysis of data. KKI: Contributing to write the manuscript. MRK: Designing the study method and the questionnaire, conducting the study, interpreting the results. All authors read and approved the final manuscript.

Acknowledgement
The authors would like to thank the Research Development Center of Sina Hospital for their technical assistance.

References

1. Spencer YC, Niemann CU: Anesthesia for Abdominal Organ Transplantation. In Miller's Anesthesia Volume 2. 7th edition. Edited by Miller RD. Philadelphia: Elsevier Churchill Livingstone; 2010:2155–2183.
2. Atkins JL: Effect of sodium bicarbonate preloading on ischemic renal failure. Nephron 1986, 44:70–74.
3. Ballina JC, Vidal MC, Puche RC: Renal concentrating ability of rats fed a sodium bicarbonate enriched diet. Acta Physiol Pharmacol Latinoam 1984, 34:65–68.
4. Forsythe SM, Schmidt GA: Sodium bicarbonate for the treatment of lactic acidosis. Chest 2000, 117:260–267.
5. Lindinger MI, Franklin TW, Lands LC, Pedersen PK, Welsh DG, Heigenhauser GJ: NaHCO(3) and KHCO(3) ingestion rapidly increases renal electrolyte excretion in humans. J Appl Physiol 2000, 88:540–550.
6. Mathisen O, Raeder M, Kiil F: Mechanism of osmotic diuresis. Kidney Int 1981, 19:431–437.
7. Minich DM, Bland JS: Acid-alkaline balance: role in chronic disease and detoxification. Altern Ther Health Med 2007, 13:62–65.
8. Kaye AD, Riopelle JM: Intravascular fluid and electrolyte physiology. In Miller's Anesthesia Volume 2. 7th edition. Edited by Miller RD. Philadelphia: Elsevier Churchill Livingstone; 2010:1705–1737.
9. O'Malley CM, Frumento RJ, Hardy MA, Benvenisty AI, Brentjens TE, Mercer JS, Bennett-Guerrero E: A randomized, double-blind comparison of lactated ringer's solution and 0.9% NaCl during renal transplantation. Anesth Analg 2005, 100:1518–1524.
10. Khajavi MR, Etezadi F, Moharari RS, Imani F, Meysamie AP, Khashayar P, Najafi A: Effects of normal saline vs. lactated ringer's during renal transplantation. Ren Fail 2008, 30:535–539.
11. Hadimioglu N, Saadawy I, Saglam T, Ertug Z, Dinckan A: The effect of different crystalloid solutions on acid-base balance and early kidney function after kidney transplantation. Anesth Analg 2008, 107:264.
12. O'Malley CMN, Frumento RJ, Bennett-Guerrero E: Intravenous fluid therapy in renal transplant recipients: results of a U.S. survey. Transplant Proc 2002, 34:3142–3145.
13. Cowen RE, Jackson BT, Grainger SL, Thompson RPH: Effects of anesthetic agents and abdominal surgery on hepatic blood flow. Hepatology 1991, 14:1161–1166.
14. Puyana JC: Resuscitation of hypovolemic shock. In Textbook of critical care Volume 2. 5th edition. Edited by Fink MP, Abraham E, Vincent JL, Kochanek PM. Pennsylvania: Elsevier Saunders; 2005:1933–1944.
15. Martin G, Bennett-Guerrero E, Wakeling H, Mythen MG, el-Moalem H, Robertson K, Kucmeroski D, Gan TJ: A prospective, randomized comparison of thromboelastographiccoagulation profile in patients receiving lactated Ringer's solution, 6% hetastarch in a balanced-saline vehicle, or 6% hetastarch in saline during major surgery. J Cardiothorac Vasc Anesth 200, 16:441–446.
16. Stewart PA: Modern quantitative acid–base chemistry. Can J Physiol Pharmacol 1983, 61:1444–1461.
17. Fencl V, Leith DE: Stewart's quantitative acid–base chemistry: applications in biology and medicine. Respir Physiol 1993, 91:1–16.
18. Scheingraber S, Rehm M, Sehmisch C, Finsterer U: Rapid saline infusion produces hyperchloremic acidosis in patients undergoing gynecologic surgery. Anesthesiology 1999, 90:1265–1270.
19. McFarlane C, Lee A: A comparison of plasmalyte 148 and 0.9% saline for intra-operative fluid replacement. Anesthesia 1994, 49:779–781.
20. Carlier M, Squifflet J, Pirson Y, Grimbomont B, Alexandre GP: Maximal hydration during anesthesia increases pulmonary arterial pressures and improves early function of human renal transplants. Transplantation 1982, 34:201–204.
21. Kellum JA: Clinical review: reunification of acid–base physiology. Crit Care 2005, 9:500–507.
22. Gan TJ, Bennett-Guerrero E, Phillips-Bute B, Wakeling H, Moskowits DM, Olufolabi Y, et al: Hextend, a physiologically balanced plasma expander for large volume use in major surgery: a randomized phase ш clinical trial – hextends study group. Anesth Analg 1999, 88:992–998.
23. Wilcox CS: Regulation of renal blood flow by plasma chloride. J Clin Invest 1983, 71:726–735.
24. Wilcox CS, Peart WS: Release of renin and angiotensin 2 into plasma and lymph during hyperchloremia. Am J Physiol 1987, 253:F734–F741.
25. Modi MP, Vora KS, Parikh GP, Shah VR: A comparative study of impact of infusion of ringer's lactate solution versus normal saline on acid–base balance and serum electrolytes during live related renal transplantation. Saudi J Kidney Dis Transpl 2012, 23:135–137.
26. Othman MM, Ismael AZ, Hammouda GE: The impact of timing of maximal crystalloid hydration on early graft function during kidney transplantation. Anesth Analg 2010, 110:1440–1446.
27. Stafford-Smith M, Shaw A, Aronson S: Renal function monitoring. In Miller's Anesthesia Volume 2. 7th edition. Edited by Miller RD. Philadelphia: Elsevier Churchill Livingstone; 2010:1443–1475.

Evaluation of the antinociceptive and anti-inflammatory effects of essential oil of *Nepeta pogonosperma* Jamzad et Assadi in rats

Taskina Ali[1,2]*, Mohammad Javan[2], Ali Sonboli[3] and Saeed Semnanian[2]

Abstract

Background and the purpose of study: Concerning the different effects of essential oils from Nepeta genus on the central nervous system including pain killing effect, this study was designed to evaluate the antinociceptive and anti-inflammatory effects of essential oil of *Nepeta pogonosperma* Jamzad et Assadi *(NP)*, a recently identified species.

Methods: Air-dried aerial parts of *NP* were hydrodistillated and GC-MS analysis of obtained essential oil was conducted. Total 24 male Wister rats weighing 225 ± 25 gm were studied. Essential oil of *NP* was administered intraperitoneally at the doses of 50 mg/kg, 100 mg/kg and 200 mg/kg for the experimental groups. Control rats received equal volume (2 ml/kg) of normal saline. Antinociception was assessed by tail flick test (after 30 minutes) and formalin test (for further 60 minutes). Then the animal was sacrificed and the paw edema was measured using a water plethysmometer.

Results: 4aα,7α,7aβ-nepetalactone and 1,8-cineole were found as the main concentrated components of *NP* essential oil. All the doses of *NP* showed antinociception. NP 200 mg/kg reduced the pain sensation in tail flick ($p < 0.01$) and formalin test ($p < 0.001$ in both phases). In paw edema test, NP 100 and 200 mg/kg significantly reduced the inflammation ($p < 0.01$ and $p < 0.05$).

Conclusion: This study reveals that the essential oil of *NP* may minimize both the acute and chronic forms of nociception and may have potent role against inflammation, but the dose should be maintained precisely to obtain the intended effect.

Keywords: Nociception, *Nepeta pogonosperma*, Formalin test, Tail flick test, Essential oil, Inflammation

Introduction

Nepeta L. (from Lamiaceae) contains about 300 species, which are distributed in central and southern Europe and in near East, central and southern Asia also. Within them Iran is one of the centers of origin of this genus with 75 species and approximately 53% endemics [1]. The diversity, species richness and variation as well as chemical properties have led to much research into this genus. The extracts of many *Nepeta* species are used in domestic medicine. *N. cataria* L., commonly known as catnip, is the most intensively studied species [2], which is used as a fortifier, a disinfectant and a cure for colds. The extracts of some species are also used because of their diuretic properties and slight bacteriostatic activity, and also in ointments to heal skin disorders of eczema type [3]. Some of the species are widely used in folk medicine because of their expectorant, antiseptic, antitussive, antiasthmatic and febrifuge activities [4-6]. The beverages and infusion prepared from the aerial parts of *Nepeta crispa* Willd. were traditionally used as sedative, relaxant, carminative and also restorative tonic for nervous and respiratory disorders [7]. It has also been shown to have antimicrobial (*N. meyeri*) and anxiolytic (*N. persica*) properties [8].

* Correspondence: taskinadr@gmail.com
[1]Department of Physiology, Bangabandhu Sheikh Mujib Medical University, Dhaka, Bangladesh
[2]Department of Physiology, Faculty of Medical Sciences, Tarbiat Modares University, Tehran, Iran
Full list of author information is available at the end of the article

One of these *Nepeta* plants of Iran is *Nepeta pogonosperma* Jamzad et Assadi, which was identified as new species in 1984 [6]. The essential oil composition of its aerial parts has been reported [9]. The main components of its essential oil were 4aα, 7α, 7aβ-Nepetalactone (57.6%) and 1,8-cineol (26.4%). The dried aerial parts of other species of *Nepeta* were also shown to contain both of these components in different proportion in their essential oil [7,10].

The most important constituent of the essential oil of this *Nepeta* species, 1, 8-cineol, an oxygenated monoterpene, showed inhibitory effect on carrageenan induced paw edema and cotton-pellet induced granuloma in rats [11]. It has also been stated that this terpenoid oxide has strong inhibitory effect on cytokine production in cultured human lymphocytes and monocytes [12]. Moreover, its steroid sparing capacity in bronchial asthma was also determined [13]. A recent report on the essential oil of *Rosmarinus officinalis* L. (a endemic plant in Mexico), which contains 8.58% 1,8-cineole, showed a dose dependent antinociceptive effect in rat model [14]. In addition different isomers of Nepetalactones were reported to have considerable sedative and analgesic activity. 4aα, 7α, 7aβ-Nepetalactone, the key constituent of *Nepeta ceasarea* Boiss, was suggested to have a specific opioid receptor agonistic activity [15]. Again the catnip oil prepared from *Nepeta cataria* showed to have 40% nepetalactone, which was responsible for significant increase in the hexobarbital sleeping time in mice [16].

Different species of Nepeta genus are reported to contain antinociceptive and anti-inflammatory effects. In an study on *Nepeta cataria* essential oil showed of having 79.27% of nepetalactone which might be responsible for its potent antinociceptive and anti-inflammatory activity in mice model [17]. Moreover, extract and fractions from *Nepeta sibthorpil* have been reported to have anti-inflammatory activity in carrageenan induced paw edema model in rat [18]. Recently we reported the analgesic and anti-inflammatory effects of *Nepeta crispa* Willd. in animal models [19]. On the basis of these diversified biological activities of the *Nepeta* species and their use in folk medicine, this study was designed to evaluate antinociceptive and anti-inflammatory effects of a newly introduced species, *Nepeta pogonosperma*. We evaluated the antinociceptive effect in both acute and chronic pain models and also investigated its anti-inflammatory activity in an animal paw edema model.

Materials and methods
Plant materials
The aerial flowering parts of *Nepeta pogonosperma* Jamzad & Assadi were collected from its wild locality in Qazvin province on 20 May, 2008. The plant was identified by A. Sonboli and a voucher specimen (MPH-1917)

was deposited in herbarium of Medicinal Plants and Drugs Research Institute (MPH) of Shahid Beheshti University, Tehran, Iran.

Air-dried aerial parts (100 g) of *Nepeta pogonosperma* were subjected to hydrodistillation using a Clevenger-type apparatus. The essential oil was dried over anhydrous sodium sulfate and stored in sealed vials. The oil was stored at 4°C until the time of analysis and tests. GC-MS analysis of the essential oil was conducted on a Thermoquest-Finnigan Trace GC-MS system equipped with a fused silica DB-1 capillary column (60 m × 0.32 mm i.d., film thickness 0.25 μm). Helium was used as the carrier gas at the constant flow of 1.1 ml/min. The oven temperature was 60°C rising to 250°C at a rate of 5°C/min, then held at 250°C for 10 min; transfer line temperature, 250°C; split ratio was 1/50. The quadrupole mass spectrometer was scanned over the 45–465 amu with an ionizing voltage of 70 eV and an ionization current of 150 μA. The injector and detector (FID) temperatures were kept at 250°C and 280°C, respectively. Retention indices (RI) for all constituents were calculated according to Van den Dool approach, using *n*-alkanes ($C_6 - C_{24}$) as standards and the essential oil on a DB-1 column under the same chromatographic conditions. The identification of the components was made based on comparison of their mass spectra with those of the internal computer reference mass spectra libraries (Wiley 7.0), as well as by comparison of their retention indices with data published.

Animals
Twenty four (24) male Wister rats weighing 225 ± 25 g obtained from the Pasteur Institute, Karaj, Iran, were used. They were housed in plexiglass cages as 6 animals per cage with room temperature $24 \pm 2°C$ under a 12 hour light/dark cycle and had free access to water and pellet. The rats were accustomed to the laboratory condition for 4 days before commencement of the experiments. Efforts were made to minimize the number of animals used and their sufferings. All research and animal care procedures were performed according to the international guidelines on the use of laboratory animals and on the basis of codes for ethics in animal research in Tarbiat Modares University

Drug administration
Animals were treated intraperitoneally (i.p.) with normal saline for the control group or the essential oil of *Nepeta pogonosperma* at the doses of 50, 100 or 200 mg/kg for the experimental groups. The doses were selected based on our previous report on the antinociceptive effects of *N. crispa* [19]. An equal volume of injection of essential oil or normal saline (200 μl/100 g of body weight) was applied for all animals.

Tail-flick test

Acute antinociceptive effect was assessed based on the method introduced by D'Amour and Smith [20] using a tail-flick apparatus (Harvard Apparatus). The baseline latency was obtained using the mean of similar three consecutive measurements. Normal saline (for control rats) or essential oil (for experimental groups) were injected i.p. immediately after the third pre-drug measurement. Again, test latency was determined after 30 minutes of saline or oil administration (mean of 3 measurements). To minimize tissue damage, a maximum latency of 10 seconds was imposed. Antinociceptive effect was calculated as percent of maximum possible effect (% MPE), as follows [21]:

$$\% \ MPE = [(TL - BL)/(CT - BL)] \times 100$$

TL = Test latency; BL = Baseline latency; CT = Cut-off time.

Formalin test

The formalin test was carried out in a plexiglass observation box, with a mirror placed under the floor (at a 45° angle) to allow a clear view of the paws. Immediately after the recording of the 3rd latency time of the tail flick test, 50 μl of 2% formalin was injected subcutaneously into the plantar aspect of the rat's right hind paw. The animal was then placed in the observation cage and pain behaviors were recorded for 60 minutes. Nociception was rated using a modification of the original formalin test protocol [22]. Briefly, the pain scoring measurements were as follows: 0 = normal weight bearing on the injected paw; 1 = limping during locomotion or resting the paw lightly on the floor; 2 = elevation of the injected paw; and 3 = licking or biting of the injected paw. The first 5 minutes was considered as early phase and minutes 16 to 60 were considered as the late phase of formalin test [23]. The different behavioral parameters including jerking, flexing and licking were took out from the records as total counts per 5 minutes or total duration in seconds per 5 minutes, respectively.

Anti-inflammatory test

Anti-inflammatory effects of the essential oil were determined by the formalin-induced paw edema model. The amount of paw edema caused by intra-plantar injection of 2% formalin was used as an indicator of inflammation severity. Following 60 minutes of recording the pain behaviors (about 90 minutes after the i.p administration of the essential oil or saline), the animal was sacrificed. Then the volume of the animals' right and left hindpaws were measured using a water plethysmometer as mentioned by Fereidoni et al. 2001 [24]. Right paw volume was subtracted by left paw volume to obtain the net edema volume.

The rats were not tested more than once and all the experiments were carried out in between 9:00 and 15:00, to minimize the possible influence of circadian changes on rat behavior.

Statistical analysis

Data obtained for different pain behavior and edema were scrutinized using one way analysis of variance (ANOVA) followed by the Tukey post-hoc test. The results are expressed as mean ± S.E.M and $p < 0.05$ was considered as significant difference of means.

Results

Essential oil composition

Although, the main components of *Nepeta pogonosperma* essential oil were reported to be 1,8-cineole and 4aα,7α,7aβ-nepetalactone, concerning the percentage variations in previous reports and the seasonal and local variations in the component of different plants, we analyzed the composition of essential oil applied in this study. Hydrodistilled essential oil of aerial parts of *NP* gave pale yellow oil and forty-one components were identified representing 97.5% of the total oil. Essential oil compounds are presented in Table 1, where compounds are listed in order of their elution on the DB-1 column. The main components of the oil were 4aα,7α,7aα–nepetalactone (14.5%) and 1,8- cineole (31.2%) followed by α-terpineol (5.4%), (E)-α-bisabolene (5.4%), terpinen-4-ol (4.8%), linalool (4.5%) and β-pinene (3.5%).

Tail-flick test

The effects of 50, 100 and 200 mg/kg doses of *NP* essential oil on acute pain were evaluated using tail flick test. As evaluated at 30 minutes post injection, 50 mg/kg dose of NP did not produce any significant analgesia, but the doses of 100 and 200 mg/kg of NP reduced the acute thermal pain significantly ($p < 0.01$ and $p < 0.001$, respectively). The percentage of maximum possible effect (% MPE) of all the doses were compared to that of the control and presented in Figure 1.

Formalin test

The effects of systemic i.p. administration of different doses of the essential oil of *NP* on the early and late phases of formalin test were observed. In both phases the pain behaviors were separately analyzed as total jerking frequency, licking duration and flexing duration.

As it is mentioned in Figure 2, in the first phase of formalin test 50, 100 and 200 mg/kg doses of NP reduced the jerking frequency ($p < 0.001$, in all doses), flexing duration ($p < 0.05$, $p < 0.05$, $p < 0.01$, respectively) and licking duration ($p < 0.05$, $p < 0.001$, $p < 0.001$, respectively), significantly.

Table 1 Essential oil composition of *Nepeta pogonosperma*

Compound	RI	%
α-thujene	925	0.3
α-pinene	933	1.4
Sabinene	968	0.7
β-pinene	**974**	**3.5**
Myrcene	983	0.7
isobutyl 2-methylbutanoate	993	0.5
isobutyl isovalerate	995	0.9
p-cymene	1017	2.7
1,8-cineole	**1030**	**31.2**
γ-terpinene	1050	0.4
trans-sabinene hydrate	1059	2.1
cis-linalool oxide	1064	0.3
Linalool	**1089**	**4.5**
2-methylbutyl 2-methylbutanoate	1093	0.7
2-methylbutyl isovalerate	1096	0.3
4-acetyl-1-methyl-1-cyclohexene	1112	0.8
trans-pinocarveol	1129	0.8
Pinocarvone	1144	0.8
δ-terpineol	1153	3.1
terpinen-4-ol	**1167**	**4.8**
α-terpineol	**1179**	**5.4**
Geraniol	1240	0.5
4aβ-7α-7aα-nepetalactone	1325	0.3
4aα-7α-7aα-nepetalactone	**1336**	**14.5**
4aα-7α-7aβ-nepetalactone	1346	0.3
4aβ-7α-7aβ-nepetalactone	1361	0.5
geranyl acetate	1364	3.1
β-bourbonene	1383	0.8
trans-caryophyllene	1417	1.1
(E)-β-farnesene	1447	0.7
α-humulene	1450	0.8
germacrene D	1475	0.2
(E)-α-bisabolene	**1493**	**5.2**
caryophyllene-oxide	1573	2.7
humulene epoxide	1597	0.9
Monoterpene hydrocarbons		9.7
Oxygenated monoterpens		72.2
Sesquiterpene hydrocarbons		8.8
Oxygenated sesquiterpenes		3.6
Others		3.2
Total identified (35 comp.)		**97.5%**

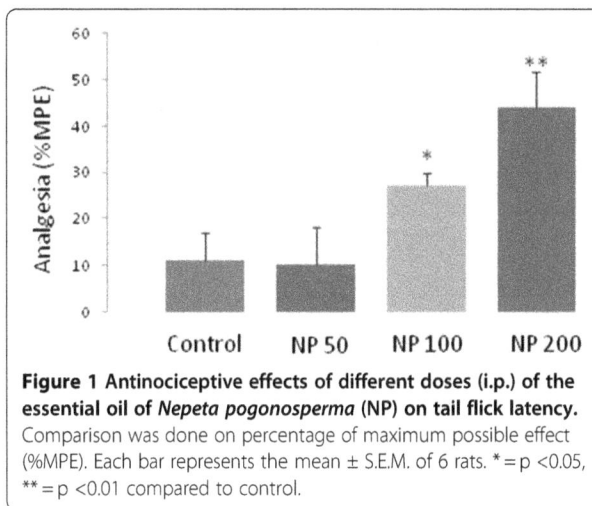

Figure 1 Antinociceptive effects of different doses (i.p.) of the essential oil of *Nepeta pogonosperma* (NP) on tail flick latency. Comparison was done on percentage of maximum possible effect (%MPE). Each bar represents the mean ± S.E.M. of 6 rats. * = p <0.05, ** = p <0.01 compared to control.

Again in the late phase of formalin test, as it is mentioned in Figure 3, all the doses of NP reduced the jerking frequency (p <0.001, in all doses), the flexing duration (p <0.001, p <0.01, p <0.001, respectively) and licking duration (p <0.01, p <0.05, p <0.001, respectively), significantly.

Anti-inflammatory effect
The amount of edema for formalin injected paw was measured at the end of formalin test. As illustrated in Figure 4, all the doses of the oil showed anti-inflammatory effect in the paw edema model though it was significant only in 100 (p <0.01) and 200 (p <0.05) mg/kg of doses of NP.

Discussion
The management of pain is probably one of the most common and yet most difficult aspects in medical practice. Many improved analgesics and anti-inflammatory agents have been developed, but there is considerable opportunity for conceptual innovation.

We used heat induced and formalin induced pain model for evaluating antinociceptive and formalin induced paw edema model for anti-inflammatory effect of *Nepeta pogonosperma* in experimental rats. Our data demonstrated that the essential oil of this plant elicited potent antinociceptive effects in rats subjected to both the acute thermal (tail-flick) and chronic or persistent formalin pain stimuli and strong anti-inflammatory effect to formalin induced paw edema model.

The Tail flick test is one of the most appropriate techniques to assess the acute somatosensory pain transmission by stimulating thermoreceptors in experimental animal model [25]. King *et al* (1997) showed that this test is sensitive to centrally acting analgesics and

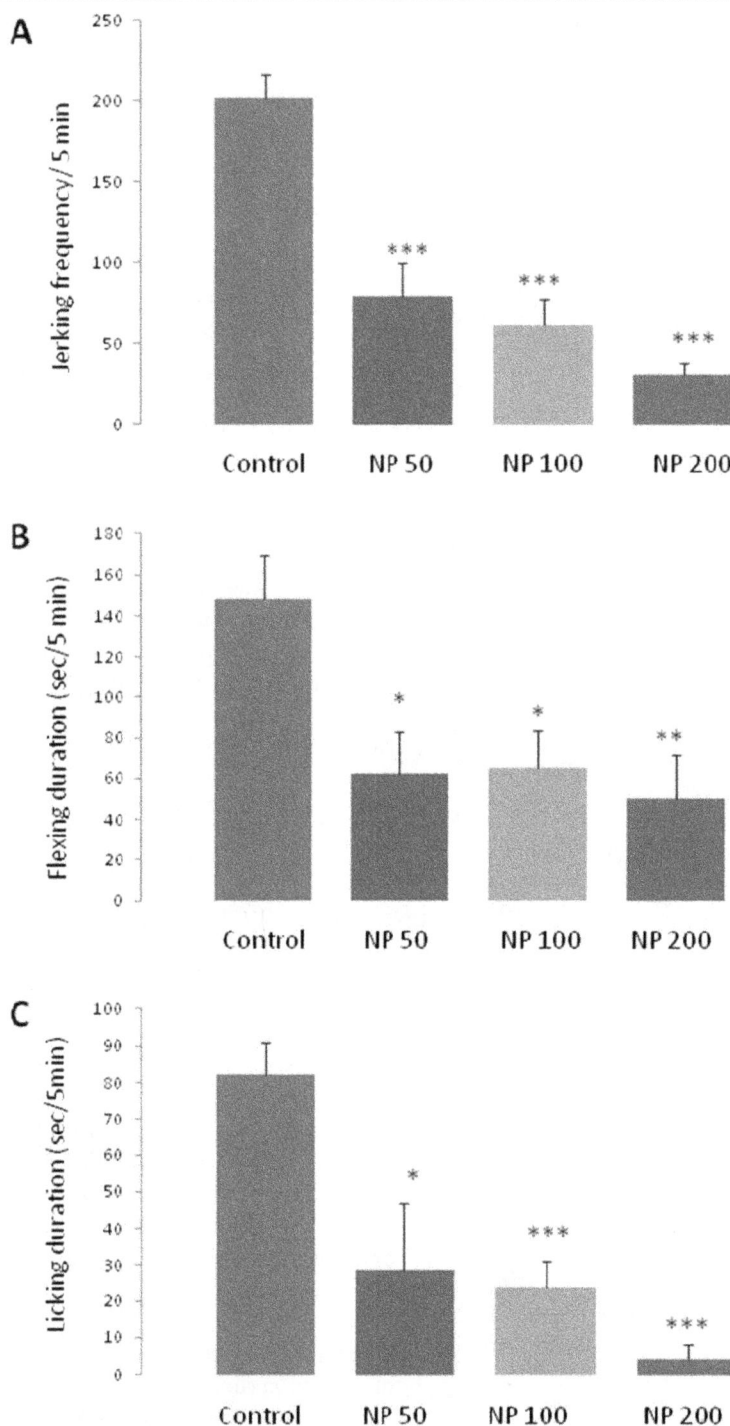

Figure 2 Antinociceptive effects of different doses of the essential oil of *Nepeta pogonosperma* (NP) in the early phase of formalin test (minutes 0 – 5). NP doses reduced different pain behaviors including jerking (**A**), flexing (**B**) and licking (**C**). Each bar symbolizes for mean ± S.E. M. for 6 rats. * = p <0.05, ** = p <0.01, *** = p <0.001 compared to control.

supraspinal systems facilitated this tail flicking response which was inhibited by a low dose of morphine [26]. Since our results mentioned potent analgesia in higher two doses of NP in tail flick test, it may be commented that the effective component(s) of this essential oil exerts its antinociceptive effect by modulating the pain transmission in the central nervous system.

Formalin test is one of the appropriate methods for producing and quantifying the chemical pain in the rat model. Pain intensity in this test is dependent on some

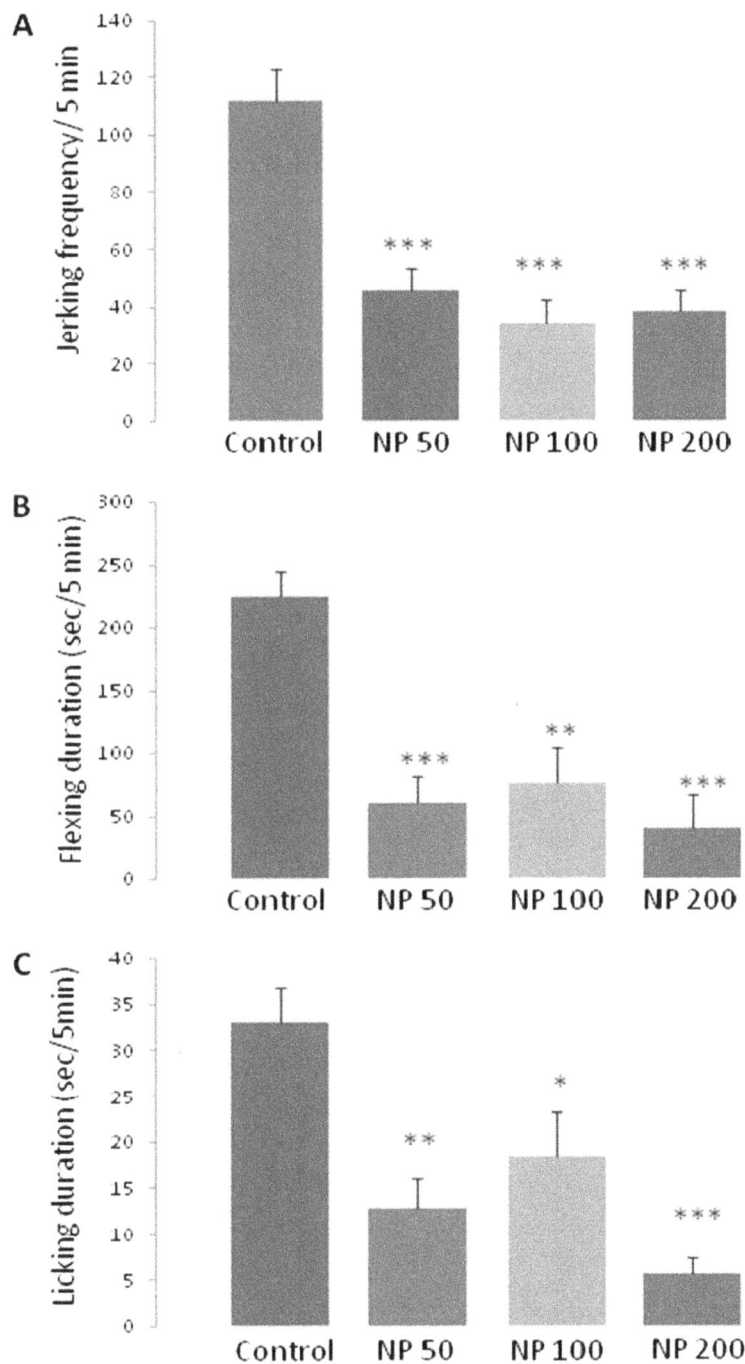

Figure 3 Antinociceptive effect of different doses of the essential oil of *Nepeta pogonosperma* (NP) in the late phase of formalin test (**minutes 16 – 60**). NP doses reduced all pain behaviors including jerking (**A**), flexing (**B**) and licking (**C**). Each bar symbolizes for mean ± S.E.M. for 6 rats. * = p <0.05, ** = p <0.01, ***p <0.001 compared to control.

objective behavioral categories and the observations are converted to numerical values [22]. Subcutaneous injection of formalin induces hindpaw inflammation, which leads to a response characterized by jerking, flexing followed by licking of the affected hindlimb. This characteristic response is considered to be a central nociceptive model, and has been associated with increased levels of chemical mediators in tissue fluids. The level of pain in this model is sensitive to both centrally and peripherally acting analgesics. In the present study, as the i.p. administration of different doses of the essential oil of *NP* inhibited both phases of pain response relative to controls, it may be suggested that it has both the central and peripheral antinociceptive effects. We checked for

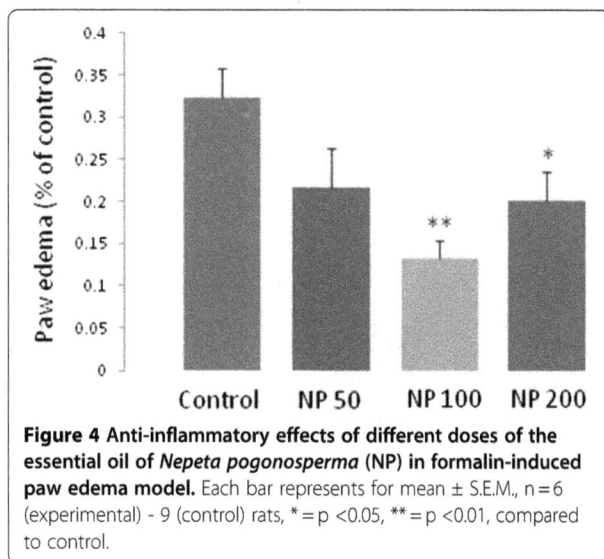

Figure 4 Anti-inflammatory effects of different doses of the essential oil of *Nepeta pogonosperma* (NP) in formalin-induced paw edema model. Each bar represents for mean ± S.E.M., n = 6 (experimental) - 9 (control) rats, * = p <0.05, ** = p <0.01, compared to control.

anti-inflammatory effect of the essential oil and observed reduced formalin induced edema. This finding proved the peripheral antinociceptive effects of the oil bye ameliorating the formalin induced inflammation. Comparing the antinociceptive and anti-inflammatory effects of the lower dose (50 mg/kg), again makes the central analgesic effect plausible. In the other word, the dose which did not produce anti-inflammatory effect exerted significant analgesic effect.

Similar to the previous report [9], NP essential oil contained 1, 8-cineole and 4aα, 7α, 7aβ-Nepetalactone as two major constituent. It has been suggested by many investigators that 1, 8-cineole, the most important constituent of *NP* essential oil has potent antinociceptive [14] and anti-inflammatory activity [11,12]. In addition, Aydin and colleagues (1998) suggested that 4aα, 7α, 7aβ-Nepetalactone, might be responsible for the significant analgesic activity and marked sedation in a rat model. They also recommended this nepetalactone might have specific opioid receptor subtype agonist activity [15]. Again in a behavioral study on rats a significant decrease in performance was observed following i.p. administration of nepetalactone enriched fraction [16]. Furthermore the nepetalactone isomers were suggested to be the responsible component of the anti-nociceptive and anti-inflammatory actions of *Nepeta cataria* L. var. citriodora (Becker) Balb. [17]. Moreover, the essential oil of *Nepeta crispa* Willd. which contained 20.3% 4aα, 7α, 7aβ-Nepetalactone and 47.9% 1,8-cineole, showed strong antibacterial, antifungal, antinociceptive and antiinflammatory activity [19,21]. This finding may support the potent anti-inflammatory activity observed in our present experiment. In a previous study, the analgesic activity of the essential oil of *Nepeta italica* L. was showed to be correlated with the amount of 1, 8-cineole [27]. In a

recent animal study, cineole has been recommended to reveal an antinociceptive activity comparable to that of morphine in thermal analgesic stimuli [28]. Hence, both of the components of *NP* essential oil, the 4aα, 7α, 7aβ-Nepetalactone and 1, 8-cineole, may be responsible for our experimental findings.

Conclusion

In conclusion, it may be recommended that the essential oil of *Nepeta pogonosperma* may minimize both the acute and chronic forms of nociception and may have potent role against inflammation, but the dose should be maintained precisely to obtain the intended effect. Although, further experimental study is needed to elucidate the exact component and mechanism responsible for these effects.

Competing interests
The authors declare that they have no competing interests.

Authors' contribution
TA performed the experiments and prepared the draft of manuscript; MJ and SS designed and supervised the study and finalized the MS; AS prepared the plant materials and measured its components. All authors read and approved the final manuscript.

Acknowledgements
The work was done at the Department of Physiology, faculty of Medicine, Tarbiat Modares University, Tehran, Iran. The authors are grateful to the Iranian Society of Physiology and Pharmacology (ISPP) and Tarbiat Modares University, Tehran, Iran for supporting Dr. Taskina Ali with a scholarship and financial support of the research project.

Author details
[1]Department of Physiology, Bangabandhu Sheikh Mujib Medical University, Dhaka, Bangladesh. [2]Department of Physiology, Faculty of Medical Sciences, Tarbiat Modares University, Tehran, Iran. [3]Department of Biology, Medicinal Plants and Drugs Research Institute, Shahid Beheshti University, Tehran, Iran.

References
1. Jamzad Z, Ingrouille M, Simmonds M: **Three new species of Nepeta (Laminaceae) from Iran.** *Taxon* 2003, **52**:92–98.
2. Grognet J: **Catnip, its uses and effects, past & present.** *Can Vet J* 1990, **31**:455–456.
3. Javidnia K, Miri R, Safavi F, Azarpira A, Shafiee A: **Composition of the essential oil of Nepeta persica Boiss from Iran.** *Flavour Fragr J* 2002, **17**:20–22.
4. Baser KHC, Kirimer N, Kerkcuoglu M, Demirci B: **Essential oil of Nepeta species in Turkey.** *Chem Nat Comp* 2000, **36**:356–359.
5. Newall CA, Anderson LA, Phillipson JD: *Herbal Medicines, a Guide for Health Care Professionals.* London: Pharmaceutical Press; 1996:154.
6. Jamzad Z, Assadi M: **New species of Nepeta and Ajuga.** *Ind Jf Botany* 1984, **2**:95–103.
7. Mozaffarian V: *A dictionary of Iranian plant names.* Tehran: Farhang Moaser; 1996.
8. Joudi L, Bibalani GH: **Exploration of medicinal species of Fabaceae, lamiacea and Asteraceae families in Ilkhji region, eastern Azerbaijan province (Northwestern Iran).** *J Med Plant Res* 2010, **4**:1081–1084.
9. Sefidkon F, Akbari-nia A: **Essential oil composition of Nepeta pogonosperma Jamzad et Assadi from Iran.** *J Essent Oil Res* 2003, **15**:327–328.
10. Javidnia K, Miri R, Safavi F, Azarpira A, Shafiee A: **Composition of the essential oil of Nepeta persica Boiss. from Iran.** *Flav Frag J* 2002, **17**:20–22.

11. Santos FA, Rao VS: **Antiinflammatory and antonociceptive effects of 1,8-cineole a terpenoid oxide present in many plant essential oils.** *Phytother Res* 2000, **14**:240–244.

12. Juergens UR, Engelen T, Racké K, Stöber M, Gillissen A, Vetter H: **Inhibitory activity of 1,8-cineole (eucalyptol) on cytokine production in cultured human lymphocytes and monocytes.** *Pulm Pharmacol Ther* 2004, **17**:281–287.

13. Juergens UR, Dethlefsen U, Steinkamp G, Gillissen A, Repges R, Vetter H: **Anti-inflammatory activity of 1,8-cineole (eucalyptol) in bronchial asthma: a double-blind placebo-controlled trial.** *Respir Med* 2003, **97**:250–256.

14. Martínez AL, González-Truzano ME, Pellicer F, López-Muñoz FJ, Navarrete A: **Antonociceptive effect and GC/MS analysis of** *Roamarinus officinalis* **L. essential oil from its aerial parts.** *Planta Med* 2009, **75**:508–511.

15. Aydin S, Beis R, OztÜrk Y, Baser KH: **Nepetalactone: a new opioid analgesic from** *Nepeta caesarea* **Boiss.** *J Pharm Pharmacol* 1998, **50**:813–817.

16. Harney JW, Barofsky IM: **Behavioral and toxicological studies of cyclopentanoid monoterpenes from** *Nepeta cataria. Lloydia* 1978, **41**:367–374.

17. Ricci EL, Toyama DO, Lago JHG, Romoff P, Kirsten TB, Reis-Silva TM, Bernardi MM: **Anti-nociceptive and anti-inflammatory actions of** *Nepeta cataria* **L. var. citridora (Becker) Balb. essenmtial oil in mice.** *J Health Sci Inst* 2010, **28**:289–293.

18. Miceli N, Taviano MF, Giuffrida D, Trovato A, Tzakou O, Galati EM: **Anti-inflammatory activity of extract and fractions from** *Nepeta sibthorpil* **Bentham.** *J Ethnopharmaco* 2004, **97**:261–266.

19. Ali T, Javan M, Sonboli A, Semnanian S: **Antinociceptive and anti-inflammatory activities of essential oil of** *Nepeta crispa* **Willd. in experimental rat models.** *Nat Prod Res*, 2012, **26**:1529–34.

20. D'Amour FE, Smith DL: **A method for determining loss of pain sensation.** *J Pharmacol Exo Ther* 1941, **72**:74–79.

21. Satarian L, Javan M, Fatollahi Y: **Epinephrine inhibits analgesic tolerance to intrathecal administrated morphine and increase the expression of calcium-calmodulin-dependent protein kinase II∞.** *Neurosci Lett* 2008, **430**:213–217.

22. Dubisson D, Dennis SG: **The formalin test: a quantitative study of the analgesic effects of morphine, meperidine and brain stem stimulation in rats and cats.** *Pain* 1997, **4**:161–174.

23. Damaj MI, Glassco W, Aceto MD, Martin BR: **Antinociceptive and pharmacological effects of metanicotine, a selective nicotinic agonist.** *J Pharmacol Exp Ther* 1999, **291**:390–398.

24. Fereidoni M, Ahmadiani A, Semnanian S, Javan M: **An accurate and simple method for measurement of paw edema.** *J Pharmacol Toxicol Methods* 2000, **43**:11–14.

25. Björkman R: **Central antinociceptive effects of non-steroidal antiinflammatory drugs and paracetamol. Experimental studies in the rat.** *Acta Anaesthesiol Scand Suppl* 1995, **103**:1–44.

26. King TE, Joynes RL, Grau JW: **Tail-Flick test: II. The role of supraspinal systems and avoidance learning.** *Behav Neurosci* 1997, **111**:754–767.

27. Aydin S, Demir T, Oztürk Y, Baser KH: **Analgesic activity of** *Nepeta italica* **L.** *Phytother Re* 1999, **13**:20–23.

28. Liapi C, Anifandis G, Chinou I, Kourounakis AP, Theodosopoulos US, Galanopoulou P: **Antinociceptive properties of 1,8-Cineole and beta-pinene, from the essential oil of** *Eucalyptus camaldulensis* **leaves, in rodents.** *Planta Med* 2007, **73**:1247–1254.

Natural gums as sustained release carriers: development of gastroretentive drug delivery system of ziprasidone HCl

Rajamma AJ[1], Yogesha HN[2] and Sateesha SB[2*]

Abstract

Background: Objective of this study is to show the potential use of natural gums in the development of drug delivery systems. Therefore in this work gastro retentive tablet formulations of ziprasidone HCl were developed using simplex lattice design considering concentration of okra gum, locust bean gum and HPMC K4M as independent variables. A response surface plot and multiple regression equations were used to evaluate the effect of independent variables on hardness, f_{lag} time, floating time and drug release for 1 h, 2 h, and 8 h and for 24 h. A checkpoint batch was also prepared by considering the constraints and desirability of optimized formulation to improve its *in vitro* performance. Significance of result was analyzed using ANOVA and $p < 0.05$ was considered statistically significant.

Results: Formulation chiefly contains locust bean gum found to be favorable for hardness and floatability but combined effect of three variables was responsible for the sustained release of drug. The *in vitro* drug release data of check point batch (F8) was found to be sustained well compared to the most satisfactory formulation (F7) of 7 runs. The 'n' value was found to be between 0.5 and 1 suggesting that release of drug follows anomalous (non-fickian) diffusion mechanism indicating both diffusion and erosion mechanism from these natural gums. Predicted results were almost similar to the observed experimental values indicating the accuracy of the design. *In vivo* floatability test indicated non adherence to the gastric mucosa and tablets remain buoyant for more than 24 h.

Conclusions: Study showed these eco-friendly natural gums can be considered as promising SR polymers.

Keywords: Okra gum, Locust bean gum, Ziprasidone HCl, Gastro retentive tablet, Simplex lattice design, *In vivo* floatability

Introduction

The use of naturally occurring hydrophilic biocompatible polymeric materials has been focused in recent research activity in the design of oral controlled release dosage forms [1]. Natural gums are among the most popular hydrophilic polymers because of their cost-effectiveness and regulatory acceptance [2,3]. The use of naturally occurring plant-based pharmaceutical excipients has become very important in the development of controlled release dosage forms, because of their ability to produce a wide range of material based on their properties and molecular weight [4]. Plant based materials can be modified to meet the requirements of drug delivery systems and thus can compete with the synthetic excipients available in the market [5].

Okra gum and locust bean gum are water soluble thickening agents which have not been much studied for their pharmaceutical applications [6]. Okra gum, obtained from the fruits of *Hibiscus esculentus* L. (Moench), Malvaceae, is a polysaccharide consisting of D-galactose, L-rhamnose and L-galacturonic acid [7]. Locust bean gum (LBG) is a neutral plant galactomannan extracted from the seed (kernels) of the carob tree *Ceratonia siliqua* L. fabaceae [8]. The okra gum and LBG shows a synergistic gelation in acidic pH [9,10] and in combination with HPMC K4M forms an original gelation which has an excellent buoyancy and useful for oral gastro retentive formulations.

* Correspondence: sbsateesh@gmail.com
[2]Department of Pharmaceutics, Acharya & BM Reddy College of Pharmacy, Soladevanahally Hesaraghatta road, Bangalore 560090, India
Full list of author information is available at the end of the article

Ziprasidone HCl is an antipsychotic agent used in the treatment of schizophrenia [11]. The systemic bioavailability of ziprasidone administered intramuscularly is 100%, or 60%, administered orally with food. Drug reaches peak plasma concentration in 6 to 8 h after oral administration with an elimination half life of 7 h. This drug is more soluble in acidic pH and its solubility decreases with increasing pH owing to its pKa (~6) value [12]. The beneficial delivery system would be gastroretentive drug delivery systems which remain in the gastric region for several hours and significantly prolong the gastric residence time of drugs [13]. Hence, the goal has been set to evaluate the potential of Okra gum and LBG in combination with HPMC K4 for gastro retentive drug delivery system of ziprasidone HCl using simplex lattice design (SLD).

Materials and methods

Ziprasidone HCl (Sanofi Aventis Pharma, Ltd, India) was received as a gift sample. HPMC K4M, okra gum (okra seeds, market), locust bean gum (Sigma Aldrich, Germany), and polyvinyl pyrollidone (Sisco research laboratories Pvt. Ltd) were purchased. All other chemicals used in the study were of analytical grade. Stat-ease Design-Expert® software was used to design the formulation.

Okra gum (pod mucilage)

The fresh *A. esculentus* fruits were collected and washed with water. The fruits were crushed and soaked in water for 5–6 h, boiled for 30 min and left to stand for 1 h to allow complete release of the mucilage. The mucilage was separated using a multi layer muslin cloth and was precipitated by adding acetone (three times the volume of filtrate). The precipitate obtained was collected, dried in an oven at 40°C, and passed through a sieve #80 to obtain discrete powder [14].

Simplex lattice design

A simplex lattice design was adopted to optimize the formulation variables of gastro retentive drug delivery system of ziprasidone HCl [15]. The simplex lattice design for a 3-component system is represented by an equilateral triangle in 2-dimensional space (Figure 1). In this design, 3 factors were evaluated by changing their concentrations simultaneously and keeping their total concentration constant. Seven batches (F1-F7) of tablet formulations were prepared, one at each vertex (A, B, C), one at the halfway point between vertices (AB, BC, AC), and one at the center point (ABC). Each vertex represents a formulation containing the maximum amount of 1 component, with the other 2 components at a minimum level. The halfway point between the 2 vertices represents a formulation containing the average

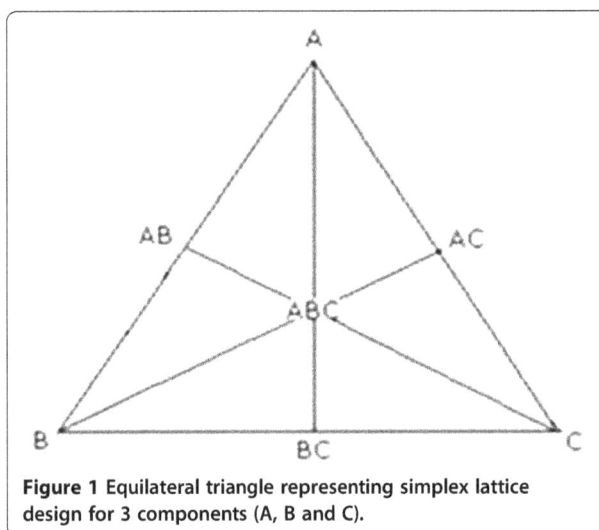

Figure 1 Equilateral triangle representing simplex lattice design for 3 components (A, B and C).

of the minimum and maximum amounts of the 2 ingredients. The center point represents a formulation containing one third of each ingredient.

Concentrations of HPMC K4M (A), okra gum (B) and LBG (C) were selected as independent variables. Hardness (kg/cm^2), floating lag time (f_{lag} time, sec), drug release for 1 h (%), drug release for 2 h (%), drug release for 8h (%) and drug release for 24 h (%) were taken as response values (Dependent variables). The response values obtained were analyzed using multiple regression analysis to find out their relationship with the factors used.

Formulation of gastroretentive matrix tablets

Weighed quantity of drug, polymers, effervescent combination and diluent (Table 1) were passed through sieve #80, mixed and triturated in a mortar for a period of 10min to obtain uniform mixture. Powder was lubricated with magnesium stearate and talcum powder for 3min. Lubricated

Table 1 Formulations of ziprasidone HCl according to simplex lattice design

Ingredients	Formulation code*							
	F1	F2	F3	F4	F5	F6	F7	F8
Ziprasidone HCl	20	20	20	20	20	20	20	20
HPMC K4M	33.3	100	-	-	16.7	16.7	66.7	74.6
Okra gum	33.3	-	-	100	16.7	66.7	16.7	15.3
Locust bean gum	33.3	-	100	-	66.7	16.7	16.7	12.4
Sodium bicarbonate	40	40	40	40	40	40	40	40
Tartaric acid	10	10	10	10	10	10	10	10
Poly vinyl pyrrolidone	15	15	15	15	15	15	15	15
Magnesium stearate	1	1	1	1	1	1	1	1
Talc	1	1	1	1	1	1	1	1
Lactose Q.S	200	200	200	200	200	200	200	200

*All values are in mg.

powder mass was compressed with 10-station Rimek Minipress RSB-1 tablet punching machine using 8 mm concave punches. The dimensional specifications were measured using thickness gauge (Okimoto); weight variation test was conducted as per pharmacopoeia of India specifications. Hardness of the tablet was measured using Pfizer type hardness tester.

Drug content estimation

Standard calibration curve of ziprasidone HCl was constructed using UV-Visible spectrophotometer (Shimadzu-1700, Kyoto, Japan). Drug solution was prepared in methanol at the concentration range of 10 µg/mL to 50 µg/mL, sonicated, filtered using 0.45 µ (Millipore) membrane filter. The drug content of standard drug solution and tablet formulation was measured at 318 nm against methanol as a blank solution [16]. This method was found to have good repeatability, reproducibility and relative standard deviation (RSD) was not more than 2%. The working curve equation for ziprasidone HCl was $y=0.011x$ with correlation coefficient value, $r^2 = 0.999$.

In vitro floatability

An *in vitro* floatability [17] of the formulation was determined by placing weighed tablet matrices in the USP dissolution testing apparatus II, in 900 ml of simulated gastric fluid (0.1N HCl, 0.2% NaCl) enzyme free at 37±0.5°C, rotated at 75 rpm.

The time required for the tablet to rise to the surface and float was determined as f_{lag} time. Floating time was the time, during which the tablet floats (including f_{lag} time) in simulated gastric fluid dissolution medium [18].

Swelling index

The extent of swelling was measured in terms of percent weight gain by the tablet [19]. Each tablet formulation was kept in a beaker containing 100 mL of simulated gastric fluid; the tablet was withdrawn, blotted with tissue paper and reweighed. Then for every 1 h, weights of the tablets were noted and the process was continuous till the end of 6 h. The percentage weight gain by the tablet was calculated using the formula

$$SI = \{(Mt - Mo)/Mo\} \times 100,$$

where, SI is swelling index, Mt is the weight of tablet at time "t", and Mo is the weight of tablet at time "t"=0.

Dissolution studies

The release rate of ziprasidone HCl from floating matrix tablets were determined using USP XXIV dissolution apparatus (TDT-08T, Electrolab) Type-II (paddle) method for 24 h. Study was carried out using 900 ml of simulated gastric fluid (0.1 N HCl, 0.2% NaCl) enzyme free,

at 37± 0.5°C at 75 rpm. Aliquot volume of 5 ml was withdrawn from the dissolution apparatus hourly for 24 h and the samples were replaced with fresh prewarmed dissolution medium. The withdrawn samples were suitably diluted with methanol, filtered and drug content was determined using UV-spectrophotometer.

Kinetic modeling on drug release profile

The dissolution profile of most satisfactory formulation of 7 runs and a check point batch (F8) were evaluated using mathematical models to describe the kinetics of the drug-release. The kinetics of drug release was evaluated for Higuchi, Korsmeyer-peppas, first order and zero order models to check the phenomena controlling the drug release from tablets [20,21]. The goodness of fit was evaluated using the correlation coefficient values (r^2).

Statistical analysis

The statistical assessment of simplex lattice design responses were performed using ANOVA and by applying the Student-t test. Model terms are significant if the calculated 't' value is less than the critical value of 't' (0.05).

In vivo floatability

The *in vivo* floatability of F8 formulation loaded with barium sulphate was investigated by radiographic images (X-ray photographs) of rabbit's stomach for specific period of time. Healthy rabbit weighing approximately 2.3 Kg was used to assess *in vivo* floating behaviour. The animal was fasted for 12 h and X-ray photograph was taken to ensure absence of radio opaque material in the stomach. The rabbit were made to swallow barium sulphate loaded tablet formulation with 30 ml of water. During the experiment rabbit were not allowed to eat but water was provided. At predetermined time intervals the radiograph of abdomen was taken to locate the formulation [22].

The preclinical study protocol was approved by Institutional Animal Ethical Committee, (Proposal No. IAEC/NCP/56/10) Nargund College of Pharmacy (NCP), Bangalore, Karnataka, India. Experiments were conducted according to the guidelines of committee for the "Purpose of Control and Supervision of Experiment on Animals" (CPCSEA).

Results and discussion
Formulation

The drug release characteristics were varied according to the types and proportion of matrix forming polymers in the formulation. HPMC K4M was selected as a hydrophilic matrixing agent [23]. LBG and Okra gum were considered as gelling agents they impart sufficient integrity to the tablets and works as release modifiers. Okra gum is insoluble in gastric pH but enormously swells which helps in retarding the drug release. Sodium

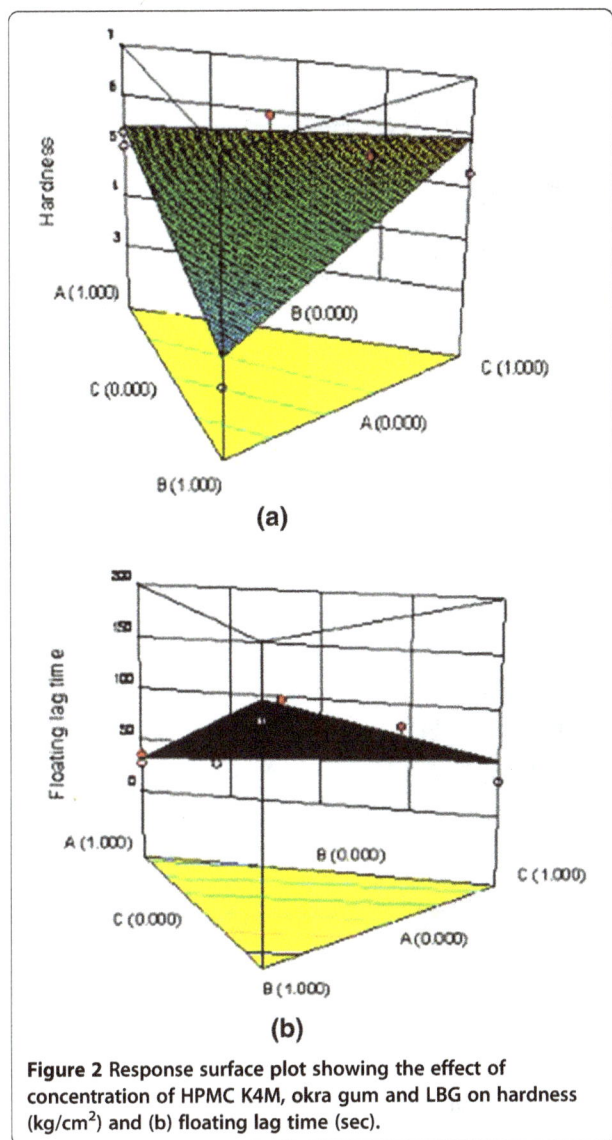

Figure 2 Response surface plot showing the effect of concentration of HPMC K4M, okra gum and LBG on hardness (kg/cm^2) and (b) floating lag time (sec).

bicarbonate generates CO_2 gas in the presence of tartaric acid upon contact with dissolution medium. The gas generated is trapped and protected within the gel (formed by hydration of HPMC K4 M), thus decreasing the density of the tablet [24]. As the density of the tablet falls below 1 (density of water), the tablet becomes buoyant.

Simplex lattice design

The general equation for the response based SLD for three components system consisting terms for pure component and mixtures of component [25].

$$R = B_0 + b_1 A + b_2 B + b_3 C \qquad (1)$$

where, R is the response variable and A, B and C are the proportions of formulation components. b_0 is the arithmetic mean response of the 7 runs and b_1, b_2 and b_3 are estimated coefficient for the factor A, B and C respectively. The coefficients can be calculated from the responses of 'R' using a multiple regression equation. The fitted equations relating the hardness, f_{lag} time, and drug release for 1h, drug release for 2 h, drug release for 8h and drug release for 24 h to the transformed factor were used to draw conclusions after considering the magnitude of coefficient and the mathematical sign it carries (i.e., positive or negative).

Effect of independent variables on hardness

$$R1 \ (Hardness) = 5.44^*A + 3.54^*B + 5.90^*C \qquad (2)$$

Although the statistical results infers {'F' value of 3.04 and 'p' value of 0.1370 (< 0.05)} the linear model equation is not significant for hardness, the values of regression coefficient infers, the concentration of HPMC K4M

Table 2 Characterization of ziprasidone HCl gastroretentive formulation

Formulation code	Responses (Dependent variables)					
	Hardness (kg/cm^2)	f_{lag} time (sec)	Drug release for 1 h (%)	Drug release for 2 h (%)	Drug release for 8 h (%)	Drug release for 24 h (%)
F1	6.52± 0.33	92.0± 5.19	4.86± 0.63	9.29± 0.81	27.39± 0.63	80.50± 0.83
F2	5.04±0.55	27.0± 5.29	11.31± 0.47	21.05± 0.23	89.39± 0.46	-
F3	5.24± 0.45	32.66± 3.51	4.39± 0.39	8.02± 0.40	25.69± 0.40	82.36± 0.39
F4	3.00± 0.37	137.0± 27.87	10.13± 0.60	14.79± 0.59	31.67± 0.45	85.45± 0.60
F5	5.66± 0.42	88.66± 14.57	4.93± 0.82	6.60± 0.40	30.55± 1.89	87.75± 1.03
F6	4.24± 0.38	136.0± 16.09	4.83± 0.80	6.56± 0.34	31.05± 0.44	82.26±0.41
F7	5.16±0.29	43.33± 13.79	5.61± 1.00	8.52± 0.61	31.31± 0.61	95.98± 0.47
F8	5.68± 0.52	37.33± 4.16	8.70± 0.41	14.83± 0.63	47.53± 0.87	97.58± 0.63

[a]All values are mean of 3 readings ± SD.

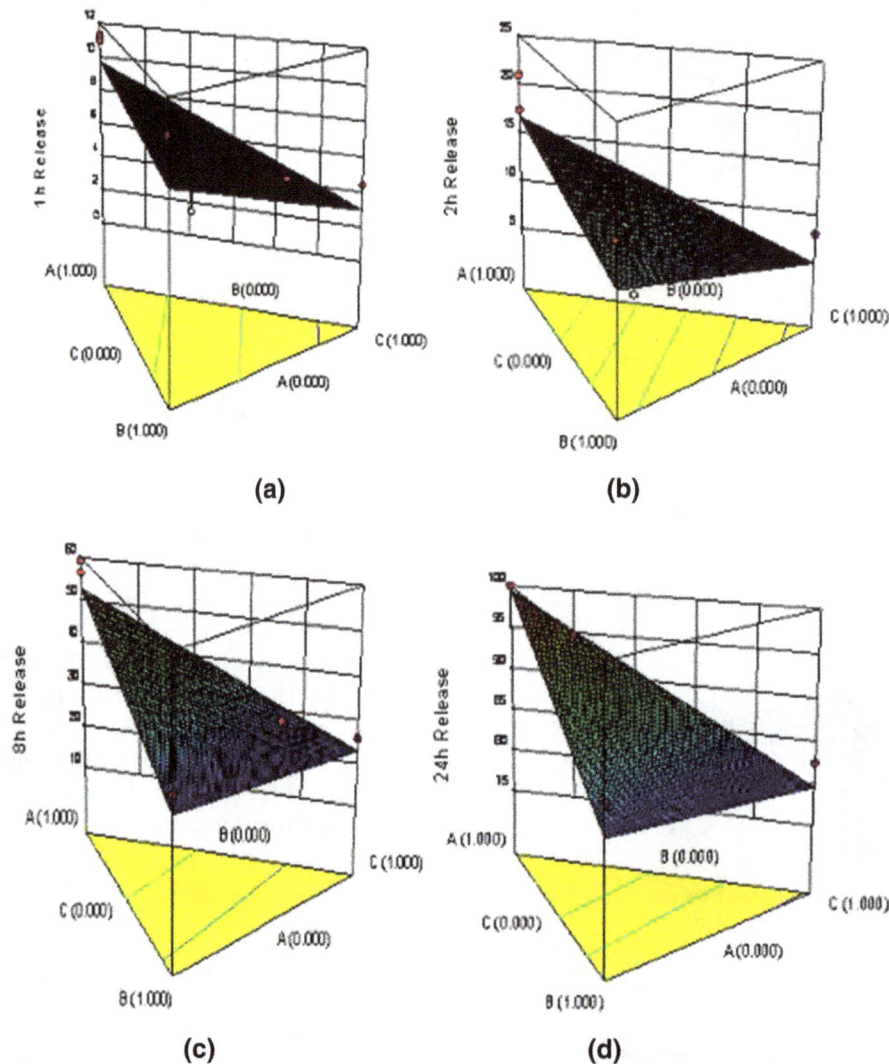

Figure 3 Response surface plot showing the effect of concentration of HPMC K4M, okra gum and LBG on % drug release for (a) 1 h, (b) 2 h, (c) 8 h and (d) 24 h respectively.

(A) and LBG (C) has equally contributed for the hardness (Figure 2a). Because HPMC K4M (A) and LBG (C) has sufficient cohesiveness and fibrous integrity makes them to undergo binding and contributed for hardness [26].

Effect of independent variables on f_{lag} time

$$R2 \ (f_{lag} \ time) = 32.58^*A + 54.92 * B + 52.51 * C \quad (3)$$

The linear equation for f_{lag} time indicates that the factor 'A' has more significant effect on f_{lag} time than 'B'

Table 3 Summary of ANOVA table for dependent variables from simplex lattice design

Source (Linear mixture)	Sum of squares	Degree of freedom	Mean square	'F' value	Probability 'p' value
Hardness	4.12	2	2.06	3.04	0.1370
f_{lag} time	12739.02	2	6369.51	16.63	0.0062*
1 h drug release	37.79	2	18.90	3.30	0.1218
2 h drug release	117.80	2	58.90	3.13	0.1315
8 h drug release	947.0	2	473.50	8.20	0.0264*
24 h drug release	432.98	2	216.49	14.19	0.0087*

*$p < 0.05$ indicate model terms are significant.

Table 4 Coded quantities of the check point batch "F8" and their desirability

Constraints

Name	Goal	Lower limit	Upper Limit	Lower weight	Upper weight	Importance
HPMC K4M	Is in range	0	1	1	1	3
Okra gum	Is in range	0	1	1	1	3
LBG	Is in range	0	1	1	1	3
Floating lag time	Minimize	27	137	1	1	3
8h release	Minimize	25.69	59.39	1	1	3
24h release	Maximize	80.5	100	1	1	3
Solutions (Desirability 0.642)						
A		B	C	f_{lag} time (sec)	8h release	24 h release
0.946		-	0.054	33.66	51.26	98.45

and 'C' (Figure 2b). This is further evident with the model terms for f_{lag} time being significant with 'F' value of 16.63 and 'p' value of 0.0062 (< 0.05) on a linear model. Floating lag time was found to increase at higher level of okra gum and decreases as the level of HPMC K4M increases. This is due to high swelling property of the later. Hence, a higher proportion of HPMC K4M is important in the formulation to decrease the f_{lag} time. This is also evident from the results of swelling index determination (221.95 to 257.15 (%) for F1 to F7 at the end of 6 h). Swelling index increases with increase in concentration of HPMC K4M signifying its importance for decrease in f_{lag} time [27].

Effect of independent variables on drug release

The magnitude of coefficients observed for 1, 2, 8 and 24 h release obtained from the results of multiple linear regression analysis is expressed in equations 4, 5, 6 and 7 respectively. The release rate and percentage drug release for the 7 batches (F1 to F7) showed a wide variation (i.e., 80 to 95%) as shown in Table 2. Formulation F2 prepared using only HPMC K4M, exhausted before 8h and fails to sustain the drug release till 24 h. This highest value of percentage release observed in initial hours is due to low value of both the independent variables (B and C), thus weakening the gel strength.

Drug release for 1h and 2h

R3 (Drug relese for 1 h)
$$= 9.75^{*}A + 7.52^{*}B + 2.97^{*}C \qquad (4)$$

R4 (Drug release for 2 h)
$$= 16.80^{*}A + 10.47^{*}B + 5.07^{*}C \qquad (5)$$

The equations 4 and 5 infer that the 'A' has more favorable effect on increase in drug release and the factor 'B' and 'C' in retarding drug release for 1 and 2 h. Although, the model terms are not significant {'p' value of

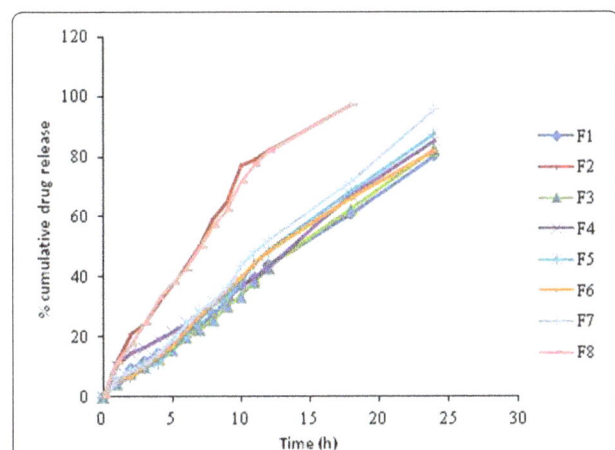

Figure 4 Comparative release profiles of ziprasidone HCl gastroretentive formulations.

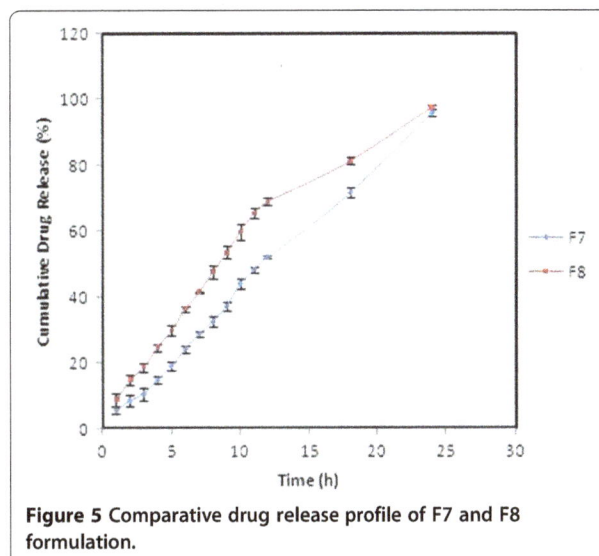

Figure 5 Comparative drug release profile of F7 and F8 formulation.

Table 5 Comparison of experimented and predicted values of check point batch "F8"

Parameter	Predicted values	Experimented values
Hardness (kg/cm²)	5.46	5.68 ± 0.52
Floating lag time (sec)	33.66	37.33 ± 4.16
% Drug release at 8 h	51.26	47.53 ± 0.87
% Drug release at 24 h	98.45	97.58 ± 0.63

[a]All values are mean of 3 readings ± SD.

0.1218 and 0.1315 (<0.05) for 1 h and 2 h drug release} it is understood that the water solubility of HPMC helps in increasing drug release and the water insolubility but the swellability of LBG and okra gum is responsible for it [28]. Optimum concentration of HPMC must be there in the formulation for immediate release of drug at initial hours.

Drug release for 8h and 24h

Concentration of HPMC K4M has important role in enhancing the drug release for 8 and 24 h and reverse is true with concentration of okra gum and LBG. As the concentration of okra gum and LBG increases, it causes an increase in viscosity of the swollen gel matrix, which decreases the water diffusion in to the core layer. Decrease in hydration of matrix contributes more hindrance for drug diffusion and consequently decrease in release rate [29]. This can be further elucidated with the help of response surface plot (Figure 3).

$$R5 \ (\text{Drug release for 8 h}) = 52.87^*A + 27.64^*B + 22.86^*C \qquad (6)$$

$$R6 \ (\text{Drug release for 24 h}) = 99.53^*A + 82.02^*B + 79.55^*C \qquad (7)$$

The model terms for *R5* (8 h release) and *R6* (24 h release) were found to be significant with an '*F*' value of 8.20 and 14.19, and '*p*' value of 0.0264 and 0.0087 (< 0.05) respectively. These results clearly indicate that the percentage drug release is strongly dependent on all the selected independent variables. This equation infers that the judicious combination of HPMC K4M, okra gum and LBG is necessary [30] to control and sustain the drug release for 24 h. Table 3 shows the results of the analysis of variance (ANOVA), which was performed to identify insignificant factors.

Based on this analysis, formulation F7 was arbitrarily selected as an optimized batch which releases the drug satisfactorily till the end of 24 h in spite of its high f_{lag} time of 43.33 ± 13.79 sec. In order to overcome the drawbacks of F7 formulation a checkpoint batch F8 prepared by considering the constraints and desirability to improve (Table 4) its *in vitro* performance. The experimental results of formulation F8 for f_{lag} time, total floating time and swelling index were found to be 37.33 ± 4.16sec, > 24 h and 204.0 ± 5.30% (up to 6 h) respectively. The *in vitro* drug release data was found to be sustained well compared to the most satisfactory formulation (F7) of 7 runs (Figure 4 and Figure 5). Predicted results were almost similar to the observed experimental values indicates the accuracy of the design (Table 5). All formulations were found to be buoyant for more than 24 h.

Kinetic modeling on drug release profile

The release profile and kinetics of drug release are important because they correlate the *in vitro* and *in vivo* drug responses by comparing results of pharmacokinetics and dissolution profile patterns [31]. Hence, the cumulative drug release results of F7 and F8 formulation were fixed into various mathematical models and the results are shown in Table 6.

The drug release pattern of formulation (F7) was found to be highly linear, and close to infinity as indicated by their high regression value as $r^2 = 0.993$. Therefore it was ascertained that the drug permeation from these formulation could follow either near zero or zero order kinetics.

The *in vitro* drug release pattern of F8 showed the highest regression value ($r^2 = 0.989$) for Koresmeyar-peppas model. The 'n' value was found to be between 0.5 and 1 suggesting that release of drug follows anomalous (non-fickian) diffusion mechanism. Release kinetics may be following both diffusion and erosion mechanism from these natural gums [32].

In vivo floatability

In vivo floatability studies conducted for F8 showed that the tablet formulation did not adhere to the gastric mucous and floated in the gastric fluid for more than 24h. To make the tablet X-ray opaque barium sulphate was incorporated into the tablet. The amount of barium sulphate (2mg per tablet) was low enough to enable the tablet to float, at the same time it was sufficient to

Table 6 Kinetic modeling of drug dissolution profiles

Formulation code	Zero order		First order		Higuchi		Koresmeyar- peppas	
	r^2	k	r^2	k	r^2	k	r^2	n
F7	0.993	4.089	0.878	0.056	0.948	23.50	0.982	0.954
F8	0.934	4.107	0.936	0.066	0.981	24.76	0.989	0.819

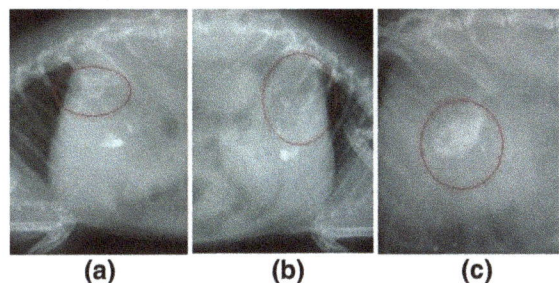

Figure 6 X-ray photographs showing floating ability of F8 formulation at different time interval (a) 6 h, (b) 12 h and (c) 24 h.

ensure visibility by X-ray. This was evident by the X-ray photographs taken at 6 h, 12 h & 24 h (Figure 6).

Conclusions

Ziprasidone HCl gastroretentive tablet is developed using naturally occurring plant based polymers showed desirable high-drug content, optimal hardness, floatability, swelling index and adequate release characteristics. The systematic formulation approach using simplex lattice design in the study helped in understanding the effect of formulation variables. The use of plant-based polymeric can be a good replacement for synthetic polymers in the development of controlled release dosage forms, because plant based materials can be modified to meet the requirements of drug delivery systems. Formulations prepared by such renewable and eco-friendly plant resources can be considered as promising SR polymers substances to bring about sustained release action, supported by more elaborated research in this aspect.

Competing interests
The authors declare that they have no competing interest.

Authors' contributions
SB is involved in design of research protocol, statistical assessment of all the results and drafted the manuscript. AJ is participated in the development of formulation and *in vitro* evaluation of formulation. HN has collected and prepared the Okra gum for formulation use and carried out the *in vivo* floatability test of the formulation. All authors read and approved the final manuscript.

Acknowledgement
We are thankful to Sanofi Aventis Pharma, Ltd. India, for providing drug sample. We are grateful to Principal, Acharya and BM Reddy College of Pharmacy, Bangalore, India, and Nargund Research Foundation, Bangalore, India, for providing research facilities. We also wish to thank Prof. CRM Setty and Prof. Binay Sankar for manuscript edition.

Author details
[1]Department of Pharmacognosy, KLE University's College of Pharmacy, Bangalore 560010, India. [2]Department of Pharmaceutics, Acharya & BM Reddy College of Pharmacy, Soladevanahally Hesaraghatta road, Bangalore 560090, India.

References

1. Gande S, Rao YM: Sustained-release effervescent floating matrix tablets of baclofen: Development, optimization and *in vitro-in vivo* evaluation in healthy human volunteers. *DARU J Pharm Sci* 2011, **19**(3):202–209.
2. Varshosaz J, Tavakoli N, Eram SA: Use of natural gums and cellulose derivatives in production of sustained release Metoprolol tablets. *Drug Deliv* 2006, **13**:113–119.
3. Bhardwaj TR, Kanwar M, Gupta A: Natural gums and modified natural gums as sustained-release carriers. *Drug Dev Ind Pharm* 2000, **26**:1025–1038.
4. Perepelkin KE: Polymeric materials of the future based on renewable plant resources and biotechnologies. Fibres, films, plastics. *Fibre Chem* 2005, **37**:417–430.
5. Lam KS: New aspects of natural products in drug discovery. *Trends Microbiol* 2007, **15**:279–289.
6. McChesney JD, Venkataraman SK, Henri JT: Plant natural products. Back to the future or into extinction? *Phytoche* 2007, **68**:2015–2022.
7. Üner M, Altinkurt T: Evaluation of Honey locust (Gleditsia triacanthos Linn) gum as sustaining material in tablet dosage forms. *I I Farmaco* 2004, **59**(7):567–573.
8. Dakia P, Blecker C, Robert C, Whatelet B, Paquot M: Composition and physicochemical properties of Locust bean gum extracted from whole seeds by acid or water dehulling pre-treatment. *Food Hyd* 2008, **22**:807–818.
9. Jaleh V, Naser T, Fatemeh K: Use of Hydrophilic Natural Gums in Formulation of Sustained-release Matrix Tablets of Tramadol Hydrochloride. *AAPS Pharm Sci Tech* 2006, **7**(1):E1–E7.
10. Pollard M, Kelly R, Fischer P, Windhab E, Eder B, Amadò R: Investigation of molecular weight distribution of LBG galactomannan for flours prepared from individual seeds, mixtures, and commercial samples. *Food Hyd* 2008, **22**:1596–1606.
11. Gunasekara NS, Spencer CM, Keating GM: Ziprasidone: a review of its use in schizophrenia and schizoaffective disorder. *Drugs* 2002, **62**(8):1217–1251.
12. Preskorn SH: Pharmacokinetics and therapeutics of acute intramuscular ziprasidone. *Clin Pharmacokinet* 2005, **44**(11):1117–1133.
13. Kumar S, Nagpal K, Singh SK, Mishra DN: Improved bioavailability through floating microspheres of Lovastatin. *DARU J Pharm Sci* 2011, **19**(1):57–64.
14. Emeje MO, Isimi CY, Kunle OO: Evaluation of Okra gum as a dry binder in Paracetamol tablet formulations. *Continental J Pharm Sci* 2007, **1**:15–2.
15. Alves MM, Antonov YA, Gonçalves MP: The effect of structural features of Gelatin on its thermodynamic compatibility with Locust bean gum in aqueous media. *Food Hyd* 1999, **13**:157–166.
16. Kumar YA, Anitha M, Hemanth A, Srinivas S: Development of rapid UV Spectrophotometric method for the estimation of Ziprasidone hydrochloride in bulk and formulations. *Dig J Nanomater Bios* 2010, **5**(1):279–283.
17. Shweta A, Javed A, Alka A, Roop K, Sanjula B: Floating Drug Delivery Systems: A Review. *AAPS Pharm Sci Tech* 2005, **6**(3):E372–E390.
18. Sateesha SB, Prakash Rao B, Rajamma AJ, Nargund LVG: Gastro retentive Orlistat microspheres: Formulation, characterization and *in vitro* evaluation. *Diss Tech* 2011, **18**(3):72.
19. Arza RA, Gonugunta CS, Veerareddy PR: Formulation and evaluation of swellable and floating gastroretentive Ciprofloxacin hydrochloride Tablets. *AAPS Pharm Sci Tech* 2009, **10**(1):220–226.
20. Faith A, Chaibva, Sandile MM, Khamanga, Roderick B, Walker: Swelling, erosion and drug release characteristics of Salbutamol sulfate from Hydroxypropyl methylcellulose-based matrix tablets. *Drug Dev Ind Pharm* 2010, **36**(12):1497–1510.
21. Sateesha SB, Rajamma AJ, Narode MK, Vyas BD: Influence of Organic Acids on Diltiazem HCl Release Kinetics from Hydroxypropyl Methyl Cellulose Matrix Tablets. *J Young Pharm* 2010, **2**(3):229–233.
22. Whitehead L, Fell JT, Collet JH, Sharma HL, Smith AM: An *in vivo* demonstrating prolonged gastric retention. *J Controlled Release* 1998, **55**:3–12.
23. Atul K, Ashok KT, Narendra KJ, Subheet J: Formulation and *in vitro, in vivo* evaluation of extended-release matrix tablet of Zidovudine: influence of combination of hydrophilic and hydrophobic matrix formers. *AAPS Pharm Sci Tech* 2006, **7**(1):E1–E9.
24. Safaa S, Gamal E, Viviane FN, Ahmed NA: Optimization of Acyclovir oral tablets based on gastroretention technology: Factorial design analysis

and physicochemical characterization studies. *Drug Dev Ind Pharm* 2011, **37**(7):855–867.

25. Dasharath MP, Natvarlal MP, Nitesh NP, Pranav DJ: **Gastroretentive Drug Delivery System of Carbamazepine: Formulation Optimization Using Simplex Lattice Design: A Technical Note.** *AAPS Pharm Sci Tech* 2007, **8**(1):E1–E5.

26. Gonzalez YM, Ghaly ES: **Modified drug release of Poloxamer matrix by including water-soluble and water-insoluble polymer.** *Drug Dev Ind Pharm* 2010, **36**(1):64–71.

27. Toti US, Aminabhavi TM: **Modified Guar Gum Matrix Tablet for Controlled Release of Diltiazem Hydrochloride.** *J Control Rel* 2004, **95**:567–571.

28. Vishal Gupta N, Shivakumar HG: **Preparation and characterization of superporous hydrogels as gastroretentive drug delivery system for Rosiglitazone maleate.** *DARU J Pharm Sci* 2010, **18**(3):200–210.

29. Syed Nisar Hussain S, Sajid A, Muhammad Akram C, Muhammad Sajid Hamid A, Rehman N, Sattar B: **Formulation and evaluation of natural gum-based sustained release matrix tablets of Flurbiprofen using response surface methodology.** *Drug Dev Ind Pharm* 2009, **35**(12):1470–1478.

30. Sharma AK, Keservani RK, Dadarwal SC, Choudary Y, Ramteke V: **Formulation and *in vitro* characterization of cepodoxime proxetil gastroretentive microballoons.** *DARU J Pharm Sci* 2011, **19**(1):33–40.

31. Bravo SA: ***In vitro* studies of Diclofenac sodium controlled-release from biopolymeric hydrophilic matrices.** *J Pharm Pharm Sci* 2002, **5**(3):213–219.

32. Nagarwal RC, Ramesh C, Nagarwal, Devendra N, Ridhurkar J, Pandit: ***In vitro* release kinetics and bioavailability of gastroretentive Cinnarizine hydrochloride Tablet.** *AAPS Pharm Sci Tech* 2010, **11**(1):294–03.

Cost-effectiveness of adding-on new antiepileptic drugs to conventional regimens in controlling intractable seizures in children

Zahra Gharibnaseri[1], Abbas Kebriaeezadeh[1,2], Shekoufeh Nikfar[1,3]*, Gholamreza Zamani[4] and Akbar Abdollahiasl[1]

Abstract

Background and purpose of the study: Intractable seizures are a subgroup of epileptic disorders challenging the physicians' skills to become controlled. Showing resistance towards common pharmacotherapy, they demand newer antiepileptic drugs acquired at higher costs. 0.06% of children around the world are estimated to suffer from epilepsy and its consequences. The aim of the present study has been to evaluate the cost-effectiveness of these drugs in the treatment of intractable seizures in children.

Methods: Clinical and cost data were collected from medical and cost records preserved at a neurologist office and a referral pharmacy respectively. Based on the new AED which are accessible in Iran, regimens were categorized into eight groups. The first group consisting of conventional AEDs was considered as comparator and the effectiveness of other groups was compared with it. Incremental Cost-effectiveness Ratio (ICER) of adding-on each new antiepileptic drug was calculated in terms of Rials per consequence (Rls/consq) and compared with each other. Furthermore ICER of the regimens was compared with the GDP per capita (Gross Domestic Product) of the year (2010).

Results: the ICER of the adding-on regimens range from negative values for Gabapentin, Levetiracetam and Zonisamide to low values for Lamotrigine (~ 6.4 million Rials/consequence [mil Rls/consq]) and Oxcarbazepine (~7.7 mil Rls/consq) and followed by high values for Topiramate (~21 mil Rls/consq) and Vigabatrin (~43.7 mil Rls/consq) considering the three months of remaining on regimen. By increasing the limit of remaining time to six months, the previously mentioned regimens persist on negative values. However Oxcarbazepine (~28.7 mil Rls/consq) and Lamotrigine (~13.8 mil Rls/consq) show a steep increase. Topiramate (~23.6 mil Rls/consq) displays a less change. Opposite to other regimens, the ICER value of Vigabatrin (~17.26 mil Rls/consq) has shown an important increase.

Major conclusions: Adding-on new antiepileptics to conventional regimens are cost-effective and justified considering the GDP per capita.

Keywords: Cost-effectiveness, New antipiletics, Intractable seizures, Children, Incremental cost-effectiveness ratio

Introduction

Epilepsy is defined as a neurological disorder of brain portrayed by persisting predisposition to develop epileptic seizures [1]. A proportion of 6 over 1,000 children around the world are estimated to suffer from epilepsy and its psychological, social and intellectual development

* Correspondence: shekoufeh.nikfar@gmail.com
[1]Department of Pharmacoeconomics and Pharmaceutical Administration, Faculty of Pharmacy, Tehran University of Medical Sciences, Tehran, Iran
[3]Food and Drug Laboratory Research Center, Ministry of Health and Medical Education, Tehran, Iran
Full list of author information is available at the end of the article

consequences [2]. Known as one of the most common neurological disorders worldwide, epilepsy has several treatment options. However pharmacotherapy remains the mainstay [3]. Since 1993 a high increase in emerging antiepileptic drugs (AEDs) has been observed [4]. The Anatomical Therapeutic Chemical (ATC) classification system of World Health Organization (WHO) collaborating center identifies 45 medicinal substances used in the treatment of epilepsy. Among which 13 are approved and prescribed in Iran. A common style of classifying AEDs is based on the year of introduction to the market.

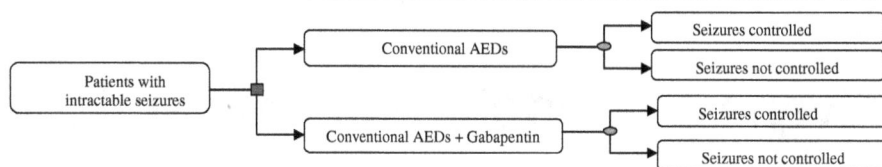

Figure 1 Sample of model used to compare the effectiveness of adding-on Gabapentin to conventional regimen.

In this perspective, AEDs fall into two categories. Conventional AEDs including Carbamazepine, Ethosuximide, Phenytoin, Phenobarbital, Primidone and Valproate and the newer AEDs including Gabapentin, Levetiracetam, Lamotrigine, Oxcarbazepine, Topiramate, Vigabatrin, Zonisamide. It should be noticed that financial supports are devoted to pharmaceuticals comprised in essential drugs list of Iran [5], resulting in the high prescription of them [6]. While the first generation of AEDs prescribed as monotherapy shows promising results in almost 70% of patients with epilepsy, polytherapy or adding-on newer AEDs is demanded by the rest of the epileptic patients whom are believed to meet intractable seizures [7].

In general, selecting an AED is performed on the basis of many factors including relative efficacy, drug-drug interactions, tolerability and cost [8]. The acquisition costs of newer AEDs are generally higher than the older; nevertheless there superiority in controlling seizures has to be established. Dealing with restricted budget, clinicians and decision-makers are interested in Pharmacoeconomics studies, which measure and balance costs and clinical outcomes of alternative medications. In spite of this, there is a tragic lack of literature on this issue in Iran; however a few of them that have been published in recent years could provide valuable information for decision making [9]. Furthermore, owing to the pharmacogenetics effect and the diversity of genotypes, applying effectiveness data across different countries is difficult [10].

The aim of this study was to compare cost-effectiveness of newer AEDs being added to conventional regimens in treating intractable seizures in children.

Methods

This study has been conducted in a cross sectional manner. Clinical data was obtained from medical records of patients archived at the office of a physician with well established expertise in pediatric neurology. Patients with seizures not being responsive to two or three conventional AEDs were included in the study [11]. Cases of nonepileptic seizures and misdiagnosis were excluded. Regimens were categorized into eight groups. The first group consisting in conventional AEDs was considered

as comparator and the effectiveness of other groups were compared with it. Each of the new antiepileptic drugs along with the regimen composed of conventional AEDs was incorporated into a model resulting in seven decision trees (sample shown in Figure 1).

An additional model comparing regimens composed of conventional AEDs and any of the seven new AEDs with the same assumptions mentioned above was set up in order to evaluate the cost-effectiveness of adding-on new AEDs in general (Figure 2).

Regarding the fact that either the inability of a regimen in controlling seizures or the inappropriate safety profile are the main reasons of switching the regimen by the clinical specialist, thus remaining on a regimen has been viewed as an acceptable indicator of effectiveness and safety for regimens. Receiving approval by the clinician, remaining on a regimen for three months and more was regarded as effectiveness endpoint (desired consequence).

The proportion of seizure controlled patients to all the patients incorporated into the model was assumed as the effectiveness of the related regimen. The effectiveness of regimens was calculated for both arms within each model. Next the effectiveness of add-on regimens was subtracted from the comparator's regimen effectiveness.

$$\Delta E = E_{add-on} - E_{comparator}$$

Cost data was primarily obtained from the referral pharmacy of Tehran (Sizdah-e-Aban Pharmacy). Given the perspective of our study has been that of the patients, latest sales price were collected and split in two sets. The first set made up of the maximum prices consisting of brand name drugs that at most cases are imported and the second set comprised of the minimum prices which belong to the generic drugs. As availability of drugs has been the only determinant factor in purchasing drugs, an average of these prices was computed. Considering the variety of the dosage forms, standardizing the daily dose of each drug was necessary in order to compare the cost of each regimen. This was managed by calculating the prescribed daily dose (PDD) of each drug as an average of all the existing doses reported in the records.

$$average\ PDD = \frac{(dose\ 1 \times frequency\ of\ dose\ 1) + (dose\ 2 \times frequency\ of\ dose\ 2)}{frequency\ of\ dose\ 1 + frequency\ of\ dose\ 2}$$

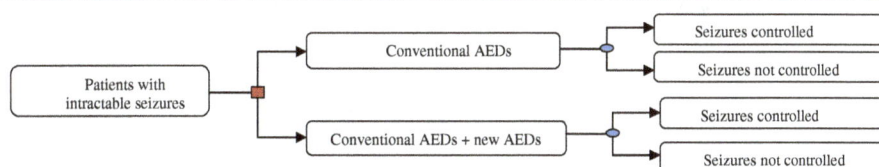

Figure 2 Decision tree of adding-on new AEDs to conventional regimens.

For example if Valproate was prescribed as 900 mg/day in two records and 600 mg/day in one record the weighted average of PDD would equal 800 mg/day. PDD of each AED was subsequently multiplied by the price of 1 mg of each drug -obtained by dividing the average price by the potency of the dosage form- as well as 365 days of year for further comparison with the GDP (Gross Domestic Product) per capita, resulting in the cost of each regimen. The cost of the comparator group (conventional AEDs) has not been calculated due to being mentioned in both arms of the decision trees. In other words the difference of costs of regimens (ΔC) was simplified as followed:

$$\Delta C = C_{Conventional+new\,AED} - C_{conventional} = C_{new\,AED}.$$

In order to compare the cost effectiveness of add-on regimens the incremental cost-effectiveness ratio (ICER) was calculated as:

$$ICER = \frac{\Delta C}{\Delta E}$$

[12].

The final step was comparing the ICER of each new AED as add-on therapy with the GDP per capita of Iran, as a measure for assessing the cost-effectiveness of different regimens.

It should be noted that all costs are reported as Rials (Rls) (1 United States of America' Dollar (USD) ~ 10,000 Rls; 1 Euro ~ 15,000 Rls) in year 2010.

Sensitivity analysis was performed at three cost levels (medium, average and maximum) and the model was re-run with an effectiveness endpoint of six months.

Results
57 patients were approved with intractable seizures giving access to 284 records of regimens. The distribution of patients has been depicted (Table 1).

ICERs regarding at least 3 months of maintenance
Table 2 shows the incremental cost-effectiveness ratio of adding-on new AEDs in three months with average prices, ranges from negative values for Gabapentin, Levetiracetam and Zonisamide indicating them as dominated regimens to positive values for Vigabatrin (ICER ~

43.7 mil Rls/consq), Topiramate (ICER ~ 21 mil Rls/consq), Oxcarbazepine (ICER ~ 7.7 mil Rls/consq) and Lamotrigine (ICER ~ 6.3 mil Rls/consq).

ICERs regarding the overall effect of adding-on new AEDs
The incremental cost-effectiveness ratio of adding any of the new AEDs shows a positive value of 37 million Rials per a desired consequence. Changing the effectiveness endpoint from three to six months raises the ICER value to 42.4 mil Rls/consq (Table 3).

Comparison with GDP per capita
As depicted in Figure 3 all new AEDs excluding Levetiracetam, Gabapentin and Zonisamide fall under the GDP per capita curve. It is noteworthy that Lamotrigine, Oxcarbazepine and Topiramate keep a distance from the curve while Vigabatrin and new AEDs point stand close to the line.

Sensitivity analysis
Taking the case of two other price levels, can cause changes in the ICER values (Figure 4). Increasing the prices ends in falling the ICER of the new AEDs group out of the very cost-effectiveness area (> GDP per capita). Decreasing the prices, results in the enhancement of cost-effectiveness of Topiramate comparing to the GDP per capita level, followed by improvement of the cost-effectiveness of the new AEDs.

Table 1 Distribution of patients with intractable seizures

		No.	% of total
Sex	Male	32	56.14
	Female	25	43.86
Age	0–3 years	13	22.8
	3–6 years	20	35.09
	6–13 years	23	4.35
	13–19 years	1	1.75
Epilepsy type	Idiopathic	13	21.6
	Symptomatic	44	77.6
	Partial	27	57.36
	Generalized	9	15.78
	Mixed	21	36.84

Table 2 Cost-effectiveness comparison of newer AEDs in three months at average prices

Regimen	ΔE	ΔC	ICER (Rials per consequence)
conventional AEDs+ Gabapentin	−0.52	1525051	Dominated
conventional AEDs+ Lamotrigine	0.13	826145	6354964
conventional AEDs+ Levetiracetam	−0.52	1732229	Dominated
conventional AEDs+ Oxcarbazepine	0.15	1149750	7665000
conventional AEDs+ Topiramate	0.36	7553771	20982698
conventional AEDs+ Vigabatrin	0.15	6560510	43736733
conventional AEDs+ Zonisamide	−0.52	1445400	Dominated

Note: the regimen solely composed of old AEDs is assumed as the comparator regimen.

Table 3 Cost-effectiveness comparison of adding-on new AEDs in three and six months at average prices

Endpoint	ΔE	ΔC (Rials)	ICER
3 months	0.08	2970408	37130101
6 months	0.07	2970408	42434402

By the limit time of six months, Gabapentin, Levetiracetam and Zonisamide still show negative values. Oxcarbazepine (ICER ~ 28.7 mil Rls/consq) turns out to exhibit dramatic changes in the cost-effectiveness due to striking decrease in effectiveness, followed by Topiramate (ICER ~ 23.6 mil Rls/consq). The increase for Lamotrigine (ICER ~ 13.8 mil Rls/consq) has been less considerable. Opposite to the previous regimens Vigabatrin (ICER ~ 17.3 mil Rls/consq) has shown a substantial decrease.

Discussion

The results confirm that adding-on new AEDs to conventional regimens in controlling intractable seizures in children is cost-effective comparing to regimens composed entirely of conventional AEDs. However choosing certain AEDs added to the conventional regimen especially in long term requires extra consideration. Given the general advantages of monotherapy against polytherapy, physicians' preference could be driven towards monotherapy by cost-effective regimens including newer AEDs such as Oxcarbazepine, Lamotrigine and Topiramate.

Since the value that Iranian society recognize for health outcomes is unknown, interpreting the results express complicacy [13]. WHO guidelines recommend comparing the cost-effective ratio (CER) with the GDP per capita of the country [14]. The GDP per capita of Iran reported by the International monetary fund (2010) has been US$ 4400 [15] (~ 44 mil Rls). It should be noted that changes in any factor that modify the calculated costs such as exchange rates, prices and etc. can result in a different cost-effectiveness comparison. There lays a vast difference between these amounts and the

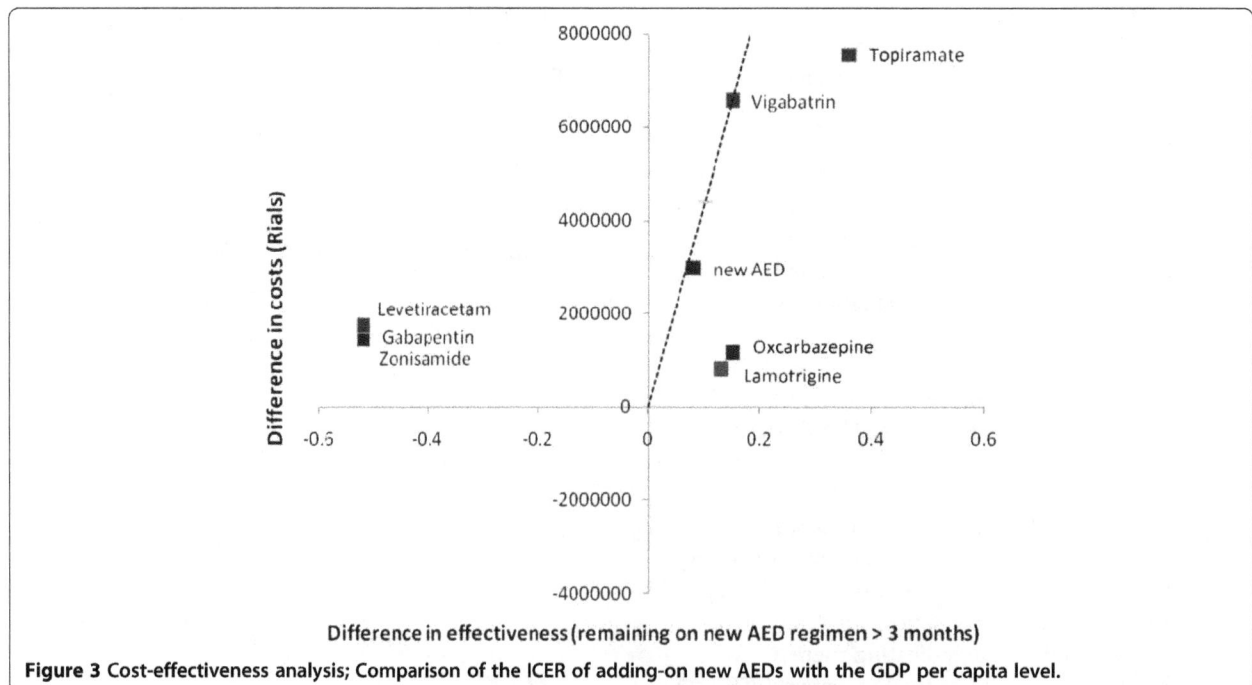

Figure 3 Cost-effectiveness analysis; Comparison of the ICER of adding-on new AEDs with the GDP per capita level.

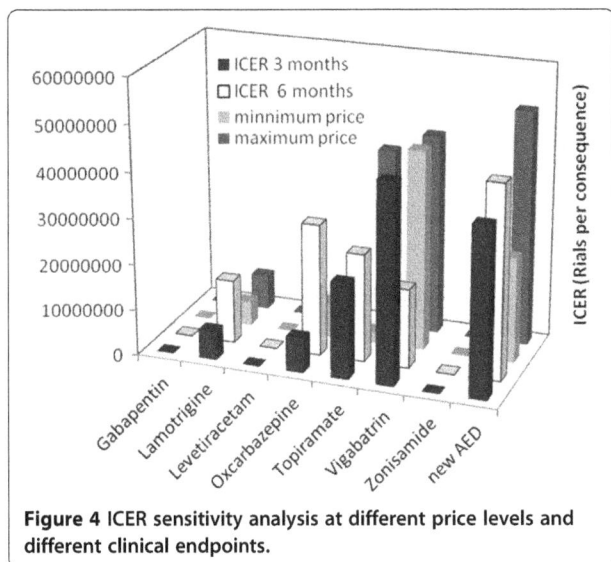

Figure 4 ICER sensitivity analysis at different price levels and different clinical endpoints.

ICER value of most regimens, allowing the prescription of the newer AEDs in large numbers. In spite of this, by considering the six months of retention as the desirable consequence, the ICER values of Oxcarbazepine at three price levels and Topiramate at the maximum price exceed the GDP per capita levels requiring more observation on their prescription. This is due to noticeable decrease in the efficacy of regimen.

If a specific regimen is causative of unacceptable side effects or is not efficient, the patient would have been quickly switched to an alternative regimen. Therefore retention rates of different regimens are appropriate indices for effectiveness. In addition actual clinical data used in this study instead of receiving abstract information by clinicians, improves realization of the results. While the study has much strength, cost and medical databanks not being available accounts for limitations through the study.

Collecting clinical data from a referral but single center can be responsible for undesirable bias in the results. Indirect costs such as costs pertaining to side effects and clinical visits were not included in this economic evaluation and different types of epilepsy were not separated due to the low number of patients.

Our results are quite different from Frew's study that has demonstrated the newer and older antiepileptic drugs different in cost terms while equal in efficacy term [16]. This conflict arises from the different target group. Similarly, Knoester's and Connek's studies confirmed the use of older AEDs for patients newly diagnosed epilepsy while not included refractory patients [2,17]. Some studies such as Boon et al. have shown the favorableness of surgery in refractory patients compared with conservative treatment [18]. In general due to methodological issues comparing different studies is not always possible

[19] and using standardized approach is suggested for further researches.

Conclusion

Adding-on new antiepileptics to conventional regimens is cost-effective and justified considering the GDP per capita. Among the new adding-on AEDs prescribed in Iran, Lamotrigine shows the best results in terms of cost-effectiveness in treating children with intractable seizures. As the same, Oxcarbazepine and Topiramate fall under the GDP per capita level, while Vigabatrin stands close to the standard. However, other adding-on medications; Gabapentin, Levetiracetam and Zonisamide; in treating the target population appears not to be cost-effective due to less effectiveness compared with older AEDs.

Competing interests
The authors declare that they have no competing interests.

Authors' contribution
ZG conceived and implemented the strategy, collected clinical and cost data, analyzed data and drafted paper, AK conceived the strategy of study and supervised the project, SN gave consultation on designing the study, conceived the strategy of study, revised the article and supervised the project, GZ gave consultation on designing the study and provided clinical data, AA gave consultation on designing the study and building the model. All authors read and approved the final manuscript.

Acknowledgment
This study was the outcome of PharmD student's thesis and was supported by student thesis grant from Tehran University of Medical Sciences.

Author details
[1]Department of Pharmacoeconomics and Pharmaceutical Administration, Faculty of Pharmacy, Tehran University of Medical Sciences, Tehran, Iran. [2]Department of Toxicology and Pharmacology Faculty of Pharmacy, Tehran University of Medical Sciences, Tehran, Iran. [3]Food and Drug Laboratory Research Center, Ministry of Health and Medical Education, Tehran, Iran. [4]Department of Pediatrics, Faculty of Medicine, Tehran University of Medical Sciences, Tehran, Iran.

References
1. Fisher RS, Emde Boas WV, Blume W, Elger C, Genton P, Lee P, Engel J: **Epileptic seizures and epilepsy: definitions proposed by the international league against epilepsy (ILAE) and the international bureau for epilepsy (IBE).** *Epilepsia* 2005, 46(4):470–472.
2. Connock M, Frew E, Evans B, Bryan S, Cummins C, Fry-Smith A, Li Wan Po A, Sandercock J: **The clinical effectiveness and cost-effectiveness of newer drugs for children with epilepsy, a systematic review.** *Health Technol Assess* 2006, 10:7.
3. Hawkins N, Epstein D, Drummond M, Wilby J, Kainth A, Chadwick D, Sculpher M: **Assessing the cost-effectiveness of new pharmaceuticals in epilepsy in adults: the results of a probabilistic decision model.** *Med Decis Making* 2005, 25:493–510.
4. Malphrus AD, Wilfong AA: **Use of the newer antiepileptic drugs in pediatric epilepsies.** *Curr Treat Options Neurol* 2007, 9:256–267.
5. Nikfar S, Kebriaeezadeh A, Majdzadeh R, Abdollahi M: **Monitoring of National Drug Policy (NDP) and its standardized indicators; conformity to decisions of the national drug selecting committee in Iran.** *BMC Int Health Hum Rights* 2005, 10(5(1)):5.
6. Abdollahiasl A, Nikfar S, Abdollahi M: **Pharmaceutical market and health system in the middle eastern and central asian countries: time for**

innovations and changes in policies and actions. *Arch Med Sci* 2011, **7**(3):365–367.

7. Elger CE, Schmidt D: **Modern management of epilepsy: a practical approach.** *Epilepsy Behav* 2008, **12**:501–539.

8. Asconape JJ: **The selection of antiepileptic drugs for the treatment of epilepsy in children and adults.** *Neurol Clin* 2010, **28**:843–852.

9. Nikfar S, Khatibi M, Abdollahiasl A, Abdollahi M: **Cost and utilization study of antidotes: an Iranian experience.** *Int J Pharmacol* 2011, **7**(1):46–49.

10. Ferraro TN, Buono RJ: **The relationship between the pharmacology of antiepileptic drugs and human gene variation: an overview.** *Epilepsy Behav* 2005, **7**:18–36.

11. Zamani G: **Treatment plan for intractable seizures.** *Iran J Pediatr* 2003, **13**(1):83–89.

12. Kochhar P, Suvarna V, Duttagupta S, Sarkar S: **Cost-effectiveness study comparing cefoperazone-sulbactam to a three-drug combination for treating intraabdominal infections in an Indian health-care setting.** *Value Health* 2008, **11**(Suppl 1):S33–8.

13. Ament A, Baltussen R: **The interpretation of results of economic evaluation: explicating the value of health.** *Heal Econ* 1997, **6**:625–635.

14. World Health Organization: *CHOosing Interventions that are Cost Effective (WHO-CHOICE).* Available at October 2010. http://www.who.int/choice/costs/CER_levels/en/.

15. *International Monetary Fund:Currency units per SDR.* Available at October 2010. http://www.imf.org/external/pubs/ft/weo.

16. Frew EJ, Sandercock J, Whitehouse WP, Bryan S: **The cost-effectiveness of newer drugs as add-on therapy for children with focal epilepsies.** *Seizure* 2007, **16**:99–112.

17. Knoester PD, Deckers CLP, Termeer EH, Boendermaker AJ, Kotsopoulos IA, de Krom MC, Keyser T, Renier WO, Hekster YA, Severens HL: **A cost-effectiveness decision model for antiepileptic drug treatment in newly diagnosed epilepsy patients.** *Value Health* 2007, **10**(3):173–182.

18. Boon P, D'Have D, Van Walleghem P, Michielsen G, Vonck K, Caemaert J, De Reuck J: **Direct medical costs of refractory epilepsy incurred by three different treatment modalities; a prospective assessment.** *Epilepsia* 2002, **43**(1):96–102.

19. Beghi E, Atzeni L, Garattini L: **Economic analysis of newer antiepileptic drugs.** *CNS Drugs* 2008, **22**(10):861–875.

Large scale screening of commonly used Iranian traditional medicinal plants against urease activity

Farzaneh Nabati[1], Faraz Mojab[2], Mehran Habibi-Rezaei[3], Kowsar Bagherzadeh[1], Massoud Amanlou[1,4] and Behnam Yousefi[5*]

Abstract

Background and purpose of the study: *H. pylori* infection is an important etiologic impetus usually leading to gastric disease and urease enzyme is the most crucial role is to protect the bacteria in the acidic environment of the stomach. Then urease inhibitors would increase sensitivity of the bacteria in acidic medium.

Methods: 137 Iranian traditional medicinal plants were examined against Jack bean urease activity by Berthelot reaction. Each herb was extracted using 50% aqueous methanol. The more effective extracts were further tested and their IC_{50} values were determined.

Results: 37 plants out of the 137 crude extracts revealed strong urease inhibitory activity (more than 70% inhibition against urease activity at 10 mg/ml concentration). Nine of the whole studied plants crude extracts were found as the most effective with IC_{50} values less than 500 μg/ml including; *Rheum ribes*, *Sambucus ebulus*, *Pistachia lentiscus*, *Myrtus communis*, *Areca catechu*, *Citrus aurantifolia*, *Myristica fragrans*, *Cinnamomum zeylanicum* and *Nicotiana tabacum*.

Conclusions: The most potent urease inhibitory was observed for *Sambucus ebulus* and *Rheum ribes* extracts with IC_{50} values of 57 and 92 μg/ml, respectively.

Keywords: Urease inhibitor, Iranian traditional medicinal plants, *Sambucus ebulus*, *Rheum ribes*, Screening of natural products

Introduction

Ureases (urea amidohydrolases, EC (3.5.1.5) are a group of widespread enzymes in nature, classified as the most proficient enzymes (with proficiency more than 10^{14}), stand as protagonist in biochemistry for several reasons. Urease was the first ureolytic enzyme obtained and named in the late nineteenth century, with landmark significance in enzymology as the first enzyme crystallized (in 1926 by Sumner) to approve the proteinous nature of the enzymes [1]. Also, as ascertained by Dixon et al. in 1975, urease was the first enzyme shown to possess nickel ions in its active site, essential for activity [2]. Since its substrate; urea is pervasively available in nature, urease was important to provide organisms with nitrogen in the form of ammonia for growth [3]. Despite the diversity in the molecular structures of urease, the amino acid sequences of the active sites are principally similar in all of the known them and consequence of this fact is the same catalytic mechanism. The active sites are always located in α subunits and contain the binuclear nickel centre, in which the Ni–Ni distances range from 3.5 to 3.7 Angstrom [4].

Urease as the most characteristic feature of *Helicobacter pylori* constitutes 5–10% of the bacteria's proteins. *H. pylori* a microaerophilic, gram-negative spiral bacterium which was first detected in 1984 by Marshall et al, is one of the most common chronic bacterial pathogens in humans [5]. Approximately more than 50% of people in the world are infected with it, and its prevalence is significantly higher in developing countries in compare with the developed ones. *H. pylori* infection is an important etiologic impetus usually leading to chronic gastritis, gastro duodenal ulcer and low grade gastric mucosa-associated lymphoid tissue lymphoma. Epidemiological data show

* Correspondence: dr.yousefi@gmail.com
[5]School of Advanced Medical Technologies, Tehran University of Medical Sciences, Tehran, Iran
Full list of author information is available at the end of the article

Table 1 Urease inhibitory activity of plants extract at concentration of 10 mg/ml

	Scientific name	Plant family	Common name in English	Common name in Persian	Part used in traditional	Inhibition (%)
1.	*Abrus precatorius*	Fabaceae	Paternoster Seed	Cheshm-e khorus	Seed	9.21 ± 0.04
2.	*Acacia Senegal*	Fabaceae	Gum Arabic	Samgh-e arabi	Gum	12.81± 0.09
3.	*Acanthophyllum squarrosum*	Asparagaceae	Soap Root	Chubak	Root	14.15 ± 0.02
4.	*Alpinia officinarum*	Zingiberaceae	Galangal	Khulanjan	Rhizome	41.75 ± 0.05
5.	*Althaea officinalis*	Malvaceae	Hollyhoch	Khatmi	Flower	20.94 ± 0.06
6.	*Alyssum homolocarpum*	Brassicaceae	Madword & Pepper Weed	Qodume	Seed	13.57± 0.12
7.	*Amaranthus lividus*	Amaranthaceae	Cock's Comb Seed	Tokhm-e tajkhorus	Seed	17.48 ± 0.11
8.	*Anethum graveolins*	Apiaceae	Dill Seed	Tokhm-e shevid	Seed	37.50 ± 0.03
9.	*Apium graveolens*	Apiaceae	Celery Seed	Tokhm-e karafs	Seed	2.43 ± 0.01
10.	*Aquilaria sinensis*	Thymelaeaceae	Agarwood	Udeqamari	Fruit	32.03 ± 0.08
11.	*Arctium Lappa*	Asteraceae	Burdock Root	Bâbââdam	Root	19.99 ± 0.08
12.	*Areca catechu*	Arecaceae	Betel Nuts	Fufel	Fruit	96.67 ± 0.01
13.	*Artemisia absinthium*	Asteraceae	Worm Wood	Afsantin	Herb	52.50 ± 0.06
14.	*Artemisia dracunculus*	Asteraceae	Tarragon	Tarkhon	Leaf	57.53 ± 0.03
15.	*Asperugo procumbens*	Boraginaceae	German Madwort	Bâdranjbuye	Herb	12.43 ± 0.02
16.	*Astragalus arbusculinus*	Fabaceae	Sarcocola	Anzarut	Gum	17.68 ± 0.06
17.	*Astragalus gossypinus*	Fabaceae	Gum Tragacanth	Katirâ	Gum	1.33 ± 0.02
18.	*Bambusa vulgaris*	Poaceae	Golden Bamboo	Tabâshir sadaf	Secretions	12.81 ± 0.04
19.	*Brassica nigra*	Brassicaceae	Mustard	Khardel	Seed	27.63 ± 0.01
20.	*Calendula officinalis*	Asteraceae	Marigold	Hamishe bahar	Flower	0.16 ± 0.06
21.	*Calendula* sp.	Asteraceae	Marigold	Hamishe bahar	Flower	8.21 ± 0.07
22.	*Camellia sinensis*	Theaceae	Green Tea	Châ(y)-e sabz	Leaf	89.40 ± 0.02
23.	*Camellia sinensis*	Theaceae	Green Tea	Châyeparsefid	Twig	90.45 ± 0.01
24.	*Cannabis sativa*	Cannabaceae	Hemp Seed	Shâhdane	Seed	9.71 ± 0.02
25.	*Capsicum annuum*	Solanaceae	Red Pepper	Felfel-e qermez	Fruit	99.01 ± 0.01
26.	*Carthamus tinctorius*	Asteraceae	Saf	Golrang	Flower	50.78 ± 0.04
27.	*Cassia angustifolia*	Fabaceae	Senna	Sena	Leaf	3.29 ± 0.03
28.	*Celosia cristata*	Amaranthaceae	Cockscomb	Gol-e halva	Flower	82.55 ± 0.03
29.	*Centaurea* sp.	Asteraceae	Centaurea	Gol-e gandom	Flower	70.33 ± 0.02
30.	*Chenopodium botrys*	Amaranthaceae	Lamb's Quarter	Dermane-e torki	Herb	15.13 ± 0.04
31.	*Cichorium intybus*	Asteraceae	Chicory	Kâsni	Herb	40.55 ± 0.04
32.	*Cinchona officinalis*	Rubiaceae	Cinchona	Gne gne	Bark	67.03 ± 0.02
33.	*Cinnamomum camphora*	Lauraceae	Camphre	Kâfur	Camphor	10.14 ± 0.08
34.	*Cinnamomum cassia*	Lauraceae	Cassia	Salikhe	Bark	91.19 ± 0.02
35.	*Cinnamomum zeylanicum*	Lauraceae	Cinnamon	Darchin	Bark	84.22 ± 0.05
36.	*Citrus aurantifolia*	Rutaceae	Limu Fruit	Limu ammâni	Fruit	99.02 ± 0.02
37.	*Citrus aurantium*	Rutaceae	Bitter Orange Peel	Khalâl-e nârenj	Rind	1.43 ± 0.05
38.	*Citrus bigardia*	Rutaceae	Orange	Gol-e nârenj	Twig	24.31 ± 0.03
39.	*Colchicum macrophyllum*	Colchicaceae	Colchicum Corms	Suranjan	Corm	9.44 ± 0.08

Table 1 Urease inhibitory activity of plants extract at concentration of 10 mg/ml *(Continued)*

40.	*Commiphora molmol*	Burseraceae	Myrrh	Morr-e Makki	Gum	8.22 ± 0.04
41.	*Crataegus microphylla*	Rosaceae	Hawthorn	Sorkhe valik	Flower	82.19 ± 0.03
42.	*Curcuma zedoaria*	Zingiberaceae	Zedoary	Zorombad	Seed	4.70 ± 0.06
43.	*Cuscuta epithymum*	Convolvulaceae	Hellweed	Aftimun	Herb	9.66 ± 0.01
44.	*Cymbopogon*	Poaceae	Lemongrass	Putar	Root	14.02 ± 0.03
45.	*Descureania*	Brassicaceae	Flixweed Seed	Khakshir	Seed	21.81 ± 0.01
46.	*Diplotaenia damavendica*	Apiaceae	Diplotaenia	Gozal	Seed	12.59 ± 0.06
47.	*Doronicum bracteatum*	Asteraceae	Doronicum	Darunj-e aqrabi	Herb	10.73 ± 0.01
48.	*Dracaena cinnabari*	Asparagaceae	Dragon Blood	Khone siyavosh	Gum	49.49 ± 0.13
49.	*Dracocephalum*	Lamiaceae	Moldavian Balm	Badrashbi	Twig	3.95 ± 0.01
50.	*Echinophora platyloba*	Apiaceae	Echinophora	Khosharize	Herb	17.48 ± 0.01
51.	*Echium amoenum*	Boraginaceae	Ox tongue Flower	Gol-e gâvzabân	Flower	31.66 ± 0.02
52.	*Elaeagnus angustifolia*	Elaeagnaceae	Oleaster	Senjed	Fruit	4.67 ± 0.14
53.	*Elaeagnus angustifolia*	Elaeagnaceae	Oleaster	Gol-e senjed	Flower	27.45 ± 0.01
54.	*Elettaria cardamomum*	Zingiberaceae	Cardamon	Hel sabz	Fruit	13.16 ± 0.04
55.	*Elletaria cardamomum*	Zingiberaceae	Cardamon	Hel sefid	Fruit	6.80 ± 0.07
56.	*Elletaria cardamomum*	Zingiberaceae	Cardamon	Hel siyah	Fruit	5.78 ± 0.071
57.	*Equisetum arvense*	Equisetaceae	Horse Tail	Dom-e asb	Stem	52.35 ± 0.05
58.	*Eruca sativa*	Brassicaceae	Rocket	Tokhm-e mandâb	Seed	13.28 ± 0.05
59.	*Eucalyptus* sp.	Myrtaceae	Eucalyptus	Okaliptus	Leaf	47.92 ± 0.01
60.	*Euphorbia* sp.	Euphorbiaceae	Euphorbia	Gav kosh	Herb	68.94 ± 0.03
61.	*Ferula assa-foetida*	Umbelliferae	Assa-Foetid	Anqoze	Gum	34.07 ± 0.04
62.	*Helicteres isora*	Malvaceae	Screw Tree Pod	Bahmanpich	Fruit	8.18 ± 0.02
63.	*Heracleum persicum*	Apiaceae	Cow Parsnip Friut	Golpar	Fruit	10.27 ± 0.02
64.	*Hibiscus gossypifolius*	Malvaceae	Rose Mallow	Chay-e Makki	Herb	96.28 ± 0.02
65.	*Humulus lupulus*	Cannabaceae	Hops	Râzak	Twig	54.85 ± 0.02
66.	*Hypericum perforatum*	Hypericaceae	St.John's Wort	Alaf-e chay	Herb	97.99 ± 0.02
67.	*Juglans regia*	Juglandaceae	Walnut Shell	Pust-e vasat-e gerdo	Septum	93.62 ± 0.01
68.	*Juglans regia*	Juglandaceae	Walnut Shell	Pust-e gerdo	Rind	1.27 ± 0.06
69.	*Juniperus Sabina*	Cupressaceae	Sabine	Abhal	Fruit	19.63 ± 0.01
70.	*Lactuca sativa*	Asteraceae	Lettuce	Tokhm-e Kâhu	Seed	2.93 ± 0.04
71.	*Lawsonia inermis*	Lythraceae	Henna	Hana	Leaf	54.00 ± 0.06
72.	*Levisticum officinalis*	Apiaceae	Lovage	Anjadân romi	Seed	10.00 ± 0.06
73.	*Linum usitatissimum*	Linaceae	Lineseed	Tokhm-e katan	Seed	2.71 ± 0.18
74.	*Malabaila secacule*	Apiaceae	Parsnip	Dogho	Root	18.18 ± 0.04
75.	*Malva sylvestris*	Malvaceae	Common Mallow	Gol-e panirak	Flower	14.15 ± 0.05
76.	*Matricaria chamomilla*	Asteraceae	Chamomile	Bâbon-e shirazi	Herb	87.21 ± 0.01
77.	*Melissa officinalis*	Lamiaceae	Balm	Barangbu	Herb	46.22 ± 0.05

Table 1 Urease inhibitory activity of plants extract at concentration of 10 mg/ml *(Continued)*

78.	*Mentha spicata*	Lamiaceae	Mint	NaAna	Leaf	93.89 ± 0.01
79.	*Myristica fragrans*	Myristicaceae	Nutmeg	Joz-e buya	Fruit	78.19 ± 0.01
80.	*Myrtus communis*	Myrtaceae	Myrtle	Murd	Leaf	72.99 ± 0.01
81.	*Nasturdium officinalis*	Brassicaceae	Watercress	Boolâgoti	Leaf	74.00 ± 0.03
82.	*Nerium Oleander*	Apocynaceae	Nerium	Gol-e kharzahre	Flower	84.62 ± 0.01
83.	*Nicotiana Tabacum*	Solanaceae	Tobacco	Tutun	Leaf	52.77 ± 0.03
84.	*Nicotiana tabacum*	Solanaceae	Tobacco	Tutun	Stem	75.26 ± 0.05
85.	*Nymphaea alba*	Nymphaeaceae	White Lotus	Gol-e nilofar	Flower	97.86 ± 0.01
86.	*Ocimum basilicum*	Lamiaceae	Basil	Reyhan-e banafsh	Leaf	19.61 ± 0.05
87.	*Ocimum basilicum*	Lamiaceae	Basil	Reyhan-e sabz	Leaf	0.41 ± 0.01
88.	*Oenothera biennis*	Onagraceae	Evening Star	Gol-e maghrebi	Flower	3.95 ± 0.04
89.	*Olea europea*	Oleaceae	Olive Leaf	Barg-e zyton	Leaf	72.30 ± 0.01
90.	*Orchis latifolia*	Orchidaceae	Oriental Salp	SaAlab-e panjei	Root	18.90 ± 0.02
91.	*Orchis mascula*	Orchidaceae	Male Orchis	SaAlab-e qolvei	Root	3.16 ± 0.04
92.	*Papaver Rhoeas*	Papaveraceae	Corn Poppy	Pust-e shaghayegh	Rind	27.25 ± 0.12
93.	*Papaver Rhoeas*	Papaveraceae	Corn Poppy	Gol-e shaghayegh	Flower	97.50 ± 0.01
94.	*Papaver somniferum*	Papaveraceae	Opium Poppy	Khashkhash	Seed	4.79 ± 0.03
95.	*Papaver somniferum*	Papaveraceae	Opium Poppy	Khashkhash	Fruit	35.95 ± 0.02
96.	*Passiflora caerulea*	Passifloraceae	Passion Flower	Gol-e sâAty	Flower	46.90 ± 0.008
97.	*Pelargonium graveolens*	Geraniaceae	Geranium	Barg-e atr	Leaf	92.19 ± 0.01
98.	*Pelargonium graveolens*	Geraniaceae	Rose Pelargonium	Gol-e atr	Flower	96.87 ± 0.02
99.	*Pterocarpus rubra*	Fabaceae	Mukwa	Sandal-e sorkh	Bark	91.75 ± 0.01
100.	*Petroselinum hortense*	Apiaceae	Parsley Seed	Tokhm-e jafari	Seed	50.35 ± 0.03
101.	*Pistachio lentiscus*	Anacardiaceae	Lentisk Pistache	Mastaki	Gum	92.37 ± 0.01
102.	*Pistacia vera*	Anacardiaceae	Pistachio Nut Shell	Pust-e peste	Rind	97.71 ± 0.01
103.	*Plantago major*	Plantaginaceae	Great Plantain	Bârhang	Seed	4.69 ± 0.11
104.	*Polyporus officinalis*	Fomitopsidaceae	White Agaric	Ghariqun	Fungi	19.97 ± 0.06
105.	*Portulaca oleracea*	Portulacaceae	Common Purslane Seed	Tokhm-e khorfe	Seed	7.19 ± 0.03
106.	*Prunus persica*	Rosaceae	Peach	Barge-e holo	Fruit	9.47 ± 0.11
107.	*Punica granatum*	Lythraceae	Pomegranate Flower	Golnar	Flower	99.90 ± 0.01
108.	*Punica granatum*	Lythraceae	Pomegranate	Golnar	Rind	99.90 ± 0.01
109.	*Quercus infectoria*	Fagaceae	Oak Gall	Qolqaf	Gall	53.97 ± 0.02
110.	*Quercus infectoria*	Fagaceae	Oak Fruit Hull	Jaft	Rind	98.84 ± 0.02
111.	*Rheum ribes*	Polygonaceae	Rhubarb	Rivâs	Root	98.93 ± 0.01
112.	*Rosa centifolia*	Rosaceae	Damask Rose	Gol-e sorkh	Flower	97.51 ± 0.01
113.	*Rosa foetida*	Rosaceae	Rosa Lutea	Gol-e zard	Flower	89.19 ± 0.023
114.	*Rosmarinus angustifolia*	Lamiaceae	Pine Rosemary	Rozmary-e aklilaljabal	Leaf	22.51 ± 0.02
115.	*Rubia tinctorium*	Rubiaceae	Madder Root	Ronas	Root	37.31 ± 0.02
116.	*Ruta graveolens*	Rutaceae	Rue	Sodab	Leaf	27.91 ± 0.04
117.	*Saccharum officinarum*	Poaceae	Sugar Cane	Shekar-e sorkh	Mann	35.04 ± 0.06
118.	*Salix aegyptiaca*	Salicaceae	Aegyption Willow	Bidmeshk	Flower	17.05 ± 0.02
119.	*Salix* sp.	Salicaceae	Whitewillow	Pust-e bid	Bark	38.10 ± 0.01

Table 1 Urease inhibitory activity of plants extract at concentration of 10 mg/ml *(Continued)*

120.	*Salvia hydrangea*	Lamiaceae	Mountain Sage	Gol-e arune	Flower	91.09 ± 0.01
121.	*Salvia macrosiphon*	Lamiaceae	Willd Sage Seeds	Thokhm-e marv	Seed	2.86 ± 0.04
122.	*Sambucus ebulus*	Adoxaceae	Dwarf Elder	Tarâsit	Fruit	99.70 ± 0.01
123.	*Santalum album*	Santalaceae	Sandalwood	Sandal-e sefid	Bark	58.69 ± 0.02
124.	*Satureja hortensis*	Lamiaceae	Savory Seed	Tokhm-e marze	Seed	35.77 ± 0.04
125.	*Scrophularia striata*	Scrophulariaceae	Striata Figwort	Mokhallace	Stem& Flower	16.47 ± 0.05
126.	*Sinapis alba*	Brassicaceae	White Mustard	Khardal-e sefid	Seed	39.77 ± 0.06
127.	*Spinacia oleracea.*	Amaranthaceae	Spinach Seed	Tokhm-e esfenaj	Seed	19.76 ± 0.04
128.	*Taraxacum sp.*	Asteraceae	Dandelion	Ghasedak	Flower	14.83 ± 0.01
129.	*Thymus kotschyanus*	Lamiaceae	Kotschyam Thyme	Avishan	Herb	17.94 ± 0.01
130.	*Tilia platyphyllos*	Malvaceae	Linden	Zirfun	Leaf & Flower	25.79 ± 0.01
131	*Trigonella foenum-graecum*	Fabaceae	Fenugreek Seed	Tokhm-e shanbalile	Seed	44.02 ± 0.02
132.	*Triticum sativum*	Poaceae	Wheat	Sabos-e ghandom	Husk	16.14 ± 0.04
133.	*Tussilago farfara*	Asteraceae	Colt/s-foot	Pakhari	Herb	69.08 ± 0.01
134.	*Veratrum album*	Melanthiaceae	White Hellebore	Kharbogh	Leaf	96.85 ± 0.06
135.	*Verbascum georgicum*	Scrophulariaceae	Mullein	Dom-e gav	Leaf	30.40 ± 0.03
336.	*Verbascum sp.*	Scrophulariaceae	Mullein	Marg-e mâhi	Fruit	0.82 ± 0.05
137.	*Ziziphus vulgaris*	Rhamnaceae	Jujube	Annâb	Fruit	26.34 ± 0.01
138.	Hydroxyurea	————————	————————	———————	Reference compound	100 ± 0.01

that high *H. pylori* infection rate, result in the incidence of gastric cancer and adenocarcinoma [6,7]. Urease catalyzes the hydrolysis of urea to produce ammonia and carbon dioxide, and the most crucial role is to protect the bacteria in the acidic environment of the stomach [8]. It has been also reported that ammonia and monochloramine, which is a reaction product of ammonia and hypochlorous acid, exhibit potent toxicity in gastric epithelium [9]. Moreover, it has been demonstrated that *H. pylori* lacking urease activity are incapable of causing infection in animal models. Thus, it is most likely that urease is essential for bacterial colonization and perhaps the pathogenesis of related disease in vivo.

World Health Organization (WHO) has categorized *H. pylori* as a class 1 carcinogen [10]. Fortunately, its eradication with antibiotics can result in ulcer healing, prevent peptic ulcer recurrence and reduce the prevalence of gastric cancer in high-risk populations. However, it is not always successful because of its resistance to one or more antibiotics and other factors such as poor patient compliance, undesirable side effects of the drugs and significant cost of combination therapy [11]. Wolle et. al. reported that approximately 20% of the patients undergoing antibiotics therapy would experience therapeutic failure [12]. In developing countries, since the application of antibiotics is still under a poor management as a whole, there is a growing need for finding new anti-*H. pylori* agents that can hopefully eradicate the invasion

and presence of survived *H. pylori* strains to avoid relapse of gastric ulcer. Hence, a considerable variety of studies involving tests for medicinal plants showing antimicrobial activity and discrepant susceptibility test results are available due to variations in the methods and conditions used for its susceptibility testing.

One of the best sources of new substances to treat *H. pylori* is natural products and their derivatives [13]. Variety of techniques such as synthesizing [6], and also molecular modeling and virtual screening methods [14,15] have been applied to find possible urease inhibitors. The biological activity of plant-derived substances may be considered as a source of new anti-*H. pylori* drugs come from different classes of compounds and are characterized by the diversity of their structures. Therefore, almost all traditional Iranian herbal medicines that are used as remedies and sold as medicines to manage different diseases were screened to discover possible plant-derived urease inhibitors.

Methods

Materials

Sodium nitroprusside (sodium pentacyanonitrosyloferrate III) and urease (EC 3.5.1.5) from Jack beans were purchased from Sigma (St. Louis, MO, USA). All other chemicals were of analytical reagent grade from Merck. Deionized water was used in all experiments. Potassium

Table 2 IC$_{50}$ and medicinal uses of most active plants

	Scientific name	Effects & medicinal uses	IC$_{50}$ (µg/ml)	Std. Error log IC$_{50}$
1.	*A. catechu*	Anthelmintic, gastric tonic	216	0.01
2.	*C. cristata*	Styptic, depurative, sedative, constipating, antibacterial, febrifuge,	6175	0.68
3.	*C. annuum*	Anti flatulence, gout, gastric tonic, paralysis	751	0.14
4.	*C. aurantifolia*	Appetitive, anti-flatulence, analgesic	432	0.06
5.	*C. cassia*	Gastric tonic, anti-spasmodic, anti-flatulence	867	0.05
6.	*C. microphylla*	Anti-flatulence, gastric tonic	665	0.14
7.	*C. sinensis*	Anti-bacterial, anti diarrhea, diuretic, astringent, reduce cholesterol	579	0.04
8.	*C. zeylanicum*	Gastric tonic, anti-flatulence, 'anti-spasmodic	361	0.02
9.	*C. sinensis*	Anti-diarrhea, diuretic, astringent, anti-bacterial, reduce cholesterol	1314	0.04
10.	*Cetaurea* sp.	Anti-inflammatory, astringent, emmenagogue, sedative	5152	0.05
11.	*H. gossypifolius*	Analgesic, anti-tussive, demulcent, diuretic, febrifuge, highly emollient, slightly laxative and odontalgic, anti-inflammations and laryngitis,	819	0.01
12.	*H. perforatum*	Astringent, analgesic, anti-inflammator, anti-anxiety aphrodisiac	3509	0.10
13.	*J. regia*	Anti-inflammatory, astringent, anti-spasmodic	1271	0.08
14.	*M. chamomilla*	Anti-inflammation, appetitive, and aids digestion and sleep, acts as a diuretic and nerve tonic.	3188	0.02
15.	*M. fragrans*	Anti-flatulence appetitive 'anti-spasmodic' antiseptic, analgesic, anti-inflammatory	215	0.15
16.	*M. spicata*	Analgesic, Anti-spasmodic, anti-flatulence	7822	0.17
17.	*M. communis*	Antiseptic, disinfectant, expectorant, deodorizer	170	0.04
18.	*N. officinale*	Diuretic, expectorant, purgative, hypoglycemic, odontalgic, stimulant, tonic and stomachic	2055	0.19
19.	*N. alba*	Astringent, antiseptic, anesthetic, aphrodisiac, sedative, used for gastrointestinal disorders and jaundice	820	0.19
20.	*N. Oleander*	Dermatitis, abscesses, eczema, psoriasis, sores, warts, corns, ringworm, scabies, herpes, skin cancer, asthma, dysmenorrheal, epilepsy, malaria,	9877	0.26
21.	*N. tabacum*	Anti-spasmodic, diuretic, sedative, sialagogue	473	0.15
22.	*O. europea*	Hypotensive, diuretic, hypoglycemic	2857	0.06
23.	*P. granatum*(Rind)	Hypoglycemic, anti-cancer, anthelmintic	1484	0.10
24.	*P. granatum* (Flower)	Hypoglycemic, anti-cancer, anthelmintic	1331	0.11
25.	*P. graveolens*	Anti-inflammatory, antiseptic, aromatherapy, astringent, anti- cancer, sedative	976	0.03
26.	*P. graveolens*	Analgesic, anti-Bacterial, anti-Depressant, anti-inflammatory, antiseptic, astringent, diuretic, insect repellent, refreshing, relaxing, sedative, styptic, tonic	1242	0.14
27.	*P. lentiscus*	Antibacterial	121	0.03
28.	*P. Rhoeas*	Anodyne, emmenagogue, emollient, expectorant, hypnotic, sedative, tonic	5636	0.04
29.	*P. rubra*	Astringent, tonic	930	0.06
30.	*P. vera*	Aphrodisiac, anti-anxiety	4687	0.12
31.	*Q. infectoria*	Gingivitis, infectoria, anti-diabetic, anti-tremorine, local anesthetic, antiviral, antibacterial, antifungal.	1214	0.12
32.	*R. centifolia*	Anti-inflammatory, antispasmodic, aphrodisiac, astringent, depurative, laxative, analgesic, appetitive	544	0.07
33.	*R. foetida*	Heart diseases, digestive, skin diseases, muscular pains, anti-parasite	2441	0.19
34.	*R. ribes*	Appetitive, astringent, anti bacteria, anti depressive and used to treat diabetes, hemorrhoids, ulcer, diarrhea	92	0.06
35.	*S. hydrangea*	anti-flatulence, astringent, anti-spasmodic	2960	0.11
36.	*S. ebulus*	Anti-inflammatory, antinociceptive, anti-cancer, anti-angiogenic, anti-oxidative	57	0.05
37.	*V. album*	Analgesic, anthelmintic, cathartic, emetic, expectorant, hypnotic	1037	0.07
38.	hydroxyurea		37	0.02

phosphate buffer (100 mM), pH 7.6 was prepared in distilled water.

The studied plants were collected from local medicinal herb shops, Tehran, Iran (June 2010) and were identified by one of our authors of the presented article (F. Mojab). The authenticated samples were deposited in the Herbarium of Shahid Beheshti University of Medical Sciences.

Extract preparation
10 g of air-dried and powdered plant material was extracted in 10 ml, 50:50 methanol: water at room temperature for 24 hrs. The resulting liquid extract was filtered and concentrated to dryness under reduced pressure. The dry extracts were stored at -20°C till used [16].

Determination of urease activity
All extracts were tested for urease inhibitory at concentration of 10 mg/ml by the modified spectrophotometric method developed by Berthelot reaction [17]. For herbal extracts that were proven to exert significant inhibition and also for positive controls, inhibitory assays were performed. The plant extracts were tested in a concentration range of 0 to 10 mg/ml. Hydroxyurea was used as standard inhibitor.

The solution assay mixture consisted of urea (30 mM) and (100 μl) crud extract with a total value of 950 μl. The reactions were initiated by the addition of 50 μl of urease enzyme solution in phosphate buffer (100 mM, pH 7.6, 1 mg/ml). Urease activity was determined by measuring ammonia concentration after 15 minutes of enzymatic reaction. The ammonia was determined using 500 μl of solution A (contained 5.0 g phenol and 25 mg of sodium nitroprusside in 500 ml of distilled water) and 500 μl of solution B (contained of 2.5 g sodium hydroxide and 4.2 ml of sodium hypochlorite 5% in 500 ml of distillated water) at 37°C for 30 minutes. The absorbance was read at 625 nm. Activity of uninhibited urease was designated as the control activity of 100%.

Data processing
The extent of the enzymatic reaction was calculated based on the following equation:

$$I(\%) = [1-(T/C)] * 100$$

Where I (%) is the inhibition of the enzyme, T (test) is the absorbance of the tested sample (plant extract or positive control in the solvent) in the presence of enzyme, C (control) is the absorbance of the solvent in the presence of enzyme. Data are expressed as mean ± standard error (SD) and the results were taken from at least three times.

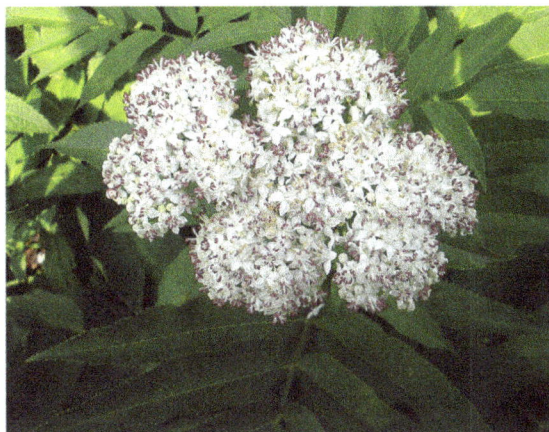

Figure 1 *Sambucus ebulus* in flowering stage [19].

Determination of IC$_{50}$ values
IC$_{50}$ values (concentration of test compounds that inhibits the hydrolysis of substrates by 50%) were determined by studying the extracts urease inhibitory activity at their different concentrations in comparison to their individual positive control employing spectrophotometric measurement. IC$_{50}$ values were obtained from dose-response curves by linear regression, using Graphpad software, prism 5.

Results and discussion
Medicinal plants as an appropriate and renewable source of active chemical compounds can be used as templates to discover new lead compounds. Doxorubicin, vincristine, and taxol, are examples of these herbal compounds which are clinically applied. According to the literature, 50% of commercially presented medicines in 1985 was from herbal origins [18]. Gastrointestinal diseases, especially gastric, duodenal and peptic ulcer, arise from different factors, in particular microbial agent *H. pylori*.

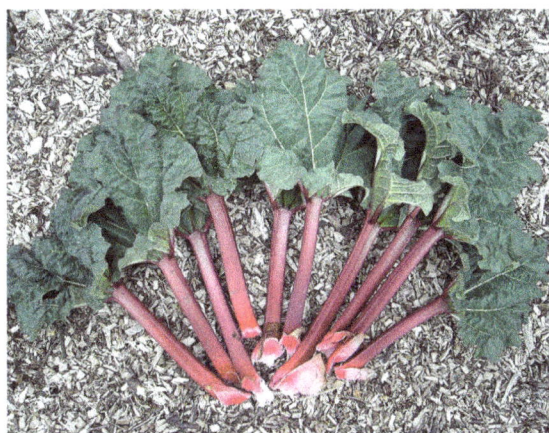

Figure 2 *Rheum ribes* leaf [21].

Common multi-drug therapies not only have side effects, but are also expensive. On the other hand, the probability of drug resistance occurrence and disease retrogression is quite concerning. Already reported studies have shown that herbal compounds have the ability to prevail this microbe. Among the studied herbal essences and extracts, many did not exceed the study level due to production limits, toxicity and impossibility of drug form preparation. Majority of the researches have focused on ways to inhibit the bacteria growth or it's elimination from the culture, while a few has particularly concerned inhibition of urease enzyme which is responsible for the bacteria defense system against the stomach very acidic medium.

Specific inhibition or reduction of urease enzyme activity would result in an increased sensitivity of the bacteria in acidic medium and therefore it's natural elimination by stomach acidic condition or the body immune system.

In the presented study, urease enzyme inhibition potency of 137 herbal extracts was investigated from which 37 extracts have shown inhibitory activity up to more than 70% in the concentration of 10 mg/ml (Table 1). Further examinations and IC_{50} determination revealed that *Sambucus ebulus, Rheum ribes, Pistachia lentiscus, Myrtus communis, Myristica fragrans, Areca catechu, Cinnamomum zeylanicum, Citrus aurantifolia* and *Nicotiana tabacum* extracts inhibit urease enzyme in concentrations less than 500 µg/ml. It should also be mentioned that *C. zeylanicum, M. chamomilla* and *M. spicata* are already used as gastrointestinal remedies and this research has proved that these herbs can inhibit urease activity and prevent gastric upsets. Names of the studied plants and the 37 final more active extracts are presented in Table 2. As it is shown, the most potent urease inhibitory was observed for *S. ebulus* and *R. ribes* with IC_{50} values less than 100 µg/ml.

S. ebulus (Figure 1) is a native perennial herb of the Adoxaceae family [19]. It has been prescribed in traditional medicines for the treatment of inflammatory reactions, such as hemorrhoid, bites and sore-throat. In addition, *S. ebulus* has been shown to have anti-inflammatory, antinociceptive, anti-cancer, anti-angiogenic and anti-oxidative activities. Ebulitin, ebulin 1, flavonoid, anthocyanin and other components have been isolated from *S. ebulus* and identified as active ingredients of biological and pharmacological activities [20]. The anti-*H. pylori* effect of the *S. ebulus* extract was observed by using the agar dilution method [13].

R. ribes (Figure 2) is a hardy perennial, cultivated in some temperate countries for its edible red leaf stalks [21]. It is used to treat diabetes, hemorrhoids, ulcer, diarrhea, and expectorant activity reported. The efficacy and safety of a hydroalcohlic extract of *R. ribes* in treatment of mild to moderate major depression disorder has been

investigated and the observations show some anti depressive effects. The methanolic extract of *R. ribes* have demonstrated anti-ulcer activity comparable with standard drugs cimetidine [22].

According to strong inhibitory activity of the herbs presented in Table 2, simultaneous application of theses herbs and the medicines prescribed in gastrointestinal disease therapies would fasten the treatment. Additionally, isolation of active compounds and further investigation of each isolated compound against urease activity would lead to new chemical structures which may have the potency to inhibit urease activity.

Competing interests

There are no other conflicts of interest related to this publication.

Authors' contributions

All authors contributed to the concept and design, making and analysis of data, drafting, revising and final approval. MA and BY are responsible for the study registration. FM is responsible for plants identification and collection. FN and KB carried out plant extraction and enzymatic tests and drafted manuscript. MHR, FN, MA and BY participated in collection and/or assembly of data, data analysis, interpretation and manuscript writing. All authors read and approved the final manuscript.

Acknowledgements

We would like to thank Fereshteh Keyghobadi for her cooperation in the practical herbal testes. The financial supports of the Research Council of the Tehran University of Medical Science, University of Tehran and Iran National Science Foundation (INSF) are gratefully acknowledged.

Author details

[1]Department of Medicinal Chemistry, Faculty of Pharmacy, Tehran University of Medical Sciences, Tehran, Iran. [2]Department of Pharmacognosy, School of Pharmacy, Shahid Beheshti University of Medical Sciences, Tehran, Iran. [3]School of Biology, College of Science, University of Tehran, Tehran, Iran. [4]Medicinal Plants Research Center, Tehran University of Medical Sciences, Tehran, Iran. [5]School of Advanced Medical Technologies, Tehran University of Medical Sciences, Tehran, Iran.

References

1. Jabri E, Lee MH, Hausinger RP, Karplus PA: **Preliminary crystallographic studies of urease from jack bean and from Klebsiella aerogenes.** *J Mol Biol* 1992, **227**:934–937.
2. Todd MJ, Hausinger RP: **Purification and characterization of the nickel-containing multicomponent urease from Klebsiella aerogenes.** *J Biol Chem* 1987, **262**:5963–5967.
3. Koper TE, El-Sheikh AF, Norton JM, Klotz MG: **Urease-encoding genes in ammonia-oxidizing bacteria.** *Appl Environ Microbiol* 2004, **70**:2342–2348.
4. Krajewska B, Ureases I: **Functional, catalytic and kinetic properties: A review.** *J Mol Catal B: Enzym* 2009, **59**:9–21.
5. Owen RJ: **Bacteriology of *Helicobacter pylori*.** *Baillieres Clin Gastroenterol* 1995, **9**:415–446.
6. Kosikowska P, Berlicki L: **Urease inhibitors as potential drugs for gastric and urinary tract infections: a patent review.** *Expert Opin Ther Pat* 2011, **21**:945–957.
7. Mobley HL, Hu LT, Foxal PA: ***Helicobacter pylori* urease: properties and role in pathogenesis.** *Scand J Gastroenterol Suppl* 1991, **187**:39–46.
8. Stingl K, Altendorf K, Bakker EP: **Acid survival of *Helicobacter pylori*: how does urease activity trigger cytoplasmic pH homeostasis?** *Trends Microbiol* 2002, **10**:70–74.
9. Dekigai H, Murakami M, Kita T: **Mechanism of Helicobacter pylori-associated gastric mucosal injury.** *Dig Dis Sci* 1995, **40**:1332–1339.
10. Forman D: ***Helicobacter pylori* and gastric cancer.** *Scand J Gastroenterol Suppl* 1996, **215**:48–51.

11. O'Connor A, Gisbert JP, McNamara D, O'Morain C: **Treatment of Helicobacter pylori infection.** *Helicobacter* 2011, **1**(16 Suppl):53–58.

12. Wolle K, Malfertheiner P: **Treatment of** *Helicobacter pylori*. *Best Pract Res Clin Gastroenterol* 2007, **21**:315–324.

13. Yesilada E, Gurbuz I, Shibata H: **Screening of Turkish anti-ulcerogenic folk remedies for anti-*Helicobacter pylori* activity.** *J Ethnopharmacol* 1999, **66**:289–293.

14. Azizian H, Nabati F, Sharifi A, Siavoshi F, Mahdavi M, Amanlou M: **Large-scale virtual screening for the identification of new *Helicobacter pylori* urease inhibitor scaffolds.** *J Mol Model* 2011, **3**:1–11.

15. Azizian H, Bahrami H, Pasalar P, Amanlou M: **Molecular modeling of** *Helicobacter pylori* **arginase and the inhibitor coordination interactions.** *J Mol Graph Model* 2010, **28**:626–635.

16. Gennaro AR: *Remington's Pharmaceutical Sciences*. Pennsylvania: Mack Publishing Company; 1985:1516.

17. Nabati F, Habibi-Rezaei M, Amanlou M, Moosavi-Movahedi AA: **Dioxane enhanced immobilization of urease on alkyl modified nano-porous silica using reversible denaturation approach.** *J Mol Catal B: Enzym* 2011, **70**:17–22.

18. Lipp FJ: **The efficacy, history, and politics of medicinal plants.** *Altern Ther Health Med* 1996, **2**:36–41.

19. Wikipedia contributors: *"Danewort" Wikipedia, The Free Encyclopedia*. http://en.wikipedia.org/wiki/Danewort, (accessed September 25, 2012).

20. Shokrzadeh M, Saravi S: **The chemistry, pharmacology and clinical properties of** *Sambucus ebulus*: **a review.** *J Med Plants Res* 2010, **4**:95–103.

21. Wikipedia contributors: *"Rheum" Wikipedia, The Free Encyclopedia*. http://en.wikipedia.org/wiki/Rheum_(plant), (accessed September 25, 2012).

22. Sindhu RK, Kumar P, Kumar J, Kumar A, Arora S: **Investigations into the anti-ulcer activity of** *Rheum ribes* **linn leaves extracts.** *Int J Pharm Pharm Sci* 2010, **2**:90–92.

Inhibition of HIV and HSV infection by vaginal lactobacilli *in vitro* and *in vivo*

Rezvan Zabihollahi[1], Elahe Motevaseli[2], Seyed Mehdi Sadat[1], Ali Reza Azizi-Saraji[1], Sogol Asaadi-Dalaie[1] and Mohammad Hossein Modarressi[2*]

Abstract

Background and the purpose of the study: The cervico-vaginal mucosa which is populated with microflora (mostly includes lactobacilli) is the portal of entry for sexually transmitted pathogens.

Methods: The *in vitro* anti-viral effect of vaginal and non-vaginal lactobacillus was evaluated using single cycle HIV-1 replication and HSV-2 plaque reduction assays. The XTT proliferation assay was used to monitor the cellular toxicity. The *in vivo* anti-HSV-1 activity was evaluated in BALB/c mouse model by monitoring skin lesion and immune response development.

Results and major conclusion: DMEM culture supernatant of *L. Gasseri* and *L. fermentum* (PH 7.3) did not show toxic effect but inhibited 50% of HIV replication at 12 and 31% concentrations, respectively. Co-culture of *L. gasseri* (1000 CFU/ target cell) showed mild cytotoxicity but inhibited 68% of HIV replication. The supernatant of *L. crispatus* inhibited 50% of HSV replication at 4% and also co-culture of *L. gasseri, L. rhamnosus* and *L. crispatus* revokes almost all of the HSV multiplication. Culture supernatants of *L. gasseri* and *L. crispatus* had significant virucidal effect against the HIV and HSV and inhibited HSV infection in a stage before viral entry to the target cells. Alive *L. gasseri* cells showed high potential for inhibiting HSV-1 infection *in vivo* condition. Current data indicates that lactobacilli supernatant encompasses components with neutralizing activity against HIV and HSV and it would be a determinant factor for viral diseases transmission and promising lead for anti-viral probiotic design.

Keywords: HIV, HSV, Sexually transmitted disease, Lactobacillus

Introduction

The cervico-vaginal mucosa is the portal of entry for sexually transmitted pathogenic microorganisms. In child-bearing age healthy females, the vaginal protective mucosa is populated with microflora that mostly includes lactobacilli. Vaginal health is positively associated with dominance of lactobacilli over pathogenic anaerobes [1]. Bacterial vaginosis (BV) is a situation with an imbalance of the vaginal microbial flora and is not caused by specific pathogenic microorganisms [2]. Reduction, absence or lack of antimicrobial properties (production of acid and H_2O_2) of lactobacilli and their replacement by anaerobic microbes such as *Gardnerella vaginalis* may be seen in BV [3].

Increasing data indicate that lacking lactobacilli or abnormal vaginal flora facilitates the transmission of viral sexually transmitted diseases (STD) [4]. There are some data reporting that HIV seropositivity correlates with BV independent of other behavior variabilities [5,6]. Recent prospective investigations demonstrated the association between vaginal flora alterations and the acquisition of Human immunodeficiency virus (HIV) infection [7]. Also, reduction in vaginal flora lactobacillus content was identified as a predisposing factor for infection of human papillomavirus (HPV) and herpes simplex virus type (HSV) [8-10]. Recent studies have revealed that abnormal vaginal flora triggers the shedding of HSV and cytomegalovirus (CMV) in women genital tract [11,12]. On the other hand genital herpes infection is a major risk factor for acquisition and transmission of HIV via sexual contact [13,14]. Moreover, HIV copy number in female genital-tract discharge inversely correlates with lactobacilli counts in bacterial flora [15].

* Correspondence: modaresi@sina.tums.ac.ir
[2]School of Medicine, Tehran University of Medical Sciences (TUMS), Tehran, Iran
Full list of author information is available at the end of the article

Therefore lactobacilli exhibit an important role for viral infections in both the female health protection as well as reducing the risk of infection transmission to a healthy man. *In vitro* studies have disclosed that hydrogen peroxide production by *L. acidophilus* strain displays a virucidal effect against HIV-1 [16]. Additionally, it has been reported that pre-incubation with different lactobacillus strains reduces the infection titer of vesicular stomatitis virus (VSV) [17]. However the inhibition mechanism of lactobacilli against viral infections is poorly understood, but nevertheless metabolic products such as lactic acid, H_2O_2 and bacteriocins are possible mediators to account for the protection against viruses. These factors might act against viral particles by inactivation, epithelial cell attachment competition, mucin gel preservation or maintaining the appropriate innate immune response [18-20].

In spite of the clinical and epidemiological studies, the *in vitro* anti-viral activity of these probiotic bacteria in cell culture environment has not been investigated in detail. The purpose of this study is to evaluate anti-HIV and HSV activity of vaginal lactobacilli *in vitro* and *in vivo* conditions and determine the possible mode of action.

Materials and methods

Lactobacilli strains and growth condition

Vaginal lactobacilli strains; *L. crispatus ATCC33820*, *L. gasseri ATCC33323*, *L. rhamnosus GG* and *L. fermentum ATCC14931* were used in this study as well as the non-vaginal ones; *L. acidophilus LA-5* (Hansen company, USA), *L. paracasei subsp. Casei ATCC25302*, *L. acidophilus NCFM* and *L. casei CRL431* (Hansen company, USA). All bacteria were stored at −70°C in 85% de Man- Rogosa-Sharpe (MRS) supplemented with 15% glycerol. Lactobacilli were inoculated from frozen glycerol vials onto MRS broth and incubated at 37°C for 48hs under anaerobic conditions [21]. Plating of serial lactobacilli 10-fold dilutions in MRS-agar was used to determine the colony forming units (CFU) titer. Colony counting was carried out after 48hs of incubation.

Culture supernatant

Lactobacilli were harvested from fresh MRS culture by centrifuging at 3×10^3 g and the pellet was washed with DMEM twice to eliminate the remnants MRS. Working stokes were prepared in DMEM (2×10^9 CFU/ml) and stored at 4°C. These working stokes were freshly (no more than 2 weeks) used for experiments. To prepare the culture supernatant (CS), lactobacilli (3.6×10^8 CFU) were inoculated onto each well of 6-wells plates containing 6 ml of high glucose DMEM and incubated for 20hs in a CO_2 incubator. Culture supernatant (neutral pH phase) was harvested by clarification of the medium with 0.22 µm filters and used freshly for each experiment.

Cell culture and transfection

HEK293T (Human emberionic kidney), Hela (Cervix cancer) and vero (African green monkey kidney) cell lines were cultured in Dulbecco's Modified Eagle Medium (DMEM, Gibco, USA) supplemented with 10% fetal bovine serum (FBS, Gibco, USA), 5 mM glutamine. The cells medium was supplemented with penicillin (100 IU/ml) and streptomycin (100 µg/ml) in particular experiments. HEK293T cells were transfected using polyfect transfection reagent (Qiagen, USA). Transfection was performed according to the manufacturer's protocol in 6-wells plates [22].

Viruses

Single cycle replicable (SCR) HIV-1 (NL4-3) and HSV-2 viruses were used in this study. Plasmid mixture (2 µg) of PmzNL4-3 [23], pSPAX.2 and pMD2G was cotransfected into the HEK293T cells to prepare VSV surface glycoprotein (VSVG) pseudotyped SCR HIV-1 [24]. Virus containing supernatant was harvested and pooled 24, 48 and 72hs post transfection.

Vero cells were infected to supply the HSV-2 virus stokes. The Cells were seeded onto 6-wells plates (4.5×10^5 cells/well) and incubated for one day to reach 98% of confluence. One milliliter of virus supernatant was used to infect cells in each well and unbound virions were removed after 2hs. Virus containing supernatants were harvested and pooled every 24hs after infection until day 4.

HIV and HSV virus containing supernatants were clarified using 0.22 µm filters and 10mins centrifuging at 10^4 g. Viruses were stored at −70°C and assessed for infectious titer using replication and plaque reduction assays.

HIV replication assay

Single cycle replication assay was used to evaluate the inhibitory activity against replication of VSVG psudotyped SCR HIV-1 virions [24,25]. Hela cells were seeded in 96-wells plates (6×10^3 cells/well) and maintained for 24hs in antibiotic free medium. Lactobacilli cells or supernatant were added into the wells 2hs before infection. Cells were infected with SCR HIV-1 virions (600 ng P24) and incubated for 20hs to accelerate the virions adsorption [22]. After virus entry, the cells were washed two times with DMEM to remove unbound viral particles. Cells were fed with antibiotic containing medium and incubated for additional 48 hrs. Plates were centrifuged for 15mins at 3×10^3 g and P24 content of the cells supernatant was evaluated using P24 capture ELISA (Biomerieux, France).

HSV plaque reduction assay

The inhibitory effect of lactobacilli against multiplication of HSV was investigated using plaque reduction assay. Vero cells were placed into the 24-wells culture plates

(Nunc, Denmark) at density of 4×10^5 cells per well and incubated for 24hs (in antibiotic free medium) to reach at least 98% of confluence. The cell monolayer was infected with 50pfu of HSV and washed after 1hs to remove unbound virions. The cell monolayer were then overlaid with DMEM supplemented by 1.5% of methylcellulose, 5% FBS and antibiotics. After 72hs, the overlay medium was removed and the cells were washed twice with DMEM and fixed by methanol. The formed plaques were counted after staining with 0.5% crystal violet.

Time-of-addition study

The inhibitory effect of *L. gasseri* and *L. crispatus* supernatant against different intervals of HSV replication was examined according to the previously described procedure with some minor modifications [26]. Vero cells monolayer was prepared by seeding the cells into 24-well plates (Nunc, Denmark) as describe above. Then, 20% concentration of *L. gasseri* and *L. crispatus* CS were added into the cells environment before (–6 and –2 hs), during (0 hs) or after (2 and 6 hs) time course of HSV-2 infection. Afterwards, the procedures similar to plaque reduction assay section were performed except that cell monolayer was washed twice by DMEM to eliminate the lactobacilli supernatant in pre-infection (–6, –2 and 0hs) groups. In other groups the lactobacilli CS was added after infection (2 and 6hs) and the concentration was kept constant until the end of the test.

Virucidal assay

The direct effect of *L. gasseri* and *L. crispatus* CS on HSV and HIV infectivity was evaluated by using virucidal assay. Different concentrations (2, 20 and 50%) of CSs were mixed thoroughly with HSV (5×10^3 pfu) and HIV (1.2×10^3 P24) virions, in final volume of 10 µl. The mixtures were incubated at 37°C for 2hs and then the fresh medium (90 µl) was added to each tube. Residual virus infectivity was determined by plaque reduction and HIV replication assays as described above.

In vivo anti-HSV assay

Animal consisted of pathogen-free, female BALB/c mice with 6–8 weeks of age-average 20 g of weight (purchased from Pasteur Institute of Iran, Iran) were handled according to the guidelines of the national institute of health guide and care for use of laboratory animal, Iran. The skin of BALB/c mice was shaved in right flank and scratched by needle (gauge 22). The naked and scratched skin was infected with 10^4 pfu of HSV-1 virions. Alive lactobacilli suspension (10^5 CFU in 20 µl of PBS) was added immediately after infection. Mice were maintained for six weeks and then evaluated for skin lesions and weight loss. The acyclovir cream (5%) was used as positive control. The immune response against HSV was also monitored by extracting the spleen cells and investigating their proliferative response to HSV antigens. Total spleen cells were treated with lysis buffer to remove red blood cells. Cell suspension was adjusted to 5.1×10^6 cells per milliliter and cultured (120 µl) in each well of 96-well plates with 10^3 pfu of inactivated HSV for 72hs. Phytohemagglutinin-A (PHA 7 µg/ml; Gibco, USA) was used as control. The proliferation of the cells was measured by addition of 50 µl of XTT (sodium 3_-[1-(phenylaminocarbonyl)- 3,4-tetrazolium]-bis(4-methoxy-6-nitro)benzene sulfonic acid; Roche, Germany) into each well. The plates were incubated at 37°C for 2hs and then read at test and references wavelengths of 450 and 630 nm, respectively.

Cytotxicity assay

The toxicity of lactobacilli cells and supernatant for Vero and Hela cells was determined using XTT (Roche, Germany) proliferation assay as previously is described. Vero cells were cultured in 96-wells plates (6×10^3/well) (Nunc, Denmark) contain lactobacilli cells (6×10^7 CFU/ml) and CS. Bacterial cells were removed after 1 hr and antibiotic containing medium was added into the wells. After 72hs, the medium was discarded and the cells were subsequently rinsed with phosphate buffered saline (PBS). To study the effect of lactobacilli cells and supernatant on Hela cells viability, HIV replication assay plates were subjected to the proliferation assay directly after washing cells with PBS. The XTT reagent (40 µl/well) was added into the plates and incubated at 37°C for additional 3hs. The optical densities (OD) were measured using enzyme immunoassay reader (stat fax2100, Awareness, USA) at test and reference wavelengths of 450 nm and 630 nm respectively.

Results and discussion
Anti-viral activity of lactobacilli supernatant

The DMEM culture supernatant (CS) of lactobacilli (pH of 7.3) was used to appraise the overall anti-HIV and HSV activity (Table 1). Virus multiplication was significantly decreased by all lactobacilli CS, although to different extents. *L. gasseri*, *L. fermentum*, *L. acidophilus* and *L. crispatus* inhibited 50% of HIV-1 virions replication at 12, 31, 46 and 48% concentration, respectively. Parallel experiments were performed to investigate the anti-HSV-2 activity of lactobacilli CS using plaque reduction assay. Lactobacilli CSs showed very high activity for inhibition of HSV virions replication. *L. crispatus* CS inhibited plaques formation by 50% in the very low concentration (4%) that reveals noteworthy anti-HSV activity of this strain. Other lactobacilli also showed moderate to strong anti-HSV activity. *L. gasseri*, *L. acidophilus*, *L. rhamnosus* and *L. casei* inhibited the HSV replication with IC_{50} value of 11,

Table 1 The antiviral activity of lactobacilli supernatant

Lactobacilli strain	Antiviral activity (%)			
	HIV-1 Inhibitory		HSV-2 Inhibitory	
	IC$_{50}$ (v/v)	CC$_{50}$ (v/v)	IC$_{50}$ (v/v)	CC$_{50}$ (v/v)
L. crispatus	48.5 ± 4.4	NT	4.2 ± 1.7	NT
L. acidophilus (Hansen co.)	46.3 ± 8.3	NT	>50	NT
L. paracasei subsp. Casei	≥50	NT	43.1 ± 3.6	NT
L. rhamnosus	≥50	NT	17.7 ± 6.3	NT
L. fermentum	31.7 ± 4.1	≥50	>50	≥50
L. casei (Hansen co.)	≥50	NT	19.3 ± 1.6	NT
L. gasseri	12.2 ± 3.5	47.4 ± 2.1	11.2 ± 3.3	≥50
L. acidophilus	≥50	NT	14.9 ± 5.2	NT

IC$_{50}$ is a concentration (v/v) which is able to inhibit 50% of virus multiplication; CC$_{50}$ is a concentration (v/v) which is 50% toxic for target cells; *NT*, Not toxic.

14, 17 and 19%. *L. crispatus* showed significant inhibitory activity for HSV but was not effective for inhibition of HIV replication. This finding emphasizes the anti-HSV active components of this strain inhibit HSV in a specific manner.

The cytotoxicity results showed that the CS from vaginal and non-vaginal lactobacilli had no toxicity for target cells. This indicates the safety of these strains and selective activity of their CS for reducing of viral replication rather than cellular proliferation.

Moderate anti-HIV and strong anti-HSV activity of the lactobacilli supernatants demonstrate that the lactobacilli CS encompass molecules with considerable specific activity for inhibition of viral replication. These data also revealed notably difference between the anti-viral activity of vaginal and non-vaginal strains (Table 1). The anti-viral activity of lactobacilli due to disinfectant activity of MRS culture supernatants was previously reported

[16,27]. Although in this study the neutral pH lactobacilli supernatant of lactobacilli in DMEM showed no cytotoxicity but significant anti-viral activity implying the presence of active compounds rather than disinfectant activity.

The anti-viral activity of co-cultured lactobacilli

The potential of lactobacilli for inhibition of HSV-2 and HIV-1 replication was studied by co-culturing the lactobacilli with cells. Lactobacilli were added into the cells environment considering physiological concentration in vaginal environment (100 CFU/cell) one hour before infection and removed by washing after viral adhesion to the cells. Antibiotics were added to the medium after infection to eradicate any growth of bacteria after viral entry. The cytotoxicity of lactobacilli was investigated in a parallel experiment. The vaginal lactobacilli strains (*L. gasseri*, *L. crispatus* and *L. rhamnosus*) showed higher

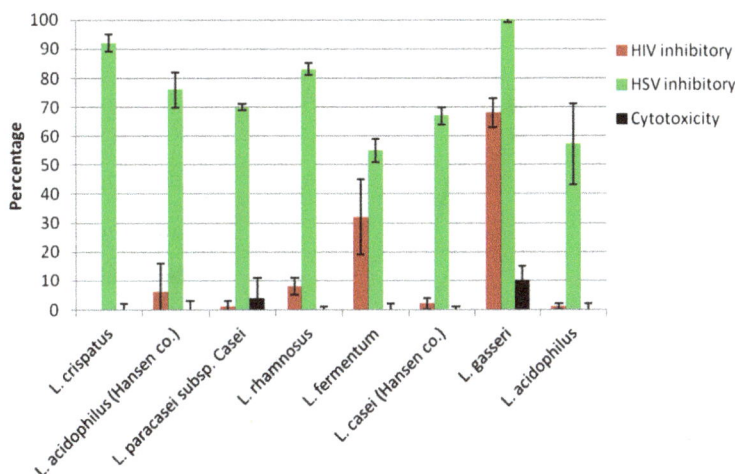

Figure 1 The anti-viral potential of lactobacilli co-culture against HSV-2 and HIV infection in co-cultures. Lactobacilli were added to the cells environment one hour before infection and removed by washing after viral adhesion to the cells. Cells were fed with antibiotic containing medium after infection.

Table 2 The virucidal effect of lactobacilli supernatant

Lactobacillus Strain	HIV virucidal effect (%)			HSV-2 virucidal effect (%)		
	2%v/v	20%v/v	50%v/v	2%v/v	20%v/v	50%v/v
L. crispatus	1.1 ± 0.5	8.5 ± 0.6	14.3 ± 3.3	15.6 ± 8.7	28.6 ± 3.9	76.4 ± 7.2
L. gasseri	4.3 ± 1.7	7.3 ± 1.5	15.4 ± 1.4	0.7 ± 0.2	6.3 ± 1.7	24.7 ± 3.2
L. rhamnosus	0.1 ± 0.02	2.1 ± 0.09	11.8 ± 0.01	4.2 ± 0.9	15.6 ± 2.1	38.3 ± 4.5

potential for inhibition of HSV virion (Figure 1). *L. gasseri* blocked almost all of HSV virions infection however *L. crispatus* and *L. rhamnosus* inhibited this virus by 93 and 84 percent, respectively. Approximately 68 and 31% of HIV inhibition was observed by *L. gasseri* and *L. fermentum* co-culture, whereas little inhibition was shown by other lactobacilli strains investigated in this study. Our results demonstrated that presence of vaginal lactobacilli significantly reduces viral entry to the target cells although the non-vaginal ones were apparently lesser potent. All of investigated vaginal strains were active for blocking HSV however only two strains (*L. gasseri* and *L. fermentum*) had anti-HIV activity.

Mode of anti-viral activity

Acording to the virucidal assay *L. crispatus* and *L. gasseri* inactivated 74 and 24%of HSV virions in 50% concentration, respectively (Table 2). The remarkable virucidal activity of lactobacilli CS is in consistent with the protective effect of lactobacilli against HSV and HIV virion in co-culture condition (Figure 1), suggesting that lactobacilli may secrete bacteriocins or other sort of molecules with viral neutralization activity. This mode of anti-viral activity is rather different from previously reported ones (due to H_2O_2 and H^+ secretion) [27] since

CS used in this study was in neutral pH and had no toxic effect for target cells.

The culture supernatants of *L. gasseri* and *L. crispatus* (20%) were added at different intervals (before, during, and after) of HSV infection. The results showed that *L. gasseri* and *L. crispatus* CS restrain HSV infection when added −6 and -2hs before virion inoculation by 75 and 83%, respectively (Figure 2). However, the inhibitory rate declined to 40 and 65% or less when *L. gasseri* and *L. crispatus* CSs and virions were simultaneously added. This data indicated that the lactobacilli supernatants affect the initial stage of HSV-2 infection. The lactobacilli products may inhibit HSV through disturbing the adhesion of virions to the cells or neutralizing the viral particles. This is a fairly new proposed mode of anti-viral activity for lactobacilli which is different from held belief that lactobacilli inactivate viral particles by lowering PH and disinfectant agent secretion [27].

The in vivo anti-HSV activity

The anti-HSV-1 activity of *L. crispatus* and *L. gasseri*, strains with highest potential *in vitro* experiments, was studied in BALB/c mice model. Alive *L. gasseri* cells showed significant activity for protecting mice against HSV-1 virions infection. As it can be seen in Figure 3, *L. gasseri* treated mice raised normal hairs while comparative

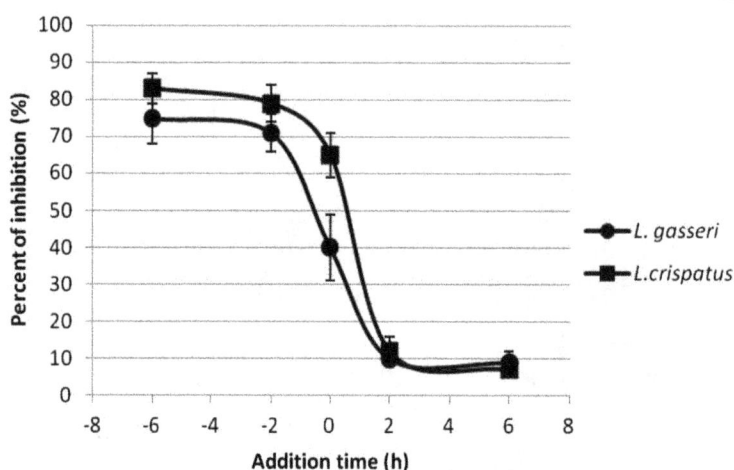

Figure 2 The inhibitory effect of *L. gasseri* and *L. crispatus* culture supernatants against different stages of HSV-2 infection. Culture supernatants (20%v/v) were added at different periods (before, during, and after) of HSV infection. The cells were washed twice by DMEM to eliminate lactobacilli supernatants prior to the inoculation of virions for pre-infection (−6, −2 and 0 h) groups.

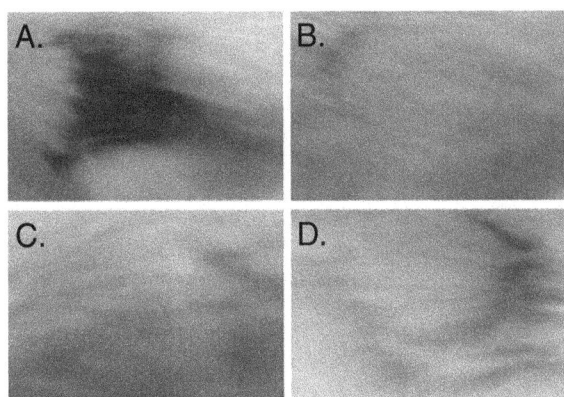

Figure 3 Skin lesions 6 weeks after cutaneous infection of HSV-1 in BALB/c mice. The shaved and scratch skin of right flank was infected with 10^4pfu of HSV-1 and the development of skin lesions was monitored after 6 weeks. The hair loss in the site of infection was clearly seen in infected mice (**A**) in comparison with ones treated with acyclovir cream (5%) (**B**). *L. gasseri* treated mice raised normal hairs (**C**) while comparative hair loss can be seen in *L. crispatus* (**D**).

hair loss can be seen in *L. crispatus* and control groups. The 6.5 and 8.8 g of weight loss was just observed in mice which received *L. crispatus* or no treatment, respectively (Table 3). To prove the inhibitory activity of *L. gasseri* against HSV infection the lymphocyte cells were extracted from mice spleen and evaluated for proliferation response to HSV antigens. Spleen cells from Acyclovir and *L. gasseri* treated mice showed no response to viral antigens with stimulation index (SI) values of 1.01 and 1.05 (Table 3). These data indicates that immune cells were not exposed to HSV antigens which unequivocally show inhibition of establishment of infection. The findings of this study lead to the conclusion that *L. gasseri* cells have comparable potential for inhibition of HSV infection *in vivo* condition to Acyclovir.

Conclusion

The results of the present study reveal the anti-HSV and HIV effect of lactobacilli by production of anti-viral molecules and other possible mechanisms. Infection was significantly reduced with no cytotoxicity if HSV and

Table 3 The *in vivo* anti-HSV activity of lactobacilli

Lactobacilli strain	Disease progress		Immune response	
	Weight loss (g)	Hairless area (cm²)	Lymphocyte proliferation (OD)	Stimulation index (SI)
L. crispatus	6.5 ± 0.4	1.7 ± 0.6	1.684 ± 0.43	1.9 ± 0.2
L. gasseri	0 ± 0.1	0.07 ± 0.2	0.876 ± 0.12	1.05 ± 0.3
Negative control	8.8 ± 0.3	4.1 ± 0.3	1.882 ± 0.62	2.1 ± 0.1
Acyclovir	0 ± 0.2	0.09 ± 0.01	0.793 ± 0.31	1.01 ± 0.2

HIV were cultured in the presence of living lactobacilli cells. The presence of lactobacilli cells was not necessary for inhibitory activity since virus replication is also inhibited in the presence of neutral pH supernatants. Vaginal lactobacilli strains were able to inhibit the first stages of HSV infection. The anti-viral activity of lactobacilli cells in the midst of herpes virus binding to the target cell was strain-dependent. *L. gasseri* showed inhibitory activity against HIV virions among investigated lactobacilli in this study. Numerous mechanisms may be involved in the inhibitory effect of lactobacilli against HSV and HIV such as: interfering with the early steps of virus infection, viral particle neutralizing and secretion of compounds with the ability of blocking the intracellular events of virus replication. The *in vivo* experiment confirmed the anti-viral activity of lactobacilli in mouse models. Potent lactobacilli could be promising probiotic candidates for protection against HSV and HIV or other viruses infections transmission.

Competing interest

The authors who have taken part in this study declare that they do not have anything to disclose regarding conflict of interest with respect to this manuscript.

Authors' contributions

RZ: Central contributions to conception, design and performing the experiments. Drafting and revising the manuscript. EM: Substantial contributions to conception, design and a part of experiments. SMS: Substantial contributions to conception, Analysis and interpretation of data and revising the article. ARA-S: Acquisition of data. SA-D: Acquisition of data. MHM: Corresponding author. Analysis and interpretation of data, revising the article. All authors read and approved the final manuscript.

Acknowledgement

This study was performed in Pasteur institute of Iran. This project was financially supported by Pasteur institute of Iran.

Author details

[1]Hepatitis and AIDS department, Pasteur institute of Iran, Tehran, Iran. [2]School of Medicine, Tehran University of Medical Sciences (TUMS), Tehran, Iran.

References

1. Martin HL, Richardson BA, Nyange PM, Lavreys L, Hillier SL, Chohan B, Mandaliya K, Ndinya-Achola JO, Bwayo J, Kreiss J: Vaginal lactobacilli, microbial flora, and risk of human immunodeficiency virus type 1 and sexually transmitted disease acquisition. *J Infect Dis* 1999, **180**:1863–1868.
2. Donders G: Diagnosis and management of bacterial vaginosis and other types of abnormal vaginal bacterial flora: a review. *Obstet Gynecol Surv* 2010, **65**:462–473.
3. Barrons R, Tassone D: Use of Lactobacillus probiotics for bacterial genitourinary infections in women: a review. *Clin Ther* 2008, **30**:453–468.
4. Brotman RM, Erbelding EJ, Jamshidi RM, Klebanoff MA, Zenilman JM, Ghanem KG: Findings associated with recurrence of bacterial vaginosis among adolescents attending sexually transmitted diseases clinics. *J Pediatr Adolesc Gynecol* 2007, **20**:225–231.
5. Cohen CR, Duerr A, Pruithithada N, Rugpao S, Hillier S, Garcia P, Nelson K: Bacterial vaginosis and HIV seroprevalence among female commercial sex workers in Chiang Mai, Thailand. *AIDS* 1995, **9**:1093–1097.
6. Sewankambo N, Gray RH, Wawer MJ, Paxton L, McNaim D, Wabwire-Mangen F, Serwadda D, Li C, Kiwanuka N, Hillier SL, Rabe L,

Gaydos CA, Quinn TC, Konde-Lule J: **HIV-1 infection associated with abnormal vaginal flora morphology and bacterial vaginosis.** *Lancet* 1997, **350**:546–550.

7. Atashili J, Poole C, Ndumbe PM, Adimora AA, Smith JS: **Bacterial vaginosis and HIV acquisition: a meta-analysis of published studies.** *AIDS* 2008, **22**:1493–1501.

8. Cherpes TL, Meyn LA, Krohn MA, Hillier SL: **Risk factors for infection with herpes simplex virus type 2: role of smoking, douching, uncircumcised males, and vaginal flora.** *Sex Transm Dis* 2003, **30**:405–410.

9. Watts DH, Fazzari M, Minkoff H, Hillier SL, Sha B, Glesby M, Levine AM, Burk R, Palefsky JM, Moxley M, Ahdieh-Grant L, Strickler HD: **Effects of bacterial vaginosis and other genital infections on the natural history of human papillomavirus infection in HIV-1-infected and high-risk HIV-1-uninfected women.** *J Infect Dis* 2005, **191**:1129–1139.

10. Nagot N, Ouedraogo A, Defer MC, Vallo R, Mayaud P, Van de Perre P: **Association between bacterial vaginosis and Herpes simplex virus type-2 infection: implications for HIV acquisition studies.** *Sex Transm Infect* 2007, **83**:365–368.

11. Cherpes TL, Melan MA, Kant JA, Cosentino LA, Meyn LA, Hillier SL: **Genital tract shedding of herpes simplex virus type 2 in women: effects of hormonal contraception, bacterial vaginosis, and vaginal group B Streptococcus colonization.** *Clin Infect Dis* 2005, **40**:1422–1428.

12. Ross SA, Novak Z, Ashrith G, Rivera LB, Britt WJ, Hedges S, Schwebke JR, Boppana AS: **Association between genital tract cytomegalovirus infection and bacterial vaginosis.** *J Infect Dis* 2005, **192**:1727–1730.

13. Zuckerman RA, Lucchetti A, Whittington WL, Sanchez J, Coombs RW, Zuniga R, Magaret AS, Wald A, Corey L, Celum C: **Herpes simplex virus (HSV) suppression with valacyclovir reduces rectal and blood plasma HIV-1 levels in HIV-1/HSV-2-seropositive men: a randomized, double-blind, placebo-controlled crossover trial.** *J Infect Dis* 2007, **196**:1500–1508.

14. Corey L, Wald A, Celum CL, Quinn TC: **The effects of herpes simplex virus-2 on HIV-1 acquisition and transmission: a review of two overlapping epidemics.** *J Acquir Immune Defic Syndr* 2004, **35**:435–445.

15. Sha BE, Zariffard MR, Wang QJ, Chen HY, Bremer J, Cohen MH, Spear GT: **Female genital-tract HIV load correlates inversely with Lactobacillus species but positively with bacterial vaginosis and Mycoplasma hominis.** *J Infect Dis* 2005, **191**:25–32.

16. Klebanoff SJ, Coombs RW: **Viricidal effect of Lactobacillus acidophilus on human immunodeficiency virus type 1: possible role in heterosexual transmission.** *J Exp Med* 1991, **174**:289–292.

17. Botic T, Klingberg TD, Weingartl H, Cencic A: **A novel eukaryotic cell culture model to study antiviral activity of potential probiotic bacteria.** *Int J Food Microbiol* 2007, **115**:227–234.

18. Reid G: **Probiotic Lactobacilli for urogenital health in women.** *J Clin Gastroenterol* 2008, **42**(Suppl 3 Pt 2):S234–S236.

19. Reid G, Dols J, Miller W: **Targeting the vaginal microbiota with probiotics as a means to counteract infections.** *Curr Opin Clin Nutr Metab Care* 2009, **12**:583–587.

20. McGroarty JA: **Probiotic use of lactobacilli in the human female urogenital tract.** *FEMS Immunol Med Microbiol* 1993, **6**:251–264.

21. Martin MC, Pant N, Ladero V, Gunaydin G: *Krogh Andersen K, Alvarez B, Martinez N, Alvarez MA, Hammarstrom L.* Appl Environ Microbiol: Marcotte H. Integrative expression system for delivery of antibody fragments by lactobacilli; 2011.

22. Zabihollahi R, Vahabpour R, Hartoonian C, Sedaghati B, Sadat SM, Soleymani M, Ranjbar M, Fassihi A, Aghasadeghi MR, Memarian HR, Salehi M: **Evaluation of the in vitro antiretroviral potential of some Biginelli-type pyrimidines.** *Acta Virol* 2012, **56**:11–18.

23. Rezaei A, Zabihollahi R, Salehi M, Moghim S, Tamizifar H, Yazdanpanahi N, Amini G: **Designing a non-virulent HIV-1 strain: potential implications for vaccine and experimental research.** *Journal of research in medical sciences* 2007, **12**:227–234.

24. Zabihollahi R, Sadat SM, Vahabpour R, Aghasadeghi MR, Memarnejadian A, Ghazanfari T, Salehi M, Rezaei A, Azadmanesh K: **Development of single-cycle replicable human immunodeficiency virus 1 mutants.** *Acta virologica* 2011, **55**:15–22.

25. Sadat SM, Zabihollahi R, Vahabpour R, Azadmanesh K, Javadi F, Siadat SD, Memarnejadian A, Parivar K, Khanahmad Shahreza H, Arabi Mianroodi R, Hekmat S, Aghasadeghi MR: *Designing and biological evaluation of single-cycle replicable HIV-1 system as a potential vaccine strategy. 20th*

European Congress of Clinical Microbiology and Infectious Diseases. Austria: Clinical Microbiology and Infection; 2010:S334.

26. Yang CM, Cheng HY, Lin TC, Chiang LC, Lin CC: **Acetone, ethanol and methanol extracts of Phyllanthus urinaria inhibit HSV-2 infection in vitro.** *Antiviral Res* 2005, **67**:24–30.

27. Conti C, Malacrino C, Mastromarino P: **Inhibition of herpes simplex virus type 2 by vaginal lactobacilli.** *J Physiol Pharmacol* 2009, **60**(Suppl 6):19–26.

9

Genistein abrogates G2 arrest induced by curcumin in p53 deficient T47D cells

Puji Astuti[1*], Esti D Utami[2], Arsa W Nugrahani[3] and Sismindari Sudjadi[4]

Abstract

Background: The high cost and low level of cancer survival urge the finding of new drugs having better mechanisms. There is a high trend of patients to be "back to nature" and use natural products as an alternative way to cure cancer. The fact is that some of available anticancer drugs are originated from plants, such as taxane, vincristine, vinblastine, pacitaxel. Curcumin (diferuloylmethane), a dietary pigment present in *Curcuma longa* rizhome is reported to induce cell cycle arrest in some cell lines. Other study reported that genistein isolated from *Glycine max* seed inhibited phosphorylation of cdk1, gene involved during G2/M transition and thus could function as G2 checkpoint abrogator. The inhibition of cdk1 phosphorylation is one of alternative strategy which could selectively kill cancer cells and potentially be combined with DNA damaging agent such as curcumin.

Methods: T47D cell line was treated with different concentrations of curcumin and genistein, alone or in combination; added together or with interval time. Flow Cytometry and MTT assay were used to evaluate cell cycle distribution and viability, respectively. The presence of apoptotic cells was determined using acridine orange-ethidium bromide staining.

Results: In this study curcumin induced G2 arrest on p53 deficient T47D cells at the concentration of 10 μM. Increasing concentration up to 30 μM increased the number of cell death. Whilst genistein alone at low concentration (≤10 μM) induced cell proliferation, addition of genistein (20 μM) 16 h after curcumin resulted in more cell death (89%), 34% higher than that administered at the same time (56%). The combination treatment resulted in apoptotic cell death. Combining curcumin with high dose of genistein (50 μM) induced necrotic cells.

Conclusions: Genistein increased the death of curcumin treated T47D cells. Appropriate timing of administration and concentration of genistein determine the outcome of treatment and this method could potentially be developed as an alternative strategy for treatment of p53 defective cancer cells.

Keywords: Cell cycle, p53, Curcumin, Genistein, G2 arrest

Background

Most of chemotherapeutic drugs such as etoposide, cisplastin, doxorubicin and camptotechin induce DNA damage on cancer cells. These DNA (deoxy nucleid acid) damaging agents arrest or delay cell cycle progression, allowing time for DNA repair. This mechanism of repair functions to ensure that division only occur on cells carrying complete DNA, not mutated or damage. If the damage is beyond repair, the cells may permanently enter cellular senescence or undergo apoptosis [1,2]. The mechanism of cell cycle arrest is mediated by ATM (ataxia telangiectasia-mutated protein kinase) or ATR (ATM and Rad3-related protein kinase) through the activation of Ser/Thr kinases checkpoint kinase 1 (Chk1) and checkpoint kinase 2 (Chk2). The activation of Chk1 and Chk2 in turn modulates phosphorylation events such as phosphorylation of cdc25 phosphatases which normally activate cdk1 in G2/M boundary and result in cell cycle arrest at the G2/M or S phase [3]. Based on oncologic point of view, this mechanism of repair is beneficial to normal cells in that they have mechanism to reduce toxic effect of the chemotherapeutic agents. However, this system of protection limits the efficacy of chemotherapy on cancer cells.

* Correspondence: p.astuti@gmail.com
[1]Pharmaceutical Biology Department, Faculty of Pharmacy, Universitas Gadjah Mada, Yogyakarta, Indonesia
Full list of author information is available at the end of the article

In responds to DNA damaging agents, cell cycle arrest on G1 phase depends on tumor suppressor protein p53. Normal cells carrying wild type p53 are able to arrest at G1, S and G2 phase, whilst cells having defect on p53 gene, which occur on >50% of tumor, would progress through S phase and arrest at G2 phase [4-6]. Any agents which capable of abrogating cell cycle arrest at G2 phase would induce premature entry into mitosis, with cells still carry damaged DNA and resulting in apoptosis. Inducing mitotic catastrophe in G2 arrested cell can be used as a strategy to selectively kill tumor cell lacking functional p53, and at the same time provide opportunities for normal cells to survive.

Although conventional chemotherapy using DNA damaging agents resulting in tumor cell death, the deleterious side effects are well known. Furthermore, the high cost of treatment urges the finding of selective agents with more affordable price. Currently, there is trend of patients to use natural medicine as an alternative therapy against cancer. The fact that some of available anticancer drugs such as taxan, vincristine, vinblastine and pacitaxel are medicinal plant origin, provide great opportunities to effectively use natural compounds to treat cancer. A lot of studies have been conducted to examine the potential of natural compounds against cancer with one of example is curcumin.

Curcumin (diferuloylmethane) is dietary pigment and presence as major compound in *Curcuma longa rizhome*. This compound has a potential to be developed as anticancer agent and was in phase II clinical trials [7,8]. Curcumin was reported to be cytotoxic and inactive in normal and primary cells. In mouse embryonic fibroblast line C3H/10 T1/2, rat embryonic fibroblasts, and human foreskin fibroblast, curcumin did not induce cell death, whereas in cancer cells it stimulated cell death through mechanism of apoptosis [8-12]. Curcumin also induced cell cycle arrest in colorectal tumor line HCT116, medulloblastoma and human acute promyelocytic leukemia HL-60 [12-14]. The ability to induce cell death increased with addition of piperine, the major compound of *Piper nigrum* L) which reportedly increase the bioavailability of curcumin [14-17].

The activity of curcumin as anticancer agent can be increased by combination with compounds having effect as G2 checkpoint abrogator. Flavonoid is natural polyphenolic compounds potential to be developed as anticancer agents [18,19]. Isoflavonoid genistein was found to be active in pancreatic cells by modulating cell cycle and inhibition of angiogenesis [20,21]. Following administration of irinotecan, this compound inhibited phosphorylation of cdk1 mediated by wee1 kinase, a negative regulator of cdk1 kinase activity [22]. Inhibition of cdk1 phosphorylation could be a potential strategy to abrogate G2 checkpoint activation [23].

Methods
Materials
Genistein was obtained from Sigma, curcumin was kindly given by Dr. Hilda Ismail, 86% purity by HPLC (High Pressure Liquid Chromatography). They were dissolved in ethanol absolute, divided into aliquots, and stored frozen at $-20°C$.

Cell lines and culture conditions
T47D (Human ductal breast epithelial tumor cell line) was cultured in RPMI 1640 media supplemented with 10% Fetal Bovine Serum (Gibco) 2% Penicillin - Streptomycin (Gibco), dan 0.5% Fungizon (Gibco), 2% Sodium bicarbonate (Gibco) and HEPES (4-(2-hydroxyethyl)-1-piperazineethanesulfonic acid) (Invitrogen). Cell lines were maintained at 37°C in a humidified incubator containing 5% CO_2.

Cell cycle analysis
Treated cells were harvested using trypsine and washed three times with 1×PBS. Cell pellets were resuspended with 500 μl staining solution (40 μg/ml propidium iodide (Sigma) and 500μg/ml RNase A (Sigma), covered with aluminium foil and incubated at 37°C for 30 minutes. Cells were analysed using FACS (Fluorescence Activated Cell Sorting) Calibur (BD).

Viability assay
A hundred μl of media containing $5x10^3$ cells was added to 96-well plate and incubated for 48 hours until 70% – 80% confluent. Curcumin was added alone or in combination with genistein, added together or in interval time. Cells were incubated at 37°C in CO_2 incubator. Following the treatment, cells were gently washed with 1X PBS (Phosphate Buffer Saline), and 100 μl of MTT (3-(4,5-Dimethylthiazol-2-yl)-2,5-diphenyltetrazolium bromide) 0.5 mg/ml was added to the well. The cells were incubated for 4 hours at 37°C and the reaction was stopped by adding 100 μl SDS (sodium dodecyl sulfate) 10%. The plates were incubated overnight and read in microplate reader (Bio-Rad) at 595 nm.

Apoptotic assay
T47D cells were plated onto 6 well plate containing coverslip and treated with curcumin, genistein or in combination as indicated. Following the treatment, the cells on coverslip were treated with ethidium bromide-acridine orange and the cells were analysed under fluorescence microscope (Carl Zeiss).

Results
Curcumin induced G2 arrest in T47D cells
To study the mechanism of action of curcumin in vitro, we have tested the effect of increasing concentration of

Table 1 Cell cycle distribution of T47D cells after treatment of different concentration of curcumin overnight

Treatment	Sub G1 (%)	G1 (%)	S (%)	G2 (%)
Control	2.32	37.23	27.88	25.34
10 µM curcumin	1.26	22.74	19.30	44.13
20 µM curcumin	12.78	22.13	13.79	37.43
30 µM curcumin	14.28	28.38	11.39	39.57

curcumin in inducing G2 arrest in T47D cells. The cells were treated at different concentration of curcumin and incubated overnight. As shown in Table 1 and Figure 1, curcumin at 10 µM induced G2 arrest in T47D cells. The cells showed a strong block in the G2/M phase of the cell cycle (reaching 44% compared with 25% in the untreated controls). Increasing the concentration up to 30 µM did not significantly increase G2/M population. Instead, it appeared a marked sub-G1 peak (from 2% in control cells to 12% at 20 µM and 14% at 30 µM of treated cells), because of the presence of dead cells. Adding curcumin at low as 5 µM did not induce cell cycle arrest (data not shown). These data demonstrate that curcumin at 10 µM arrest T47D cells at G2/M with little cytotoxicity.

Genistein abrogated G2 arrest induced by curcumin

In an attempt to discover natural compounds that disrupt G2 checkpoint in cancer cells, we used genistein, an inhibitor of cdk1 phosphorylation [22]. We examine the ability of different concentration of genistein in modulating G2 arrest induced by curcumin. Firstly, we

activated the G2 checkpoint by adding curcumin at the concentration of 10 µM overnight. Sixteen hours after DNA damage, the cells were treated with different concentration of genistein for another 24 hours. The cells were harvested and the cell cycle distribution was analysed. Indeed, as shown in Table 2 and Figure 2, genistein at concentration of 20 µM abrogated the G2/M block induced by curcumin, decreasing G2/M population from 28% in curcumin only treated cells to 6% in combination with 20 µM genistein. Increasing concentration of genistein up to 50 µM did not significantly reduce the shift of G2/M population. The G2/M population only decreased to 10% in combination with 50 µM genistein. Combination of curcumin with genistein increased the subG1 population which represents dead cells, from 2% to 44% (20 µM genistein) and 47% (50 µM genistein).

Addition of genistein following G2 arrest induced by curcumin resulted in more cell death

To check the effect of combination of genistein with curcumin on cell viability, we treated the cells with curcumin, genistein and in combination with various interval times by means of MTT assay. The experiments were performed in three replicates. Previously we found that curcumin at concentration of 10 µM induced G2/M arrest with little toxicity. In this experiment we confirmed the finding that treatment curcumin at given concentration retained the viability of cells of 83.66%. An attempt to increase the sensitivity of this compound in inducing cell death is conducted by addition of genistein. Table 3 shows that genistein alone at low concentration of 5 and

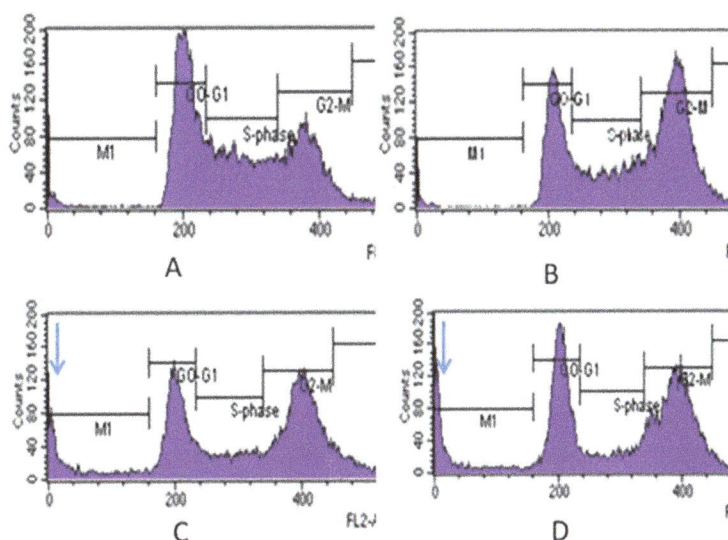

Figure 1 Cell cycle analysis of T47D cell using flowcytometry after treatment with different concentration of curcumin. T47D cells were plated onto 6 well plate and treated overnight with (**A**) control untreated cells, (**B**) 10 µM curcumin, (**C**), 20 µM curcumin and (**D**) 30 µM curcumin. Arrow indicated the presence of sub G1 population.

Table 2 Cell cycle distribution of T47D cells after treatment of 10 μM curcumin overnight followed by 20 μM genistein or 50 μM genistein

Treatment	Sub G1 (%)	G1 (%)	S (%)	G2 (%)
Control	8.51	48.85	11.13	18.52
10 μM curcumin	2.71	31.12	18.86	28.22
10 μM curcumin + 20 μM genistein	44.25	39.66	5.72	6.44
10 μM curcumin + 50 μM genistein	47.47	29.17	6.76	10.14

10 μM induced cell proliferation as compared to control, reaching 191.80% and 171.22% respectively. Increasing concentration to 20 μM maintained the viability of 90.41%, whereas high concentration of 50 μM induced 61.28% cell death. In this study we found that genistein (20 μM) which was added 16 hours after 10 μM curcumin resulted in more cell death, from 83.66% viability in curcumin only treated cells to only 10.88% in combination. Adding higher concentration of genistein (50 μM) only slightly increased the percentage of cell death (8.48%). Interestingly, in this study we found that adding genistein following DNA damage induced by curcumin produced more cell death (89.12%) compared to adding at the same time (56.51%). The effect of inducing cell death by combination of curcumin and genistein were confirmed by observing the morphology of the cells after treatment with curcumin or in combination with genistein using ethidium bromide and acridine – orange double staining under fluoresence microscope. The presence of apoptotic cells were shown as orange to red population as compared to healthy green cell population [24]. As shown in Figure 3, only few dead cells were observed in curcumin only treated cells. However, combining curcumin with genistein resulted in high accumulation of apoptotic cells. Combination with high concentration of genistein induced the presence of necrotic cells, as appear as a form of debris (Figure 3).

Discussion

Conventional chemotherapeutics have been widely applied in treatment against various type of cancer. The effectiveness of these therapies depends on their ability to kill proliferating cancer cells by damaging their DNA and inducing apoptosis. The cell responds to DNA damage to induce cell cycle arrest at any stage, ensuring the damage is repaired prior to enter subsequent phase of cell cycle [25]. This mechanism of control is function to maintain genetic integrity, with the failure of repair resulted in mutations and eventually cell death. However, these agents convey some drawbacks in which they developed resistance to DNA damage-induced cell killing and they are also toxic to actively proliferating normal cells.

One of the characteristics of tumor growth is uncontrolled cell proliferation as a result of loss in normal cell cycle control. Currently there is an increasing of interest to target cell cycle in effort to find targeted anticancer therapies [26-29]. In fact >50% of human cancer have

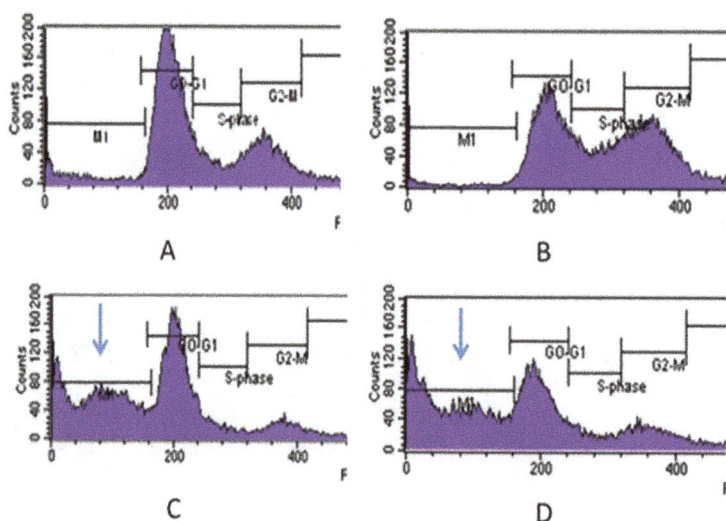

Figure 2 Cell cycle analysis of T47D cell using flowcytometry after treatment with curcumin and genistein. T47D cells were plated onto 6 well plate and treated with (**A**) control untreated cells, (**B**) 10 μM curcumin, (**C**), 10 μM curcumin overnight followed by 20 μM genistein and (**D**) 10 μM curcumin overnight followed by 50 μM genistein. Arrow indicated the presence of subG1 population.

Table 3 Persentage of cell viability following the administration of curcumin, genistein and combination (n =3)

No	Treatment	% viability ± SE
1	Curcumin 10 µM	83.66 ± 8.24
2	Genistein 5 µM	191.80 ± 8.94
3	Genistein 10 µM	171.22 ± 6.63
4	Genistein 20 µM	90.41 ± 2.13
5	Genistein 50 µM	38.72 ±3.99
6	Curcumin 10 µM + Genistein 20 µM*	10.88 ± 1.85
7	Curcumin 10 µM + Genistein 50 µM*	2.40 ± 0.59
8	Curcumin 10 µM + Genistein 20 µM**	43.49 ± 4.90
9	Curcumin 10 µM + Genistein 50 µM**	15.83 ± 0.88

** Curcumin and genistein were added at the same time. * Genistein was added 16 hours after the addition of curcumin. These data represent minimal two independent experiments.

loss in the tumor suppressor gene p53. This gene is an essential component for apoptosis induction in response to DNA damage and also a component of cell cycle checkpoint. The loss of p53 resulted in cell reliance on G2 phase checkpoint in response to DNA damage inducing agent which easily can be bypassed by adding G2 phase checkpoint inhibitors to induce aberrant mitosis and eventually increased cell death [30,31].

In Indonesia, there is a high trend of using herbal medicine in promoting health with some of the herbal materials commonly used are curcuma rizhome (*Curcuma longa* L) and soy bean (*Glycin max*) which contain bioactive compound of curcumin and genistein, respectively. The bioactivities of these natural products have been widely reported [13,15,21,32]. In this study we tested the combined effects of genistein with curcumin in inhibiting the growth of cancer cells. As was seen in T47D cells, curcumin induces G2 phase arrest, similar as reported by others [12,13] and genistein abrogated the G2 checkpoint controls induced by curcumin. The combination of the two agents reduced cell viability up to seven fold, in comparison of adding the agent alone. Since many of cancers have

defective of checkpoint control due to the loss of p53 gene, further deregulation of this mechanism of control can result in increased apoptotic cell death.

In this study we demonstrated the success of applying strategies to deliver a more cancer-specific cytotoxic treatment by synthetic lethality targeting p53 defective cancer cells. These synthetic lethality strategies are currently being used to search new drugs or targets within specific tumor types such as inhibition of Chk1 in p53 mutant cancers to achieve better outcomes [33,34]. Using this strategy, reduced side effects and better outcomes could be achieved since doses of chemotherapeutic agents can be reduced at least twofold [35-37]. In this study we showed the selectivity of synthetic lethality strategy by targeting the loss of function of p53 and application of DNA damage inducing agent. In T47D, p53 deficient cells, survival of the cells following DNA damage are dependent on activation of the Chk1 pathway to induce G2 cell cycle arrest and DNA repair. Disruption of this Chk1-dependent pathway by genistein can selectively sensitize cells to exit G2 phase before the damage are repaired and eventually the cells undergo apoptosis. In this study we demonstrated that adding combination of curcumin followed by genistein on T47D cells showed greater cell death, indicating the importance of appropriate timing of administration in inducing cell death. Similar study was reported by Tse et al. [38], when combining topoisomerase I posion and checkpoint inhibitor 7-hydroxystaurosporine in human colon cancer. Sequential treatment of SN-38 followed by UC-01, a Chk1 inhibitor, resulted in enhanced apoptosis in p53 mutant cells, and this was proven to be effective in p53 mutant but to lesser degree in p53 intact cells.

Collectively, these studies provide a new insight in using naturally derived agents to treat cancer with selective methods to achieve better outcomes. This approach is based on understanding that in the synthetic lethal strategy targeting p53 defective cells, the loss of stress response mechanism can reduce cell viability. This

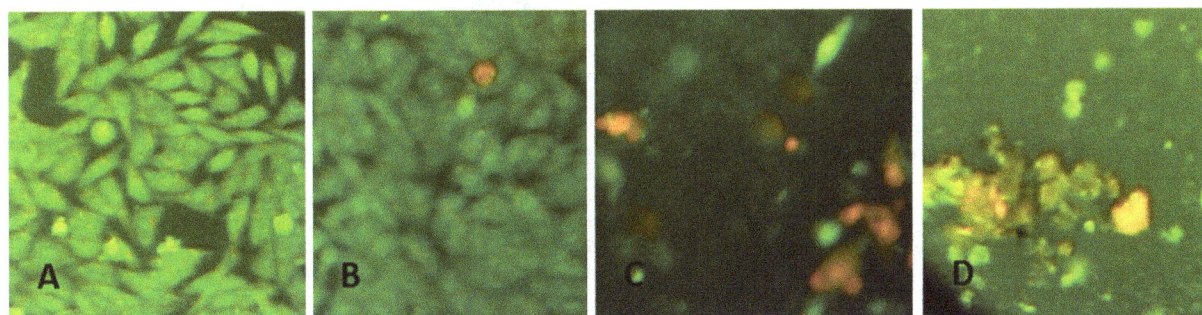

Figure 3 Morphology of cells treated with curcumin, genistein or in combination. T47D cells were plated onto 6 well plate and treated with (**A**) control cells, (**B**) 10 µM curcumine only, (**C**) curcumin (10 µM) was added overnight followed by treatment with genistein (20 µM), (**D**) curcumin (10 µM) was added overnight followed by treatment with genistein (50 µM).

response of mechanisms, when combined with the loss of compensatory systems can generate complete loss of cell viability [33,39].

Conclusions

In this study we demonstrated that genistein increased the death of curcumin treated T47D cells. We showed that the inhibition of checkpoint pathway is generated by genistein and the selectivity is achieved by the loss of p53 function in T47D cells and application of curcumin. Since the main active compounds used in this study are natural product origin, it is expected that this study could support the rational of using traditional medicines for maintaining health. Appropriate use of these natural products could help cancer patients in using alternative therapies with scientific evidence based medicines.

Competing interest
The authors declare that there is no conflict of interest related to this publication.

Authors' contributions
PA contributes to the concept, design, data acquisition, analysis and interpretation; preparation of the manuscript and approval of final article. EDU contributes to data acquisition and analysis, preparation of the manuscript and approval of final article. Part of the data was collected for her master thesis. AWN participated in data acquisition and analysis and helped to draft the manuscript. SS participated in the design and coordination, preparation of the manuscript. All authors read and approved the final manuscript.

Acknowledgements
This work was performed with Hibah Berkualitas Prima Faculty of Pharmacy UGM 2011. We are grateful to Dr. Hilda Ismail for the donation of curcumin used in these experiments.

Author details
[1]Pharmaceutical Biology Department, Faculty of Pharmacy, Universitas Gadjah Mada, Yogyakarta, Indonesia. [2]Pharmacy Department, Faculty of Medicinal and Health Sciences, Universitas Jenderal Soedirman, Purwokerto, Indonesia. [3]Sekolah Tinggi Ilmu Farmasi (STIFAR), Pharmacy Foundation, Semarang, Indonesia. [4]Pharmaceutical Chemistry Department, Faculty of Pharmacy, Universitas Gadjah Mada, Yogyakarta, Indonesia.

References
1. Kastan BM, Bartek J: Cell-cycle checkpoints and cancer. Nature 2004, 432:316–323.
2. Eastman A: Cell cycle checkpoints and their impact on anticancer therapeutic strategies. J Cell Biochem 2004, 91:223–231.
3. Lukas J, Lukas C, Bartek J: Mammalian cell cycle checkpoints: signaling pathways and their organization in space and time. DNA Repair (Amst) 2004, 3:997–1007.
4. Levine AJ: p53, the cellular gatekeeper for growth and division. Cell 1997, 88:323–331.
5. Wang Y, Li J, Booher RN, Kraker A, Lawrence T, Leopold WR, Sun Y: Radiosensitization of p53 Mutant Cells by PD0166285, a Novel G2 Checkpoint Abrogator. Cancer Res 2001, 61:8211–8217.
6. Eastman A, Kohn EA, Brown MK, Rathman J, Livingstone M, Blank DH, Gribble DW: A Novel Indolocarbazole, ICP-1, Abrogates DNA Damage induced Cell Cycle Arrest and Enhances Cytotoxicity: Similarities and Differences to the Cell Cycle Checkpoint Abrogator UCN-011. Mol Cancer Ther 2002, 1:1067–1078.
7. Sharma RA, Gescher AJ, Steward WP: Curcumin: the story so far. Eur J Cancer 2005, 41:1955–1968.
8. Chauhan DP: Chemotherapeutic potential of curcumin for colorectal cancer. Curr Pharm 2002, 8:1695–1706.
9. Jiang MC, Yang-Yen HF, Yen JJ, Lin JK: Curcumin induces apoptosis in immortalized NIH 3 T3 and malignant cancer cell lines. Nutr Cancer 1996, 26:111–120.
10. Karunagaran D, Rashmi R, Kumar TR: Induction of apoptosis by curcumin and its implications for cancer therapy. Curr Cancer Drug Targets 2005, 5:117–129.
11. Song G, Mao YB, Cai QF, Yao LM, Ouyang GL, Bao SD: Curcumin induces human HT-29 colon adenocarcinoma cell apoptosis by activating p53 and regulating apoptosis-related protein expression. Braz J Med Biol Res 2005, 38:1791–1798.
12. Tan TW, Tsai HR, Lu HF, Lin HL, Tsou MF, Lin YT, Tsai HY, Chen YF, Chung JG: Curcumin-induced cell cycle arrest and apoptosis in human acute promyelocytic leukemia HL-60 cells via MMP changes and caspase-3 activation. Anticancer Res 2006, 26(6B):4361–4371.
13. Jiang Z, Jin S, Yalowich JC, Brown KD, Rajasekaran B: The Mismatch Repair System Modulates Curcumin Sensitivity through Induction of DNA Strand Breaks and Activation of G2-M Checkpoint. Mol Cancer Ther 2010, 9(3):558–568.
14. Elamin MH, Shinwari Z, Hendrayani SF, Al-Hindi H, Al-Shail E, Khafaga Y, Al-Kofide A, Aboussekhra A: Curcumin inhibits the Sonic Hedgehog signaling pathway and triggers apoptosis in medulloblastoma cells. Mol Carcinog 2010, 49(3):302–314.
15. Anand P, Kunnumakkara AB, Newman RA, Aggarwal BB: Bioavailability of Curcumin: Problems and Promises. Mol Pharm 2007, 4(6):807–818.
16. Anand P, Thomas SG, Kunnumakkara AB, Sundaram C, Harikumar KB, Sung B, Tharakan ST, Misra K, Priyadarsini IK, Rajasekharan KN, Aggarwal BB: Biological activities of curcumin and its analogues (Congeners) made by man and Mother Nature. Biochem Pharmacol 2008, 76(11):1590–1611.
17. Kakarala M, Brenner DE, Korkaya H, Cheng C, Tazi K, Ginestier C, Liu S, Dontu G, Wicha MS: Targeting breast stem cells with the cancer preventive compounds curcumin and piperine. Breast Cancer Res Treat 2010, 122(3):777–785.
18. Li W, Fan J, Bertino JR: Selective sensitization of retinoblastoma protein-deficient sarcoma cells to doxorubicin by flavopiridol-mediated inhibition of cyclin-dependent kinase 2 kinase activity. Cancer Res 2001, 61(6):2579–2582.
19. Li Y, Ahmed F, Ali S, Philip PA, Kucuk O, Sarkar FH: Inactivation of nuclear factor kappaB by soy isoflavone genistein contributes to increased apoptosis induced by chemotherapeutic agents in human cancer cells. Cancer Res 2005, 65(15):6934–6942.
20. Buchler P, Reber HA, Buchler MW, Friess H, Lavey RS, Hines OJ: Antiangiogenic activity of genistein in pancreatic carcinoma cells is mediated by the inhibition of hypoxia-inducible factor-1 and the down-regulation of VEGF gene expression. Cancer 2004, 100(1):201–210.
21. Banerjee S, Zhang Y, Ali S, Bhuiyan M, Wang Z, Chiao PJ, Philip PA, Abbruzzese J, Sarkar FH: Molecular evidence for increased antitumor activity of gemcitabine by genistein in vitro and in vivo using an orthotopic model of pancreatic cancer. Cancer Res 2005, 65(19):9064–9072.
22. Papazisis KT, Kalemi TG, Zambouli D, Geromichalos GD, Lambropoulos AF, Kotsis A, Boutis LL, Kortsaris AH: Synergistic effects of protein tyrosine kinase inhibitor genistein with camptothecins against three cell lines in vitro. Cancer Lett 2006, 233(2):255–264.
23. Leijen S, Beijnen JH, Schellens JH: Abrogation of the G2 checkpoint by inhibition of Wee-1 kinase results in sensitization of p53-deficient tumor cells to DNA-damaging agents. Curr Clin Pharmacol 2010, 5(3):186–191.
24. Baskić D, Popović S, Ristić P, Arsenijević NN: Analysis of cycloheximide-induced apoptosis in human leukocytes: fluorescence microscopy using annexin V/propidium iodide versus acridin orange/ethidium bromide. Cell Biol Int 2006, 30(11):924–932.
25. Medema RH, Macůrek L: Checkpoint control and cancer. Oncogene 2012, 31(21):2601–2613.
26. Hanahan D, Weinberg RA: Hallmarks of cancer: the next generation. Cell 2011, 144:646–674.
27. Zhang C, Yan Z, Painter CL, Zhang Q, Chen E, Arango ME, Kuszpit K, Zasadny K, Hallin M, Hallin J, Wong A, Buckman D, Sun G, Qiu M, Anderes K, Christensen JG: PF-00477736 mediates checkpoint kinase 1 signaling

pathway and potentiates docetaxel-induced efficacy in xenografts. *Clin Cancer Res* 2009, **15**:4630–4640.

28. Hagimori K, Fukuda T, Hasegawa Y, Omura S, Tomoda H: **Fungal malformins inhibit bleomycin-induced G2 checkpoint in Jurkat cells.** *Biol Pharm Bull* 2007, **30**(8):1379–1383.

29. Warrener R, Beamish H, Burgess A, Waterhouse NJ, Giles N, Fairlie D, Gabrielli B: **Tumor cell-selective cytotoxicity by targeting cell cycle checkpoints.** *FASEB J* 2003, **17**:1550–1552.

30. Mukhopadhyay UK, Senderowicz AM, Ferbeyre G: **RNA silencing of checkpoint regulators sensitizes p53-defective prostate cancer cells to chemotherapy while sparing normal cells.** *Cancer Res* 2005, **65**:2872–2881.

31. Ma CX, Janetka JW, Piwnica- Worms H: **Death by releasing the breaks: CHK1 inhibitors as cancer therapeutics.** *Trends Mol Med* 2011, **17**:88–96.

32. Wu AH, Ziegler RG, Nomura AM, West DW, Kolonel LN, Horn-Ross PL, Hoover RN, Pike MC: **Soy intake and risk of breast cancer in Asians and Asian Americans.** *Am J Clin Nutr* 1998, **68**(Suppl 6):1437S–1443S.

33. Gabrielli B, Brooks K, Pavey S: **Defective cell cycle checkpoints as targets for anti-cancer therapies.** *Front Pharmacol* 2012, **3**(9):1–6.

34. Kuiken HJ, Beijersbergen RL: **Exploration of synthetic lethal interactions as cancer drug targets.** *Future Oncol* 2010, **6**:1789–1802.

35. Blasina A, Hallin J, Chen E, Arango ME, Kraynov E, Register J, Grant S, Ninkovic S, Chen P, Nichols T, O'Connor P, Anderes K: **Breaching the DNA damage checkpoint via PF-00477736, a novel small-molecule inhibitor of checkpoint kinase1.** *Mol Cancer Ther* 2008, **7**:2394–2404.

36. Tse AN, Rendahl KG, Sheikh T, Cheema H, Aardalen K, Embry M, Ma S, Moler EJ, Ni ZJ, Lopes De Menezes DE, Hibner B, Gesner TG, Schwartz GK: **CHIR-124, a novel potent inhibitor of Chk1, potentiates the cytotoxicity of topoisomerase I poisons invitro and invivo.** *Clin Cancer Res* 2007, **13**:591–602.

37. Zabludoff SD, Deng C, Grondine MR, Sheehy AM, Ashwell S, Caleb BL, Green S, Haye HR, Horn CL, Janetka JW, Liu D, Mouchet E, Ready S, Rosenthal JL, Queva C, Schwartz GK, Taylor KJ, Tse AN, Walker GE, White AM: **AZD7762, a novel checkpoint kinase inhibitor, drives checkpoint abrogation and potentiates DNA-targeted therapies.** *Mol Cancer Ther* 2008, **7**:2955–2966.

38. Tse A, Schwartz G: **Potentiation of cytotoxicity of topoisomerase I poison in human colon carcinoma cells by concurrent and sequential treatment with the checkpoint inhibitor 7-hydroxystaurosporine involves disparate mechanisms resulting in different pharmacological endpoints.** *Cancer Res* 2004, **64**:6635–6644.

39. Kaelin WG Jr: **The concept of synthetic lethality in the context of anticancer therapy.** *Nat Rev Cancer* 2005, **5**:689–698.

10

In vitro α-glucosidase inhibitory activity of phenolic constituents from aerial parts of *Polygonum hyrcanicum*

Fahimeh Moradi-Afrapoli[1,2], Behavar Asghari[3], Soodabeh Saeidnia[4], Yusef Ajani[5], Mobina Mirjani[1], Maryam Malmir[4], Reza Dolatabadi Bazaz[6], Abbas Hadjiakhoondi[1,4], Peyman Salehi[3], Mattias Hamburger[7] and Narguess Yassa[1,4*]

Abstract

Background and the purpose of the study: The early stage of diabetes mellitus type 2 is associated with postprandial hyperglycemia. Hyperglycemia is believed to increase the production of free radicals and reactive oxygen species, leading to oxidative tissue damage. In an effort of identifying herbal drugs which may become useful in the prevention or mitigation of diabetes, biochemical activities of *Polygonum hyrcanicum* and its constituents were studied.

Methods: Hexane, ethylacetate and methanol extracts of *P. hyrcanicum* were tested for α-glucosidase inhibitory, antioxidant and radical scavenging properties. Active constituents were isolated and identified from the methanolic extract in an activity guided approach.

Results: A methanolic extract from flowering aerial parts of the plant showed notable α-glucosidase inhibitory activity ($IC_{50} = 15$ μg/ml). Thirteen phenolic compounds involving a cinnamoylphenethyl amide, two flavans, and ten flavonols and flavonol 3-O-glycosides were subsequently isolated from the extract. All constituents showed inhibitory activities while compounds 3, 8 and 11 ($IC_{50} = 0.3$, 1.0, and 0.6 μM, respectively) were the most potent ones. The methanol extract also showed antioxidant activities in DPPH ($IC_{50} = 76$ μg/ml) and FRAP assays (1.4 mmol ferrous ion equivalent/g extract). A total phenol content of 130 mg/g of the extract was determined by Folin-Ciocalteu reagent.

Conclusion: This study shows that *P. hyrcanicum* contains phenolic compounds with in vitro activity that can be useful in the context of preventing or mitigating cellular damages linked to diabetic conditions.

Keywords: *Polygonum hyrcanicum*, Polygonaceae, α-Glucosidase, Antioxidant, Cinnamoylphenethyl amide, Flavonoid

Introduction

The early stage of diabetes mellitus type 2 is associated with postprandial hyperglycemia due to impaired after-meal acute insulin secretion. Hyperglycemia is believed to increase the production of free radicals and reactive oxygen species, leading to oxidative tissue damage and diabetic complications such as nephropathy, neuropathy, retinopathy, and memory impairment [1]. Glucosidases are a group of digestive enzymes which break down the dietary carbohydrates into simple monosaccharides. Glucosidase inhibitors such as acarbose reduce the rate of carbohydrate digestion and delay the carbohydrate absorption from the digestive tract. Therefore, they have a potential to prevent the development of type 2 diabetes mellitus by lowering the after-meal glucose levels [2].

Polygonum species are valuable medicinal plants which possess interesting biological activities such as anti-inflammation [3], cardiovascular protection [4], neuro-protection [5], and mitigation of biochemical processes involved in age-related neurodegenerative disorders such as Alzheimer's [6] and Parkinson's disease [7]. It is

* Correspondence: yasa@sina.tums.ac.ir
[1]Department of Pharmacognosy, Faculty of Pharmacy, Tehran University of Medical Sciences, Tehran, Iran
[4]Medicinal Plants Research Centre, Faculty of Pharmacy, Tehran University of Medical Sciences, Tehran, Iran
Full list of author information is available at the end of the article

believed that these beneficial effects are, at least in part, due to antioxidant and radical scavenging properties of the plant. Moreover, some *Polygonum* species were reported to possess glucosidase inhibitory properties. Phenylpropanoid glycosides of *P. sachalinense* [8] and tannins of *P. cuspidatum* [9] were subsequently identified as active compounds.

Polygonum hyrcanicum is an endemic species that grows widely in northern areas of Iran [10]. In folk medicine of the Turkmen Sahra region (southeast of the Caspian Sea), decoctions made from aerial parts of the plant are used for the treatment of liver problems, anemia, hemorrhoids, and kidney stones [11]. To our knowledge, no biological or phytochemical investigation has been carried out with this species. To explore the plant's properties with respect to potential prevention or mitigation of cellular damages linked to diabetic conditions, different extracts of *P. hyrcanicum* were tested for α-glucosidase inhibitory, antioxidant and radical scavenging properties. Active constituents were isolated and identified from the methanolic extract.

Material and methods
General
Column chromatography was carried out using silica gel (230–400 mesh) obtained from Merck (Germany), RP-18 (230–400 mesh) and Sephadex LH-20 procured from Fluka (Switzerland). Pre-coated silica gel 60 F_{254} plates and silica gel 60 RP-18 $F_{254}S$ plates (Merck, Germany) were used for TLC. Spots were observed under UV at 254 and 366 nm and spraying with anisaldehyde-H_2SO_4 reagent (Sigma-Aldrich Chemie, Germany) and heating at 120°C for 5 min. HPLC separations were performed on a Knauer Wellchrom system connected to a photodiode array detector (Smart line system, Germany). ^1H and ^{13}C NMR spectra were measured on a Bruker Avance DRX 500 spectrometer operating at 500 MHz for ^1H and 125 MHz for ^{13}C using a 5 mm PABBO probehead. α-glucosidase (EC 3.2.1.20, from baker's yeast, 77 U/mg), p-nitrophenyl-α-d-glucopyranoside, vitamin E 97% and 2, 2-diphenyl-picrylhydrazyl (DPPH) were obtained from Sigma-Aldrich Chemie (Germany). Sodium carbonate, $FeCl_3$, sodium acetate, ferrous sulfate [$FeSO4.7H2O$], gallic acid, 2, 4, 6-tripyridyl-s-triazine (TPTZ) solution, and Folin-Ciocalteu reagent were all obtained from Merck (Germany).

Plant materials
Aerial parts of *Polygonum hyrcanicum* Rech. f. at full flowering stage were collected in September 2008 near the village of Veresk (Mazandaran Province) in the north of Iran. The plant material was identified by the forth co-author. A voucher specimen (6729-TEH) has been deposited at the Herbarium of the Faculty of Pharmacy, Tehran University of Medical Sciences.

Extraction and isolation
Shade-dried aerial parts of the plant (1200 g) were cut to small pieces and macerated with n-hexane, ethyl acetate, and methanol, successively, at room temperature (3×48 hours with each solvent). The extracts were concentrated under reduced pressure, then freeze dried, resulting in dry extracts of hexane (14 g), ethyl acetate (12 g), and methanol (150 g).

Methanol extract (150 g) of *P. hyrcanicum* was suspended in ethyl acetate and divided into an ethyl acetate–soluble portion (ESP, 15 g) and methanol–soluble portion (MSP, 135 g). The ESP was applied to normal phase silica gel column chromatography (5×45 cm) and eluted with CHCl3, CHCl3:EtOAc (6:4, 2:8), EtOAc, and MeOH, successively. Seven fractions (ESP_{1-7}) were collected. ESP_3 (375 mg) and ESP_5 (190 mg) were purified on a Sephadex LH-20 column eluted with MeOH:EtOAc (2:1), to afford compounds **1** (12 mg) and **2** (4 mg), respectively. ESP_6 (450 mg) was separated on a Sephadex LH-20 column eluted with MeOH:EtOAc (4:1) to give sub-fractions ESP_{6-1}–ESP_{6-6}. ESP_{6-2} (42 mg) was subjected to RP chromatography on an RP-18 column eluted with a step gradient of aqueous MeOH (MeOH 40% to 100%). Compounds **3** (11 mg) and **4** (2 mg) were obtained. Compounds **5** (3.5 mg) and **6** (5.5 mg) were purified from ESP_{6-3} (52 mg) by an RP-18 column eluted with aqueous MeOH (50% to 100%). ESP_{6-4} (19 mg) and ESP_{6-5} (28 mg) were separately chromatographed on an RP-18 column eluted with water:MeOH (1:1) to give compounds **7** (5 mg) and **8** (5 mg), respectively.

A portion of the MSP (20 g) was applied to an RP-18 silica gel column eluted with a step gradient of water: MeOH (8:2, 7:3, 5:5, 3:7, 0:10), yielding seven sub-fractions (MSP1–MSP7). Compound 9 (5.6 mg) was obtained by semi-preparative HPLC of MSP3 (128 mg) on an RP-18 column (250×20 mm, 7 μm). Water (solvent A) and MeOH (solvent B) were used as mobile phase (0–20 min, 40% B; 20–21 min, 40–50% B; 21-31 min, 50% B; 31–45 min, 50–60% B; 45–46 min, 60–100% B; 46-51 min, 100% B; flow rate of 4 ml/min). Subfraction MSP4 (596 mg) was separated on a Sephadex LH-20 column (MeOH) into four fractions (MSP4-1–MSP4-4). Semi-preparative RP-18 HPLC of MSP4-2 with water (solvent A) and MeOH (solvent B) as the mobile phase (0–30 min, isocratic elution with 50% B; 30–35 min, 100% B, lasting for 5 minutes; flow rate: 4 ml/min) yielded pure **10** (5.4 mg) and **11** (11 mg). MSP_{4-4} was separated on a Sephadex LH-20 column (MeOH) to give compound **12** (7.5 mg). Compound **13** (17 mg) was purified from MSP_5 (1.148 g) by chromatography on a Sephadex LH-20 column eluted with MeOH–water (8:2) followed by RP-18 chromatography (aqueous MeOH 20–100%). The purified compounds were identified using spectroscopic methods (^1H and ^{13}C NMR, 2D NMR involving COSY, HSQC, and HMBC) and comparison with literature data. The NMR spectra of compound 4 were previously recorded only in acetone-d6 and no ^{13}C-NMR data have been reported for compound 5 up to now.

Compound **4**: 1 H NMR (DMSO-d6, 500 MHz); $\delta = 7.45$ (*brs*, H-2'), 7.43 (*d*, $J = 8.1$ Hz, H-6'), 6.92 (*d*, $J = 8.1$ Hz, H-5'), 6.45 (*brs*, H-8), 6.25 (*brs*, H-6), 5.66 (*brs*, H-1"), 4.74 (br d, J = 4.1 Hz, H-3"), 4.38 (*brs*, H-2"), 4.17 (*dd*, J = 11.7, 3.5 Hz, H-5"), 3.96 (*dd*, J = 11.7, 6.4 Hz, H-5"), 3.81 (*m*, H-4"), 2.13 (*s*, CH3), 1.98 (*s*, CH3); 13 C NMR (DMSO- d6, 125 MHz); $\delta = 178.0$ (C-4), 170.2, 170.5 (COO), 164.5 (C-7), 161.7 (C-5), 157.6 (C-2), 156.7 (C-9), 149.0 (C-4'), 145.5 (C-3'), 133.7 (C-3), 121.5 (C-6'), 121.0 (C-1'), 116.1 (C-2'), 115.6 (C-5'), 108.4 (C-1"), 103.9 (C-10), 99.2 (C-6), 94.0 (C-8), 82.4 (C-4"), 79.4 (C-2"), 79.7 (C-3"), 63.5 (C-5"), 20.7, 20.5 (CH3)

Compound **5**: 1 H NMR (MeOD, 500 MHz); $\delta = 7.47$ (*brs*, H-2'), 7.44 (*d*, $J = 8.2$ Hz, H-6'), 6.88 (*d*, $J = 8.2$ Hz, H-5'), 6.37 (*brs*, H-8), 6.19 (*brs*, H-6), 5.72 (br s, H-1"), 4.81(*d*, $J = 3.8$, H-3"), 4.44 (*brs*, H-2"), 3.70 (*d*, $J = 3.8$, H-4"), 3.53 (2 H, H-5"), 2.80 (*s*, CH3); 13 C NMR (MeOD, 125 MHz); $\delta = 179.4$ (C-4), 172.4 (COO), 166.3 (C-7), 163.1 (C-5), 159.6 (C-2), 158.5 (C-9), 149.6 (C-4'), 146.3 (C-3'), 135.0 (C-3), 123.2 (C-1'), 123.0 (C-6'), 117.3 (C-5'), 116.0 (C-2'), 109.8 (C-1"), 105.7 (C-10), 99.9 (C-6), 94.8 (C-8), 86.8 (C-4"), 81.3 (C-3"), 81.2 (C-2"), 62.5 (C-5"), 20.9 (CH$_3$).

Sugar analysis
Sugar moieties of glycoside structures were detected by GC-MS analysis after acid hydrolysis and derivatization with L-cysteine methyl ester and silylation [12].

α-Glucosidase inhibition assay
α-Glucosidase inhibitory activities were evaluated according to the chromogenic method described by McCue et al. (2005), with some modifications [13]. The enzyme solution contained 20 µl α-glucosidase (0.5 unit/ml) and 120 µl 0.1 M phosphate buffer (pH 6.9). *p*-Nitrophenyl-α-D-glucopyranoside (5 mM) in the same buffer (pH 6.9) was used as a substrate solution. Ten microliters of test samples, dissolved in DMSO at various concentrations, were mixed with enzyme solution in microplate wells and incubated for 15 min at 37°C. Twenty microliters of substrate solution were added and incubated for an additional 15 min. The reaction was terminated by adding 80 µl of 0.2 M sodium carbonate solution. Absorbance of the wells was measured with a microplate reader at 405 nm, while the reaction system without plant extracts was used as control. The system without α-glucosidase was used as blank, and acarbose was used as positive control. Each experiment was

conducted in triplicate. The enzyme inhibitory rates of samples were calculated as follows:

$$\text{Inhibition\%} = [(\text{control absorption} - \text{sample absorption}) / \text{control absorption})] \times 100.$$

The IC$_{50}$ values of samples were calculated and reported as the mean ± standard deviation (SD) of three experiments.

DPPH free radical scavenging activity
The antioxidant activities of the extracts were determined with the DPPH assay according to an established protocol [14]. Extract solutions of 500, 250, 100, and 50 µg/ml were prepared in methanol. Each test tube contained 1 ml of the samples and 2 ml freshly prepared DPPH solution of 40 µg/ml in methanol. Negative control tubes were the same as the test tubes, except that they did not include DPPH. Absorbance of the mixtures were recorded at 517 nm after 30 minutes, against the blank covets of DPPH solution. Vitamin E was used as a positive control. All samples were assayed in triplicate and IC$_{50}$ values were calculated.

FRAP assay
Antioxidant activities of plant extracts were evaluated by monitoring their ferric-reducing abilities [15]. Freshly prepared FRAP reagent contained 5 ml FeCl3 (20 mM) plus 5 ml of a 10 mM TPTZ solution in 40 mM HCl and 50 ml of 300 mM acetate buffer (pH = 3.6). One hundred microliters of the samples, dissolved in methanol at various concentrations, were mixed with 3 ml FRAP reagent and incubated at 37°C for 10 minutes; the absorptions at 593 nm were recorded. A calibration curve was generated in the range of 125–750 µM ferrous sulfate (FeSO$_4$.7H2O). Vitamin E was used as a positive control and the results were expressed as mmol ferrous ion equivalent per gram of extracts.

Determination of total phenolic content
Total phenolic contents of extracts were assessed using Folin-Ciocalteu reagent [16]. The reagent was diluted 10-fold with distilled water. Two hundred microliters of appropriate dilutions of extracts were added to 1.5 ml reagent and allowed to stand at room temperature for 5 minutes. Sodium bicarbonate solution (1.5 mL, 60 g/L) was added to the mixture and stored at room temperature for an additional 90 minutes; absorptions at 725 nm were recorded. Known concentrations of gallic acid (0–100 µg/ml in methanol) were applied as standard samples and a calibration curve was created. Total phenolic contents were expressed as mg of gallic acid equivalents (GAE) per gram of dry extracts.

Table 1 *In vitro* activities and total phenol content of *P. hyrcanicum* extracts

Sample	α-Glucosidase inhibition IC$_{50}$(μg/ml)	DPPH assay IC$_{50}$(μg/ml)	FRAP assay (mmol ferrous ion equivalent/g)	Total phenol content (mg gallic acid equivalent/g)
Hexane extract	56.20 ± 1.2	1000<	trace	trace
EtOAc extract	42.30 ± 0.9	146.6 ± 5.2	0.54 ± 0.21	20.30 ± 2.5
MeOH extract	15.30 ± 0.5	76.00 ± 3.4	1.37 ± 0.42	135.00 ± 4.4
Vitamin E	-	14.12 ± 0.9	2.40 ± 0.76	-
Acarbose	8.70 ± 1.1	-	-	-

Result and discussion

Sequential extraction of the aerial parts of *P. hyrcanicum* yielded 1.0% of hexane, 0.8% of ethyl acetate, and 12.5% of methanol extracts, respectively. The methanol extract of P.

hyrcanicum showed noticeable α-glucosidase inhibitory activity (IC$_{50}$ = 15.3 μg/ml), whereas the ethyl acetate and hexane extracts only caused moderate inhibition. Acarbose (IC$_{50}$ = 8.7 μg/ml) was used as a positive control (Table 1).

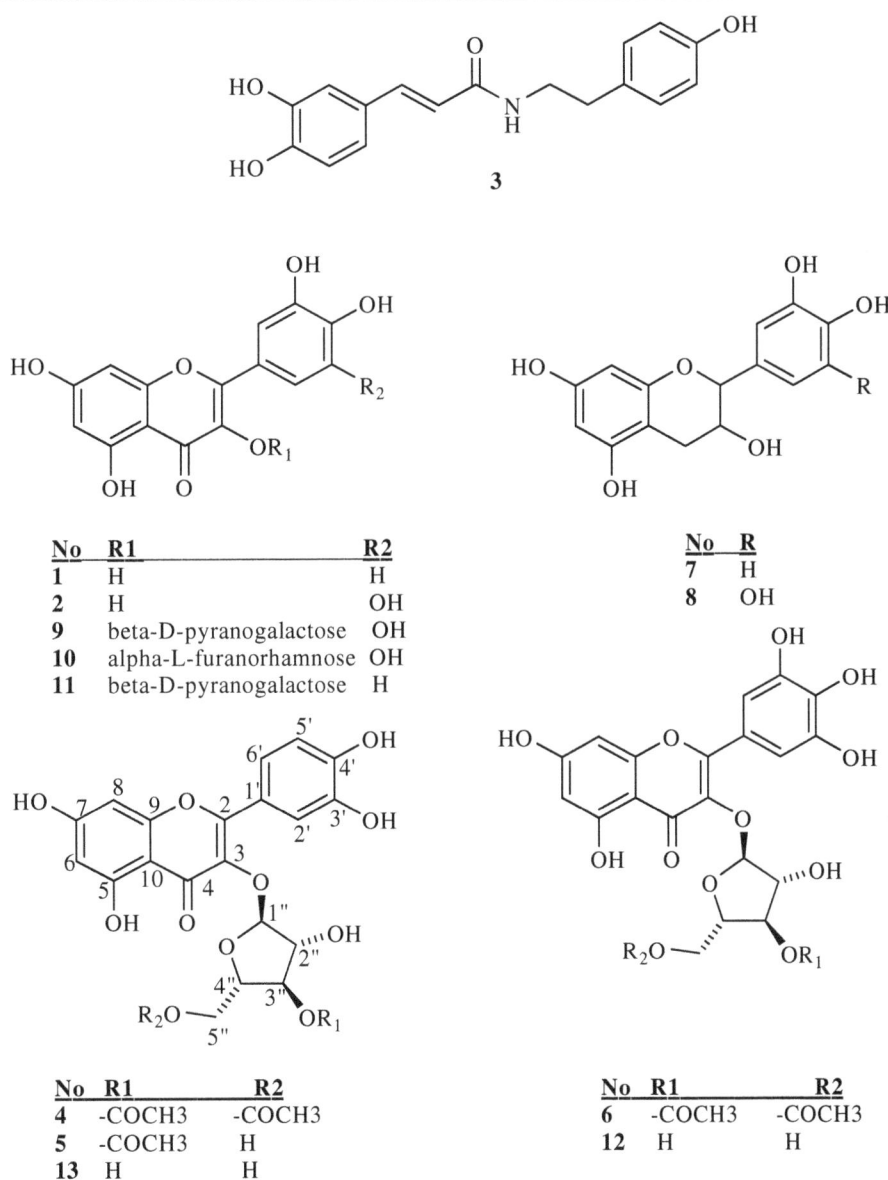

No	R1	R2
1	H	H
2	H	OH
9	beta-D-pyranogalactose	OH
10	alpha-L-furanorhamnose	OH
11	beta-D-pyranogalactose	H

No	R
7	H
8	OH

No	R1	R2
4	-COCH3	-COCH3
5	-COCH3	H
13	H	H

No	R1	R2
6	-COCH3	-COCH3
12	H	H

Figure 1 Structures of the phenolic constituents 1-13 isolated from the methanolic extract of *Polygonum hyrcanicum* Comparisons of the spectroscopic data with literature [21,26] led to the identification of sugar moiety of compounds 4, 5, 6, 12, 13.

In vitro enzyme-inhibitory assay-guided fractionation of methanol extract resulted in the purification of 13 phenolic compounds as the active constituents. Based on NMR data, the purified compounds were identified as quercetin (**1**) [17], myricetin (**2**) [17], N-trans-caffeoyl-tyramine (**3**) [18], quercetin 3-O-α-L-(3",5"-diacetyl-arabinofuranoside) (**4**) [19], quercetin 3-O-α-L-(3"-acetyl-arabinofuranoside) (**5**) [20], myricetin 3-O-α-L-(3",5"-diacetyl-arabinofuranoside) (**6**) [21], (+) catechin (**7**) [22], (-) gallocatechin (**8**) [22], myricetin 3-O-β-D-galactopyranoside (**9**) [23], myricetin 3-O-α-L-rhamnopyranoside (myricitrin) (**10**) [23], quercetin 3-O-β-D-galactopyranoside (**11**) [24], myricetin 3-O-α-L-arabinofuranoside [21] (**12**), and quercetin 3-O-α-L-arabinofuranoside (avicularin) (**13**) [25] (Figure 1). GC analysis of sugars obtained from hydrolysis of compounds 4, 5, 6, 12, and 13 and comparison with the authentic sample resulted in the detection of L-arabinose (RT = 24.3 min).

The sugar moiety of compounds 9 and 11 were confirmed to be D-galactose (RT = 31.1 min) and compound 10 was verified to have an L-rhamnose (RT = 26.7 min). All the compounds were isolated from P. hyrcanicum for the first time. Compounds 4, 5, and 6 are rare flavonoids with mono- or diacetylglycosyl moieties which have not been detected in the *Polygonum* genus up to now.

Subsequently, α-glucosidase inhibitory activities of phenolic compounds 1–13, isolated from the methanolic extract, were evaluated. The results are reported in Table 2. All constituents showed interesting inhibitory activities while compounds 3, 8 and 10 (IC50 = 0.3, 1.0, and 0.6 μM, respectively) were the most potent ones. The α-glucosidase inhibitory activities of compounds **4**, **5**, **6**, and **12** have not been reported in the literature

previously. Comparing the IC_{50} values of tested flavonoids shows that hydroxyl substitution affects the inhibitory activity so that increasing number of free phenolic groups results in higher activity.

Since oxidative stress is considered as a key factor in the pathogenesis of diabetic complications, antioxidant properties of the extracts were also studied. DPPH radical scavenging activity and ferric reducing power of P. hyrcanicum extracts are summarized in Table 1. The methanolic extract showed noticeable antioxidant activities in both DPPH (IC_{50} = 76.0 μg/ml) and FRAP (1.4 mmol ferrous ion equivalent/g) assays compared to vitamin E (IC_{50} = 14.1 μg/ml, FRAP value of 2.4 mmol ferrous ion equivalent/g) as the positive control. The ethyl acetate extract was a moderate antioxidant, while the hexane extract was not active at the concentrations tested. The antioxidant properties were in accord with the total phenol content of the extracts (Table 1). Methanol and ethyl acetate extracts contained 135.0 mg and 20.3 mg gallic acid equivalent/g, respectively, and the hexane extract was free of phenolic constituents.

Conclusion

In the perspective of identifying traditional herbal drugs which might be useful in preventing or mitigating cellular damages related to diabetes, we carried out the first study of the Persian edible plant, P. hyrcanicum. The methanolic extract, in particular, showed promising α-glucosidase, antioxidant, and radical scavenging activities and thirteen phenolic compounds were purified in an activity-guided approach. All the isolated compounds (IC_{50} = 0.3–7.6 μM) were more potent than the positive control acarbose (IC_{50} = 13.5 μM). This study suggests that P. hyrcanicum is a promising source of active compounds that can prevent the development of diabetes mellitus type 2 and its complications. While these *in vitro* results are of a preliminary nature, further investigation of P. hyrcanicum, in particular, *in vivo* pharmacological testing of the methanolic extract is warranted. These studies will provide a more in depth picture on the potential of this interesting traditional Persian plant.

Competing interests
No conflict of interest has been declared.

Authors' contribution
M-AF. Performed plant preparation, extraction, isolation and identification of plant substances and drafted the manuscript. AB. Determined inhibitory activity of the enzyme. SS. Advised separation of plant substances by HPLC. AY. Did the botanical studies and identified scientific name of the Plant. MM. Carried out antioxidant assays and total phenol content of the extracts. MM. Was engaged in phytochemical investigations and helped in isolation of substances. DR. Advised on NMR techniques of isolated compounds. HA. Advised antioxidant assays and edited the article. SP. Advised inhibitory activity determination of the enzyme. HM. Advised sugar analysis and edited the article. YN. Conceived the study and edited the manuscript. All authors read and approved the final manuscript.

Table 2 α-Glucosidase inhibitory activity (IC$_{50}$) of phenolic compounds 1-13

No	Compounds	IC$_{50}$ (μM)
1	Quercetin	3.3 ± 2.0
2	Myricetin	1.3 ± 0.6
3	N-trans-Caffeoyl-tyramine	0.3 ± 0.3
4	Quercetin 3-O-α-L-(3",5"-diacetyl-arabinofuranoside)	4.9 ± 1.5
5	Quercetin 3-O-α-L-(3"-acetylarabinofuranoside)	4.8 ± 1.9
6	Myricetin 3-O-α-L-(3",5"-diacetyl-arabinofuranoside)	5.8 ± 2.8
7	(+) Catechin	6.6 ± 3.5
8	(-) Gallocatechin	1.0 ± 0.3
9	Myricetin 3-O-β-D-galactopyranoside	4.8 ± 0.8
10	Myricitrin	0.6 ± 0.2
11	Quercetin 3-O-β-D-galactopyranoside	6.7 ± 3.0
12	Myricetin 3-O-α-L-arabinofuranoside	4.2 ± 2.9
13	Avicularin	7.6 ± 0.9
	Acarbose	13.5 ± 1.7

Acknowledgements

The research is supported by a Tehran University of Medical Sciences and Health Services grant (No. 56-8516). Special thanks go to Orlando Fertig and Samad N. Ebrahimi for sugar analysis at the University of Basel.

Author details

[1]Department of Pharmacognosy, Faculty of Pharmacy, Tehran University of Medical Sciences, Tehran, Iran. [2]Department of Pharmacognosy, Faculty of Pharmacy, Mazandaran University of Medical Sciences, Sari, Iran. [3]Department of Phytochemistry, Medicinal Plants and Drugs Research Institute, Shahid Beheshti University, Tehran, Iran. [4]Medicinal Plants Research Centre, Faculty of Pharmacy, Tehran University of Medical Sciences, Tehran, Iran. [5]Institute of Medicinal Plants, ACECR, Tehran, Iran. [6]Department of Medicinal Chemistry, Faculty of Pharmacy, Tehran University of Medical Sciences, Tehran, Iran. [7]Department of Pharmaceutical Sciences, University of Basel, Basel, Switzerland.

References

1. Maritim AC, Sanders RA, Watkins JB: **Diabetes, oxidative stress, and antioxidants: a review.** *J Biochem Mol Toxic* 2003, **17**:24–38.
2. Liu L, Deseo MA, Morris C, Winter KM, Leach DN: **Investigation of α-glucosidase inhibitory activity of wheat bran and germ.** *Food Chem* 2011, **126**:553–561.
3. Bralley EE, Greenspan P, Hargrove JL, Wicker L, Hartle DK: **Topical anti-inflammatory activity of** *Polygonum cuspidatum* **extract in the TPA model of mouse ear inflammation.** *J Inflamm* 2008, **5**:1–7.
4. Yim TK, Wu WK, Pak WF, Mak DHF, Liang SM, Ko KM: **Myocardial protection against ischaemia-reperfusion injury by a** *Polygonum multiflorum* **extract supplemented 'Dang-Gui decoction for enriching blood', a compound formulation, ex vivo.** *Phytother Res* 2000, **14**:195–199.
5. Wang T, Gu J, Wu PF, Wang F, Xiong Z, Yang YJ, et al: **Protection by tetrahydroxystilbene glucoside against cerebral ischemia: involvement of JNK, SIRT1, and NF-κB pathways and inhibition of intracellular ROS/RNS generation.** *Free Radical Bio Med.* 2009, **47**:229–240.
6. Um MY, Choi WH, Aan JY, Kim SR, Ha TY: **Protective effect of** *Polygonum multiflorum* **Thunb on amyloid β-peptide 25-35 induced cognitive deficits in mice.** *J Ethnopharmacol* 2006, **104**:144–148.
7. Li X, Matsumoto K, Murakami Y, Tezuka Y, Wu Y, Kadota S: **Neuroprotective effects of** *Polygonum multiflorum* **on nigrostriatal dopaminergic degeneration induced by paraquat and maneb in mice.** *Pharmacol Biochem Behav* 2005, **82**:345–352.
8. Fan P, Terrier L, Hay AE, Marston A, Hostettmann K: **Antioxidant and enzyme inhibition activities and chemical profiles of** *Polygonum sachalinensis* **F.Schmidt ex Maxim (Polygonaceae).** *Fitoterapia* 2010, **81**:124–131.
9. Tang W, Shen Z, Yin J: **Inhibitory activity to glycosidase of tannins from** *Polygonum cuspidatum.* *Tianran Chanwu Yanjiu Yu Kaifa* 2006, **18**:266–268.
10. Mozaffarian V: *A dictionary of Iranian plant names.* Tehran: Farhang Moaser; 2007.
11. Ghorbani A: **Studies on pharmaceutical ethnobotany in the region of Turkmen Sahra, north of Iran: (Part 1): General results.** *J Ethnopharmacol* 2005, **102**:58–68.
12. Chai XY, Xu ZR, Ren HY, Shi HM, Lu YN, Li FF, et al: **Itosides A-I, new phenolic glycosides from** *Itoa orientalis.* *Helv Chim Acta* 2007, **90**:2176–2185.
13. McCue P, Kwon YI, Shetty K: **Anti-amylase, anti-glucosidase and anti angiotensin I converting enzyme potential of selected foods.** *J Food Biochem* 2005, **29**:278–294.
14. Yassa N, Razavi Beni H, Hadjiakhoondi A: **Free radical scavenging and lipid peroxidation activity of the Shahani black grape.** *Pak J Biol Sci* 2008, **11**:1–4.
15. Benzie IF, Strain JJ: **The ferric reducing ability of plasma (FRAP) as a measure of "antioxidant power": the FRAP assay.** *Anal Biochem* 1996, **239**:70–76.
16. Al-Farsi M, Alasalvar C, Morris A, Baron M, Shahidi F: **Comparison of antioxidant activity, anthocyanins, carotenoids, and phenolics of three native fresh and sun-dried date (***Phoenix dactylifera* L.) varieties grown in Oman.** *J Agr Food Chem* 2005, **53**:7592–7599.
17. Shen CC, Chang YS, Hott LK: **Nuclear magnetic resonance studies of 5,7-dihydroxyflavonoids.** *Phytochem* 1993, **34**:843–845.
18. Santos LP, Boaventura MA, de Oliveira AB, Cassady JM: **Grossamide and N-trans-caffeoyltyramine from** *Annona crassiflora* **seeds.** *Planta Med* 1996, **62**:76.
19. Chin YW, Kim J: **Three new flavonol glycosides from the aerial parts of** *Rodgersia podophylla.* *ChemI Pharml Bull* 2006, **54**:234–236.
20. Takemoto T, Miyase T: **Studies on constituents of** *Boehmeria tricuspis* **Makino.** *I. Yakugaku Zasshi* 1974, **94**:1597–1602.
21. Torres-Mendoza D, González J, Ortega-Barría E, Heller MV, Capson TL, McPhail K, et al: **Weakly antimalarial flavonol arabinofuranosides from** *Calycolpus warszewiczianus.* *J Nat Prod* 2006, **69**:826–828.
22. Lee SS, Wang JS, Chen KCS: **Chemical constituents from the roots of** *Zyziphus jujube* **Mill. Var. spinosa (I).** *J Chinese Chem Soc* 1995, **42**:77–82.
23. Zhang Y, Zhang Q, Wang B, Li L, Zhao Y: **Chemical constituents from** *Ampelopsis grosseden ta ta.* *JCPS* 2006, **15**:2.
24. Lin HY, Kuo YH, Lin YL, Chiang W: **Antioxidative Effect and Active Components from Leaves of** *Lotus* **(***Nelumbo nucifera***).** *J Agr Food Chem* 2009, **57**:6623–6629.
25. Gohar A, Gedara SR, Baraka HN: **New acylated flavonol glycoside from** *Ceratonia siliqua* L. seeds. *J Med Plants Res* 2009, **3**:424–428.
26. Young-Won C, Song Won, Young Choong K, Sang Zin C, Kang Ro L, Jinwoong K: **Hepatoprotective flavonolglycosides from aerial parts of** *Rodgersia podophylla.* *Planta Med* 2004, **70**(6):576–577.

GC-MS analysis of insecticidal essential oil of flowering aerial parts of *Saussurea nivea* Turcz

Sha Sha Chu[1], Guo Hua Jiang[2] and Zhi Long Liu[1*]

Abstract

Background: Several species from *Saussurea* have been used in the traditional medicine, such as *S. lappa*, *S. involucrate*, and *S. obvallata*. There is no report on medicinal use of *S. nivea*. The aim of this research was to determine chemical composition and insecticidal activity of the essential oil of *S. nivea* Turcz (Asteraceae) aerial parts against maize weevils (*Sitophilus zeamais* Motschulsky) for the first time.

Results: Essential oil of *S. nivea* flowering aerial parts was obtained by hydrodistillation and analyzed by gas chromatography–mass spectrometry (GC-MS). A total of 43 components of the essential oil of *S. nivea* were identified. The principal compounds in the essential oil were (+)-limonene (15.46%), caryophyllene oxide (7.62%), linalool (7.20%), α-pinene (6.43%), β-pinene (5.66%) and spathulenol (5.02%) followed by β-eudesmoll (4.64%) and eudesma-4,11-dien-2-ol (3.76%). The essential oil of *S. nivea* exhibited strong contact toxicity against *S. zeamais* with an LD_{50} value of 10.56 μg/adult. The essential oil also possessed fumigant toxicity against *S. zeamais* with an LC_{50} value of 8.89 mg/L.

Conclusion: The study indicates that the essential oil of *S. nivea* flowering aerial parts has a potential for development into a natural insecticide/fumigant for control of insects in stored grains.

Keywords: Saussurea nivea, Sitophilus zeamais, Contact toxicity, Fumigant, Essential oil composition

Background

The maize weevil (*Sitophilus zeamais* Motschulsky) is one of the major pests of stored grains and grain products in the tropics and subtropics [1]. Infestations not only cause significant losses due to the consumption of grains; they also result in elevated temperature and moisture conditions that lead to an accelerated growth of molds, including toxigenic species [2]. Currently, control of stored product insects relies heavily on the use of synthetic insecticides and fumigants, which has led to problems such as disturbance of the environment, increasing application costs, pest resurgence, pest resistance to pesticides and lethal effects on non-target organisms in addition to direct toxicity to the users [3]. Thus, there is a considerable interest in developing natural products that are relatively less damaging to mammalian health and the environment than existing conventional pesticides, as alternatives to non-selective

synthetic pesticides to control the pests of medical and economic importance [4,5]. In recent years, various workers have been concentrating their efforts on the search for natural products as an alternative to conventional insecticides and fumigants, as well as the re-evaluation of traditional botanical pest control agents [5]. Essential oils or their constituents may provide an alternative to currently used fumigants/pesticides to control stored-food insects. Investigations in several countries confirm that some plant essential oils not only repel insects, but possess contact and fumigant toxicity against stored product pests as well as exhibited feeding inhibition or harmful effects on the reproductive system of insects [5,6]. In addition, it has been shown that essential oils have antibacterial and antinematicidal activities [7-14].

During the screening program for new agrochemicals from Chinese medicinal herbs and wild plants, the essential oil of *Saussurea nivea* Turcz (synonym: *Himalaiella nivea*; *Aplotaxis nivea*; *Saussurea deltoidea var. nivea*; and *Saussurea crispa*) [15] flowering aerial parts was found to possess strong insecticidal toxicity against the

* Correspondence: zhilongliu@cau.edu.cn
[1]Department of Entomology, China Agricultural University, Haidian District, Beijing 100193, China
Full list of author information is available at the end of the article

grain storage insect, *S. zeamais*. *Saussurea* is a genus of about 300 species of flowering plants in the family Asteraceae, native to cool temperate and arctic regions of Asia, Europe, and North America. Many species of *Saussurea* were used in traditional medicine such as *S. lappa*, *S. involucrate*, and *S. obvallata*. For example, *S. involucrata* aerial parts have long been used in traditional Chinese medicine for the treatment of rheumatoid arthritis, cough with cold, stomachache, dysmenorrhea, and altitude sickness, and have antiinflammatory, cardiotonic, abortifacient, anticancer, and antifatigue actions [16]. However, there is no report on medicinal use of *S. nivea*. *S. nivea* is an herbaceous perennial plant distributed mainly in the north of China (Beijing, Hebei, Liaoning, Gansu, Ningxia, Shaanxi, Shanxi Province and Inner Mongolia) and Korea [16]. The aqueous extract of this plant was used to control insect pests by the local farmer [17]. Five constituent compounds (quercetin-3-*O*-β-*D*-glucoside, kaempferol-3-*O*-β-*D*-glucoside, α-amyrin, β-sitosterol, hentiantane) have been isolated from the ethanol extract of *S. nivea* [17]. However, a literature survey has shown that there is no report on the volatile constituents and insecticidal activity of *S. nivea*; thus we decided to investigate the chemical constituents and insecticidal activities of the essential oil of *S. nivea* aerial parts against grain storage insect for the first time.

Materials and methods
Plant material
The aerial parts of *S. nivea* at flowering state were collected in August 2009 from Xiaolongmen National Forest Park (39.48° N latitude and 115.25° E longitude, Mentougou District, Beijing 102300). The sample was air-dried and identified by Dr. Liu, Q.R. (College of Life Sciences, Beijing Normal University, Beijing 100875, China) and a voucher specimen (ENTCAU-Compositae-10014) was deposited at the Department of Entomology, China Agricultural University (Beijing 100193). The sample was ground to a powder using a grinding mill (Retsch Mühle, Germany). Each 600 g portion of powder was mixed in 1,800 ml of distilled water and soaked for 3 h. The mixture was then boiled in a round-bottom flask, and steam distilled for 6–8 h. Volatile essential oil from distillation was collected in a flask. Separation of the essential oil from the aqueous layer was done in a separatory funnel, using *n*-hexane. The solvent was evaporated using rotary evaporator (BUCHI Rotavapor R-124, Switzerland). The sample was dried over anhydrous Na_2SO_4 and kept in a refrigerator (4°C) for subsequent experiments.

Insects
The maize weevils (*S. zeamais*) were obtained from laboratory cultures in the dark in incubators at 29-30 °C and 70-80% relative humidity and were reared on whole wheat at 12-13% moisture content in glass jars (diameter 85 mm, height 130 mm). Unsexed adult weevils used in all the experiments were about one week old. All containers housing insects and the petri dishes used in experiments were made escape proof with a coating of polytetrafluoroethylene (Fluon, Blades Biological, UK).

Gas chromatography–mass spectrometry
The essential oil of *S. nivea* was subjected to GC-MS analysis on an Agilent system consisting of a model 6890 N gas chromatograph, a model 5973 N mass selective detector (EIMS, electron energy, 70 eV), and an Agilent ChemStation data system. The GC column was an HP-5 ms fused silica capillary with a 5% phenylmethylpolysiloxane stationary phase, film thickness of 0.25 μm, a length of 30 m, and an internal diameter of 0.25 mm. The GC settings were as follows: the initial oven temperature was held at 60 °C for 1 min and then heated at 180 °C at a rate of 10 °C/min, held for 1 min, and then heated to 280 °C at 20 °C/min and held for 15 min. The injector temperature was maintained at 270 °C. The sample (1 μl) was injected neat, with a split ratio of 1: 10. The carrier gas was helium at flow rate of 1.0 mL min^{-1}. Spectra were scanned from 20 to 550 m/z at 2 scans s^{-1}. Most constituents were identified by gas chromatography by comparison of their retention indices with those of the literature or with those of authentic compounds available in our laboratories. The retention indices were determined in relation to a homologous series of *n*-alkanes (C_8–C_{24}) under the same operating conditions. Further identification was made by comparison of their mass spectra with those stored in NIST 08 and Wiley 275 libraries or with mass spectra from literature [18]. Component relative percentages were calculated based on normalization method without using correction factors.

Contact toxicity by topical application
Range-finding studies were run to determine the appropriate testing concentrations of the essential oil of *S. nivea*. A serial dilution of the essential oil (5.0%-15.0%, 5 concentrations) was prepared in *n*-hexane. Aliquots of 0.5 μl per insect were topically applied dorsally to the thorax of the weevils, using a Burkard Arnold microapplicator. Controls were determined using 0.5 μl *n*-hexane per insect. Ten insects were used for each concentration and control, and the experiment was replicated six times. Both the treated and control weevils were then transferred to glass vials (10 insects/vial) with culture media and kept in incubators at 29-30°C and 70-80% relative humidity. Mortality was observed after 24 h. The insects were considered dead if appendages did not move when probed with a camel brush. The observed mortality data were corrected for control

Drug Conception, Design and Manufacturing

Table 1 Chemical constituents of essential oil derived from *Saussurea nivea* flowering aerial part

Compounds	RI*	Peak Area (%)
α-Pinene	939	6.43
β-Pinene	981	5.66
(+)-Limonene	1027	15.46
Benzeneacetaldehyde	1036	0.39
γ-Terpinene	1057	2.32
cis-Linalool oxide	1076	0.99
Linalool	1094	7.20
Phenylethyl Alcohol	1116	0.14
Nopinone	1142	0.48
Camphor	1146	0.56
Sabina ketone	1154	0.48
Borneol	1167	1.37
4-Terpineol	1175	1.05
p-Cymen-8-ol	1179	0.58
α-Terpineol	1188	1.77
Geraniol	1253	1.61
Nonanoic acid	1283	0.66
Chavibetol	1362	0.79
Copaene	1374	0.35
trans-β-Damascenone	1382	0.94
β-Bourbonene	1387	0.23
Dodecanal	1407	0.14
(Z)-Caryophyllene	1409	2.14
α-Cedrene	1411	0.13
Caryophyllene	1420	2.74
Germacrene D	1478	0.45
Geranyl acetone	1453	0.77
α-Caryophyllene	1454	1.85
γ-Muurolene	1473	0.79
α-Amorphene	1479	1.43
α-Curcumene	1483	1.34
β-Ionone	1487	2.09
α-Muurolene	1500	0.89
δ-Cadinene	1523	1.97
Dihydroactinolide	1538	2.07
α-Calacorene	1546	0.42
Spathulenol	1578	5.02
Caryophyllene oxide	1583	7.62
Isoaromadendrene epoxide	1594	1.19
Widdrol	1597	2.62
β-Eudesmol	1648	4.64
Eudesma-4,11-dien-2-ol	1691	3.76
γ-Costol	1732	2.87
Total		96.38
Monoterpenoids		45.96

Table 1 Chemical constituents of essential oil derived from *Saussurea nivea* flowering aerial part (Continued)

Sesquiterpenoids	47.97
Others	2.47

*RI, retention index as determined on a HP-5MS column using the homologous series of n-hydrocarbons.

mortality using Abbott's formula. Results from all replicates were subjected to probit analysis using the PriProbit Program V1.6.3 to determine LD_{50} values [19].

Fumigant toxicity bioassay
Range-finding studies were run to determine the appropriate testing concentrations of S. nivea essential oil. The fumigant toxicity of S. nivea essential oil was determined by used the method of Liu and Ho [1] with some modifications. A Whatman filter paper (diameter 2.0 cm) was placed on the underside of the screw cap of a glass vial (diameter 2.5 cm, height 5.5 cm, volume 24 ml). Ten microliters of the essential oil (5.39-20.00%, 6 concentrations) was added to the filter paper. The solvent was allowed to evaporate for 15 s before the cap was placed tightly on the glass vial (with 10 unsexed insects) to form a sealed chamber. The vials were upright and the Fluon (ICI America Inc) coating restricted the insects to the lower portion of the vial to prevent them from the treated filter paper. They were incubated at 27-29°C and 70-80% relative humidity for 24 h. Mortality of insects was observed. The insects were considered dead if appendages did not move when probed with a camel brush. The observed mortality data were corrected for control mortality using Abbott's formula. Results from all replicates were subjected to probit analysis using the PriProbit Program V1.6.3 to determine LC_{50} values [19].

Results and discussions
The yellow essential oil yield of S. nivea flowering aerial parts was 0.11% (V/W) and the density of the concentrated essential oil was determined as 0.81 g/ml. A total of 46 components of the essential oil were identified, accounting for 96.38% of the total oil. The principal compounds in the essential oil of S. nivea flowering aerial parts were (+)-limonene (15.46%), caryophyllene oxide (7.62%), linalool (7.20%), α-pinene (6.43%), β-pinene (5.66%) and spathulenol (5.02%) followed by β-eudesmol (4.64%) and eudesma-4,11-dien-2-ol (3.76%) (Table 1). Monoterpenoids represented 14 of the 43 compounds, corresponding to 45.96% of the whole oil while 23 of the 43 constituents were sesquiterpenoids (47.97% of the crude essential oil).

The essential oil of S. nivea flowering aerial parts exhibited contact toxicity against S. zeamais adults with an LD_{50} value of 10.56 μg/adult (Table 2). When compared with the positive control pyrethrum extract [20], the

**Table 2 Contact toxicity (CT) and fumigant toxicity (FT) of
Saussurea nivea essential oil against *Sitophilus zeamais*
adults**

Treatment	LD$_{50}$ (μg/adult) LC$_{50}$ (mg/L air)	95% FL	Slope ± SE	Chi square (χ^2)
CT *S. nivea*	10.56	9.75–11.32	3.41 ± 0.35	16.22
Pyrethrum extract*	4.29	3.86–4.72	-	-
FT *S. nivea*	8.89	7.91–9.73	2.86 ± 0.30	13.37
MeBr**	0.67	-	-	-

* from Wang et al. [20]. ** from Liu and Ho [1].

essential oil demonstrated 2.5 times less toxic against *S. zeamais*. However, compared with the other essential oils in the literature, the essential oil of *S. nivea* flowering aerial parts possessed stronger contact toxicity against *S. zeamais* adults, e.g. essential oils of *Artemisia lavandulaefolia, A. sieversiana, A. capillaries, A. mongolica, A. vestita* and *A. eriopoda* (LD$_{50}$ = 55.2 μg/adult, 113.0 μg/adult, 106.0 μg/adult, 87.9 μg/adult, and 50.6 μg/adult, 24.8 μg/adult, respectively) [21-24], essential oil of *Schizonpeta multifida* (30.2 μg/adult) [25], essential oil of *Illicium simonsii* fruits (LD$_{50}$ = 112.7 μg/adult) [26] and essential oil of *Cayratia japonica* (LD$_{50}$ = 44.5 μg/adult) [27].

The essential oil of *S. nivea* flowering aerial parts possessed fumigant toxicity against the maize weevils with an LC$_{50}$ value of 8.89 mg/L (Table 2). The commercial grain fumigant, methyl bromide (MeBr) was reported to have fumigant activity against *S. zeamais* adults with an LC$_{50}$ value of 0.67 mg/L [1], thus the essential oil was 13 times less toxic to *S. zeamais* adults compared with MeBr. However, compared with fumigant activity of the other essential oils in the literature, the essential oil of *A. igniaria* exhibited stronger fumigant toxicity against *S. zeamais* adults, e.g. essential oils of *S. multifida* [25], *Kadsura heteroclite* [13], *Murraya exotica* [28], and several essential oils from Genus *Artemisa* [21-24]. Moreover, one of the main constituent compounds, (+)-limonene has been commercialized for use as flea dips and shampoos for pets as well as sprays and aerosols [29] and was used to prepare for durable insect repellent cotton fabric [30]. It has been demonstrated to possess insecticidal activity against several stored-product insects such as the cowpea weevil (*Callosobruchus maculates*), lesser grain borer (*Rhyzopertha dominica*), flat grain beetle (*C. pusillus*), rice weevil (*S. oryzae*), maize weevil (*S. zeamais*), red flour beetle (*Tribolium castaneum*) and German cockroaches (*Blattella germanica*) [31-35]. Another main constituent compound, linalool was also found to have fumigant toxicity against the triatomine bug (*Rhodnius prolixus*) [36] and houseflies with a 24 h LC$_{50}$ value of 13.6 mg/L [37]. Moreover, linalool possessed both contact and fumigant toxicity against human head louse (*Pediculus humanus*

capitis) [38] and showed a high acaricidal activity by vapor action against mobile stages of *Tyrophagus putrescentiae* [39]. The two constituent compounds were demonstrated to be a potent inhibitor of acetylcholinesterase (AChE) activity from larvae of several stored product insects [34,40,41].

The above findings suggest that fumigant activity of the essential oil of *S. nivea* flowering aerial parts is quite promising by considering the currently used fumigants are synthetic insecticides and it shows potential to develop a possible new natural fumigant/insecticide for control of stored product insects. However, for the practical application of the essential oil as novel insecticide/fumigant, further studies on the safety of the essential oil to humans and on development of formulations are necessary to improve the efficacy and stability and to reduce cost.

Conclusion

The study indicates that the essential oil of *S. nivea* flowering aerial parts has a potential for development into a new natural insecticide/fumigant for control of insects in stored grains. However, further studies on the safety of the oil in humans as well as development studies are required to optimize the efficacy and stability of this extract, and to reduce cost.

Competing interest
The authors declare that they have no competing interests.

Authors' contributions
CSS carried out collection of plant sample, participated in bioassay, and performed the statistical analysis. JGH carried out GC and GC-MS, helped to draft the manuscript. LZL MT participated in the design of the study and bioassay, and drafted the manuscript. All the authors read and approved the final manuscript.

Acknowledgements
This work was funded by the Hi-Tech Research and Development of China (2011AA10A202 and 2006AA10A209). We thank Dr. Liu QR from the College of Life Sciences, Beijing Normal University, Beijing 100875 for the identification of the investigated plant.

Author details
[1]Department of Entomology, China Agricultural University, Haidian District, Beijing 100193, China. [2]Analytic and Testing Center, Beijing Normal University, Haidian District, Beijing 100875, China.

References
1. Liu LZ, Ho SH: Bioactivity of the essential oil extracted from *Evodia rutaecarpa* Hook f. et Thomas against the grain storage insects, *Sitophilus zeamais* Motsch. and *Tribolium castaneum* (Herbst). *J Stored Prod Res* 1999, 35:317–328.
2. Magan N, Hope R, Cairns V, Aldred D: Postharvest fungal ecology: impact of fungal growth and mycotoxin accumulation in stored grain. *Eur J Plant Pathol* 2003, 109:723–730.
3. Zettler JL, Arthur FH: Chemical control of stored product insects with fumigants and residual treatments. *Crop Prot* 2000, 19:577–582.
4. Ismam MB: Plant essential oils for pest and disease management. *Crop Prot* 2000, 19:603–608.

5.   Isman MB: **Botanical insecticides, deterrents, and repellents in modern agriculture and an increasingly regulated world.** *Ann Rev Entomol* 2006, 51:45–66.

6.   Rajendran S, Srianjini V: **Plant products as fumigants for stored-product insects control.** *J Stored Prod Res* 2008, 44:126–135.

7.   Javidnia K, Tabatabaiee M, Shafiee A: **Composition and antimicrobial activity of essential oil of *Ziziphora teniur*, population Iran.** *Daru* 1996, 6:56–60.

8.   Khalighi-Sigaroodi F, Hadjiakhoondi A, Shahverdi AR, Mozaffaricen VA, Shafiee A: **Composition and antimicrobial activity of the essential oil of *Ferulago bernardii* Tomk. and M. Pimen.** *Daru* 2005, 13:100–104.

9.   Dehghan G, Solaimanian R, Shahverdi AR, Amin G, Abdollahi M, Shafiee A: **Chemical composition and antimicrobial activity of essential oil of *Ferula szovitsiana* D.C.** *Flavour Fragr J* 2007, 22:224–227.

10. Wang JH, Zhao JL, Liu H, Zhou LG, Liu ZL, Han JG, Zhu Y, Yang FY: **Chemical analysis and biological activity of the essential oils of two Valerianaceous species from China: *Nardostachys chinensis* and *Valeriana officinalis*.** *Molecules* 2010, 15:6411–6422.

11. Wang JH, Liu H, Zhao JL, Gao HF, Zhou L, Liu ZL, Chen YQ, Sui P: **Antimicrobial and antioxidant activities of the root bark essential oil of *Periploca sepium* and its main component 2-Hydroxy-4-methoxybenzaldehyde.** *Molecules* 2010, 15:5807–5817.

12. Bai CQ, Liu ZL, Liu QZ: **Nematicidal constituents from the essential oil of *Chenopodium ambrosioides* aerial parts.** *E-J Chem* 2011, 8(S1):143–148.

13. Li HQ, Bai CQ, Chu SS, Zhou L, Du SS, Liu ZL, Liu QZ: **Chemical composition and toxicities of the essential oil derived from *Kadsura heteroclita* stems against *Sitophilus zeamais* and *Meloidogyne incognita*.** *J Med Plants Res* 2011, 5:4943–4948.

14. Wang JH, Xu L, Yang L, Liu ZL, Zhou LG: **Composition, antibacterial and antioxidant activities of essential oils from *Ligusticum sinense* and *L. jeholense* (Umbelliferae) from China.** *Rec Nat Prod* 2011, 5:314–318.

15. Raab-Straube E: **Phylogenetic relationships in *Saussurea* (Compositae, Cardueae) sensu lato, inferred from morphological, ITS and *trnL-trn*F sequence data, with a synopsis of *Himalaiella* gen. nov., *Lipschitziella* and *Frolovia*.** *Willdenowia* 2003, 33:379–402.

16. Chen YL, Shih C: **Flora Reipublicae Popularis Sinicae.** *Science Press, Beijing, China* 1999, 78(2):175–177. http://www.efloras.org/florataxon.aspx?flora_id=2&taxon_id=200024432.

17. Ren YL, Yang JS: **Study on chemical constituentes of *Saussurea nivea*.** *Chin Pharm J* 2001, 36:87–89.

18. Adams RP: *Identification of essential oil components by Gas Chromatography/ Mass Spectrometry.* Carol Stream, Illinois, USA: Allured Publ. Corp; 2007.

19. Sakuma M: **Probit analysis of preference data.** *Appl Entomol Zool* 1998, 33:339–347.

20. Wang CF, Yang K, Zhang HM, Cao J, Fang R, Liu ZL, Du SS, Wang YY, Deng ZW, Zhou L: **Components and insecticidal activity against the maize weevils of *Zanthoxylum schinifolium* fruits and leaves.** *Molecules* 2011, 16:3077–3088.

21. Liu ZL, Liu QR, Chu SS, Jiang GH: **Insecticidal activity and chemical composition of the essential oils of *Artemisia lavandulaefolia* and *Artemisia sieversiana* from China.** *Chem Biodiv* 2010, 7:2040–2045.

22. Liu ZL, Chu SS, Liu QR: **Chemical composition and insecticidal activity against *Sitophilus zeamais* of the essential oils of *Artemisia capillaris* and *Artemisia mongolica*.** *Molecules* 2010, 15:2600–2608.

23. Chu SS, Liu QR, Liu ZL: **Insecticidal activity and chemical composition of the essential oil of *Artemisia vestita* from China against *Sitophilus zeamais*.** *Biochem Syst Ecol* 2010, 38:489–492.

24. Jiang GH, Liu QR, Chu SS, Liu ZL: **Chemical composition and insecticidal activity of the essential oil of *Artemisia eriopoda* against maize weevil. *Sitophilus zeamais*.** *Nat. Prod. Communications* 2012, 7:267–268.

25. Liu ZL, Chu SS, Jiang GH: **Toxicity of *Schizonpeta multifida* essential oil and its constituent compounds towards two grain storage insects.** *J Sci Food Agric* 2011, 91:905–909.

26. Chu SS, Liu SL, Jiang GH, Liu ZL: **Composition and toxicity of essential oil of *Illicium simonsii* Maxim (Illiciaceae) fruit against the maize weevils.** *Rec Nat Prod* 2010, 4:205–210.

27. Liu ZL, Yang K, Huang F, Liu QZ, Zhou LG, Du SS: **Chemical composition and toxicity of the essential oil of *Cayratia japonica* against two grain storage insects.** *J Essential Oil Res* 2012, 24:237–240.

28. Li WQ, Jiang CH, Chu SS, Zuo MX, Liu ZL: **Chemical composition and toxicity against *Sitophilus zeamais* and *Tribolium castaneum* of the essential oil of *Murraya exotica* aerial parts.** *Molecules* 2010, 15:5831–5839.

29. Prates HT, Santos JP, Waquil JM, Fabris JD, Oliveira AB, Foster JE: **Insecticidal activity of monoterpenes against *Rhyzopertha dominica* (F.) and *Tribolium castaneum* (Herbst).** *J Stored Prod Res* 1988, 34:243–249.

30. Hebeish A, Fouda MMG, Hamdy IA, El-Sawy SM, Abdel-Mohdy FA: **Preparation of durable insect repellent cotton fabric: Limonene as insecticide.** *Carbohydr Polym* 2008, 74:268–273.

31. Bekele AJ, Hassanali A: **Blend effects in the toxicity of the essential oil constituents of *Ocimum kilimandscharicum* and *Ocimum kenyense* (Labiateae) on two post-harvest insect pests.** *Phytochemistry* 2001, 57:385–391.

32. Lee BH, Choi WS, Lee SE, Park BS: **Fumigant toxicity of essential oils and their constituent compounds towards the rice weevil, *Sitophilus oryzae* (L.).** *Crop Prot* 2001, 20:317–320.

33. Tripathi AK, Prajapati V, Khanuja SPS, Kumar S: **Effect of d-limonene on three stored-product beetles.** *J Econ Entomol* 2003, 96:990–995.

34. Jang YS, Yang YC, Choi DS, Ahn YJ: **Vapor phase toxicity of marjoram oil compounds and their related monoterpenoids to *Blattella germanica* (Orthoptera: Blattellidae).** *J Agric Food Chem* 2005, 53:7892–7898.

35. Abdelgaleil SAM, Mohamed MIE, Badawy MEI, El-Arami SAA: **Fumigant and contact toxicities of monoterpenes to *Sitophilus oryzae* (L.) and *Tribolium castaneum* (Herbst) and their inhibitory effects on acetylcholinesterase activity.** *J Chem Ecol* 2009, 35:518–525.

36. Sfara V, Zerba EN, Alzogaray RA: **Fumigant insecticidal activity and repellent effect of five essential oils and seven monoterpenes on first-instar nymphs of *Rhodnius prolixus*.** *J Med Entomol* 2009, 46:511–515.

37. Palacios SM, Bertoni A, Rossi Y, Santander R, Urzua A: **Efficacy of essential oils from edible plants as insecticides against the house fly, *Musca domestica* L.** *Molecules* 2009, 14:1938–1947.

38. Yang YC, Lee SH, Clark JM, Ahn YJ: **Ovicidal and adulticidal activities of *Origanum majorana* essential oil constituents against insecticide-susceptible and pyrethroid/malathion-resistant *Pediculus humanus capitis* (Anoplura: Pediculidae).** *J Agric Food Chem* 2009, 57:2282–2287.

39. Sanchez-Ramos I, Castanera P: **Acaricidal activity of natural monoterpenes on *Tyrophagus putrescentiae* (Schrank), a mite of stored food.** *J Stored Prod Res* 2001, 37:93–101.

40. Badawy MEI, El-Arami SAA, Abdelgaleil SAM: **Acaricidal and quantitative structure activity relationship of monoterpenes against the two-spotted spider mite, *Tetranychus urticae*.** *Exp Appl Acarol* 2010, 52:261–274.

41. Ryan FM, Byrne O: **Plant-insect coevolution and inhibition of acetylcholinesterase.** *J Chem Ecol* 1988, 14:1965–1975.

Neuroprotective properties of *Melissa officinalis* after hypoxic-ischemic injury both *in vitro* and *in vivo*

Mohammad Bayat[1], Abolfazl Azami Tameh[2], Mohammad Hossein Ghahremani[3], Mohammad Akbari[1], Shahram Ejtemaei Mehr[4], Mahnaz Khanavi[5] and Gholamreza Hassanzadeh[1,6*]

Abstract

Background: Brain ischemia initiates several metabolic events leading to neuronal death. These events mediate large amount of damage that arises after some neurodegenerative disorders as well as transient brain ischemia. *Melissa officinalis* is considered as a helpful herbal plant in the prevention of various neurological diseases like Alzheimer that is related with oxidative stress.

Methods: We examined the effect of *Melissa officinalis* on hypoxia induced neuronal death in a cortical neuronal culture system as *in vitro* model and transient hippocampal ischemia as *in vivo* model. Transient hippocampal ischemia was induced in male rats by tow vessel-occlusion for 20 min. After reperfusion, the histopathological changes and the levels inflammation, oxidative stress status, and caspase-3 activity in hippocampus were measured.

Results: Cytotoxicity assays showed a significant protection of a 10 μg/ml dose of Melissa against hypoxia in cultured neurons which was confirmed by a conventional staining (P<0.05). Melissa treatment decrease caspase3 activity (P<0.05) and TUNEL-positive cells significantly (P<0.01). Melissa oil has also inhibited malon dialdehyde level and attenuated decrease of Antioxidant Capacity in the hippocampus. Pro-inflammatory cytokines TNF-α, IL-1β and HIF-1α mRNA levels were highly increased after ischemia and treatment with Melissa significantly suppressed HIF-1α gene expression (P<0.05).

Discussion: Results showed that *Melissa officinalis* could be considered as a protective agent in various neurological diseases associated with ischemic brain injury.

Keywords: *Melissa officinalis*, Ischemia, Cell death, Hippocampus, Neuron

Background

Ischemic brain injury often causes irreversible neural damage. The cascade of events leading to neuronal injury and death in ischemia includes excitotoxicity, inflammation, edema, apoptosis, and necrosis [1]. In humans and experimental animals subjected to ischemia, selective and delayed neuronal death occurs in pyramidal neurons of the hippocampal CA1 region [2]. Several studies have indicated that early and late neuronal death occurring in the neurons of cortex and hippocampus after ischemia could be both

apoptotic and necrotic cell death [3]. A special kind of cell death occurs some days after the initial ischemic insult, a phenomenon termed delayed neuronal death (DND) [4].

It is demonstrated that hypoxia-inducible factor-1α (HIF-1α), interleukin-1 β (IL-1β) and tumor necrosis factor α (TNF-α) expression increase in the rat brain during cerebral ischemia induced by different models of ischemia. In ischemic neuronal damage, inflammatory responses involving cytokines, adhesion molecules and leukocytes, are critical to the pathogenesis of tissue damage [5]. Local inflammatory responses contribute to secondary injury to potentially viable tissues could lead to clinical outcome in patients with ischemic stroke [6].

Reactive oxygen species (ROS) are a class of highly reactive molecules derived from oxygen and generated

* Correspondence: hassanzadeh@tums.ac.ir
[1]Department of Anatomy, School of Medicine, Tehran University of Medical Sciences, Tehran, Iran
[6]Department of Neuroscience, School of Advanced Medical Technology, Tehran University of Medical Sciences, Tehran, Iran
Full list of author information is available at the end of the article

by some normal metabolic processes [7]. Enhanced production of ROS and the subsequent oxidative stress have been thought to play a pivotal role in ischemia/reperfusion induced neuronal death.

Natural antioxidants in plants are well known to protect human against free radicals and prevent from some diseases. *Melissa officinalis* or Lemon balm, an herb from the Labiatae family has traditionally been used for its effects on nervous system. *Melissa officinalis* leaves contain polyphenoliccompounds, such as rosmaric acid, trimeric compounds and some flavonoids [8] that can scavenge free radicals and have antioxidant properties [9]. This may prevent apoptosis induced by oxidative stress.

Essential oils derived from herbs have strong antioxidant activity due to their high contents of phenolic compounds and tocopherols [10]. Balm oil anti-diabetic and antioxidant activity reported earlier [11]. It was reported that some component of essential oil obtained from Melissia officinalis such as monoterpene aldehydes, ketones (neral/geranial, citronellal, isomenthone, and menthone) and mono- and sesquiterpene hydrocarbons (E-caryophyllene) poses free radical scavengering properties [10].

Neuroprotective effect of this plant was investigated earlier by using an *in vitro* cellular model with PC12 cell line, which was a hydrogen peroxide induced toxicity system [7]. We have reported earlier that aqueous extract of Melissa can provide neuroprotection against ecstasy induced neurotoxicity in hippocampal primary culture [12]. Recently it has been reported that oral administration of *Melissa officinalis* can increase cell proliferation and differentiation by decreasing serum corticosterone levels as well as by increasing GABA levels in the mouse dentate gyrus [13]. Infusion of lemon balm (*Melissa officinalis*) leaf for 30 days in radiology staffs exposed to low-dose ionizing radiation (x-ray) can improve oxidative stress condition and DNA damage [9].

Although several reports have been published on *Melissa officinalis*, there is no reported information, to our knowledge, regarding the *in vivo* neuroprotection properties of this plant. Studies on neurological and neuroprotective properties of *Melissa officinalis* may demonstrate the effects of this plant on the central nervous system as well as to elucidate the mechanisms involved in the activity.

The present study was carried out to examine the protective effect of Melissa in an *in vitro* hypoxia model and also the protective ability of administration before and after ischemia followed by reperfusion in hippocampal neurons as an *in vivo* model.

Methods

Cell culturing and treatment

Primary neuronal cultures were prepared from gestation day 15 / 16 mouse embryos (Balb c) and cultured as described previously [14]. All procedures were performed in accordance with local institutional guidelines for animal care and use.

Our procedure typically yields cultures that contain > 90% neurons and < 10% supporting cells. Neuronal purity was assessed by incubation with rabbit anti-MAP2 polyclonal antibody (Abcam,1:300 dilution) overnight at 4°C, followed by FITC-labeled goat anti-rabbit antibody (Abcam, 1:1000 dilution) for 1 h at room temperature, Hoechst 33342 counterstaining (1:10000 dilution) for 10 minutes, and cover slipping in Mowiol mounting media (Sigma, Germany).

Cultures were maintained at 37°C in a humidified atmosphere containing 95% air–5% CO2 for 7 days. Prior to experiments, the medium was replaced by supplemented neurobasal medium after 24 h and changed every 3 days after.

Treatment with melissa and hypoxia

Balm Oil (B4008 Sigma, Germany) was serially diluted in serum free medium. Cultures were pretreated with Melissa for 2 h in normal incubator (95% air i.e., ~21% O2 –5% CO2 equilibrated to 37°C and 95% humidity) as normoxia incubator before their transfer in to hypoxia incubator (90% N2–5% CO2 and 5% O2 equilibrated to 37°C and 95% humidity) for 24 h [15]. After 24 h of hypoxia, cultures were removed from the hypoxic chamber, and were returned to normoxia incubator for another 4 h reperfusion period until analysis.

MTS/LDH assay

Cell membrane integrity was determined by lactate dehydrogenase (LDH) using CytoTox-ONE™ Homogeneous Membrane Integrity Assay according to the manufacturer's instructions (Promega, Germany). Two vials per experiment were treated 2 h with 2μl lysis solution containing Triton X-100 as positive control. Having no background from mediums containing Melissa was assured by reading their absorption with 492nm - 620nm filters which were near zero (Data not shown).

Cell viability was determined by MTS using One Solution Cell Proliferation Assay according to the manufacturer's instructions (Promega, Germany).

Propidium Iodide (PI) /Hoechst staining and fixation

Cell death was determined by 4 h incubation of cultures in medium containing 4 μl/ml PI (500μg/ml) (Sigma, Germany) before fixation. Viable neurons with sufficient cell membrane integration could pump PI out hence late apoptotic and necrotic cells could not do that and in this experiment are presented as PI positive neurons. Cells were then fixed with 4% formaldehyde for 15 minutes. Staining was done in darkness to prevent bleaching. A repeat count of necrotic cells was performed, the cells were kept at 4°C in PBS overnight, and then necrotic cells were again counted. This provided an index of the preservation of the PI stain after fixation. Hoechst 33342 0.1 μg/ml (Sigma, Germany) staining was done for 10 min after fixation in order to normalize PI positive neurons to the total number of nuclei in the field which were stained with Hoechst. Cells were visualized using an Axioskop 2 plus microscope (Carl Zeiss, Germany) with a 40× phase contrast water immersion objective, and images captured using an AxioCam HRc camera controlled by AxioVision software.

Preparation of *in vivo* ischemia model and drug administration

All *in vivo* experiments were performed on male Sprague–Dawley (250 to 280 g) rats. Before the induction of transient cerebral ischemia, rats were anaesthetized with chloral-hydrate (350 mg/kg, i.p.) and the body temperature was maintained at 37±0.5°C throughout the procedure with the use of a heating pad. A midline incision was made on the ventral side of the neck to expose the common carotid arteries. The common carotid arteries were isolated from vagus nerves and clamped with non-traumatic aneurysm clips [16]. Sham-operated control rats underwent the same procedure, but without common carotid artery occlusion. The surgery was accompanied by a 100% survival rate following common carotid occlusion. Carotid artery blood flow was reperfused by releasing the clips following 20 minutes occlusion. The average duration of operation was about 30 minutes.

Plant material diluted with physiological saline to obtain a final concentration of 10%. To find out the most effective dose of M. officinalis we used several dosage (50, 100, 200 and 400 mg/kg) of plant material [13]. In order to dose response data, 100 mg/kg of plant material was selected (Data not shown). 100 mg/kg Melissa was gavaged orally using the gavage needle every day for two weeks before operation as pretreatment and also continued after ischemia in different reperfusion time points. Animal groups were three: sham-operated group also considered as control, vehicle-treated group and Melissa treated group.

Caspase-3 assay

To recognize the *in vivo* neuroprotective properties of *Melissa officinalis*, we examined caspase-3-like activity at different time periods after ischemia. Fluorometric assay kit for caspase-3 activity (BD Pharmingen™) was used according to manufacturer's instruction. Rats were killed, brains were removed and both hippocampi were rapidly dissected out on ice, were minced with scissors, and homogenized in ice-cold lysis buffer containing 10 mM Tris–HCl; 10 mM NaH2PO4/NaHPO4 (pH 7.5);

130 mM NaCl; 1% TritonR-X-100; 10 mM NaPPi (sodium pyrophosphate). Lysates were centrifuged (14000 rpm, 10 min, 4°C) and the supernatants were taken and kept in –80°C for further use. Protein concentration was measured using Bradford protein assay [17]. 100 μg total protein was incubated for 1 h at 37°C with reaction buffer [40 mM HEPES (pH 7.5); 20% glycerol; 4 mM DTT] and the fluorogenic substrate Ac-DEVD-AMC [N-acetyl-Asp-Glu-Val-Asp-AMC (7-amino-4-methylcoumarin)]. The amount of 7-amino-4-methylcoumarin liberated from the Ac-DEVD-AMC fluorogenic peptide via the action of caspase-3 was measured on a spectrofluorometer with an excitation wavelength of 380 nm and an emission wavelength of 420 nm.

In situ labeling of DNA fragmentation

TUNEL methodology was used to assess neuronal cell death in the CA1 (Cornu Ammonis) region of the hippocampus. Hence it takes 2–3 days for the neuronal damage of CA1 to become morphologically obvious, cresyl violet and TUNEL staining were done at day 5 after reperfusion. Apoptosis occurring *in vivo* was assessed by TUNEL labeling [18]. An in situ cell death detection kit (Roche, Germany) was used to carry out TUNEL staining on sections according to the manufacturer's instructions. Staining was visualized with diaminobenzidine. Each group contained 7 animals and from each animal 3 sections stained. The number of surviving neurons and TUNEL-positive cells per millimeter linear length in the CA1 region [18,19] of the dorsal hippocampus was counted by an investigator who was blinded to the experimental conditions.

RT-PCR

Expression of HIF- α, TNF-α and IL1-β are increased after permanent or transient cerebral ischemia [20-23]. Although anti-inflammatory strategies to attenuate ischemic brain injury have been inadequate, we carried out to examine the gene expression of HIF-1α, IL-1β and TNF-α after ischemia and anti-inflammatory properties of *Melissa officinalis*.

After 20 minutes ischemia and two days reperfusion, animals were sacrificed by decapitation, brains were removed rapidly, and hippocampi were dissected quickly, placed in RNA later RNA Stabilization Reagent (Qiagen, Germany) over night at 4°C and finally stored at –80°C until used. Total RNA was extracted using the RNeasy Mini Spin Columns Collection Tubes (Qiagen, Germany). Reverse transcription was done using the RT-PCR technology according to manual instruction (Bioneer, South Korea). Using specific primer sets (Table 1), aliquots of cDNA were amplified by a PCR machine (Peqlab, Germany), with initial denaturation at 94°C for 5 min, followed by 30 cycles of denaturation at 94°C for 30 s,

Table 1 Primers used for RT-PCR, F, forward sequence; R, reverse sequence, and primer source

Gene	Annealing temperature (°C)	Product size (bp)	Sequence (5'–3')	accession number
HIF-1α	61	197	F TCAAGTCAGCAACGTGGAAG	[GenenBank:024359.1]
			R TATCGAGGCTGTGTCGACTG	
IL1-b	60	209	F CTGTGACTCGTGGGATGATG	[GenenBank:031512.2]
			R GGGATTTTGTCGTTGCTTGT	
TNF-α	60	209	F CTCCCAGAAAAGCAAGCAAC	[GenenBank:012675.3]
			R CGAGCAGGAATGAGAAGAGG	
GAPDH	59	161	F CATCACCATCTTCCAGGAGCGAGA	[GenenBank:017008.3]
			R CAGCGGAAGGGGCGGAGA	

annealing at variable primer-specific temperatures for 30 s, 45 s for extension at 72°C, and a further 5 min final extension at 72°C on completion of the cycles. Cycle optimization was performed for each primer set before PCR. The amplified products were subjected to 1% (W/V) agarose gel for electrophoresis, stained with ethidium bromide, then observed and photographed under an ultraviolet lamp in a gel imaging system. PCR product bands were analyzed with the ImageJ 1.440 software (National Health Institute, USA), ratios of each target gene to that of the house-keeping gene GAPDH (glyceraldehyde-3-phosphate dehydrogenase) was taken as the semiquantitative results of the samples.

Determination of Trolox Equivalent Antioxidant Capacity (TEAC)

Oxidative damage in the ischemic animals was measured by the level of antioxidant capacity in the tissue homogenates. Tissue homogenates TEAC was determined by its ability to inhibition of peroxidase-mediated formation of the 2,2'-azino-bis-3-ethylbenzthiozoline-6-sulfonate (ABTS$^{.+}$) radical [24]. 50 µL of samples were loaded onto respective wells on the 96-well microplate. 200 µL Chromagen (ABTS) (Sigma-Aldrich Inc., USA) was then added to these wells and the mixture left to react at 25°C for 6 minutes before reading the absorbance at 750 nm using the Bio-Rad Benchmark Plus Microplate Reader. The capacity of the homogenate antioxidant to inhibit ABTS oxidation was compared to the water-soluble vitamin E analogue (trolox) (Sigma-Aldrich Inc., USA). The TEAC values were determined from the trolox standard curve. Results were expressed as millimoles per trolox equivalents per liter of homogenate. TEAC values were taken as the total antioxidant capacity in the tissue homogenates samples of the animals.

Assay for thiobarbituric acid reactive substances (TBARS)

Oxidative damage in the ischemic animals was measured by the level of malondialdehyde (MDA) formed in the tissue homogenates. MDA levels in hippocampal tissue were determined according to the method of Ohkawa et al. [25]. Briefly, the hippocampus was homogenized in cold 0.1M phosphate buffer (pH 7.4) to make a 10% homogenate. Then homogenates were centrifuged for 30 min at 3000×g at 4°C. An aliquot of supernatant was added to a reaction mixture containing 100µl of 8.1% sodium dodecyl sulphate, 750µl of 20% acetic acid (pH 3.5), 750µl of 0.8% thiobarbituric acid and 300µl distilled water. Samples were then boiled for 1 h at 95°C and centrifuged at 4000×g for 10 min. The absorbance of the supernatant was measured spectrophotometrically at 532nm and results were expressed as nanomoles of MDA per mg of protein.

Statistical analysis

The values are expressed as mean ± standard deviation (SD). The results were computed statistically (Graphpad Prism 5.0) using t test.

Degrees of significance were assessed by three different rating values: $P<0.05$ = *(significant), $P<0.01$ = ** (highly significant), and $P<0.001$ = *** (extremely significant). For clarity, data in figures are expressed relative to their respective controls.

Results
Cortical neuronal viability after hypoxia

Almost all types of CNS cells appear to be vulnerable to hypoxia, including astrocytes, microglia and neurons, although regional and cellular differences with respect to exposure time may also be considerable. In a first step, we aimed to analyze the vulnerability of cortical neurons to a given hypoxia percent and exposure duration. Cell viability was assessed by lactate dehydrogenase (LDH) release in the culture supernatant and metabolic activity of cells by 3-(4,5-dimethylthiazol-2-yl)-5-(3-carboxy methoxyphenyl)-2-(4-sulfophenyl)-2H-tetrazolium) (MTS) in adherent neurons. As shown in Figure 1 hypoxia induced a significant increasein LDH activity in the supernatant. This was paralleled by a decrease in corresponding metabolic activity by MTS assay. After 24 h of 5% hypoxia

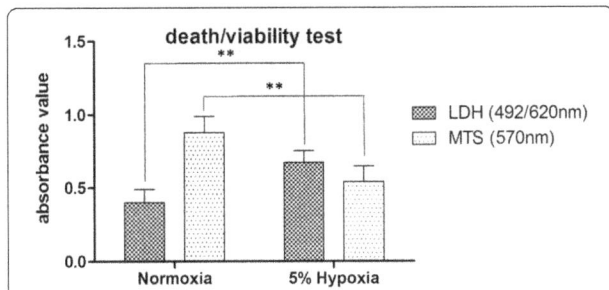

Figure 1 MTS/LDH release in normoxic and hypoxic conditions. Hypoxia induced by 5% oxygen for 24h and followed by 4h reperfusion in normal condition. Results are given in absorbance values to control groups which were all the time in normoxia condition. LDH release is increased and MTS activity is decreased significantly in hypoxic condition. **P< 0.01, vs. normoxia.

administration and 4 h reperfusion the viability of cortical neurons observed to have declined by approximately 55% (P< 0.01, vs.normoxia), as indicated by a massive increase in LDH activity. Metabolic activity was also decreased around 20% (P< 0.01, vs.normoxia), as shown by MTS absorbance in Figure 1.

Dose response of cortical neurons to M. Officinalis
In this step, we intended to see the response of cortical neurons to different concentrations of Melissa. For this purpose we did a set of LDH and MTS assays in normoxic condition in order to find the suitable dose of Melissa for further administration in hypoxic condition. As shown in Figure 2 there was no change in MTS activity or LDH release in low concentrations (5, 10 and

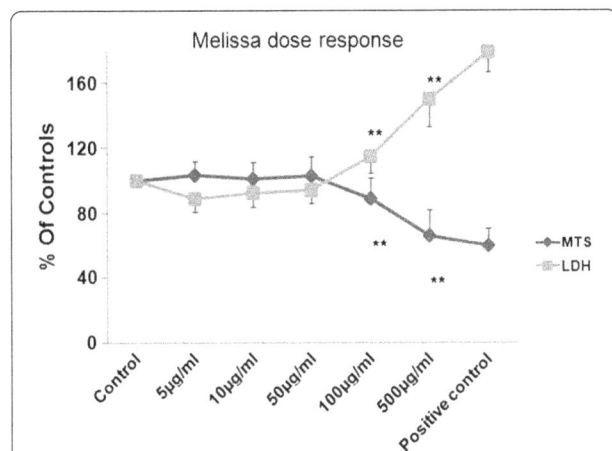

Figure 2 Melissa dose response in normoxia condition. There is no change in MTS activity or LDH release in low concentrations (5, 10 and 50 μg/ml) of Melissa in normoxic condition while higher concentrations (100 and 500 μg/ml) cause significant decrease in neuronal viability which is seen in MTS reduction and LDH increase. Results are given as a relation of both MTS and LDH values to their controls which were in normoxia condition.**P< 0.01, vs. control or normoxia.

50 μg/ml) of Melissa in normoxic condition compared to control group. But higher concentrations (100 and 500 μg/ml) were seemed to be toxic and caused significant decrease in metabolic activity (P< 0.05, vs. control) (Figure 2).

Protective effects of M. Officinalis during hypoxia *in vitro*
A 24h hypoxia exposure followed by 4h reperfusion resulted in an approximately half maximal decline in cell viability; this protocol was used for all further experiments. To recognize the protective properties of Melissa on neuronal hypoxia induced death, neurons were treated with neurobasal medium containing 10 μg/ml concentration of Melissa. As shown in Figure 3, PI positive cortical neurons increased significantly after hypoxia protocol comparing to normoxia (a and b) and single dose of Melissa significantly reduced PI positive cell count comparing to cultures exposed to hypoxia without any treatment (b and c) (P< 0.05, vs. hypoxia controls).

Caspase-3 activity assay
After 20 minutes ischemia followed byseveral time pointsof reperfusion, caspase-3like activity in the hippocampus was increased significantly (Figure 4) (P< 0.01, vs. controls animals).

At day 3 caspase-3 activity as seen in Figure 4 was at highest level. On the basis of the above mentioned result and also a recent similar study [26], we assessed the effect of *in vivo* treatment with *Melissa officinalis* on the caspase-3like protease activity at day 3of reperfusion. Treatment with 100 mg/kg of Melissa oilattenuated the increased caspase-3 like protease activity significantly (P< 0.05, vs.ischemia group) (Figure 4).

In situ labeling of DNA fragmentation
TUNEL staining revealed that many TUNEL-positive neurons were present in the hippocampal CA1 region of ischemic rats (Figure 5b). Few TUNEL-positive cells were found in the CA1 region of sham operated rats (Figure 5a). The number of TUNEL-positive cells was reduced by treatment with plant material (Figure 5c).

Cresyl violet staining revealed extensive neuronal loss in the CA1 region of ischemic rats (Figure 5e). No cell damage was evident by the cresyl violet staining in the CA1 region of sham-operated rats (Figure 5d). Hippocampal neuronal damage was decreased by treatment with 100mg/kg Melissa administration (Figure 5f).

RT-PCR
Expression of HIF- α, TNF-αand IL1-β are increased after permanent or transient cerebral ischemia [21-23]. We further examined the expression of HIF-1α, TNF-α and IL1-β after ischemia and when treated with Melissa in the ischemic rat brain. On the basis of similar studies

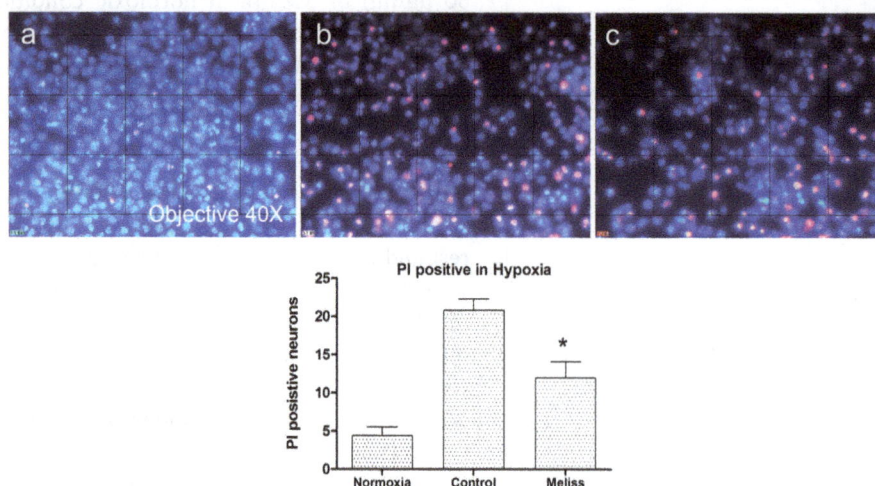

Figure 3 PI positive neurons in normoxia (a), hypoxia (b) and 10 μg/ml treatment of melissa (c). Total number of PI positive neurons is higher than hypoxic groupafter Melissa treatment (b and c). PI positive neurons (red) were counted and normalized to all cells counterstained with Hoechst (blue).*P< 0.05, vs. control.

[27,28] 2days after induction of ischemic brain injury, expression of HIF- α, TNF-α and IL1-β were measured. As shown in Figure 6, mRNA expressions of HIF-1α, TNF-α and IL1-β were up-regulated after ischemia/ reperfusion injury (p < 0.01). Melissa (100 mg/kg) treatment suppressed the expression of HIF-1α in the ischemic hippocampus (P<0.05) while TNF-α and IL1- β expression have not been decreased significantly (Figure 6).

Lipid peroxidation and antioxidant capacity

In ischemic animals, on the basis of a recent similar study, MDA level and antioxidant status in hippocampus measured at day 2of reperfusion [18]. MDA level increased after 2 days of reperfusion. In balm oil treated (100 mg/kg) ischemic animals MDA level was significantly lower than sham operated animals (P< 0.01) (Figure 7).

The antioxidant status was assessed by studying the level of TEAC in the tissue homogenates. A lowered

antioxidant defense system in ischemic animals compared to the sham operated animals is noted. At day 2 of reperfusion TEAC concentrations in tissue homogenates of ischemic animals were lower than sham operated animals. In balm oil treated (100 mg/kg) ischemic animals the level of TEAC was significantly higher than ischemic animals (p < 0.05) (Figure 7).

Discussion

Increasing evidence has indicated that production of free radicals after cerebral ischemia and reperfusion, caused oxidative stress which is involved in ischemic brain damage [29]. During ischemia and especially reperfusion, free radicals are expected to attack lipids and proteins of the cell membrane and DNA [30]. Novel therapeutic neuroprotective strategies support the applications of ROS scavengers and induction of endogenous antioxidants, such as natural antioxidants, for example plant derived

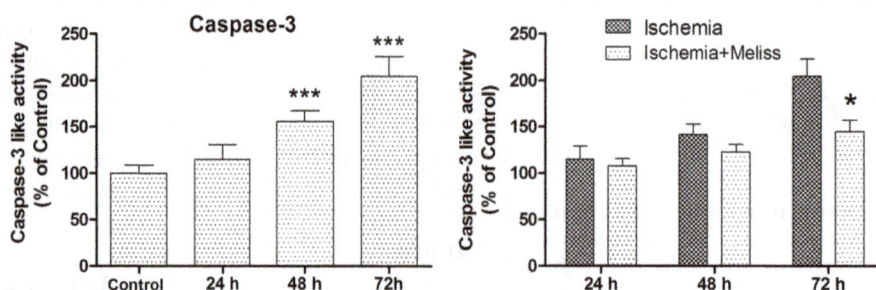

Figure 4 Caspase-3-like activity. Left: Temporal profiles of caspase-3-like activity in the hippocampus after transient ischemia. Results are given in % of control group absorbance value. Significant increase in caspase-3 activity is observed after 48h and 72h reperfusion. ***p < 0.001, vs. control animals(n=8). Right: Treatment with 100 mg/kg of *Melissa officinalis* attenuated the increased caspase-3 like protease activity. *P< 0.05, vs. ischemia group (n=11).

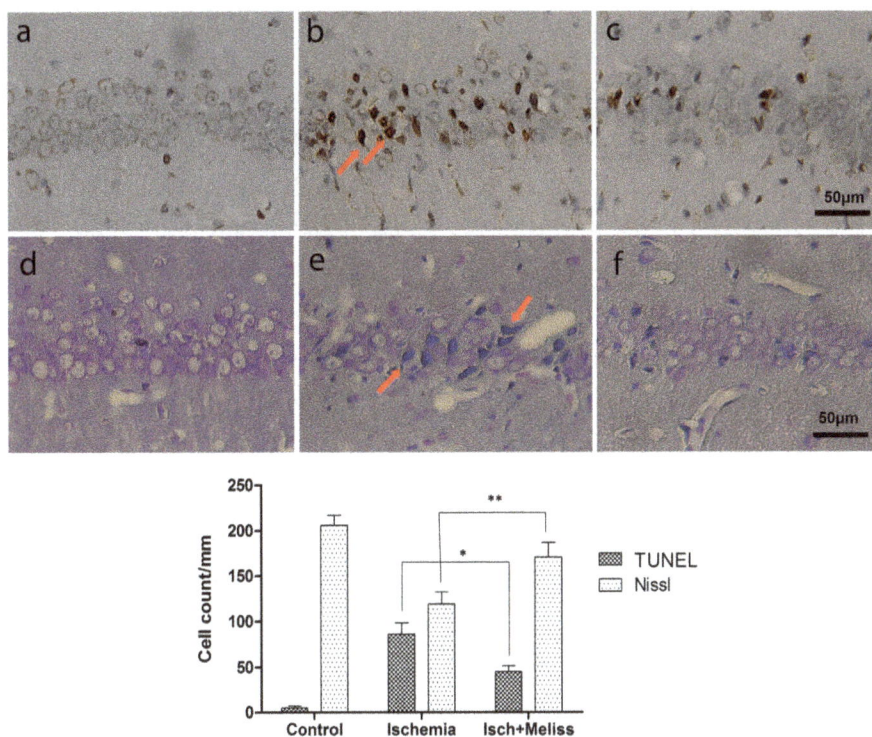

Figure 5 Micrographs of TUNEL-positive cells and cresyl-violet stained cells. Representative micrographs of TUNEL-positive cells (dark brown) (**a–c**) and cresyl-violet stained cells (**d–f**) in the hippocampal CA1 region from sham (**a** and **d**); ischemic (**b** and **e**); Melissa-treated animals (**c** and **f**) at 5 days of reperfusion. Scale bar: 50μm. Graph shows the comparison of apoptotic (TUNEL-positive) and surviving (Nissel positive) neurons between groups. *p < 0.05, **p < 0.01 compared with ischemia group (n=7).

polyphenolic compounds, for the treatment of neurodegenerative diseases [18,31,32]. It is known that some compounds of *Melissa officinalis* have antioxidant activity which is due to its free Radical Scavenging Capacity (RSC) [33]. Antioxidant activity of Melissa has previously been reported in different studies [8,33-35]. In addition it is reported that this plant has protective effect on hydrogen peroxide induced toxicity in PC12 cells which have some characteristics of neurons [7], but the protective effects in primary culture of neurons after hypoxic stress have never been reported. In this study, 24 h exposure of primary cortical neurons to 5% hypoxia followed by 4 h reperfusion reduced both cell viability and metabolic activity to around 55% and 20%, respectively. This could be considered as an approval on hypoxia system. Hoechst/PI staining of neurons showed that 10 μg/ml concentration of Melissa could significantly reduce cell death. Although, analysis of dose response results showed that high doses (100–500 μg/ml) could worsen the condition with500 μg/ml dose as half maximal inhibitory concentration (IC_{50}) of Melissa. These results suggest that some concentrations of Melissa have protective activities in neurons and may keep them safe from oxidative stress. *In vitro* results lead us to postulate the hypothesis that Melissa could have some protective

effects on neurons in the brain. Therefore, we examined its effects in ischemic model of brain injury as *in vivo* model. Investigations showed that after induction of ischemia, Caspase-3 activity in hippocampus significantly increased, and there were many TUNEL positive neurons in CA1 area. TUNEL is a common method for detecting DNA fragmentation that results from apoptotic signalling cascades. The assay relies on the presence of nicks in the DNA which can be identified by terminal deoxynucleotidyl transferase or TdT, an enzyme that will catalyse the addition of dUTPs that are secondarily labelled with a marker. It may also label cells that have suffered severe DNA damage.

Mechanisms leading to DNA fragmentation following ischemia may not be clear but a specific DNase, caspase-activated DNase (CAD) that cleaves chromosomal DNA appears to be an important enzyme in apoptotic cell death. CAD is generally found as a complex with ICAD (inhibitor of CAD) which serves to limit its DNase activity. After initiation of apoptosis signals, caspases, in particular caspase-3, cleave ICAD to dissociate CAD from ICAD, thereby allowing CAD to cleave chromosomal DNA [36]. So we investigate both caspase-3 activity and DNA fragmentation. This could suggest that Melissa provided neuroprotection against cerebral I/R injury in

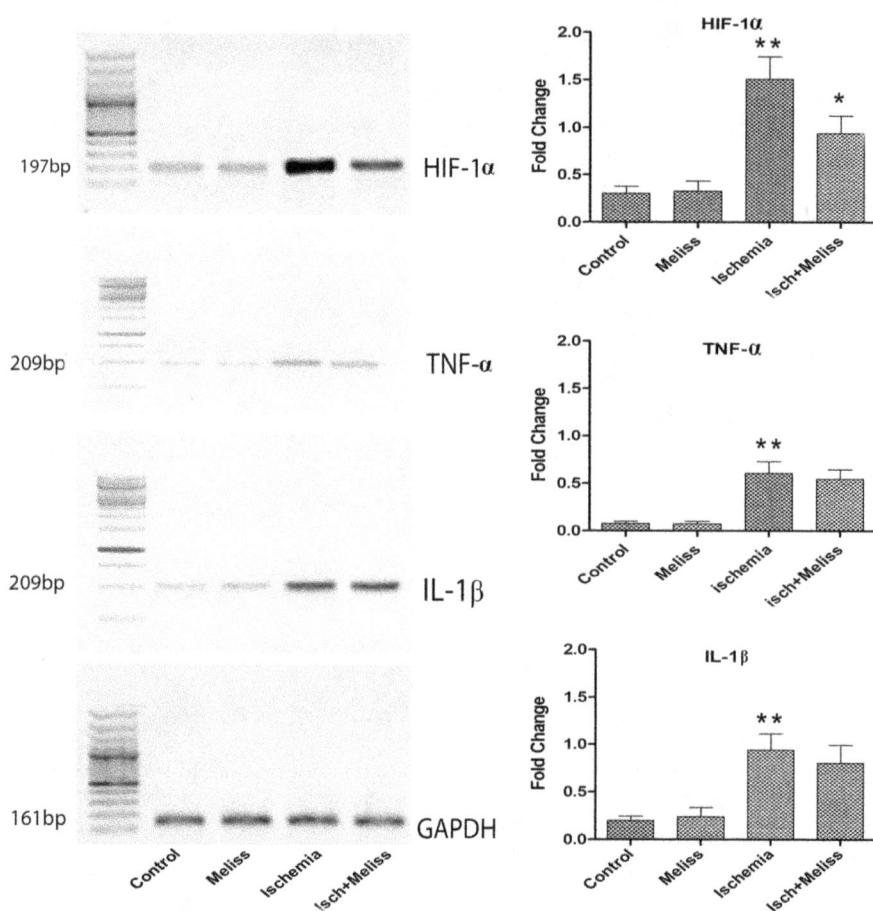

Figure 6 RT-PCR analysis of HIF-1α, TNF-α and IL-1β gene expression in the hippocampus of ischemic rats after ischemia. 100 mg/kg treatment of Melissa significantly suppressed the expression of HIF-1α in the ischemic hippocampus (P<0.05) while TNF-α and IL1-β expression have not been significantly decrease (n=8).

the rat brain. These results were consistent with our *in vitro* study and this is the first time that shows protective activity for *Melissa officinalis* after brain ischemia.

In present study, the increased MDA and decreased antioxidant defense system in the hippocampus of the

ischemic group as compared to the sham group suggests a state of enhanced oxidative stress in ischemia–reperfusion injury. Apoptotic cell death occurs in response to various stimuli including oxidative stress [37]. The brain is very vulnerable to oxidative stress due

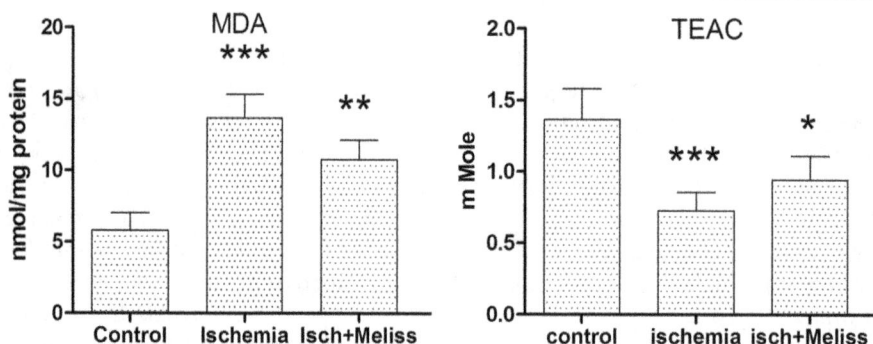

Figure 7 Lipid Peroxidation and Antioxidant Capacity. Left: Comparison of the level of MDA (left) and TEAC (right) inthe hippocampus of sham operated, ischemic and *Melissa officinalis* treated ischemic animals. Treatment with 100 mg/kg of Melissa decreased the elevated MDA levels in the hippocampus (**p < 0.01) and attenuates decrease of antioxidant status of ischemic animals (*p < 0.05) (n = 8 each).

to its high polyunsaturated fatty acid (PUFA) content, which is particularly susceptible to ROS damage [38]. During ischemia, superoxide anions and hydrogen peroxide form and cannot be readily scavenged. Lipid peroxidation (LPO) is one of the important markers of oxidative damage in the ischemic cascade as PUFA constitutes a major component of brain, which results in the formation of lipid peroxides, and may affect a variety of cellular functions involving proteins namely: receptors, signal transduction mechanisms, transport systems and enzymes [39]. Treatment of ischemic rats with Melissa significantly inhibited MDA level and attenuated decrease of antioxidant capacity in the hippocampus. It is well documented that attenuating oxidative stress is important in evolving neuroprotective strategies for enhanced neuronal survival after cerebral ischemia [18]. We suggest that some components of plant material that have antioxidative properties can attenuate oxidative damage induced by ischemic brain injury.

Ischemic brain injury induced increase in HIF-1α, IL-1β and TNF-α mRNA level, this can represent the inflammatory response of neuronal or glial cells suffering from the ischemic insult. It is demonstrated that expression of HIF-1α and HIF-1β mRNA in rat and mouse has been up-regulated in ischemic brain injury [23]. In this study, showed that the elevation of active caspase-3 expression occurred as well as HIF-1α expression after ischemic injury, and these events could be significantly suppressed by treatment with Balm oil. Hypoxia can cause HIF-1α to bind with p53 in order to stabilize it, and also activates the expression of various genes, including bax. In this study, plant material can down-regulate the transcription of HIF-1α during hippocampal ischemia and inhibit caspase-3 activation. Proinflammatory and immunomodulatory cytokines like TNF-α, IL-1β and IL-6 mRNA level increases after focal ischemia [22], implicating that these cytokines can develop ischemic brain injury. Gene expression of TNF-α and IL-1β, after cerebral ischemia is up-regulated. Treatment of ischemic animals with Melissa did not effectively inhibit mRNA expression of TNF-α and IL-1β, indicating that the inhibition of TNF-α and IL-1β might not be the neuroprotective mechanism for plant materialin ischemic brain injury.

Conclusions

In conclusion, results implicate that *Melissa officinalis* has shown protective effect on ischemic damage mediated by the inhibition of HIF-1α and oxidative stress, followed by the inhibition of apoptosis.

These results propose the potential use of *Melissa officinalis* or its constituents for central nervous system diseases and as a neuroprotective agent to prevent disorders involved with oxidative stress. Experiments are necessary to identify which of the plant components are responsible for these activities.

Competing interest
The authors have no financial interest to declare. There is no conflict of interest to declare.

Authors' contributions
GH designed the study. MB, AAT, MHG, MA, SEM, MK, performed the experiments and analyses. MB and AAT wrote the paper. All authors read and approved the final manuscript.

Acknowledgements
This study was supported by Tehran University of Medical Sciences and Health Services, Tehran, Iran (grant No. 7862-30-04-87).

Author details
[1]Department of Anatomy, School of Medicine, Tehran University of Medical Sciences, Tehran, Iran. [2]Anatomical Sciences Research Center, Kashan University of Medical Sciences, Kashan, Iran. [3]Department of Toxicology - Pharmacology, School of Pharmacy, Tehran University of Medical Sciences, Tehran, Iran. [4]Department of Pharmacology, School of Medicine, Tehran University of Medical Sciences, Tehran, Iran. [5]Department of Pharmacognosy, School of Pharmacy, Tehran University of Medical Sciences, Tehran, Iran. [6]Department of Neuroscience, School of Advanced Medical Technology, Tehran University of Medical Sciences, Tehran, Iran.

References
1. Kuroda S, Siesjo BK: Reperfusion damage following focal ischemia: pathophysiology and therapeutic windows. *Clin Neurosci* 1997, 4:199–212.
2. Petito CK, Feldmann E, Pulsinelli WA, Plum F: Delayed hippocampal damage in humans following cardiorespiratory arrest. *Neurology* 1987, 37:1281–1286.
3. Northington FJ, Ferriero DM, Graham EM, Traystman RJ, Martin LJ: Early Neurodegeneration after Hypoxia-Ischemia in Neonatal Rat Is Necrosis while Delayed Neuronal Death Is Apoptosis. *Neurobiol Dis* 2001, 8:207–219.
4. Kirino T: Delayed neuronal death in the gerbil hippocampus following ischemia. *Brain Res* 1982, 239:57–69.
5. Huang J, Upadhyay UM, Tamargo RJ: Inflammation in stroke and focal cerebral ischemia. *Surg Neurol* 2006, 66:232–245.
6. del Zoppo GJ, Becker KJ, Hallenbeck JM: Inflammation after stroke: is it harmful? *Arch Neurol* 2001, 58:669–672.
7. Lopez V, Martin S, Gomez-Serranillos MP, Carretero ME, Jager AK, Calvo MI: Neuroprotective and neurological properties of *Melissa officinalis*. *Neurochem Res* 2009, 34:1955–1961.
8. Pereira RP, Fachinetto R, de Souza Prestes A, Puntel RL, da Silva GN S, Heinzmann BM, Boschetti TK, Athayde ML, Burger ME, Morel AF, et al: Antioxidant effects of different extracts from *Melissa officinalis*, Matricaria recutita and Cymbopogon citratus. *Neurochem Res* 2009, 34:973–983.
9. Zeraatpishe A, Oryan S, Bagheri MH, Pilevarian AA, Malekirad AA, Baeeri M, Abdollahi M: Effects of *Melissa officinalis* L. on oxidative status and DNA damage in subjects exposed to long-term low-dose ionizing radiation. *Toxicol Ind Health* 2011, 27:205–212.
10. Mimica-Dukic N, Bozin B, Sokovic M, Simin N: Antimicrobial and antioxidant activities of *Melissa officinalis* L. (Lamiaceae) essential oil. *J Agric Food Chem* 2004, 52:2485–2489.
11. Chung MJ, Cho SY, Bhuiyan MJ, Kim KH, Lee SJ: Anti-diabetic effects of lemon balm (*Melissa officinalis*) essential oil on glucose- and lipid-regulating enzymes in type 2 diabetic mice. *Br J Nutr* 2010, 104:180–188.
12. Hassanzadeh GH, Pasbakhsh P, Akbari M, Shokri S, Ghahremani M, Amin GH, Kashani I, Azami Tameh A: Neuroprotective Properties of *Melissa officinalis* L. Extract Against Ecstasy-Induced Neurotoxicity. *CELL JOURNAL(Yakhteh)* 2011, 13:25–30.
13. Yoo DY, Choi JH, Kim W, Yoo KY, Lee CH, Yoon YS, Won MH, Hwang IK: Effects of *Melissa officinalis* L. (lemon balm) extract on neurogenesis associated with serum corticosterone and GABA in the mouse dentate gyrus. *Neurochem Res* 2011, 36:250–257.

14. Lorenz L, Dang J, Misiak M: **Tameh Abolfazl A, Beyer C, Kipp M: Combined 17beta-oestradiol and progesterone treatment prevents neuronal cell injury in cortical but not midbrain neurones or neuroblastoma cells.** *J Neuroendocrinol* 2009, 21:841–849.

15. Weiss J, Goldberg MP, Choi DW: **Ketamine protects cultured neocortical neurons from hypoxic injury.** *Brain Res* 1986, 380:186–190.

16. Dos-Anjos S, Martinez-Villayandre B, Montori S, Regueiro-Purrinos MM, Gonzalo-Orden JM, Fernandez-Lopez A: **Transient global ischemia in rat brain promotes different NMDA receptor regulation depending on the brain structure studied.** *Neurochem Int* 2009, 54:180–185.

17. Bradford MM: **A rapid and sensitive method for the quantitation of microgram quantities of protein utilizing the principle of protein-dye binding.** *Anal Biochem* 1976, 72:248–254.

18. Liang HW, Qiu SF, Shen J, Sun LN, Wang JY, Bruce IC, Xia Q: **Genistein attenuates oxidative stress and neuronal damage following transient global cerebral ischemia in rat hippocampus.** *Neurosci Lett* 2008, 438:116–120.

19. Zhang DL, Zhang YT, Yin JJ, Zhao BL: **Oral administration of Crataegus flavonoids protects against ischemia/reperfusion brain damage in gerbils.** *J Neurochem* 2004, 90:211–219.

20. Matrone C, Pignataro G, Molinaro P, Irace C, Scorziello A, Di Renzo GF, Annunziato L: **HIF-1alpha reveals a binding activity to the promoter of iNOS gene after permanent middle cerebral artery occlusion.** *J Neurochem* 2004, 90:368–378.

21. Chang Y, Hsiao G, Chen SH, Chen YC, Lin JH, Lin KH, Chou DS, Sheu JR: **Tetramethylpyrazine suppresses HIF-1alpha, TNF-alpha, and activated caspase-3 expression in middle cerebral artery occlusion-induced brain ischemia in rats.** *Acta Pharmacol Sin* 2007, 28:327–333.

22. Saito K, Suyama K, Nishida K, Sei Y, Basile AS: **Early increases in TNF-alpha, IL-6 and IL-1 beta levels following transient cerebral ischemia in gerbil brain.** *Neurosci Lett* 1996, 206:149–152.

23. Wiener CM, Booth G, Semenza GL: *In vivo* **expression of mRNAs encoding hypoxia-inducible factor 1.** *Biochem Biophys Res Commun* 1996, 225:485–488.

24. Miller NJ, Rice-Evans C, Davies MJ, Gopinathan V, Milner A: **A novel method for measuring antioxidant capacity and its application to monitoring the antioxidant status in premature neonates.** *Clin Sci (Lond)* 1993, 84:407–412.

25. Ohkawa H, Ohishi N, Yagi K: **Assay for lipid peroxides in animal tissues by thiobarbituric acid reaction.** *Anal Biochem* 1979, 95:351–358.

26. Su X, Zhu CL, Shi W, Ni LC, Shen JH, Chen J: **Transient global cerebral ischemia induces up-regulation of MLTKalpha in hippocampal CA1 neurons.** *J Mol Histol* 2011, 43:187–193.

27. Liu T, McDonnell PC, Young PR, White RF, Siren AL, Hallenbeck JM, Barone FC, Feurestein GZ: **Interleukin-1 beta mRNA expression in ischemic rat cortex.** *Stroke* 1993, 24:1746–1750. discussion 1750–1741.

28. Althaus J, Bernaudin M, Petit E, Toutain J, Touzani O, Rami A: **Expression of the gene encoding the pro-apoptotic BNIP3 protein and stimulation of hypoxia-inducible factor-1alpha (HIF-1alpha) protein following focal cerebral ischemia in rats.** *Neurochem Int* 2006, 48:687–695.

29. Traystman RJ, Kirsch JR, Koehler RC: **Oxygen radical mechanisms of brain injury following ischemia and reperfusion.** *J Appl Physiol* 1991, 71:1185–1195.

30. Mattson MP: **Modification of ion homeostasis by lipid peroxidation: roles in neuronal degeneration and adaptive plasticity.** *Trends Neurosci* 1998, 21:53–57.

31. Ishige K, Schubert D, Sagara Y: **Flavonoids protect neuronal cells from oxidative stress by three distinct mechanisms.** *Free Radic Biol Med* 2001, 30:433–446.

32. Mandel S, Youdim MB: **Catechin polyphenols: neurodegeneration and neuroprotection in neurodegenerative diseases.** *Free Radic Biol Med* 2004, 37:304–317.

33. Mencherini T, Picerno P, Scesa C, Aquino R: **Triterpene, antioxidant, and antimicrobial compounds from** *Melissa officinalis.* *J Nat Prod* 2007, 70:1889–1894.

34. Lopez V, Akerreta S, Casanova E, Garcia-Mina JM, Cavero RY, Calvo MI: *In vitro* **antioxidant and anti-rhizopus activities of Lamiaceae herbal extracts.** *Plant Foods Hum Nutr* 2007, 62:151–155.

35. Canadanovic-Brunet J, Cetkovic G, Djilas S, Tumbas V, Bogdanovic G, Mandic A, Markov S, Cvetkovic D, Canadanovic V: **Radical Scavenging, Antibacterial, and Antiproliferative Activities of** *Melissa officinalis* L. *Extracts. J Med Food* 2008, 11:133–143.

36. Liu Z, Zhao W, Xu T, Pei D, Peng Y: **Alterations of NMDA receptor subunits NR1, NR2A and NR2B mRNA expression and their relationship to apoptosis following transient forebrain ischemia.** *Brain Res* 2010, 1361:133–139.

37. Ramakrishnan N, McClain DE, Catravas GN: **Membranes as sensitive targets in thymocyte apoptosis.** *Int J Radiat Biol* 1993, 63:693–701.

38. Finkel T, Holbrook NJ: **Oxidants, oxidative stress and the biology of ageing.** *Nature* 2000, 408:239–247.

39. Parihar MS, Hemnani T: **Phenolic antioxidants attenuate hippocampal neuronal cell damage against kainic acid induced excitotoxicity.** *J Biosci* 2003, 28:121–128.

Preparation and evaluation of inhalable itraconazole chitosan based polymeric micelles

Esmaeil Moazeni[1], Kambiz Gilani[1*], Abdolhossein Rouholamini Najafabadi[1], Mohamad reza Rouini[2], Nasir Mohajel[1], Mohsen Amini[3] and Mohammad Ali Barghi[4]

Abstract

Background: This study evaluated the potential of chitosan based polymeric micelles as a nanocarrier system for pulmonary delivery of itraconazole (ITRA).

Methods: Hydrophobically modified chitosan were synthesized by conjugation of stearic acid to the hydrophilic depolymerized chitosan. FTIR and ^{1}HNMR were used to prove the chemical structure and physical properties of the depolymerized and the stearic acid grafted chitosan. ITRA was entrapped into the micelles and physicochemical properties of the micelles were investigated. Fluorescence spectroscopy, dynamic laser light scattering and transmission electron microscopy were used to characterize the physicochemical properties of the prepared micelles. The in vitro pulmonary profile of polymeric micelles was studied by an air-jet nebulizer connected to a twin stage impinger.

Results: The polymeric micelles prepared in this study could entrap up to 43.2 ± 2.27 µg of ITRA per milliliter. All micelles showed mean diameter between 120–200 nm. The critical micelle concentration of the stearic acid grafted chitosan was found to be 1.58×10^{-2} mg/ml. The nebulization efficiency was up to 89% and the fine particle fraction (FPF) varied from 38% to 47%. The micelles had enough stability to remain encapsulation of the drug during nebulization process.

Conclusions: In vitro data showed that stearic acid grafted chitosan based polymeric micelles has a potential to be used as nanocarriers for delivery of itraconazole through inhalation.

Keywords: Polymeric micelles, Itraconazole, Chitosan, Nebulization, Pulmonary drug delivery

Background

Invasive pulmonary fungal infection is major infectious disease among immunosuppressed patients. Difficulty of early clinical diagnosis and poor response to the common antifungal treatment result in high mortality percent of patients. In the recent years many efforts done to found an alternative drug delivery strategies for antifungal agents [1,2]. Aerosolization of antifungal agents can be used for prophylaxis against pulmonary fungal infections. High drug concentration in the site of infection, non invasive route of administration and reduce systemic toxicities are some advantages of this route of administration [3].

While amphotericin is an effective drug for treatment of fungal infections, its adverse effects reduces its potential uses and particular interest has been focused on the use of other antifungal drugs [4].

Itraconazole (ITRA), a triazole member, is a highly hydrophobic drug (water solublility ~1 ng/ml at neutral pH and 4 µg/ml at pH 1) [5] which has broad spectrum of activity against a number of fungal species [6].

Most of potent antifungal compounds like amphotericin and azoles have very low solubility. Approaches for achieving complete dissolution of ITRA often have disadvantages associated with large quantities of required excipients [7]. These strategies may cause some limitation due to the toxicity induced by high concentrations of the drug or excipients like 2-hydroxypropyl-β-cyclodexterin. Scientists have been used different strategies to obtain technologies which required lower amounts of

* Correspondence: gilani@tums.ac.ir
[1]Aerosol Research Laboratory, Department of Pharmaceutics, School of Pharmacy, Tehran University of Medical Sciences, Tehran, Iran
Full list of author information is available at the end of the article

excipients to increase the solubility. Various solid dispersion, emulsification and nanotechnology approaches have been widely used to increase the solubility of itraconazole. Akkar and Muller prepared intravenous itraconazole emulsion based on solEmuls technology. Using this technology, the drug localizes in the interfacial lecithin layer of the emulsions by homogenising a hybrid dispersion of oil droplets and drug nanocrystals in water [8]. Also Keck and Muller used modified high pressure hemogenisation technique (NANOEDGE) to prepare nanocrystals of poorly water soluble drugs like itraconazole [9]. Some studies based on evaporative precipitation into aqueous solution (EPAS) or spray freezing into liquid (SFL) techniques has been used to obtain nano itraconazole for pulmonary delivery systems [10-12]. McConville and co-workers nebulized itraconazole dispersion prepared by EPAS or SFL techniques and obtained high lung concentration in animal study [11].

Self-assembled polymeric micelles (PM) are widely investigated as an alternative choice in the development of delivery systems for poorly water soluble drugs. PMs are composed of different amphiphilic copolymers. The micelles prepared by these copolymers in the aqueous medium contain internal hydrophobic segments as drug reservoir and external hydrophilic segments as surrounding shell [13]. PMs based on chitosan, a natural biodegradable cationic polysaccharide [14], with various modification by different hydrophobic groups have been used for encapsulation of different hydrophobic drugs. Doxorubicin [15], camptothecin [16], all-trans retinoic acid [17] and paclitaxel [18] are some hydrophobic drugs that encapsulated by chitosan based polymeric micelles. There are only few reports investigating the application of inhalable polymeric micelles for delivery of all trans retinoic acid, amphotericin B and budesunide [19-21].

The ability of the modified chitosan polymeric micelles to improve ITRA solubility and pulmonary delivery of ITRA were investigated in this research. In current study, depolymerized chitosan (Mw 24 kDa) was chemically modified by stearic acid and its properties were characterized by ^{1}HNMR and FT-IR. In vitro nebulization parameters like fine particle fraction (FPF), nebulization efficiency (NE) and drug remained encapsulated in the micelles (DRE) after nebulization process were studied.

Methods
Materials
Itraconazole was kindly supplied by Hetero, India. Chitosan (Medium molecular weight, 95% deacetylated) was obtained from Primex, Iceland. Stearic acid, KCl, NaOH, glacial acetic acid, sodium nitrite, 1-ethyl-3-(3-dimethylaminopropyl) carbodiimide (EDC), diethylene amin (DEA), pyrene and all other solvents in analytical and HPLC grade were provided from Merck, Germany.

Depolymerization of chitosan
Chitosan was chemically depolymerized by sodium nitrite at room temperature according to Mao et al. pervious report [22]. Medium molecular weight chitosan was dissolved in 1% acetic acid and then appropriate amount of 0.1 M NaNO$_2$ was added at room temperature. The reaction was performed for 3 hrs under nitrogen gas. To precipitate depolymerized chitosan, the pH value of reaction was increased to about 8 with NaOH. The obtained chitosan after centrifugation was dialyzed (MWCO 8 kDa, Spectrum Laboratories, USA) against deionized water for 48 hrs and finally lyophilized (Christ, α2-4, Germany) at −80°C and 0.001 mbar pressure for 48 hrs. The molecular weight of obtained chitosan was determined by size exclusion chromatography using Knauer apparatus (Berlin, Germany) utilized with a PL Aquagel-OH Mixed column (25 mm ID 8 μm at 25°C) and a flow rate of 4 ml/min in acetate buffer medium (0.2 M acetic acid and 0.1 M sodium acetate with pH value of 4.6 ± 0.05) as diluent.

Synthesis and characterization of stearic acid grafted to depolymerized chitosan
Stearic acid grafted to depolymerized chitosan was synthesized as previously reported method [18]. Briefly, 30 ml aqueous solution of the depolymerized chitosan was prepared at concentration of 30 mg/ml. Stearic acid (50 mg/ml) and EDC (3 mol/mol stearic acid) were dissolved in absolute ethanol and the mixture was added to the chitosan solution under stirring at 80°C for 5 hrs and the reaction was stirred further 24 hrs at room temperature. The mixture then was dialyzed (8 kDa dialysis tube, Spectrum laboratories, USA) against distilled water containing 10% v/v ethanol for 48 hrs and finally the dialysis was continued against distilled water for 2 hrs. The final product was lyophilized (Christ, α2-4, Germany). FT-IR spectra were carried out using Nicolet (magna IR-550, USA) spectrometer by preparation of KBr disks. Bruker FT-500 ^{1}H NMR (Bruker, Germany) spectra were used to characterize and calculate the substitution degree of modified chitosan.

Critical micelle concentration (CMC) measurement
The fluorescence technique was used to measure the critical micelle concentration (CMC) of polymeric micelles, where pyrene was chosen as a fluorescence probe [23]. Pyrene (6×10^{-7} M) was added to each of a series of vials and then 10 ml of the modified chitosan solutions with various concentrations (250 ng/ml–2 mg/ml) were added. After 3 hrs stirring at room temperature, the fluorescence spectrum was obtained with a spectrofluorometer (Cecil

9000 series, England) and I_1 and I_3 were taken from the emission intensity of pyrene at 374 nm and 395 nm, respectively.

Preparation and characterization of ITRA micellar formulations

Different ITRA micellar formulations were prepared by film hydration procedure [18,24]. Briefly, 10 mg or 20 mg of the modified chitosan and an appropriate amount of ITRA (5% to 50% weight of the polymer) were added to 100 ml of dichloromethane in a 250 ml round-bottomed flask. The mixtures were sonicated using a bath sonicator (Starsonic60, Liarre, Italy) to obtain nearly clear dispersions, then the solvents were removed using a rotary evaporator (Buchi Rotavapor R-124, Buchi, Switzerland) at a reduced pressure at 60°C and 120 rpm to obtain thin films. To remove residual amount of the solvents, the films were placed in a vacuum oven (Memmert, VO400, Germany) at 40°C overnight. The dried thin films were hydrated with 10 ml of deionized water (Direct-Q® 3UV, Millipore, France) for 45 min at 50°C and 120 rpm.

Finally, the suspensions were sonicated for 2 min by a probe sonicator (UP400S, hielscher ultrasound technology, Germany) in ice-bath.

To measure ITRA entrapment efficiency (EE), the final dispersions were filtered through 0.22 μm Durapore® filters (MILLEX®-GV, Millipore, Ireland) and specified amounts of the filtrates were added to 8 ml of DMF:water (80:20). Measurement of ITRA concentration was carried out using an HPLC system (Waters 600E, Millipore, USA) equipped with a C18 column (4.6 mm×150 mm, 5 μm, teknokroma, Spain). The mobile phase consisting of acetonitrile, water, and diethyl amine (60:40:0.05, v/v) was delivered at a flow rate of 1 ml/min, while UV detection was utilized at 260 nm. The injection volume was 20 μl. The drug EE was calculated as a percentage value by dividing the amount of ITRA entrapped in the micelles to the initial amount of ITRA. The drug loading (DL) value obtained as percent ratio of the weight of ITRA loaded in the micelles to the total weights of the micelles. The particle size distribution and the zeta potential of polymeric micelle formulations were measured by a Zetasizer (Nano-ZS, Malvern Instruments Ltd., UK).

Nebulization efficacy of ITRA-loaded polymeric micelle formulations

Nebulization of the polymeric micelle formulations were done with an Air-jet nebulizer (Hudson®, UK). 5 ml of each formulation was placed into the nebulizer which was connected to the mouthpiece of a Twin stage impinger (TSI; Copley, UK) containing DMF/distilled water (3/1 vol.) in the stages 1 and 2. After connecting the TSI to a vacuum pump, the air flow (28.3 l/min) was

adjusted through the apparatus. Nebulization was ended when no aerosol was produced. After nebulization, the two chambers of TSI, its mouthpiece and the nebulizer were washed separately with DMF/distilled water (3/1 vol.). The total amount of the ITRA recovered from the two stages of TSI was defined as the emitted dose. Nebulization efficiency (NE) was calculated as the percentage of the ratio of the emitted dose to the initial amount of the drug poured into the nebulizer. Fine particle fraction (FPF) was determined by dividing the amount of ITRA recovered from the lower stage of TSI (fine particle dose; FPD) to the emitted dose and expressed as percentage. Drug remained encapsulated in the micelles (DRE) at the end of the nebulization process was determined with minimum change in the procedure which was used for determination of the nebulization efficiency. Briefly, distilled water was located in the upper and lower chambers of TSI. After collection of the nebulized micelles, half of the dispersion was diluted four times with DMF to determine the total amount of the drug emitted from the nebulizer. The other half was filtered through a syringe filter (0.45 μm) to separate the non-encapsulated drug. Then, the filtrate was diluted four times with DMF. The percent of ITRA remained in the micelles during nebulization was calculated by dividing the concentration of ITRA in the filtrate to the total amount of the drug emitted from the nebulizer, expressed as percentage.

In vitro release study

The in vitro release profile of ITRA from micelles were carried out by dialysis method [16].Briefly, 5 ml of each micellar formulation(5% drug percent ratio with 1 and 2 mg/ml of polymer concentration) was placed in a dialysis tube (Mwco 8 kDa, Spectrum laboratories, USA) which was immersed in 20 ml of PBS (pH 7.4) in a bath shaker at 37°C under mild agitation. At predetermined time intervals, the whole medium was taken out and the same volume of fresh medium replaced. The amount of ITRA released from the micelles was determined by the HPLC method which has been described before.

In vitro Anti fungal activity

ITRA minimal inhibitory concentration (MIC) was determined by broth macro dilution method in Sabouraud dextrose broth medium. The antifungal efficacy of two drug loaded polymeric micelle formulations prepared using 50% and 5% initial drug amount per mg of polymer weight at 2 mg/ml initial polymer concentration were tested against dissolved ITRA in DMSO. MIC was defined as the minimal concentration of the antifungal agent inhibiting visible growth of the microorganism. The concentration of ITRA used for MIC determination of each fungi varied from 4 to 0.03 μg/ml. In each tube containing 1 ml

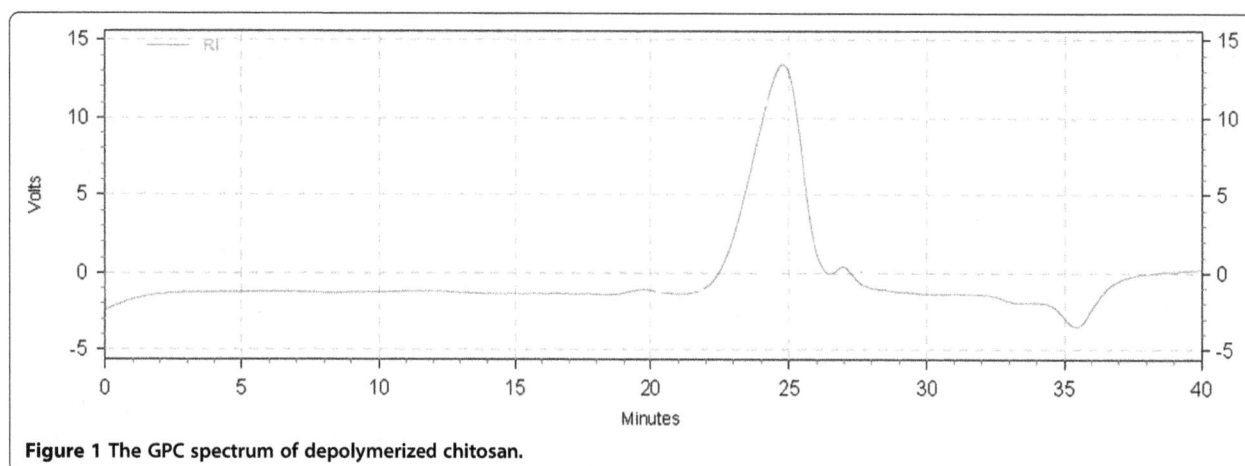

Figure 1 The GPC spectrum of depolymerized chitosan.

of broth medium and diluted ITRA formulation, 10^6 CFU of fungal organisms (*Candida albicans, Aspergillus niger, Aspergillus fumigatus*) was added as an inoculum. The tubes with total volume of approximately 1 ml in each were incubated at 25°C for 72 h. The incubation time for *Candida albicans* was 48 h. All the tests were repeated three times.

Statistical analysis

Data for all measurements were considered as mean ± standard deviation (S.D.) of three separate experiments. One-way analysis of variance (ANOVA) followed by Tukey post hoc test were used for statistical analysis of the results. The significance level was set at $p < 0.05$.

Results and discussions
Depolymerization of chitosan

Depolymerization of chitosan by $NaNO_2$ and H_2O_2 were previously investigated [22,25]. In this study, $NaNO_2$ was used and the obtained depolymerized chitosan showed good water solubility. Figure 1 shown gel permeation chromatography (GPC) spectrum of depolymerized chitosan. The data of GPC revealed that the depolymerized chitosan had number average molecular

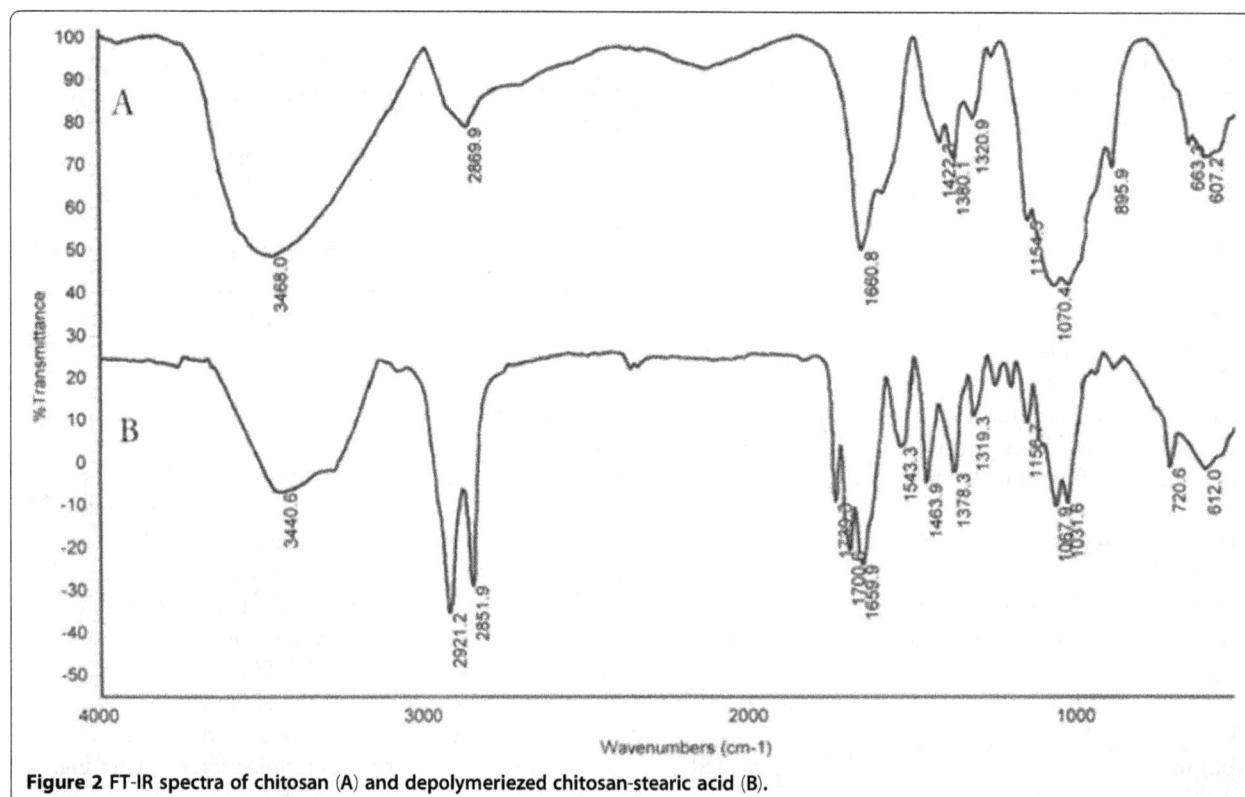

Figure 2 FT-IR spectra of chitosan (A) and depolymeriezed chitosan-stearic acid (B).

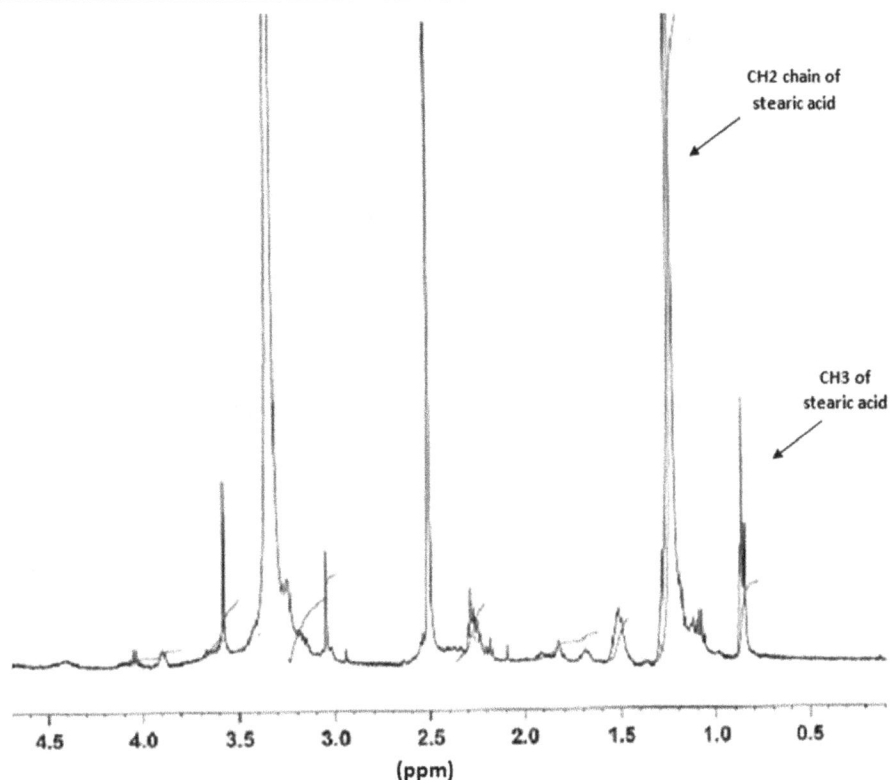

Figure 3 HNMR spectra of depolymerized chitosan grafted to stearic acid in DMSO-d6.

weight (Mn) of 9560 K, weight average molecular weight (Mw) of 14984 K and Z-average molecular weight of 24378 K with a narrow molecular mass distribution with polydispersity index (Mw/Mn) of 1.56, indicating a monodispersed chain length.

Synthesis and characterization of stearic acid grafted to depolymerized chitosan

The synthesis yield was about 41%. To confirm structural change and binding of stearic acid to the depolymerized chitosan, FT-IR and ^{1}HNMR analysis were used.

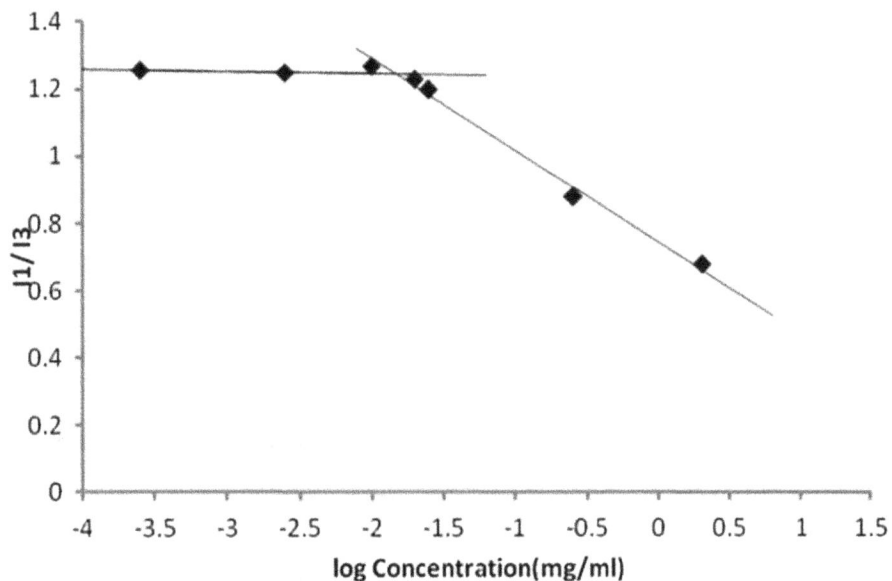

Figure 4 Intensity ratio plot of 1374/1395 versus concentration of chitosan-stearic acid.

Table 1 Physicochemical properties of the polymeric micelle formulations prepared by film hydration method (mean±SD, n=3)

DA[a]	Polymer concentration									
	1 mg/ml					2 mg/ml				
	EE% [b]	Conc. [c]	DL [d]	Size (nm)	Z.P[e] (mv)	EE%	Conc.	DL	Size (nm)	Z.P (mv)
50%	6.45±0.1	32.25±1.6	3.12±0.05	154.25±1.1	60.25±1.9	4.32±0.2	43.2±2.3	4.13±0.21	189.65±1.3	34.2±1.6
16.6%	9.94±0.6	16.51±1.1	1.62±0.10	125.75±1.7	63.25±1.7	6.03±0.4	20.03±1.4	0.99±0.07	176.71±2.6	45.31±1.8
5%	50.66±3.9	25.33±1.9	2.47±0.18	146.95±1.9	71.62±1.1	37.16±2.9	37.16±2.9	1.82±0.14	196.51±1.3	52.95±1.1
Blank micelle	-	-	-	121.37±1.1	74.28±1.8	-	-	-	168.31±1.2	58.34±1.7

[a] Drug amount per mg of polymer weight, [b] Entrapment efficiency, [c] Drug concentration in formulation(μg/ml), [d] Drug loading, [e] Zeta potential.

Compared to the IR spectrum of chitosan, the stearic acid-chitosan spectrum showed some changes according to the binding between stearic acid carboxylic group and chitosan amine (Figure 2). The increase of the C-H absorption at 2851.9 cm[-1] indicated the presence of stearic acid. Stearic acid-chitosan showed two absorptions at 1700.6 cm[-1] and 1739.3 cm[-1] that ascribed to the carbonyl zone which related to the chemical and physical binding of stearic acid and chitosan. The purity of the synthesized polymers has been studied by using FT-IR spectrum of the samples, according to the similar studies. After dialysis of stearic acid grafted to the chitosan (against distilled water containing 10% v/v ethanol for 48 hrs) the free stearic acid removed from synthesized product. To confirm this result, the results obtained from washing synthesized product with warm ethanol on the 0.45 μm filter were compared and shown similar results as well as the dialysis method. Considering the low solubility of stearic acid in water, the trace of free stearic acid molecules remained in the aqueous media might find its way to the core hydrophobic segments of the micelles, the place that is thermodynamically more suitable for these molecules. But it is possible a very low percent of free stearic acid intercalate between natural polymer chain and cannot remove completely. The FT-IR spectrum after repeat of synthesis procedures were same and shown the suitability and repeatability of our procedure.. All of these results indicated the formation of amide band and confirmed the conjugation of chitosan to stearic acid.

The ^{1}H-NMR spectra of the depolymerized chitosan grafted to stearic acid showed in Figure 3. compared with chitosan ^{1}H-NMR spectrum the triplet signals at 0.85 ppm, due to the terminal CH3 protons of stearic acid. The new peak at 1–1.5 ppm was corresponded to the CH2 chain of acyl chain. These results exhibited that stearic acid was linked to depolymerized chitosan.

The degree of substitution of the prepared modified polymer was about 61%, calculated by ^{1}HNMR method. To calculate the degree of substitution, the area under the triplet signals at 0.85 ppm was compared to the area under the peaks at 2–4 ppm, which were related to hydrogens of the depolymerized chitosan.

Critical micelle concentration (CMC) measurement

Many researches exhibited that polymeric micelles generally have lower CMC than low molar weight surfactant micelles. When pyrene is in polar media, its emission is weak and only there is an enhancement in the intensity of I_1 (the emission intensity at 374 nm), whereas no effect is seen on that of I_3 (the emission intensity at 395 nm). By formation of micelles in an aqueous solution, pyrene entered to the hydrophobic core of the micelles and the intensity of the third highest vibrational band at 395 nm (I_3) starts to strongly increase. Therefore, the changes in the intensity ratio of I_1/I_3 were used to determine the CMC of stearic acid-depolymerized chitosan micelles. The plot of the intensity ratio of I_1/I_3 versus the logarithm of the polymer concentration is exhibited in Figure 4. The interception of the two straight lines was considered as CMC of the polymer and was observed at 1.58×10^{-2} mg/ml of the polymer. This value was similar to the CMC values that were reported in the literature [26,27].

Entrapment efficiency of ITRA in the polymeric micelle formulations

The amount of drug entrapment in polymeric micelles by physical procedure is depended on several factors, including physicochemical properties of drug and block copolymers [28]. In this study, a long fatty acid chain (stearic acid) was used to entrap itraconazole as a highly hydrophobic molecule.

Table 2 Aerosolization parameters of ITRA loaded polymeric micelles at 2 mg/ml polymer concentration (mean±SD, n=3)

DA[a]	RD[b](%)	ED (μg)	FPD (μg)	FPF (%)	DRE (%)	NE (%)
50%	84.05±3.23	197.5±3.53	94.2±3.64	47.7±0.98	89.4±1.5	89.9±0.99
16.6%	80.15±1.20	92.25±4.59	39.7±3.20	43.0±1.32	95.3±1.1	88.9±0.11
5%	84.9±1.97	171±7.07	76.1±1.55	44.5±2.73	98.0±0.6	89.5±0.27

[a]Drug amount per mg of polymer weight, [b]Recovered Dose.

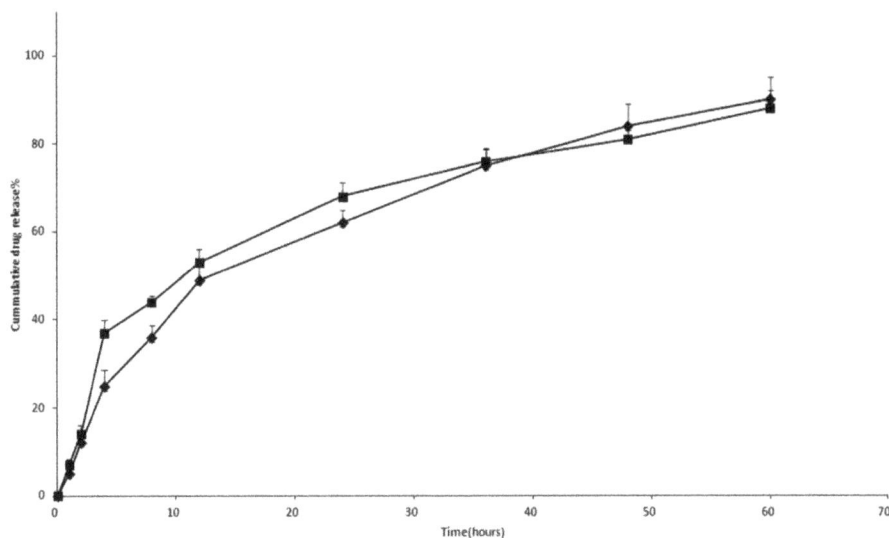

Figure 5 In vitro ITRA release profile from micelles prepared by different polymer concentration (♦) 2mg/ml and (■) 1mg/ml with same drug percent ratio (5%).

The polymeric micelles prepared in this study could entrap up to 43.2±2.27 µg/ml of ITRA (Table 1), more than 1000-fold relative to its aqueous solubility. It seemed that in the film hydration method good dispersion of the drug molecules through very thin polymer film helped to efficiently entrap ITRA. The data showed that by increasing in drug percent ratio in both concentrations of polymer the EE% decreased because the initial amount of added drug was high, however the high amount of ITRA encapsulated at both polymer concentration at 50% weight ratio of drug to the polymer.

The highest entrapment efficiency obtained by this procedure (37.16±2.91) when the polymer concentration was high (2 mg/ml) and the drug was used at the lowest percentage.

Particle size distribution measurements
The molecular weight of polymer and the properties of hydrophobic segment and drug are the most important factors influencing the size of polymeric micelles [29]. In all formulations, the mean diameters of the ITRA loaded polymeric micelles were between 120 to 200 nm with polydispersity index ranged between 0.18-0.22 (Table 1). The size of micelles increased significantly with increasing the polymer concentration. Data showed that significant change has been made with increasing ITRA to polymer weight percent from 5% to 50%, while keeping the polymer concentration constant. The more ITRA entrapped into the blank micelles, the more zeta potential was decreased (Table 1). Generally zeta potential exhibited reverse relation with the amount of ITRA entrapped into the micelles.

Nebulization of ITRA loaded polymeric micelles
For evaluation of nebulization efficacy, ITRA loaded polymeric micelle formulations were aerosolized at 28 l/min through a twin stage impinger. FPF (ratio of aerosolized particles < 6.4 µm) and the value of nebulization efficiency of the formulations are exhibited in Table 2. The results showed that polymeric micelles with different particle size had the same aerosolization properties.

These results are in accordance with our previous work on amphotericin B polymeric micelle formulations [20]. Also some reports showed that physical properties of the nebulization medium have an important role in the size distribution of the aerosolized droplets and droplets aerosolized from medium with similar properties showed the same size distribution [30]. To calculate the resistance of polymeric micelle formulations against shear force that occur in the air jet nebulizer and to evaluate the capability of these formulation to remained ITRA encapsulated during nebulization, the encapsulation efficiency of the formulations after nebulization

Table 3 Minimal inhibitory concentration of free ITRA (dissolved in DMSO) and ITRA loaded in polymeric micelles against three fungal strains (mean±SD, n=3)

ITRA in	C. albicans ATCC 10231	A. fumegatus ATCC 13073	A. niger ATCC 16404
Micelles 5%*	0.5	2	1
Micelles 50%**	0.5	2	1
DMSO	0.5	2	1

*, Micelles prepared by using 5% initial drug amount per mg of polymer weight at 2 mg/ml initial polymer concentration.
**, Micelles prepared by using 50% initial drug amount per mg of polymer weight at 2 mg/ml initial polymer concentration.

were studied. Our results showed that almost all of the formulations were stable during nebulization process (Table 2). These data suggested that polymeric micelles have good stability against shear force induced in air jet nebulizer. Similar results were observed after nebulization of amphotericin B loaded polymeric micelles [20].

In vitro release study

In vitro release profile of ITRA from formulation containing 5% drug amount per mg of polymer weight at 1 and 2 mg/ml polymer concentration exhibited in Figure 5. The release profiles showed two phase pattern. Over the first 12 hrs about 49% of the drug released from both micellar formulations. This relative rapid release behavior may be due to the drug molecules which adsorb on the outer surface of the micelles or intercalate between hydrophilic polymers. Total amount of the drug released after 60 hrs. Similar release pattern from polymeric micelles reported in some other studies [31,32]. As it shown in Figure 5 and results obtained from statistical analysis there is no significant difference between release profile of formulations.

In vitro antifungal activity

Table 3 showed the MIC of ITRA in different formulations for 3 fungal strains. The results showed that ITRA loaded polymeric micelle formulations had the same MIC values as dissolved ITRA in DMSO. The antifungal activity of the two micellar formulations was similar probably due to close proximity of the size distribution data of the formulations. The data obtained from antifungal experiments revealed that chitosan based polymeric micelles could be used for solubilization of ITRA in aquouse media with antifungal activities equal to that of organic based ITRA solutions. The micelles without drug had no significant antifungal activity.

Conclusion

Through grafting stearic acid onto depolymerized chitosan, the modified polymer can form micelles in nano size range. The data showed that stearic acid as the hydrophobic core of the micelles could entrap ITRA and increase the solubility of the drug. The size distribution of all formulations was mono modal and ranged from 120 nm to 200 nm. In vitro nebulization study of the ITRA loaded formulations showed that the stearic acid-chitosan based polymeric micelles had adequate capability as nanocarriers to deliver ITRA and can remain their stability during nebulization.

Competing interests
The authors report no conflicts of interest. The authors alone are responsible for the content and writing of the paper.

Authors' contributions
EM: Carried out synthesis studies of polymer, micelle preparation, different characterization of micelles and drafted the manuscript. KM: Supervisor and participated in the drafted the manuscript. ARN, MRR: Supervisor. NM: Carried out in vitro pulmonary studies. MA: Supervisor and participated in polymer characterization. MAB: Carried out characterization of synthesized polymer. All authors read and approved the final manuscript.

Acknowledgements
This research received no specific grant from any funding agency in the public, commercial, or not-for-profit sectors.

Author details
[1]Aerosol Research Laboratory, Department of Pharmaceutics, School of Pharmacy, Tehran University of Medical Sciences, Tehran, Iran. [2]Department of Pharmaceutics, School of Pharmacy, Tehran University of Medical Sciences, Tehran, Iran. [3]Department of Medicinal Chemistry, School of Pharmacy and Drug Design & Development Research Center, Tehran University of Medical Sciences, Tehran, Iran. [4]XRD Research Laboratory, School of Sciences, Tehran University, Tehran, Iran.

References

1. Denning DW: **Invasive aspergillosis, Clinical infectious disease.** *Chest* 1998, 26:781–803.
2. Ruchel R: **Diagnosis of invasive mycoses in severely immunosuppressed patients.** *Ann Hematol* 1993, 67:1–11.
3. Wong-Beringer A, Lambros MP, Beringer PM, Johnson DL: **Suitability of Caspofungin for Aerosol Delivery Physicochemical Profiling and Nebulizer Choice.** *Chest* 2005, 128:3711–3716.
4. Berenguer J, Ali NM, Allende MC, Lee J, Garrett K, Battaglia S, Piscitelli SC, Rinaldi MG, Pizzo PA, Walsh TJ: **Itraconazole for Experimental Pulmonary Aspergillosis: Comparison with Amphotericin B, Interaction with Cyclosporin A, and Correlation between Therapeutic Response and Itraconazole Concentrations in Plasma.** *Antimicrob Agents Chemother* 1994, 38:1303–1308.
5. Peeters J, Neeskens P, Tollenaere JP, Remoortere PV, Brewster ME: **Characterization of the interaction of 2-hydroxypropyl-ß-cyclodextrin with Itraconazole at pH 2, 4, and 7.** *J Pharm Sci* 2002, 91:1414–1422.
6. Boogaerts MA, Maertens J, Gees RVD, Bosly A, Michaux JL, Hoof AV, Cleeren M, Wostenborghs R, Beule KD: **Pharmacokinetics and Safety of a 7-Day Administration of Intravenous Itraconazole followed by a 14-Day Administration of Itraconazole Oral Solution in Patients with Hematologic Malignancy.** *Antimicrob Agents Chemother* 2001, 45:981–985.
7. Kipp JE: **The role of solid nanoparticle technology in the parenteral delivery of poorly water-soluble drugs.** *Int J Pharm* 2004, 284:109–122.
8. Akkar A, Muller RH: **Intravenous itraconazole emulsions produced by SolEmuls technology.** *Eur J Pharm Biopharm* 2003, 56:29–36.
9. Keck CM, Muller RH: **Drug nanocrystals of poorly soluble drugs produced by high pressure homogenization.** *Eur J Pharm Biopharm* 2006, 62:3–16.
10. Sinswat P, Gao X, Yacaman MJ, Williams RO, Johnston KP: **Stabilizer choice for rapid dissolving high potency itraconazole particles formed by evaporative precipitation into aqueous solution.** *Int J Pharm* 2005, 302:113–124.
11. McConville JT, Overhoff KA, Sinswat P, Vaughn JM, Frei BL, Burgess DS, Talbert RL, Peters JI, Johnston KP, Williams RO: **Targeted High Lung Concentrations of Itraconazole Using Nebulized Dispersions in a Murine Model.** *Pharm Res* 2006, 23:901–911.
12. Yang W, Tam J, Miller DA, Zhou J, McConville JT, Johnston KP, Williams RO: **High bioavailability from nebulized itraconazole nanoparticle dispersions with biocompatible stabilizers.** *Int J Pharm* 2008, 361:177–188.
13. Nishiyama N, Kataoka K: **Current state, achievements, and future prospects of polymeric micelles as nanocarriers for drug and gene delivery.** *Pharmacol Ther* 2006, 112:630–648.
14. Illum L: **Chitosan and its use as a pharmaceutical excipient.** *Pharm Res* 1998, 15:1326–1331.
15. Zhang J, Chen XG, Li Y, Liu CS: **Self-assembled nanoparticles based on hydrophobically modified chitosan as carriers for doxorubicin.** *Nanomedicine* 2007, 3:258–265.

16. Min KH, *et al*: Hydrophobically modified glycol chitosan nanoparticles-encapsulated camptothecin enhance the drug stability and tumor targeting in cancer therapy. *J Control Rel* 2008, **127**:208–218.

17. Opanasopit P, Ngawhirunpat T, Rojanarata T, Choochottiros C, Chirachanchai S: **N-Phthaloylchitosan-g-mPEG design for all-trans retinoic acid-loaded polymeric micelles.** *Eur J Pharm Sci* 2007, **30**:424–431.

18. Hu FQ, Ren GF, Yuan H, Du YZ, Zeng S: **Shell cross-linked stearic acid grafted chitosan oligosaccharide self-aggregated micelles for controlled release of paclitaxel.** *Colloids Surf B* 2006, **50**:97–103.

19. Wichit A, Tangsumranjit A, Pitaksuteepong T, Waranuch: **Polymeric Micelles of PEG-PE as Carriers of All-Trans Retinoic Acid for Stability Improvement.** *AAPS PharmSciTech* 2012, **13**:336–343.

20. Gilani K, Moazeni E, Ramezanli T, Amini M, Fazeli MR, Jamalifar H: **Development of Respirable Nanomicelle Carriers for Delivery of Amphotericin B by Jet Nebulization.** *J Pharm Sci* 2011, **100**:252–259.

21. Sahib M, Darwis Y, Peh K, Abdulameer S, Tan Y: **Rehydrated sterically stabilized phospholipid nanomicelles of budesonide for nebulization: physicochemical characterization and in vitro, in vivo evaluations.** *Int J Nanomedicine* 2011, **6**:2351–2356.

22. Mao S, Shuai X, Unger F, Simon M, Bi D, Kissel T: **The depolymerization of chitosan: effects on physicochemical and biological properties.** *Int J Pharm* 2004, **281**:45–54.

23. Du YZ, *et al*: **Preparation and characteristics of linoleic acid-grafted chitosan oligosaccharide micelles as a carrier for doxorubicin.** *Colloids Surf B* 2009, **69**:257–263.

24. Yi Y, *et al*: **A mixed polymeric micellar formulation of itraconazole: Characteristics, toxicity and pharmacokinetics.** *J Control Rel* 2007, **117**:59–67.

25. Tian F, Liu Y, Hu K, Zhao B: **Study of the depolymerization behavior of chitosan by hydrogen peroxide.** *Carbohydr Polym* 2004, **57**:31–37.

26. Jiang GB, Quan D, Liao K, Wang H: **Preparation of polymeric micelles based on chitosan bearing a small amount of highly hydrophobic groups.** *Carbohydr Polym* 2006, **66**:514–520.

27. Lee KY, Kwon IC, Kim YH, Jo WH, Jeong SY: **Preparation of chitosan self-aggregates as a gene delivery systems.** *J Control Rel* 1998, **51**:213–220.

28. Lavasanifar A, Samuel J, Kwon GS: **Poly(ethylene oxide)-block-poly(L-amino acid) micelles for drug delivery.** *Adv Drug Deliv Rev* 2002, **54**:169–190.

29. Kwon SK, Park JH, Chung H, Kwon IC, Jeong SY: **Physicochemical characteristics of self-assembled nanoparticles based on glycol chitosan bearing 5ß-cholanic acid.** *Langmuir* 2003, **19**:10188–10193.

30. Tam J, McConville J, Williams R, Johnston K: **Amorphous cyclosporin nanodispersions for enhanced pulmonary deposition and dissolution.** *J Pharm Sci* 2008, **97**:4915–4933.

31. Ye YQ, Yang FL, Hu FQ, Du YZ, Yuan H, Yu HY: **Core-modified chitosan-based polymeric micelles for controlled release of doxorubicin.** *Int J Pharm* 2008, **352**:294–301.

32. Lin J, Zhang S, Chen T, Lin S, Jin H: **Micelle formation and drug release behavior of polypeptide graft copolymer and its mixture with polypeptide block copolymer.** *Int J Pharm* 2007, **336**:49–57.

14

Structural relationships and vasorelaxant activity of monoterpenes

Tamires Cardoso Lima[1], Marcelo Mendonça Mota[1], José Maria Barbosa-Filho[2], Márcio Roberto Viana Dos Santos[1] and Damião Pergentino De Sousa[1*]

Abstract

Background and purpose of the study: The hypotensive activity of the essential oil of *Mentha* x *villosa* and its main constituent, the monoterpene rotundifolone, have been reported. Therefore, our objective was to evaluate the vasorelaxant effect of monoterpenes found in medicinal plants and establish the structure-activity relationship of rotundifolone and its structural analogues on the rat superior mesenteric artery.

Methods: Contractions of the vessels were induced with 10 μM of phenylephine (Phe) in rings with endothelium. During the tonic phase of the contraction, the monoterpenes (10^{-8} - 10^{-3}, cumulatively) were added to the organ bath. The extent of relaxation was expressed as the percentage of Phe-induced contraction.

Results: The results from the present study showed that both oxygenated terpenes (rotundifolone, (+)-limonene epoxide, pulegone epoxide, carvone epoxide, and (+)-pulegone) and non-oxygenated terpene ((+)-limonene) exhibit relaxation activity. The absence of an oxygenated molecular structure was not a critical requirement for the molecule to be bioactive. Also it was found that the position of ketone and epoxide groups in the monoterpene structures influence the vasorelaxant potency and efficacy.

Major conclusion: The results suggest that the presence of functional groups in the chemical structure of rotundifolone is not essential for its vasorelaxant activity.

Keywords: Essential oils, Terpenes, Spasmolytics, Structure-activity relationships, Cardiovascular activity

Introduction

The essential oils are natural products extracted from species of aromatic plants and exhibit a variety of biological properties [1-6]. These effects are attributed mainly to the terpenes, which are the major chemical components of these oils. The cardiovascular activity of essential oils has been reported [7-10]. Some studies showed that the main chemical components of these oils are bioactive [7,10-12].

The antihypertensive activity of some plants also has been related to the presence of terpenes. Extracts and diterpenoids of *Salvia* species have shown cardiovascular activity, such as ferruginol and 7-oxo-abieta-9,12,14-triene [13]. In another work, in normotensive anaesthetised rats, the cardiovascular effect of the essential oil of *Mentha* x *villosa* and its main constituent, rotundifolone, suggests

that hypotensive activity may result from its vasodilatory effects directly upon vascular smooth muscle [11]. Additional studies showed that the hypotensive activity of the monoterpene rotundifolone is related to decrease in heart rate and peripheral vascular resistance, probably via nonselective muscarinic receptor stimulation [14].

For these reasons, it appeared possible that terpenes found in essential oils could also have cardiovascular activity. Therefore, our objective was to verify the potential vasorelaxant effect of representative monoterpenes present in medicinal plants and to determine the relationship between the chemical structure of rotundifolone and its vasorelaxant activity to understand the influence of the functional groups present in this monoterpene. Therefore, we assessed *p*-menthane monoterpenes containing ketone groups and/or epoxy in different positions in the chemical structure. In addition, a monoterpene that does not contain these functional groups was also evaluated.

---

* Correspondence: damiao_desousa@yahoo.com.br
[1]Department of Physiology, Federal University of Sergipe, CEP 49100-000, São Cristóvão, Sergipe, Brazil
Full list of author information is available at the end of the article

Materials and methods
Chemicals and solutions
(+)-Limonene epoxide was prepared via oxidation of (+)-limonene with m-chloroperoxybenzoic acid [15]. Pulegone epoxide [16] and carvone epoxide [17] were prepared via oxidation of (+)-pulegone and (–)-carvone, respectively, using hydrogen peroxide in alkaline medium as previously described. (+)-Pulegone was purchased from Aldrich. (+)-Limonene was purchased from company Dierberger Óleos Essenciais S.A., Barra Bonita, Brazil. Rotundifolone was isolated from the essential oil of *Mentha* x *villosa* using a previously described procedure [18]. The purity of test compounds was higher than 95%. L-Phenylephrine chloride (Phe) and acetylcholine chloride (Ach) were purchase from Sigma (Sigma Chemical Co., USA). In the preparation of the stock solutions, the monoterpenes were diluted in Tyrode/cremophor (0.15% v/v) solution. Phe and Ach were diluted or in Tyrode solutions only. All stock solutions were maintained at 0°C and diluted to the desired concentration, when necessary. Cremophor (Sigma Chemical Co., USA) in used concentrations showed no effect on control experiments (data not shown).

(Composition of Tyrode's solution in mM: NaCl 158.3, KCl 4.0, $CaCl_2$ 2.0, $NaHCO_3$ 10.0, $C_6H_{12}O_6$ 5.6, $MgCl_2$ 1.05 and NaH_2PO_4 0.42).

Animals
Male Wistar normotensive rats (200 – 300 g) were obtained from colonies maintained in the Department of Physiology, Federal University of Sergipe, Sergipe, Brazil. They were maintained in a large cage under controlled conditions of temperature and lighting (lights on: 06:00–18:00 h), fed with rodent diet and tap water *ad libtum*. All procedures were approved by the Animal Research Ethics Committee of the Universidade Federal de Sergipe, Brazil (Protocol number 15/2009) and were in compliance with the Guide for the Care and Use of Laboratory Animals published by the US National Institutes of Health (NIH publication 85–23, revised 1996).

Pharmacological assays
The tissue preparation was performed as described in Menezes et al. [19]. Rats were sacrificed by exsanguination under ether aesthesia and superior mesenteric artery was removed, cleaned from connective and fat tissues and sectioned in rings (1 – 2 mm). These rings were suspended in organ baths containing 10 mL of Tyrode's solution, gassed with carbogen and maintained at 37°C under a resting tension of 0.75 g for 60 min (stabilization period). The isometric tension was recorded through a force transducer (Letica, Model TRI210, Italy) coupled to an amplifier-recorder (AVS, Brazil). Endothelium functionality of the rings was assessed by the ability of Ach (10 μM) to induce more than 70% relaxation of Phe (10 μM) tonus.

After verify the functionality of vascular endothelium, contractions of the vessels were induced with 10 μM Phe in rings with endothelium. During the tonic phase of the contraction, the monoterpenes rotundifolone, (+)-limonene epoxide, pulegone epoxide, carvone epoxide, (+)-pulegone and (+)-limonene (10^{-8} - 10^{-3}, cumulatively) were added to the organ bath. The extent of relaxation was expressed as the percentage of Phe-induced contraction.

Statistic analysis
Values were expressed as the mean ± SEM. The results were analyzed with one-way ANOVA followed by Bonferroni post-test. The potency was expressed as pD_2 value (negative logarithm of molar concentration producing the half maximum effect - E_{max}) of *in vitro* experiments were obtained by non-linear regression. All procedures were performed by using Graph Pad Prism 3.02™.

Results and discussion
Several studies have reported pharmacological effects of essential oils on the rat cardiovascular system [9-11,20,21]. However, there are few studies on bioactive compounds that contribute to the pharmacological activity of these oils. We report in this comparative study the findings on the vasorelaxant activity of six monoterpenes (Figure 1): rotundifolone (having α,β-unsaturated ketone and endocyclic epoxide groups), limonene epoxide (having only an epoxide group), pulegone epoxide (having ketone and exocyclic epoxide groups), carvone epoxide (having ketone and endocyclic epoxide groups), (+)-pulegone (having an α,β-unsaturated ketone), and (+)-limonene (non-oxygenated terpene).

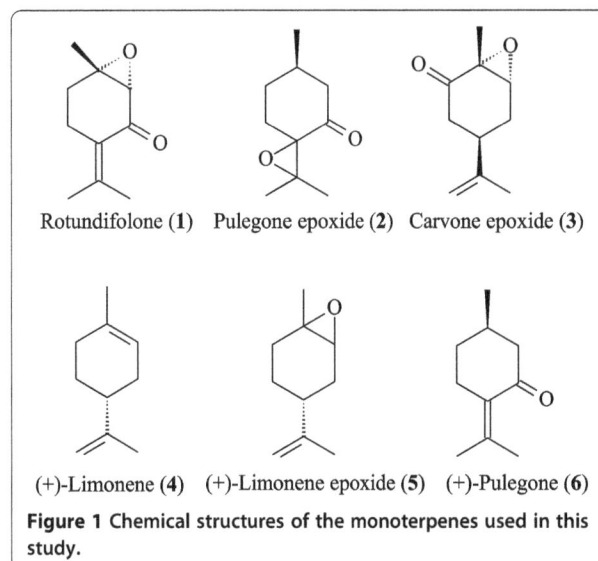

Figure 1 Chemical structures of the monoterpenes used in this study.

The investigation of the influence of the position of ketone and epoxide groups in the molecular structure was performed by comparing the rotundifolone (1) with the pulegone epoxide (2) and carvone epoxide (3). The rotundifolone showed a vasorelaxant effect in rat mesenteric artery more potent than carvone epoxide ($p < 0.01$), suggesting that the position of the ketone group influences this spasmolytic property. In addition, the pharmacological activity of rotundifolone was lower than the pulegone epoxide ($p < 0.05$). This result demonstrates that the position of epoxide group in the p-menthane structure alters the pharmacological activity. The experimental data also showed that the pulegone epoxide exhibit more significant vasorelaxant activity in comparison to carvone epoxide ($p < 0.001$), indicating that the exocyclic epoxide group contributes more to the pharmacological effect than the endocyclic epoxide group. These results confirm that the position of epoxide and ketone functional groups in molecules change the vasorelaxant activity. Comparing rotundifolone with (+)-limonene (4), these compounds showed equipotent vasorelaxant activity ($p > 0.05$). The spasmolytic activity of (+)-limonene shown in this study demonstrates that non-oxygenated terpenes present in cardioactive essential oils may contribute to this activity. (+)-Limonene epoxide (5) and (+)-pulegone (6) presented vasorelaxant activity below 50%, so it was not allowed to calculate their pD_2 (Table 1).

Similarly, the effectiveness of the tested compounds was investigated by comparing their maximum effects. The rotundifolone showed a higher pharmacological effect than (+)-pulegone ($p < 0.05$). While (+)-limonene was more effective than (+)-pulegone ($p < 0.01$) and limonene epoxide ($p < 0.01$). Carvone epoxide exhibited a maximum effect of relaxation greater than pulegone epoxide ($p < 0.01$), (+)-pulegone ($p < 0.001$), and limonene epoxide ($p < 0.001$).

Table 1 Values of pD_2 and E_{max} obtained of concentration-response curves to monoterpenes in isolated rings of rat superior mesenteric artery with functional endothelium pre-contracted with Phe (10 μM)

Monoterpenes	N	pD_2	E_{max}
Rotundifolone (1)	4	5.1 ± 0.2	71.7 ± 6.2
Pulegone epoxide (2)	4	$6.3 \pm 0.3^{a,c}$	55.5 ± 3.0
Carvone epoxide (3)	4	3.4 ± 0.3^{e}	$99.8 \pm 18.7^{***,***}$
(+)-Limonene (4)	4	5.1 ± 0.1	$84.2 \pm 4.1^{##}$
(+)-Limonene epoxide (5)	4	—	34.0 ± 2.0
(+)-Pulegone (6)	4	—	$30.3 \pm 2.3^{*}$

N = Number of experiments; pD_2 – Potency; E_{max} – Maximum Effect; [a]$p < 0.05$ vs rotundifolone and (+)-limonene; [c]$p < 0.001$ carvone epoxide, and [e]$p < 0.01$ vs rotundifolone and (+)-limonene. *$p < 0.05$ vs rotundifolone, ***$p < 0.001$ vs (+)-pulegone and limonene epoxide; **$p < 0.01$ vs pulegone epoxide, and [##] $p < 0.01$ vs (+)-pulegone and limonene epoxide.

It is described in the literature that the monoterpene terpinen-4-ol produces hypotensive effect in rats. Terpinen-4-ol is the main constituent of the essential oil of *Alpinia zerumbet* (Pers.) B. L. Burtt. & R. M. Sm. (Zingiberaceae). Lahlou *et al.* [12] proved that the hypotensive effects of the essential oil of *Alpinia zerumbet* are partially attributed to the actions of terpinen-4-ol, which was more potent than this oil. In another study, Barbosa-Filho *et al.* [22] showed that the essential oils from stem and root of the plant *Ocotea duckei* have hypotensive activity. The main chemical constituents of these oils are the terpene β-eudesmol and elemol, respectively. These reports, together with our findings, demonstrate the importance of this natural chemical class as good candidates for antihypertensive drugs.

Furthermore, studies have demonstrated that some of these terpenes exhibit depressant properties in other organic systems. Sadraei *et al.* [4] and Camara *et al.* [5] showed that both, (+)-α- and (−)-β-pinene, relax rat and guinea-pig ileum, respectively. Other studies have shown that (±)-linalool promotes spasmolytic effect in guinea-pig ileum mediated by cAMP [23], and recently Tanida *et al.* [24] demonstrated that the inhalation of (±)-linalool reduces the blood pressure mediated by the central nervous system in rats. Therefore, the hypotensive activity could originate from vasodilatory effects induced by these compounds. This possible mechanism of action was studied in citronellol, which lowers blood pressure by a direct effect on the vascular smooth muscle leading to vasodilation [25].

The biotransformation of some compounds tested is known. For example, (+)-limonene is biotransformed to several metabolites, such as (+)-limonene epoxide, carvone, and perillyl alcohol [26,27]. (+)-Limonene epoxide is one of the bioactive compounds of the present study. Carvone has ketone group which is present in the chemical structure of carvone epoxide, another evaluated compound. The monoterpene perillyl alcohol has hypotensive activity [28]. Pulegone also produces bioactive metabolites, such as menthol [29] which has vasorelaxant activity [30]. Therefore, the metabolites of (+)-limonene, pulegone, and other tested compounds should contribute to their vasorelaxant activity. In addition, the tested compounds must act by different mechanisms of action. In fact, monoterpene alcohols, aldehydes, ethers, and hydrocarbons show effects on the cardiovascular system via vasorelaxation, decreased heart rate or hypotension, among others [31]. The mechanisms of action of these compounds should be related to their metabolites.

Conclusion

The results from the present study showed that both oxygenated terpenes and hydrocarbon terpene exhibit spasmolytic activity. The absence of an oxygenated molecular structure was not a critical requirement for the molecule to be bioactive. The position of ketone and epoxide groups in the *p*-menthane structure influences the vasorelaxant potency and efficacy. Therefore, these functional groups contribute to the vasorelaxant activity of rotundifolone.

Competing interests
The authors declare that they have no competing interests.

Authors' contributions
TCL was responsible for the preparation of monoterpenes and wrote the chemical content of the manuscript; MMM evaluated the pharmacological activity of monoterpenes; JMB-F isolated and identified the rotundifolone; MRVDS interpreted and wrote the pharmacological data of the manuscript; DPDS analyzed, interpreted and corrected the structure-activity relationships data of monoterpenes. All authors read and approved the final manuscript.

Acknowledgements
We thank CNPq, CAPES and FAPITEC-SE for financial support.

Author details
[1]Department of Physiology, Federal University of Sergipe, CEP 49100-000, São Cristóvão, Sergipe, Brazil. [2]Laboratório de Tecnologia Farmacêutica, Federal University of Paraíba, Caixa Postal 5009, CEP 58051-970, João Pessoa, Paraíba, Brazil.

References
1. Mohamed AEH, El-Sayed MA, Hegazy ME, Helaly SE, Esmail AM, Mohamed NS: Chemical constituents and biological activities of *Artemisia herba-alba*. Rec Nat Prod 2010, 4(1):1–25.
2. De Almeida RN, Araújo DAM, Gonçalves JCR, Montenegro FC, De Sousa DP, Leite JR, Mattei R, Benedito MAC, Carvalho JGB, Cruz JS, Maia JGS: Rosewood oil induces sedation and inhibits compound action potential in rodents. J Ethnopharmacol 2009, 124:440–443.
3. Arruda TA, Antunes RMP, Catão RMR, Lima EO, De Sousa DP, Nunes XP, Pereira MSV, Barbosa-Filho JM, Cunha EVL: Preliminary study of the antimicrobial activity of *Mentha* x *villosa* Hudson essential oil, rotundifolone and its analogues. Rev Bras Farmacogn 2006, 16:307–311.
4. Sadraei H, Asghari GR, Hajhashemi V, Kolagar A, Ebrahimi M: Spasmolytic activity of essential oil and various extracts of *Ferula gummosa* Boiss. on ileum contractions. Phytomedicine 2001, 8:370–376.
5. Camara CC, Nascimento NR, Macedo-Filho CL, Almeida FB, Fonteles MC: Antispasmodic effect of the essential oil of *Plectranthus barbatus* and some major constituents on the guinea-pig ileum. Planta Med 2003, 69:1080–1085.
6. Compagnone RS, Chavez K, Mateu E, Orsini G, Arvelo F, Suárez AI: Composition and cytotoxic activity of essential oils from *Croton matourensis* and *Croton micans* from Venezuela. Rec Nat Prod 2010, 4:101–108.
7. Interaminense LF, Leal-Cardoso JH, Magalhães PJ, Duarte GP, Lahlou S: Enhanced hypotensive effects of the essential oil of *Ocimum gratissimum* leaves and its main constituent, eugenol, in DOCA-salt hypertensive conscious rats. Planta Med 2005, 71:376–378.
8. Lahlou S, Figueiredo AF, Magalhães PJ, Leal-Cardoso JH: Cardiovascular effects of 1,8-cineole, a terpenoid oxide present in many plant essential oils, in normotensive rats. Can J Physiol Pharmacol 2002, 80:1125–1131.
9. Cunha RM, Farias SRQ, Duarte JC, Santos MRV, Ribeiro EAN, Medeiros IA: Cardiovascular effects induced by the essential oil of *Ocotea duckei* Vattimo (Lauraceae). Biol Geral Exper 2004, 5:12–18.
10. De Siqueira RJ, Magalhães PJ, Leal-Cardoso JH, Duarte GP, Lahlou S: Cardiovascular effects of the essential oil of *Croton zehntneri* leaves and its main constituents, anethole and estragole, in normotensive conscious rats. Life Sci 2006, 78:2365–2372.
11. Lahlou S, Carneiro-Leao RF, Leal-Cardoso JH, Toscano CF: Cardiovascular effects of the essential oil of *Mentha* x *villosa* and its main constituent, piperitenone oxide, in normotensive anaesthetised rats: role of the autonomic nervous system. Planta Med 2001, 67:638–643.
12. Lahlou S, Interaminense LF, Leal-Cardoso JH, Duarte GP: Antihypertensive effects of the essential oil of *Alpinia zerumbet* and its main constituent, terpinen-4-ol, in DOCA-salt hypertensive conscious rats. Fundam Clin Pharmacol 2003, 17:323–330.
13. Ulubelen A: Cardioactive and antibacterial terpenoids from some *Salvia* species. Phytochemistry 2003, 64:395–399.
14. Guedes DN, Silva DF, Barbosa-Filho JM, Medeiros IA: Muscarinic agonist properties involved in the hypotensive and vasorelaxant responses of rotundifolone in rats. Planta Med 2002, 86:700–704.
15. Thomas AF, Bessière Y: Limonene. Nat Prod Rep 1989, 6:291–309.
16. Katsuhara J: Absolute configuration of pulegone oxide and piperitenone dioxide. J Org Chem 1967, 32:797–799.
17. Santos RB, Brocksom TJ, Brocksom U: A convenient deoxygenation of α, β epoxy ketones to enones. Tetrahedron Lett 1997, 38:745–748.
18. Almeida RN, Hiruma CA, Barbosa-Filho JM: Analgesic effect of rotundifolone in rodents. Fitoterapia 1996, 67:334–338.
19. Menezes IAC, Moreira IJA, Carvalho AA, Antoniolli AR, Santos MRV: Cardiovascular effects of the aqueous extract from *Caesalpinia ferrea*: involvement of ATP-sensitive potassium channels. Vasc Pharmacol 2007, 47:41–47.
20. Lahlou S, Leal-Cardoso JH, Magalhães PJ: Essential oil of *Croton nepetaefolius* decreases blood pressure through an action upon vascular smooth muscle: studies in DOCA-salt hypertensive rats. Planta Med 2000, 66:138–143.
21. Lahlou S, Leal-Cardoso JH, Magalhães PJ, Coelho-de-Souza AN, Duarte GP: Cardiovascular effects of the essential oil of *Croton nepetaefolius* in rats: role of the autonomic nervous system. Planta Med 1999, 65:553–557.
22. Barbosa-Filho JM, Cunha RM, Dias CS, Athayde-Filho PF, Silva MS, Cunha EVL, Machado MIL, Craveiro AA, Medeiros IA: GC-MS analysis and cardiovascular activity of the essential oil of *Ocotea duckei*. Rev Bras Farmacogn 2008, 18:37–41.
23. Lis-Balchin M, Hart S: Studies on the mode of action of the essential oil of lavender (*Lavandula angustifolia* P. Miller). Phytother Res 1999, 13:540–542.
24. Tanida M, Niijima A, Shen J, Nakamura T, Nagai K: Olfactory stimulation with scent of lavender oil affects autonomic neurotransmission and blood pressure in rats. Neurosci Lett 2006, 398:155–160.
25. Bastos JFA, Moreira IJA, Ribeiro TP, Medeiros IA, Antoniolli AR, De Sousa DP, Santos MRV: Hypotensive and vasorelaxant effects of citronellol, a monoterpene alcohol, in rats. Basic Clin Pharmacol Toxicol 2010, 106:331–337.
26. Miyazawa M, Shindo M, Shimada T: Metabolism of (+)- and (−)-limonenes to respective carveols and perillyl alcohols by CYP2C9 and CYP2C19 in human liver microsomes. Drug Metab Dispos 2002, 30:602–607.
27. Shimada T, Shindo M, Miyazawa M: Species differences in the metabolism of R-(−)- and S-(+)-limonenes and their metabolites, carveols and carvones, by cytochrome P450 enzymes in liver microsomes of mice, rats, guinea pigs, rabbits, dogs, monkeys, and humans. Drug Metab Pharmacokinet 2002, 17:507–515.
28. Saito K, Okabe T, Inamori Y, Tsujibo H, Miyake Y, Hiraoka K, Ishida N: The biological properties of monoterpenes: hypotensive effects on rats and antifungal activities on plant pathogenic fungi of monoterpenes. Mokuzai Gakkaishi 1996, 42:677–680.
29. Engel W: In vivo studies on the metabolism of the monoterpene pulegone in humans using the metabolism of ingestion-correlated amounts (MICA) approach: explanation for the toxicity differences between (S)-(−)- and (R)-(+)-pulegone. J Agric Food Chem 2003, 51(22):6589–97.
30. Johnson CD, Melanaphy D, Purse A, Stokesberry SA, Dickson P, Zholos AV: Transient receptor potential melastatin 8 channel involvement in the regulation of vascular tone. Am J Physiol Heart Circ Physiol 2009, 296(6):H1868–H1877.
31. Santos MRV, Moreira FV, Fraga BP, De Sousa DP, Bonjardim LR, Quintans-Junior LJ: Cardiovascular effects of monoterpenes: a review. Rev Bras Farmacogn 2011, 21(4):764–771.

Terpenes From the Root of *Salvia hypoleuca* Benth

Soodabeh Saeidnia[1], Mitra Ghamarinia[2], Ahmad R Gohari[1,3*] and Alireza Shakeri[2]

Abstract

Background: The genus *Salvia*, with nearly 900 species, is one of the largest members of Lamiaceae family. In the Flora of Iran, the genus *Salvia* is represented by 58 species of which 17 species are endemic. *Salvia hypoleuca* Bёnth., is one of these species growing wildly in northern and central parts of Iran. *Salvia* species are well known in folk medicine and widely used for therapeutic purposes. Literature review shows that there is no report on phytochemical investigation of the roots of *S. hypoleuca*.

Results: The separation and purification process were carried out using various chromatographic methods. Structural elucidation was on the basis of NMR and MS data, in comparison with those reported in the literature. The isolated compounds were identified as sitosteryl oleate (1), β-sitosterol (2), stigmasterol (3), manool (4), 7α-acetoxy royleanone (5), ursolic acid (6), oleanolic acid (7), 3-epicorosolic acid (8), 3-epimaslinic acid (9) and coleonolic acid (10).

Conclusions: In the present study, three sterols, two diterpenes and five triterpenes were isolated from the ethyl acetate extract of the roots of *S. hypoleuca*. As the chemotaxonomic significance, some of the isolated compounds (1–7, 9) have not been previously reported from the species *S. hypoleuca*, while the triterpenes 8 and 10 are now documented from *Salvia* genus for the first time.

Keywords: *Salvia hypoleuca*, Coleonolic acid, 7α-acetoxyroyleanone, 3-epimaslinic acid, 3-epicorosolic acid, Manool

Background

The genus *Salvia* L. (Lamiaceae), with more than 900 species throughout the world, is represented 58 species in Iran, 17 of which are endemic. Most of the species are used as herbal tea and flavoring agent by people and also used in traditional medicine as tonic, anti-rheumatoid, antimicrobial and carminative [1-3]. *Flora Orientalis* includes as many as 107 species of *Salvia* [4]. *Salvia hypoleuca* Benth., is one of these species which growing wildly in northern and central parts of Iran [1].

Literature review show that various secondary metabolites such as terpenoids, phenolic acids [5], polyphenols, flavonoids [3,6] and anthocyanins [7] have been reported from *Salvia* species. Limonene, α-pinene, β-pinene, 1,8-cineol, bicyclogermacrene, caryophyllene oxide and α-gurjunene are the main components of the essential oils of various species of *Salvia* growing wildly in Iran [8-11]. In the literature, there are several reports on phytochemical investigation of the above mentioned species.

Several sesterterpene lactones, isomeric epoxides, monolactone and hypoleuenoic acid have been reported from varies fractions of *S. hypoleuca* [12-14]. The main aromatic components of the essential oil of *S. hypoleuca* roots have been identified as hexadecanoic acid (27.4%) and viridiflorol (14.9%) [15], while germacrene D (15.1%) and β-caryophyllene (22.0%) identified as the major constituents during flowering stages [16]. A great number of diterpenes exhibited interesting biological activities *e.g.* anti-tuberculous, antitumour, antibacterial, antileishmanial and antispasmolytic, and *Salvia* species are the excellent source of diterpenoids [17]. In this study, we aim to report the isolation and identification of some sterols, diterpenoids and triterpenoids from the root extract of *S. hypoleuca* which have not been previously reported from this species.

* Correspondence: goharii_a@tums.ac.ir
[1]Medicinal Plants Research Center, Tehran University of Medical Sciences, P. O. Box 14155–6451, Tehran, Iran
[3]Medicinal Plants Research Center, Faculty of Pharmacy, Tehran University of Medical Sciences, PO Box 14155–6451, Tehran, Iran
Full list of author information is available at the end of the article

Methods

Instruments and materials

^{1}H-NMR and ^{13}C-NMR spectra were recorded on a Brucker Avance 500 DRX spectrometer $^®$ with tetramethylsilane as an internal standard and chemical shifts are given in δ (ppm). Multiple-pulse experiments (HSQC, HMBC and H-H COSY) were performed using the standard Bruker $^®$ programs. Silicagel 60 F$_{254}$ and Silicagel 60 RP-18 F$_{254}$S pre-coated plates (Merck $^®$) were used for TLC. The spots were detected by spraying with anisaldehyde-H$_2$SO$_4$ reagent followed by heating.

Plant materials

The roots of *Salvia hypoleuca* Benth., were collected from Tehran province (near to Damavand city), Iran, at flowering stage in August 2008 and dried at room temperature. Voucher specimen was deposited at the Herbarium of Complex of Academic Center for Educational and Cultural Research under number ACECR-266.

Extraction and isolation process

Dried roots of *S. hypoleuca* (900 g) were cut into small pieces and extracted with ethyl acetate at room temperature by percolation method for 72 hours and 3 times. The solvent was evaporated by rotary evaporator. The ethyl acetate extract (2 g) was fractionated by silica gel column chromatography (CC) with hexane, hexane: chloroform (9:1, 5:5), ethyl acetate and methanol, to give seven fractions (A-G). Fraction A (88 mg) was subjected to silica gel CC with hexane: ethyl acetate (19:1) to obtain compound 1 (21 mg). Fraction B (200 mg) was submitted to silica gel CC with hexane: ethyl acetate (9:1) to give compound 2 and 3 (17 and 13 mg respectively). Fraction C (134 mg) was submitted to silica gel CC with hexane: ethyl acetate (19:1) to result in six fractions (C$_1$-C$_6$). Fraction C$_5$ (14 mg) was chromatographed on silica gel CC with chloroform: ethyl acetate (19:1) to yield compound 4 (8 mg). Fraction D (126 mg) was fractionated on silica gel CC with hexane: ethyl acetate (19:1) to obtain six parts (D$_1$-D$_6$). Fraction D$_3$ (27 mg) was separated on sephadex LH$_{20}$ with methanol: ethyl acetate (7:3) to gain four fractions (D$_{31}$-D$_{34}$). Fraction D$_{33}$ (10 mg) was subjected to reverse phase (RP) silica gel CC with methanol: water (8:2) to result in compound 5 (5 mg). Fraction F (624 mg) was fractionated on silica gel CC with chloroform: methanol (19:1) to yield three parts (F$_1$-F$_3$). Fraction F$_1$ (204 mg)

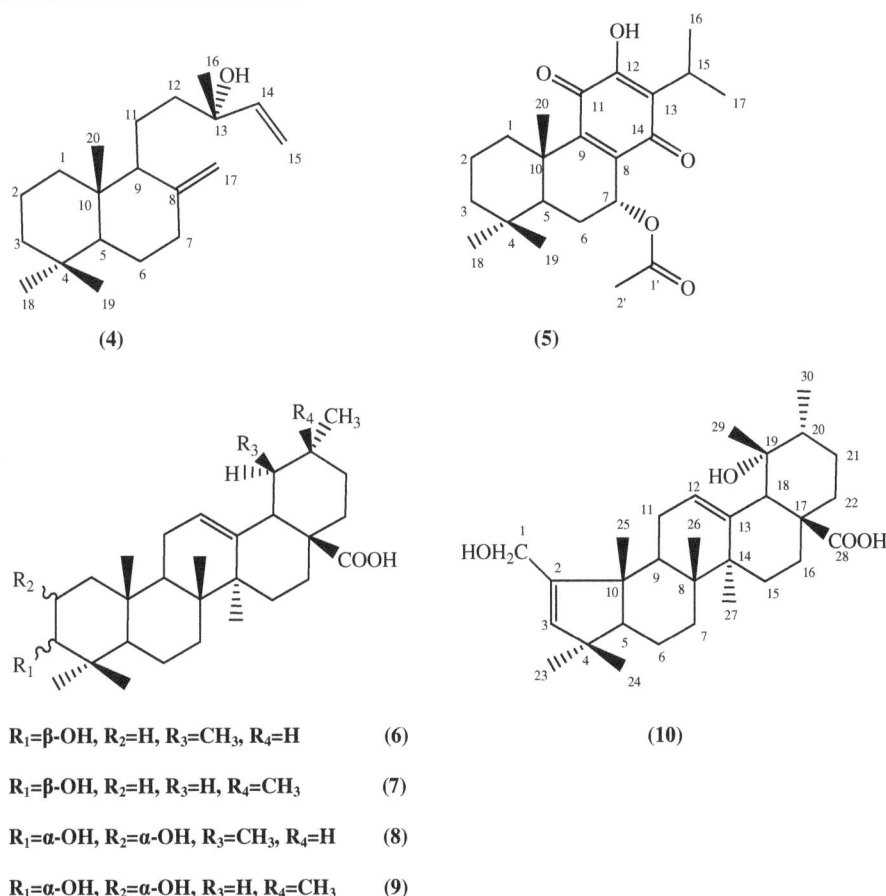

R$_1$=β-OH, R$_2$=H, R$_3$=CH$_3$, R$_4$=H (6)

R$_1$=β-OH, R$_2$=H, R$_3$=H, R$_4$=CH$_3$ (7)

R$_1$=α-OH, R$_2$=α-OH, R$_3$=CH$_3$, R$_4$=H (8)

R$_1$=α-OH, R$_2$=α-OH, R$_3$=H, R$_4$=CH$_3$ (9)

Figure 1 Structures of the isolated terpenes from the root of *Salvia hypoleuca*.

Table 1 NMR data of the compound 4 in CDCl$_3$

Carbon Number	DEPT	HSQC		HMBC	H-HCOSY
		^{1}H-NMR δ(ppm)	^{13}C-NMR δ(ppm)		
1	CH$_2$	1.00 (m, 1H)	39.07	C-5	H-1b, H-1a
		1.76 (m, 1H)			
2	CH$_2$	1.36 (m, 1H)	17.70		H-2b, H-2a
		1.55 (m, 1H)			
3	CH$_2$	1.17 (m, 1H)	42.19	C-4, C-5, C-18	H-3b, H-3a
		1.36 (m, 1H)		C-2	
4	C		33.16		-
5	CH	1.08 (brd, J=12.3 Hz, 1H)	55.58	C-4, C-6, C-7, C-18, C-20	-
6	CH$_2$	1.76 (m, 2H)	24.42		-
7	CH$_2$	1.95 (m, 1H)	38.35	C-6, C-8, C-17	-
		2.37 (brd, J=12.4 Hz, 1H)		C-5, C-6, C-8, C-9, C-17	
8	C	-	148.69		-
9	CH	1.55 (m, 1H)	57.32	C-8, C-10, C-17	-
10	C	-	39.87		-
11	CH$_2$	1.48 (m, 1H)	19.38	-	H-11b, H-11a
		1.55 (m, 1H)		C-9, C-10, C-12	
12	CH$_2$	1.27 (m, 1H)	41.43	C-16	H-12b, H-12a
		1.76 (m, 1H)		C-13, C-14	
13	C	-	73.58		-
14	CH	5.92 (dd, J=17.3,10.7 Hz, 1H)	145.29	C-13	H-15
15	CH$_2$	5.04 (d, J=10.6 Hz, 1H)	111.52	C-13	H-14
		5.20 (d, J=17.3 Hz, 1H)		C-13, C-14	
16	CH$_3$	1.27 (s, 3H)	27.66	C-12, C-14	-
17	CH$_2$	4.51 (s, 1H)	106.45	C-7, C-8, C-9	-
		4.81 (s, 1H)		C-7, C-9	
18	CH$_3$	0.79 (s, 3H)	21.71	C-3, C-4, C-5	-
19	CH$_3$	0.86 (s, 3H)	33.62	C-3, C-4, C-5, C-18	-
20	CH$_3$	0.67 (s, 3H)	14.43	C-9	-

was chromatographed on silica gel CC with chloroform: ethyl acetate (8:2) to obtain nine fractions (F$_{11}$-F$_{19}$). Fraction F$_{13}$ (30 mg) was subjected to sephadex LH$_{20}$ with methanol to result in compound 6 and 7 (7 and 5 mg, respectively). Fraction F$_{17}$ (8 mg) was submitted to sephadex LH$_{20}$ with methanol to obtain compound 8 and 9 (3 and 2 mg, respectively). Fraction F$_2$ (67 mg) was further isolated on RP silica gel CC with methanol: water (9:1) to give compound 10 (2 mg).

Results

In the present study, the ethyl acetate extract of the root of *S. hypoleuca* was used for the isolation process and structural elucidation was carried out based on spectral data. Three sterols, sitosteryl oleate (1) [18], β-sitosterol (2) [19] and stigmasterol (3) [20], two diterpenes, manool (4) [21] and 7α-acetoxyroyleanone (5) [22] together with five triterpenes, ursolic acid (6) [19], oleanolic acid (7) [23], 3-epicorosolic acid (8) [24], 3-epimaslinic acid

(9) [25] and coleonolic acid (10) [26], (Figure 1) were isolated and identified by comparison of their spectral data (^{1}H-NMR, ^{13}C-NMR, HMBC, HSQC, ^{1}H-^{1}H COSY, EI-MS) with those reported in the literature. Because these compounds were previously published from other plant sources, we do not explain the spectral assignments here. NMR data (^{1}H-NMR, ^{13}C-NMR, HMBC, HSQC and DEPT) of the compound 4 and 5 in CDCl$_3$ are shown in Tables 1 and 2 respectively. ^{13}C-NMR data of the compounds 6–10 are indicated in Table 3. Also, HMBC correlations and important assignments of the compounds 4 and 5 (H→C) are appeared in Figure 2.

The mass data of the compounds 1, 2, 3, 6 and 7 have been previously reported [27,28]. The mass of other compounds are followed: Manool (4): EIMS (70eV) m/z: 290 [M]$^+$ (8), 272 (40), 204 (20), 257 (58), 189 (28), 137 (100), 121 (48), 95 (67). 3-epicorosolic acid (8): 472 [M]$^+$ (5), 248 (100), 223 (18), 203 (61), 189 (13), 133 (20), 119 (10). 3-epimaslinic acid (9): 472 [M]$^+$ (4), 248 (100), 235

Table 2 NMR data of the compound 5 in CDCl₃

| Carbon number | DEPT | HSQC | | HMBC |
		¹H-NMR δ(ppm)	¹³C-NMR δ(ppm)	
1	CH₂	1.20 (m, 1H)	35.77	
		2.72 (brd, J=13.0 Hz, 1H)		
2	CH₂	1.58 (m, 1H)	18.80	C-10
		1.72 (dd, J=13.3,13.4 Hz, 1H)		
3	CH₂	1.21 (m, 1H)	40.97	-
		1.47 (brd, J=12.7 Hz, 1H)		C-18, C-19
4	C	-	32.96	
5	CH	1.47 (brd, J=12.7 Hz, 1H)	46.12	C-4, C-7, C-10, C-18, C-20
6	CH₂	1.60 (m, 1H)	24.61	C-5, C-10
		1.93 (d, J=14.9 Hz, 1H)		C-5, C-7, C-8, C-10
7	CH	5.92 (brs, 1H)	64.48	
8	C	-	139.45	
9	C	-	149.94	
10	C	-	39.06	
11	C	-	183.72	
12	C	-	150.75	
13	C	-	124.66	
14	C	-	185.45	
15	CH₃	3.15 (m, 1H)	24.15	C-12, C-13, C-14, C-17
16	CH₃	1.17 (d, J=7.0 Hz, 3H)	19.68	C-13, C-15, C-17
17	CH₃	1.22 (d, J=7.0 Hz, 3H)	19.86	C-13, C-15, C-16
18	CH	0.87 (s, 3H)	21.61	C-3, C-5, C-19
19	CH₃	0.87 (s, 3H)	32.96	C-3, C-5, C-18
20	CH₃	1.23 (s, 3H)	18.48	C-1, C-5, C-9, C-10
1′	C	-	169.46	
2′	CH₃	2.03 (s, 3H)	21.11	C-1′
OH-12		7.12 (s, 1H)	-	C-11, C-12, C-13

(9), 223 (12), 203 (54), 189 (15), 133 (28). coleonolic acid (10): m/z 470 [M]⁺ (7), 452 (25), 264 (18), 206 (15), 201 (35), 159 (28), 146 (50), 105 (100).

β-sitosterol: ¹³C-NMR (125 MHz, CDCl₃): δ_C (from C-1 to C-29) 37.3, 31.7, 71.8, 42.3, 140.8, 121.7, 31.9, 31.9, 50.2, 36.5, 21.1, 39.8, 42.3, 56.8, 24.3, 28.3, 56.1, 11.9, 19.8, 36.2, 18.8, 34.0, 26.1, 45.8, 29.2, 19.0, 19.4, 23.1, 12.0.

Stigmasterol: ¹³C-NMR (125 MHz, CDCl₃): δ_C (from C-1 to C-29) 37.3, 31.7, 71.8, 42.2, 140.8, 121.7, 31.9, 31.9, 50.2, 36.4, 21.1, 39.7, 42.2, 56.9, 24.4, 28.9, 56.0, 12.0, 19.4, 40.5, 21.2, 138.3, 129.3, 51.6, 31.9, 19.0, 21.1, 25.4, 12.2.

Discussion

Literature reviews show that Salvia species are important medicinal and food plants. About 200 triterpenoids have been isolated and identified from about 100 Salvia species and presented in a review article by Topcu [29]. The oleanane, and ursane triterpenes display various pharmacological activities. These triterpenes can be considered as the lead compounds for the development of new multi-targeting bioactive agents [30]. Both oleanolic and ursolic acid have been documented to protect liver against chemically induced injuries in laboratory animals via inhibition of toxicant activation and enhancement of immune systems. These two triterpenes have also been long-recognized as anti-inflammatory and anti-hyperlipidemic agents. Furthermore, anti-tumor activity has been noted from both non-toxic compounds [31].

Corosolic acid, a triterpenoid compound has been proved to have anti-diabetic effects on animal and human via enhancing glucose uptake in L6 myotubes and facilitating glucose transporters isoform 4 translocation in CHO/hIR cells. In addition, corosolic acid has been reported to inhibit the enzymatic activity of several non-receptor protein tyrosine phosphatases (PTPs) [32]. The abietane diterpene 7 α-acetoxy-royleanone, containing quinone moiety in its structure, was demonstrated to possess cytotoxic activity on cancer cell lines and also alkylating properties using the nucleophile

Table 3 ^{13}C-NMR data of the compounds 6–10

Carbon Number	8[a]	9[a]	10[b]	Carbon Number	8	9	10
1	41.94	41.69	61.4	16	24.13	23.27	27.3
2	66.49	66.50	156.1	17	48.10	46.48	-
3	78.91	78.92	135.2	18	52.63	41.04	55.3
4	38.34	38.34	42.7	19	39.04	45.89	73.5
5	48.13	48.14	64.4	20	38.84	30.67	44.4
6	18.03	18.03	18.3	21	30.61	33.83	26.6
7	32.73	32.46	35.3	22	36.70	32.46	39.0
8	39.49	39.70	42.9	23	28.48	28.48	30.3
9	47.28	47.35	43.1	24	21.81	21.79	21.9
10	38.23	38.42	51.8	25	16.47	16.33	19.1
11	23.27	22.95	27.1	26	16.98	17.13	16.5
12	125.64	122.46	129.5	27	23.74	26.07	25.5
13	138.06	143.68	140.3	28	181.95	181.95	182.2
14	42.10	41.76	43.3	29	17.10	33.05	27.7
15	27.96	27.63	29.9	30	21.16	23.58	16.5

[a] In CDCl$_3$.
[b] In CD$_3$OD.

4-(4-nitrobenzyl) pyridine [33]. Among the reported antimicrobial labdane-type diterpenes, manool is the most active, since it furnished very promising MIC values for several tested bacteria that are closely associated with periodontitis [34].

According to chemotaxonomic significance, the isolated terpenes (manool (4), 7α-acetoxy-royleanone (5), ursolic acid (6), oleanolic acid (7), 3-epimaslinic acid (9)) were previously reported from other *Salvia* species such as *S. sclarea* [21], *S. pubescens* [35], *S. lavandulifolia* [36] and *S. officinalis* [37]. To the best of our knowledge, there is no report about the presence of the above mentioned compounds from *S. hypoleuca*. The triterpene 3-epicorosolic acid (8) and coleonolic acid (10) has not been reported from *Salvia* species, while some other

genus of Lamiaceae such as *Perilla frutescens* [38] and *Coleus forskohlii* [39] contains these triterpenes.

Conclusions

In conclusion, the results of this study indicated the presence of ten terpenes and sterols in the root extract of *S. hypoleuca* as: sitosteryl oleate (1), β-sitosterol (2), stigmasterol (3), manool (4), 7α-acetoxy royleanone (5), ursolic acid (6), oleanolic acid (7), 3-epicorosolic acid (8), 3-epimaslinic acid (9) and coleonolic acid (10). Some of the isolated compounds (1–7, 9) have not been previously reported from *S. hypoleuca* and the triterpenes 8 and 10 not reported from *Salvia* genus until now. The above mentioned compounds have been recognized as

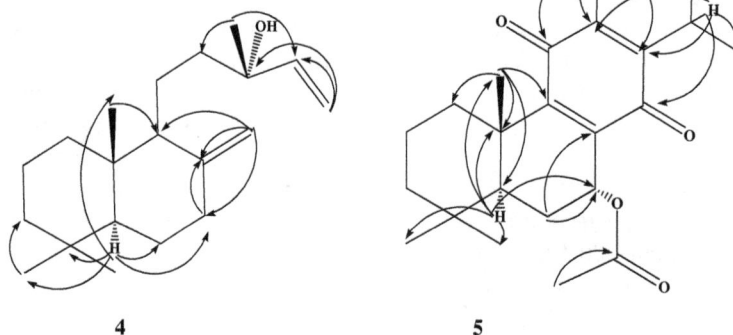

Figure 2 HMBC correlations and important assignments of the compounds 4 and 5 (H→C).

the biologically and pharmacologically active constituents from this medicinal and aromatic species of *salvia*.

Competing interests
The authors declare that they have no competing interests.

Authors' contributions
SS carried out the interpretation of the NMR data and identification of the compounds. MG carried out the isolation and purification process. ARG participated in design of the study, helped in structured elucidation and final approved of the version to be published. AS participated in drafting the manuscript and helped in isolation of the compounds. All authors read and approved the final manuscript.

Acknowledgements
This research was supported by Tehran University of Medical Sciences and Health Services grant (No. 11847). The authors wish to thank Mr. Yousef Ajani (Institute of Medicinal Plants, Jahade-Daneshgahi) for his help in collection and identification of the plant material.

Author details
[1]Medicinal Plants Research Center, Tehran University of Medical Sciences, P. O. Box 14155–6451, Tehran, Iran. [2]Department of Chemistry, Faculty of Science, Golestan University, Gorgan, Iran. [3]Medicinal Plants Research Center, Faculty of Pharmacy, Tehran University of Medical Sciences, PO Box 14155–6451, Tehran, Iran.

References
1. Hedge IC: **Labiatae**. In *Flora Iranica. Volume 151*. Edited by Rechinger KH. Graz: Akademische Druck-u Verlagsanstalt; 1986:403–480.
2. Saeidnia S, Gohari AR, Malmir M, Moradi-Afrapoli F, Ajani Y: **Tryptophan and sterols from *Salvia limbata***. *J Med Plants* 2011, **10**:41–47.
3. Lu Y, Foo LY: **Polyphenolics of *Salvia* - a review**. *Phytochemistry* 2002, **59**:117–140.
4. Tutin TG, Heywood VH, Burgess NA, Moore DM, Valentine DH, Walters SM, Webb DA: ***Salvia* L**. In *Flora Europa*. Edited by Hedge IC. Cambridge: Cambridge University Press; 1972:188–192.
5. Ulubelen A, Sönmez U, Topcu G, Johansson CB: **An abietane diterpene and two phenolics from *Salvia forskahlei***. *Phytochemistry* 1996, **42**:145–147.
6. Gohari AR, Saeidnia S, Malmir M, Hadjiakhoondi A, Ajani Y: **Flavones and rosmarinic acid from *Salvia limbata***. *Nat Prod Res* 2010, **24**:1902–1906.
7. Suzuki H, Sawada S, Watanabe K, Nagae S, Yamaguchi MA, Nakayama T, Nishino T: **Identification and characterization of a novel anthocyanin malonyltransferase from scarlet sage (*Salvia splendens*) flowers: an enzyme that is phylogenetically separated from other anthocyanin acyltransferases**. *Plant J* 2004, **38**:994–1003.
8. Amiri H: **Quantative and qualative changes of essential oil of *Salvia bracteata* Bank et Sol. in different growth stages**. *Daru* 2007, **15**(Suppl 2):79–82.
9. Sajjadi SE, Shahpiri Z: **Chemical composition of the essential oil *Salvia Limbata* C.A. mey.** *Daru* 2004, **12**(Suppl 3):94–97.
10. Ghannadi A, Samsam-shariat SH, Moattar F: **Volatile constituents of the flower of *Salvia hydrangea* DC. Ex Benth**. *Daru* 1999, **7**(Suppl 3):23–25.
11. Matloubi moghadam F, Amin GH, Safavi poorsohi E: **Composition of stembark essential oil from *Salvia macrosiphon* Boiss**. *Daru* 2000, **8**(Suppl 1):28–29.
12. Rustaiyan A, Koussari S: **Further sesterterpenes from *Salvia hypoleuca***. *Phytochemistry* 1988, **27**:1767–1769.
13. Rustaiyan A, Niknejad A, Nazarians L, Jakupovic J, Bohlmann F: **Sesterterpenes from *Salvia hypoleuca***. *Phytochemistry* 1982, **21**:1812–1813.
14. Ali MS, Ahmed W, Jassbi AR, Onocha PA: **Hypoleuenoic acid: a trans-cinnamic acid derived secondary metabolite from *Salvia hypoleuca* (Lamiaceae)**. *J Chem Soc Pak* 2005, **27**:316–319.
15. Bigdeli M, Rustaiyan A, Nadimi M, Masoudi S: **Composition of the essential oil from roots of *Salvia hypoleuca* Benth. from Iran**. *J Essent Oil Res* 2005, **17**:82–83.

16. Rustaiyan A, Komeilizadeh H, Masoudiand S, Monfared A: **Volatile constituents of three *Salvia* species grown wild in Iran**. *Flav Frag J* 1999, **14**:276–278.
17. Atta-ur-Rahman: **Studies in natural products chemistry**. *Elsevier B V* 2008, **35**:753.
18. Julien-David D, Geoffroy P, Marchioni E, Raul F, Aoude-Werner D, Miesch M: **Synthesis of highly pure (oxy) phytosterols and (oxy) phytosterol esters Part II. (Oxy)-sitosterol esters derived from oleic acid and from 9,10-dihydroxystearic acid**. *Steroids* 2008, **73**:1098–1109.
19. Gohari AR, Saeidnia S, Shahverdi AR, Yassa N, Malmir M, Mollazade K, Naghinejad AR: **Phytochemistry and antimicrobial compounds of *Hymenocrater calycinus***. *Eur Asia J Bio Sci* 2009, **3**:64–68.
20. Nasiri M, Saeidnia S, Mashinchian-Moradi A, Gohari AR: **Srerols from the red algae, *Gracilaria salicornia* and *Hypnea flagelliformis*, from Persian Gulf**. *Phcog Mag* 2011, **7**:97–100.
21. Ulubelen A, Topcu G, Eris C, Sonmez U, Kartal M, Kurucu S, Bozok-Johansson C: **Terpenoids from *Salvia sclarea***. *Phytochemistry* 1994, **36**:971–974.
22. Rodriguez B: **^{1}H and ^{13}C NMR spectral assignments of some natural abietane diterpenoids**. *Mag Res Chem* 2003, **41**:741–746.
23. Gohari AR, Saeidnia S, Hadjiakhoondi A, Abdoullahi M, Nezafati M: **Isolation and Quantificative Analysis of Oleanolic acid from *Satureja mutica* Fisch. & C. A. Mey**. *J Med Plants* 2009, **8**:65–6934.
24. Kojima H, Ogura H: **Configurational Studies on Hydroxy Groups at C-2,3 and 23 or 24 of Oleanene and Ursene-type Triterpenes by NMR Spectroscopy**. *Phytochemistry* 1989, **28**:1703–1710.
25. Mahato SB, Kundu AP: **^{13}C NMR Spectra of pentacyclic triterpenoids, a compilation and some salient features**. *Phytochemistry* 1994, **37**:1517–1575.
26. Raja Rao KV, Rao LJM, Prakasa Rao NS: **An A-Ring Contracted Triterpenoid from *Hyptis suaveolens***. *Phytochemistry* 1990, **29**:1326–1329.
27. Shahani S, Monsef-Esfahani HR, Saeidnia S, Saniee P, Siavoshi F, Foroumadi A, Samadi N, Gohari AR: **Anti-Helicobacter pylori activity of the methanolic extract of *Geum iranicum* and its main compounds**. *Z Naturforsch* 2012, **67c**:172–180.
28. Gohari AR, Hadjiakhoondi A, Sadat-Ebrahimi SE, Saeidnia S, Shafiee A: **Cytotoxic triterpenoids from *Satureja macrantha* C.A. Mey**. *Daru* 2005, **13**(4):177–181.
29. Topcu G: **Bioactive triterpenoids from *Salvia* species**. *J Nat Prod* 2006, **69**:482–487.
30. Jager S, Trojan H, Kopp T, Laszczyk MN, Scheffler A: **Pentacyclic triterpen distribution in various plants-rich sources for a new group of multi-potent plant extracts**. *Molecules* 2009, **14**:2016–2031.
31. Liu J: **Pharmacology of oleanolic acid and ursolic acid**. *J Ethnopharmacol* 1995, **49**:57–68.
32. Shi L, Zhang W, Zhou YY, Zhang YN, Li JY, Hu LH, Li J: **Corosolic acid stimulates glucose uptake *via* enhancing insulin receptor phosphorylation**. *Eur J Pharmacol* 2008, **584**:21–29.
33. Fronza M, Lamy E, Günther S, Heinzmann B, Laufer S, Merfort I: **Abietane diterpenes induce cytotoxic effects in human pancreatic cancer cell line MIA PaCa-2 through different modes of action**. *Phytochemistry* 2012, **78**:107–19.
34. Souza AB, de Souza MGM, Moreira MA, Moreira MR, Furtado NAJC, Martins CHG, Bastos JK, dos Santos RA, Heleno VCG, Ambrosio SR, Veneziani RCS: **Antimicrobial evaluation of diterpenes from *Copaifera langsdorffii* oleoresin against periodontal anaerobic bacteria**. *Molecules* 2011, **16**:9611–9619.
35. Galicia MA, Esquivel B, Sanchez AA, Cardenas J, Ramamoorthy TP, Rodriguez-Hahn L: **Abietane diterpenoids from *Salvia pubescens***. *Phytochemistry* 1988, **27**:217–219.
36. Passannantia S, Paternostroa M, Piozzi F: **Triterpene acids from *Salvia* and *Teucrium* species**. *Phytochemistry* 1983, **22**:1044–1045.
37. Brieskorn CH, Kapadia Z: **Bestandteile von *Salvia officinalis***. *Planta Med* 1980, **38**:86–90.
38. Banno N, Akihisa T, Tokuda H, Yasukawa K, Higashihara H, Ukiya M, Watanabe K, Kimura Y, Hasegawa J, Nishino H: **Triterpene acids from the leaves of *Perilla frutescens* and their anti-inflammatory and antitumor-promoting effects**. *Biosci Biotech Biochem* 2004, **68**:85–90.
39. Roy R, Vishwakarma RA, Varma N, Tandon JS: **Coleonolic acid, a rearranged ursane triterpenoid from *Coleus forskohlii***. *Tetrahedron Lett* 1990, **31**:3467–3470.

Formulation and evaluation of microsphere based oro dispersible tablets of itopride hcl

Sanjay Shah, Sarika Madan and SS Agrawal[*]

Abstract

Background: The purpose of the present work is to mask the intensely bitter taste of Itopride HCl and to formulate an Oro dispersible tablet (ODT) of the taste-masked drug by incorporation of microspheres in the tablets for use in specific populations viz. pediatrics, geriatrics and patients experiencing difficulty in swallowing.

Methods: With this objective in mind, microspheres loaded with Itopride HCl were prepared by solvent evaporation method using acetone as solvent for pH-sensitive polymer, Eudragit EPO and light liquid paraffin as the encapsulating medium. The prepared microspheres were characterized with regard to yield, drug content, flow properties, particle size and size distribution, surface features, in vitro drug release and taste. The ODTs so prepared from these microspheres were evaluated for hardness, thickness, weight variation, friability, disintegration time, drug content, wetting time, water absorption ratio, moisture uptake, in vitro dispersion, in vitro disintegration, in vitro drug release and stability.

Results: The average size of microspheres was found to be satisfactory in terms of the size and size distribution. Microspheres prepared were of a regular spherical shape. Comparison of the dissolution profiles of microspheres in different pH media showed that microspheres having drug: polymer ratio of 1:2 produced a retarding effect in simulated salivary fluid (pH 6.8) and were further used for formulation into ODTs after addition of suitable amounts of excipients such as superdisintegrant, diluent, sweetener and flavor of directly compressible grade.

Conclusions: Effective taste-masking was achieved for Itopride HCl by way of preparation of microspheres and ODTs of acceptable characteristics.

Keywords: Taste masking, Orodispersible tablets, Itopride HCl, Eudragit EPO, Superdisintegrants

Introduction

Among the different routes of administration, oral route of administration continues to be the most preferred route due to various advantages including ease of ingestion, avoidance of pain, versatility and most importantly patient compliance. The different dosage forms include tablets, capsules and oral liquid preparations. The important drawback of tablet and capsule dosage forms for pediatric and geriatric patients has been difficulty in swallowing [1]. To overcome this problem, formulators have

considerably dedicated their effort to develop a novel type of tablet dosage form for oral administration called "Oro Dispersible Tablet", (ODT) i.e., one, which disintegrates and dissolves rapidly in saliva without the need of water [2]. United States Food and Drug Administration (FDA) defined ODT as "A solid dosage form containing medicinal substance or active ingredient which disintegrates rapidly usually within a matter of seconds when placed upon the tongue [3]." The disintegration time for ODTs generally ranges from several seconds to about a min.

The two key parameters that need to be considered in the development of ODTs are taste masking of bitter drug and the disintegration time. Various taste-masking technologies have been extensively reviewed [4-6]. Solvent evaporation is a relatively simple and convenient method for the preparation of taste-masked microspheres. The drug particles are

[*] Correspondence: agrawal.shyam01@gmail.com
Delhi Institute of Pharmaceutical Sciences & Research (Formerly College of Pharmacy), University of Delhi, Pushp Vihar, Sector III, New Delhi 110017, India

Table 1 Different ratios of Drug: polymer for preparation of microspheres (mean ± SD, n = 3)

Batch	Microspheres ingredients and process parameters						Microspheres evaluation parameters *				
	Itopride HCl (mg)	Eudragit EPO (mg)	Magnesium stearate (mg)	Liquid paraffin (ml)	Acetone (ml)	Speed (RPM)	Yield (%)	Average Particle Diameter (μm)	Drug content (%)	Loading efficiency (%)	% release of drug in simulated saliva in 60 sec
A1	200	200	200	40	2.0	600	69.3 ± 1.2	186.3 ± 2.5	37.86 ± 0.5	94.65 ± 1.2	6.31 ± 0.09
A2	200	400	200	40	2.0	600	72.3 ± 1.5	197.2 ± 2.8	32.02 ± 0.2	96.09 ± 1.3	1.61 ± 0.06
A3	200	600	200	40	2.0	600	77.6 ± 2.1	202.2 ± 3.7	24.32 ± 0.3	97.28 ± 1.6	1.57 ± 0.04
A4	200	800	200	40	2.0	600	75.9 ± 1.7	278.6 ± 4.2	19.23 ± 0.1	96.15 ± 1.4	1.51 ± 0.05
A5	200	1000	200	40	2.0	600	68.3 ± 2.4	327.9 ± 3.6	16.17 ± 0.2	97.05 ± 1.3	1.43 ± 0.07

surrounded by a polymer which prevent leaching of the drug into the saliva but allow the release of the drug in the stomach. The most widely used solvent systems in solvent evaporation process are methylene chloride/water [7] and acetone/light liquid paraffin [8-11]. This technology has been applied to mask the bitter taste of therapeutic agents such as bacampicilin [8,12] pseudoephedrine [7] and cefuroxime axetil [10].

Itopride Hydrochloride is used for the management of Nonulcer dyspepsia (NUD), gastro-esophageal reflux disease (GERD), gastritis, diabetes gastro paresis and functional dyspepsia. It is a newer gastroprokinetic agent with anti cholinesterase activity as well as D_2 receptor antagonistic activity and is being used for the symptomatic treatment of various gastrointestinal motility disorders [13]. Itopride HCl is available in market in the form of immediate release tablets/capsules, for e.g. "GANATON®" sold by Abbott Laboratories (Abbott Park, Illinois). Itopride HCl is a highly water soluble and intensely bitter drug. Thus, it was envisaged to mask the taste of Itopride HCl by way of making microspheres prior to formulating ODTs with good mouth feel. To the best of our knowledge, it is the first time such an attempt has been made that would explore the rational approach of incorporating taste-masked microspheres of Itopride HCl in an orally disintegrating tablet.

Materials and methods
Materials
Itopride HCl was obtained as a gift from Ranbaxy Laboratories Ltd (Gurgaon, India). Aminoalkyl methacrylate copolymer (Eudragit EPO) was obtained as a gift from

Table 2 Taste-masked Itopride HCl microsphere ingredients, process parameters and evaluation (Mean ± SD, n = 3)

Batch	Microspheres ingredients and process parameters						Microspheres evaluation parameters			
	Itopride HCl (mg)	Eudragit EPO (mg)	Acetone (ml)	Magnesium sterate(mg)	Liquid paraffin (ml)	Speed (RPM)	(%) Yield	Average Particle Diameter(μm)	(%) Drug content	% Loading efficiency
B1	200	400	1.6	200	40	600	70.8 ± 1.3	285.5 ± 1.2	24.76 ± 0.4	99.04 ± 0.5
B2	200	400	1.8	200	40	600	81.89 ± 1.4	216.9 ± 1.7	24.05 ± 0.7	96.20 ± 0.07
B3	200	400	2.0	200	40	600	78.19 ± 1.5	197.8 ± 2.4	23.84 ± 0.3	95.36 ± 0.4
B4	200	400	2.2	200	40	600	72.6 ± 1.6	121.1 ± 1.9	23.96 ± 0.5	95.84 ± 0.2
C1	200	400	1.8	80	40	600	Batch Failed			
C2	200	400	1.8	120	40	600	61.59 ± 2.3	283.0 ± 2.6	27.56 ± 0.1	99.21 ± 0.1
C3	200	400	1.8	160	40	600	82.32 ± 2.5	238.5 ± 1.5	25.94 ± 0.2	98.58 ± 0.2
C4	200	400	1.8	180	40	600	80.18 ± 2.1	201.1 ± 3.5	24.83 ± 0.4	96.84 ± 0.4
D1	200	400	1.8	160	20	600	Batch Failed			
D2	200	400	1.8	160	30	600	73.84 ± 1.6	302.5 ± 2.4	26.17 ± 0.6	99.46 ± 0.5
D3	200	400	1.8	160	40	600	82.13 ± 1.7	264.7 ± 1.0	25.96 ± 0.7	98.66 ± 0.7
D4	200	400	1.8	160	50	600	75.58 ± 2.5	182.4 ± 3.1	25.47 ± 0.8	96.80 ± 0.3
E1	200	400	1.8	160	40	200	Batch Failed			
E2	200	400	1.8	160	40	400	84.31 ± 3.0	296.58 ± 2.2	25.36 ± 0 .7	96.35 ± 0.5
E3	200	400	1.8	160	40	600	82.11 ± 2.8	214.60 ± 3.2	25.43 ± 0.09	96.66 ± 0.3
E4	200	400	1.8	160	40	800	77.74 ± 3.2	174.64 ± 2.0	25.44 ± 0.7	96.66 ± 0.2
E5	200	400	1.8	160	40	1000	62.76 ± 2.8	128.5 ± 1.8	24.96 ± 0.4	94.48 ± 0.1

Degussa India Private Ltd (Mumbai, India). Magnesium stearate was kindly supplied by Unichem (New Delhi, India). Other excipients that were purchased included mannitol (Pearlitol, CDH (P) Ltd., New Delhi, India), sodium stearyl fumarate (ITM Chem. Pvt. Ltd. Mumbai), Nutra Sweet (Aspartame, Kawarlal and sons, Chennai, India) and crospovidone (Polyplasdone XL-10, Nanz Med Sciences Pharma Pvt. Ltd., Delhi, India). All other chemicals used in the study were of analytical grade and used as received.

Methods
Preparation of microspheres
Microspheres were prepared by the solvent evaporation method previously reported and modified for our purpose [10,12]. Firstly, Eudragit EPO was dissolved in acetone on a magnetic stirrer to obtain uniform mixing. Itopride HCl was then added to the above solution. To this mixture, magnesium stearate was added. The polymer drug solution so obtained was injected into light liquid paraffin at a low stirring speed (200–600 rpm) of mechanical stirrer for about 3 h until all the acetone evaporated. n-Hexane/petroleum ether was added to the system for hardening of the microspheres and to accelerate settling. Microspheres were separated by decantation following filtration through a Whatman filter paper (No. 41). Microspheres were then washed with *n*-hexane and the washed microspheres were dried in an oven maintained at 37°C for 24 h. Dried microspheres were stored at room temperature. Various drug: polymer ratios were selected for the formulation of microspheres (Table 1). The formulation parameters and process parameters for different batches of microspheres were evaluated (Table 2).

Characterization of Microspheres
Percentage Yield
The prepared microspheres were completely dried in an oven maintained at 37°C for 24 h and then weighed. The percentage yield of microspheres was calculated according to the following equation:

$$\% \, yield = \frac{Practical \, yield}{Theoretical \, yield} * 100 \qquad (1)$$

Drug Loading and Drug content [14]
The microspheres (100 mg) were crushed in pestle-mortar and then stirred with 100 ml 0.1 N HCl (pH 1.2) for 2 hr to ensure complete elution of drug. The readings were taken in triplicate. The Itopride HCl content of the microspheres was calculated using a standard calibration curve prepared with UV-Visible spectrophotometer at 258 nm after suitable dilution.

$$Drug \, content (\%) = \frac{Weight \, of \, drug \, in \, microspheres}{Weight \, of \, microspheres} * 100 \qquad (2)$$

$$Drug \, loading (\%) = \frac{Weight \, of \, drug \, in \, microspheres}{Weight \, of \, drug \, initially \, added} * 100 \qquad (3)$$

Evaluation of flow properties of microspheres
The prepared microspheres were evaluated for flow properties [15] including bulk density (D_b), tapped density (ρ_t), Carr's compressibility index (I) [16], Hausner ratio (H) [17] and Angle of Repose (θ).

Micromeritics of microspheres
The size distribution and average size of the microspheres were determined by sieve analysis using American society for testing of materials (ASTM) sieves. A set of 12 sieves ranging in size from 1.18 mm (# 16) to 75 microns (# 200) mounted on a sieve shaker unit was used. Amount of microspheres remaining on each sieve was then weighed and calculated [18].

Scanning Electron Microscopy Analysis of the Microspheres
The drug and microspheres were characterized further using a scanning electron microscope (JEOL JSM5200, Japan Electron Optics Ltd., Japan) after gold sputtering. Shapes and surface characteristics of the microspheres were investigated and photographed.

Thermal analysis of the microspheres
Differential scanning calorimetric (DSC) experiments were performed on Itopride Hydrochloride, Eudragit EPO and drug-loaded microspheres (Shimadzu TA 60WS, Japan). Accurately weighted samples (2–5 mg) were sealed in flat bottom aluminum pans and heated from ambient to 200°C at a rate of 10°C/min in a nitrogen atmosphere (flow rate, 10 ml/min).

Fourier-Transform IR (FTIR) studies
Fourier Transform Infrared (FTIR) scans of Itopride HCl, Eudragit EPO, Physical ad-mixture of drug plus Eudragit EPO and drug-loaded microspheres were recorded (Jasco FTIR-410, Japan). All the discs were prepared in KBr press.

In vitro release studies

In vitro drug release studies were carried out using USP XXIV dissolution apparatus II. [19]Accurately weighed Itopride HCl microspheres (equivalent to 10 mg of Itopride HCl) were added to the medium under test. The test was carried out in pH 1.2 (900 ml) and pH 6.8 phosphate buffer (900 ml) equilibrated at $37 \pm 0.5°C$. The paddle was rotated at 50 rpm. At specific times of 5, 10, 15 and 30 min, aliquots of the dissolution medium were withdrawn and which replaced with 10 ml of fresh dissolution medium. The collected samples were analyzed using UV spectrophotometer at 258 nm.

Preparation of the ODTs

Orodispersible tablets of Itopride HCl microspheres were prepared by direct compression technique using crospovidone as a superdisintegrant. The optimization of tablet disintegration is commonly done by means of the disintegration critical concentration. Below this concentration the tablet disintegration time is inversely proportional to the disintegrant concentration. Above the critical concentration, the disintegration time remains approximately constant or even increased [20]. The selected batch of microspheres were incorporated into tablets on the basis of drug loading so as to give the required dose of 50 mg/tablet. The microspheres were blended along with the other excipients (super-disintegrant, sweetener, flavor and lubricant) and processed to allow direct compression tabletting in a single punch tablet machine (Cadmach, India) using 11-mm round, convex-faced, beveled edge tooling (Panacea tools Ltd., New Delhi).

Evaluation and characterization of Tablets

Thickness of tablets was assessed using a Vernier caliper. The hardness of the tablets was determined by using Monsanto hardness tester (Pharma Chem. Machineries, India) and about 4–6 kg/cm^2 was considered adequate for mechanical stability of ODT [21]. Uniformity of weight was also determined as per Indian Pharmacopoeia (IP) [22]. As per USP 30-NF 25, friability of twenty six tablets was determined using Roche Friabilator (EI Products, India) [21]. The India Pharmacopoeia prescribes a friability <1% for good mechanical resistance.

Determination of drug content

Six tablets were crushed to a powder and powder equivalent to 10 mg Itopride HCl was taken and dissolved in 0.1 N HCl to extract the active ingredient. The solution was filtered through Whatmann filter paper (no. 41). After suitable dilution with 0.1 N HCl, the drug content was analyzed by UV spectrophotometer at 258 nm [23].

In vitro evaluation of tablets

Wetting time and water absorption ratio of tablets were determined as per method prescribed in the literature earlier [24]. Moisture uptake test was performed in conditions prescribed in literature [25]. In vitro dispersion time was measured by dropping a tablet without disc in a measuring cylinder containing 10 ml of phosphate buffer pH 6.8 (simulated saliva fluid and time required for complete dispersion of a tablet was measured. In vitro disintegration test was carried out using USP XXIV tablet disintegration test apparatus (Pharma Test, Germany) [26]. The time for disintegration of ODTs is generally less than one min and actual disintegration time that patient can experience ranges from 5–30 seconds. In-vitro Dissolution studies [27] were performed using USP XXIV Type II dissolution paddle apparatus (Lab India, DS 8000, India). The dissolution test was performed using 900 ml of 0.1 N HCl buffer at $37 \pm 0.5°C$. The speed of rotation of paddle was set at 50 rpm. Samples of commercial product GANATON and oral disintegrating tablet (F2) of Itopride HCL (equivalent to 50 mg of Itopride HCL) were introduced in the dissolution medium. The dissolution tests were carried out for 2 h with sampling time intervals of 2, 5, 10, 15, 30, 45, 60, 90 and 120 min respectively. The samples were analyzed using a double beam UV-spectrophotometer and the absorbance was recorded at 258 nm. The in-vitro dissolution studies were performed in triplicate.

In Vivo studies

Pharmacokinetic studies

ODT tablet was subjected to bioequivalence studies using albino rabbits and observed plasma concentration was plotted against the time and compared with marketed formulation GANATON.

The experiments were conducted as per CPCSEA (Committee for Prevention, Control and Supervision of Experimental Animals) guidelines. Rabbits (2.0-2.5 kg) of either sex were kept in normal housing conditions and were fed with commercially available diet, sprouted grams and cabbage. The rabbits were used in the study in accordance with a protocol approved by the Institutional ethical committee at DIPSAR protocol number: DIPSAR/IAEC/21/2010.

The rabbits were randomly divided into two groups of three rabbits each. All the rabbits were fasted for 12 h with ad libitum access to water. One group received Marketed product GANATON whereas the other group received the test formulation ODT F2. The test tablets were administered in the mouth of rabbit through intragastric tube and immediately 5 ml of water was administered to facilitate swallowing of the powder and to prevent it from sticking to the rabbit's throat while the marketed tablet was crushed prior to administration.

Table 3 Physical properties of Microspheres of Itopride HCl* (Mean ± SD, n = 3)

Formulation code	Evaluation properties					
	Angle of Repose (θ)	Bulk Density (g/cm³)	Tapped density (g/cm³)	Carr's Compressibility index (%)	Hausner's Ratio	Flowability
B2	29.35 ± 1.67	0.58 ± 0.02	0.71 ± 0.12	16.32 ± 0.55	1.56 ± 0.02	Fair
C3	27.21 ± 1.34	0.56 ± 0.15	0.67 ± 0.03	18.49 ± 0.19	1.36 ± 0.01	Good
D3	30.56 ± 1.56	0.61 ± 0.05	0.68 ± 0.04	19.57 ± 0.22	1.28 ± 0.04	Fair
E3	24.87 ± 0.89	0.52 ± 0.12	0.65 ± 0.02	14.09 ± 0.44	1.15 ± 0.02	Excellent

Blood sample (0.6 ml) was withdrawn from marginal ear vein into eppendorf tubes containing EDTA at time intervals of 5, 15, 30, 45, 60, 120 min and 4, 6, 8, 12, 16 and 24 h post administration. The blood was immediately centrifuged at 3500 rpm for 30 min at 0°C and plasma was stored at −20°C until HPTLC analysis. To 0.5 ml aliquot of plasma, 0.5 ml of ethyl acetate was added, centrifuged at 3500 rpm for 40 min at 0°C. The supernatant was separated. From this supernatant ethyl acetate was allowed to evaporate. When the samples were dried completely they were reconstituted with mobile phase (chloroform: methanol, 9:1) and kept frozen until analyzed. The plasma drug content was analyzed by HPTLC (CAMAG, Switzerland). Reconstituted sample of 1, 2, 3, 4, 5, 6, 7 and 8 µL was spotted in the bands of 4 mm width using a CAMAG microlitre syringe - volume of 100 µL, on to the precoated silica gel aluminium plate using Linomat V sample applicator. The plate was allowed to develop in linear ascending mode in CAMAG twin trough glass chamber saturated with the mobile phase. The saturation time for mobile phase was chosen at 30mins. The chromatogram run was 8 cm. The developed TLC plate was scanned on a CAMAG TLC Scanner III in the absorbance mode of 258 nm by using a deuterium lamp as a source of radiation. Pharmacokinetic parameters for Itopride following administration were determined from plasma concentration-time data. The pharmacokinetic profile of the formulation was compared with the marketed formulation administered orally to the other group of animals.

The pharmacokinetic parameters, namely, maximum plasma concentration (C_{max}) and time to reach C_{max} (T_{max}) were obtained directly from the plasma concentration–time data. The area under the plasma concentration–time curve from 0 to 24 h ($AUC_{0-24\ h}$) was calculated by the trapezoidal rule.

Stability studies

The tablets of the formulation (F2) were subjected to stability studies. During the study period of 40°C/75% RH for a specific time period up to 30 days, several parameters like hardness, friability, in vitro dispersion and drug content uniformity were evaluated at 1, 2, 3 and 4 weeks time interval for possible instability problems [28].

Results and discussion

The taste masking of Itopride HCl was carried out by coating the drug with Eudragit EPO polymer using solvent evaporation method that is not only a one step process but can be easily controlled and scaled up. Eudragit EPO was used as a taste masking agent because it dissolves at a pH of less than 5 such as in the stomach (pH 1–3) to release the drug [29]. As the polymer does not dissolve in the buccal cavity (pH 5.8-7.4), the coated drug remains intact to produce good taste masking. Magnesium stearate was used to prevent electrification and flocculation in the preparation of microspheres [9,12].

Microspheres were prepared in drug: polymer ratios 1:1, 1:2, 1:3, 1:4, 1:5 as shown in Table 1. The amount of the drug released from the microspheres in simulated salivary fluid in 60 sec was considered. When the drug/polymer ratio was increased from 1:2 to 1:3 or 1:4 or 1:5, microspheres showed almost the same drug release profile in simulated salivary fluid (1.61%, 1.57%, 1.51%

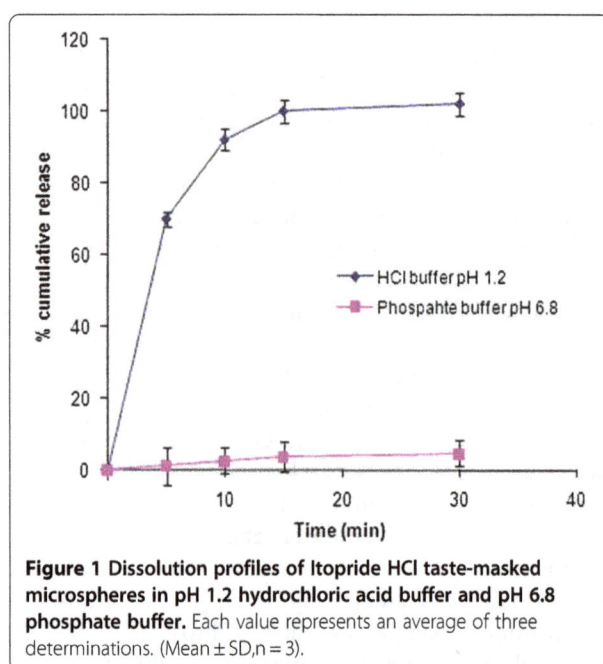

Figure 1 Dissolution profiles of Itopride HCl taste-masked microspheres in pH 1.2 hydrochloric acid buffer and pH 6.8 phosphate buffer. Each value represents an average of three determinations. (Mean ± SD,n = 3).

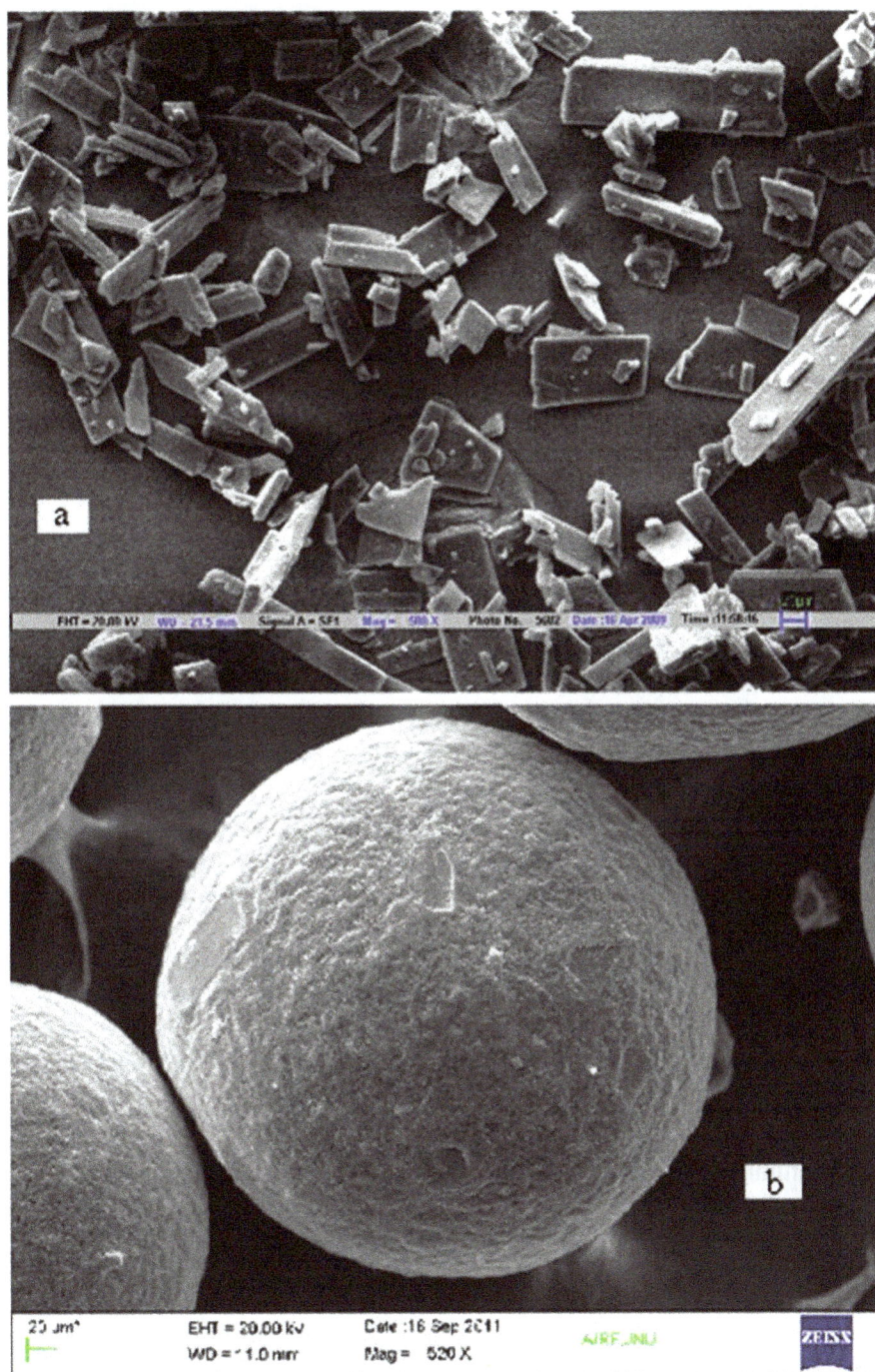

Figure 2 Scanning Electron Micrographs of a) Itopride HCl Crystals, b) Itopride HCl-loaded Microspheres (batch E3).

and 1.43%, respectively). However, if the ratio was changed from 1:2 to 1:1, a sharp increase of drug release was observed (6.31%). Therefore, the ratio 1:2 was considered to be the most suitable with respect to taste masking, and microspheres consisting of Itopride hydrochloride and Eudragit® EPO (1: 2) were further evaluated for other parameters.

The prime parameters for selection of batches were based on particle size, loading efficiency and drug content and these were evaluated (Table 2). From the average diameter (D_{av}) of microspheres determined by sieve analysis, it was found that on increasing the stirring rate, amount of acetone and liquid parafin, the mean diameter of the microspheres was found to decrease. A

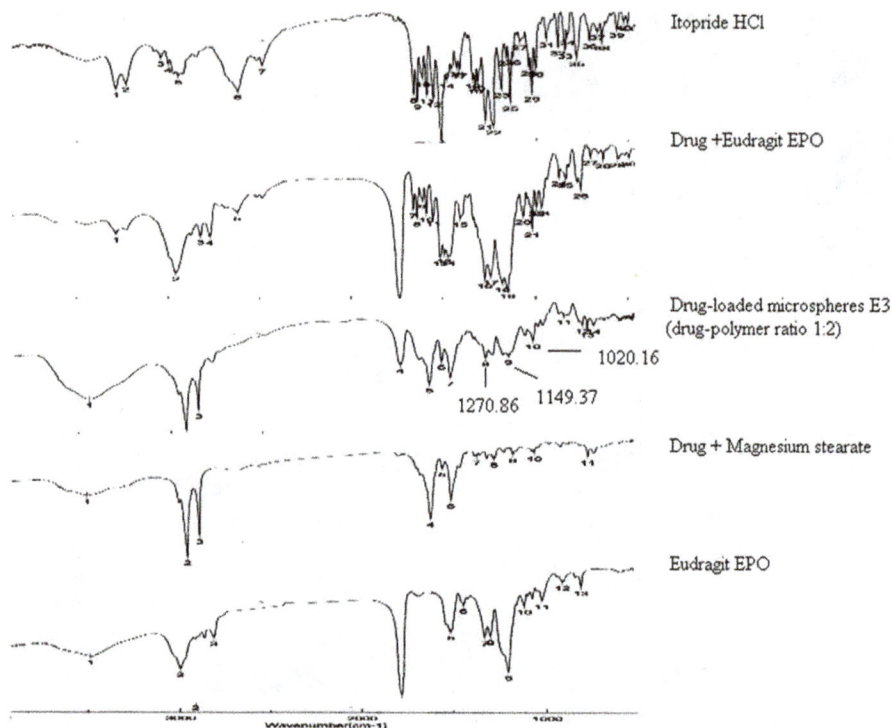

Figure 3 FTIR of Itopride HCl, Drug + Eudragit EPO, Drug-loaded microspheres E3 (drug-polymer ratio 1:2), Drug + Magnesium stearate, Eudragit EPO.

reduction in stirring speed from 600 to 200 rpm resulted in failure of batch as seen in batch E1. All microspheres varied in the size from batch to batch. Microspheres were spherical in the size range of 300–425 μm (fraction # 40/50) and 212–300 μm (# 50/70, major fraction) and microspheres of other sieve fractions 125–150 μm (# 100/120) and 125–106 μm (# 120/140) were not perfect spheres.

Further, batches of microspheres were evaluated for bulk density, tapped density, angle of repose, Carr's consolidation index and Hausner ratio. The results of powder flow properties (Table 3) clearly indicated good flow

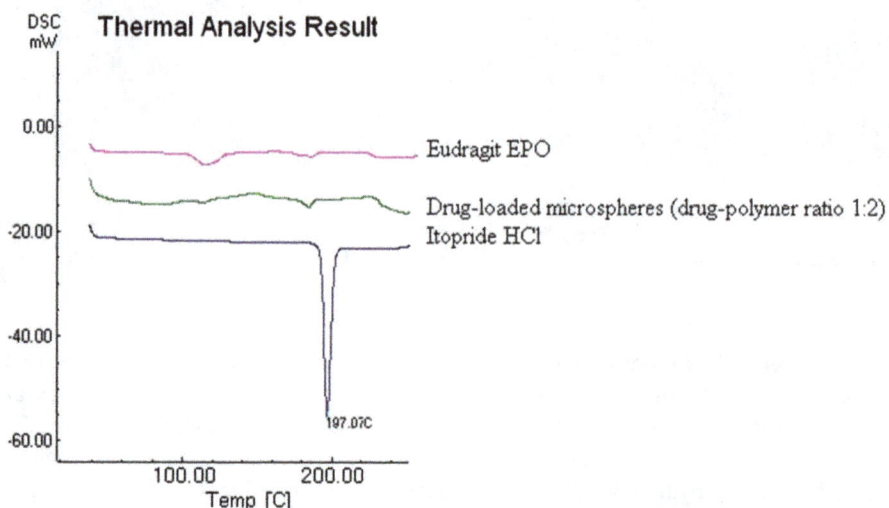

Figure 4 DSC of Eudragit EPO, Drug-loaded microspheres (drug-polymer ratio 1:2), Itopride HCl.

Table 4 Composition of Itopride HCl Orodispersible tablet formulations

Tablet ingredients (mg)/Formulation code	F-1	F-2	F-3
Microspheres containing Itopride HCl equivalent to 50 mg	196.6	196.6	196.6
Crospovidone (XL10)	20	28	40
Mannitol (Pearlitol)	173.4	165.4	153.4
Sodium stearyl fumarate	4	4	4
Aspartame	2	2	2
Talc	4	4	4
Total weight	400	400	400

characteristics for batch C3 and E3. Based upon % yield, drug content and loading efficiency, average size, flow properties and estimation of bitter taste of microspheres, batch E3 was considered to be optimum and was therefore selected for further characterization and tabletting.

Dissolution studies of Itopride HCl microspheres (Batch E3) were performed in two different pH media (pH 1.2 hydrochloric acid buffer and pH 6.8 phosphate buffer (Figure 1). Eudragit EPO is soluble in an acidic environment by formation of salts. Therefore, drug released from the microspheres very rapidly in pH 1.2 medium such that approximately 90% of the drug was released within 10 min. Drug release in pH 6.8 buffer was comparatively slower than that in pH 1.2 medium. About 2.6% drug released in 10 min in pH 6.8 medium. Eudragit EPO is insoluble at pH greater than 5 but it becomes permeable and allows the release of Itopride HCl. The gastric emptying time ranges from 32–87 min in fasted states for particles with a size in the micron range and the corresponding value is 34–75 min in fed state [30]. Therefore, it is expected that as soon as the polymer dissolves in the acidic contents of stomach, drug will be released in stomach followed by absorption from the gastrointestinal tract.

Scanning Electron Microscopy (SEM) analysis of Itopride HCl showed existence of characteristic prism like and needle like crystals as well as broad particle size distribution (Figure 2a). The structural and surface morphology of batch (E3) of microspheres having drug and polymer ratio of 1:2 showed the regularly spherical nature of microspheres with a narrow size distribution (Figure 2b) thereby confirming the encapsulation of Itopride HCl.

FTIR spectra of Itopride HCl, Eudragit EPO, physical admixture of Itopride HCl plus Eudragit EPO and drug loaded microspheres were recorded (Figure 3). FTIR spectrum of Itopride HCL showed characteristic peaks such as 1267.97 cm^{-1} for C-O-C asymmetrical ether stretching (alkyl stretching), 1028.84 cm^{-1} for C-O-C asymmetrical ether stretching (aryl ethers), 3281.29 cm^{-1} and 3226.33 cm^{-1} for NH stretching, 1631.48 cm^{-1} for NH bending, 1651.73 cm^{-1} for C = O stretching, 1147.44 cm^{-1} for C-N stretching and 2942.84 cm^{-1} and 2965.02 cm-1 for C-H. FTIR spectrum of microspheres showed some of the characteristic peaks of Itopride HCL such as 1270 cm^{-1} for C-O-C asymmetrical ether stretching (alkyl stretching), 1020 cm^{-1} for C-O-C asymmetrical ether stretching (aryl ethers), 1149 cm^{-1} for C-N stretching, thus confirming that no interaction of drug occurred with the components of the formulation. The FTIR spectrum of the physical admixture of drug plus polymer showed no significant shift or reduction in intensity of peaks of Itopride HCl at 1268.93 cm^{-1}, 3281.29 cm^{-1}, 1631.48 cm^{-1}, 1651.73 cm^{-1}, 1148 cm^{-1} and 2959.23 cm^{-1}. FTIR spectroscopic studies indicated that the drug is compatible with the polymer.

Table 5 Evaluation of Itopride HCl Orodispersible tablets* (Mean ± SD, n = 6)

Evaluation parameters/Formulation code	F-1	F-2	F-3
Weight Variation (mg)	399.8 ± 0.83	400 ± 2.34	401.2 ± 2.38
Hardness (Kg/cm^2)	4.9 ± 0.5	4.5 ± 0.7	5.7 ± 0.4
Thickness (mm)	4.22 ± 0.03	4.24 ± 0.04	4.18 ± 0.02
Friability (%)	0.74 ± 0.04	0.55 ± 0.05	0.63 ± 0.01
Drug content (%)	95.52 ± 0.07	98.38 ± 0.09	96.86 ± 0.02
Water Absorption ratio (%)	78.87 ± 1.14	84.72 ± 1.10	74.47 ± 1.81
Wetting time (sec)	32 ± 2	16 ± 1	20 ± 2
In vitro Dispersion time (sec)	18 ± 1	9 ± 1	14 ± 0.5
In vitro Disintegration time (sec)	36	18	24
Moisture uptake (%)	0.71 ± 0.13	0.75 ± 0.25	0.82 ± 0.19

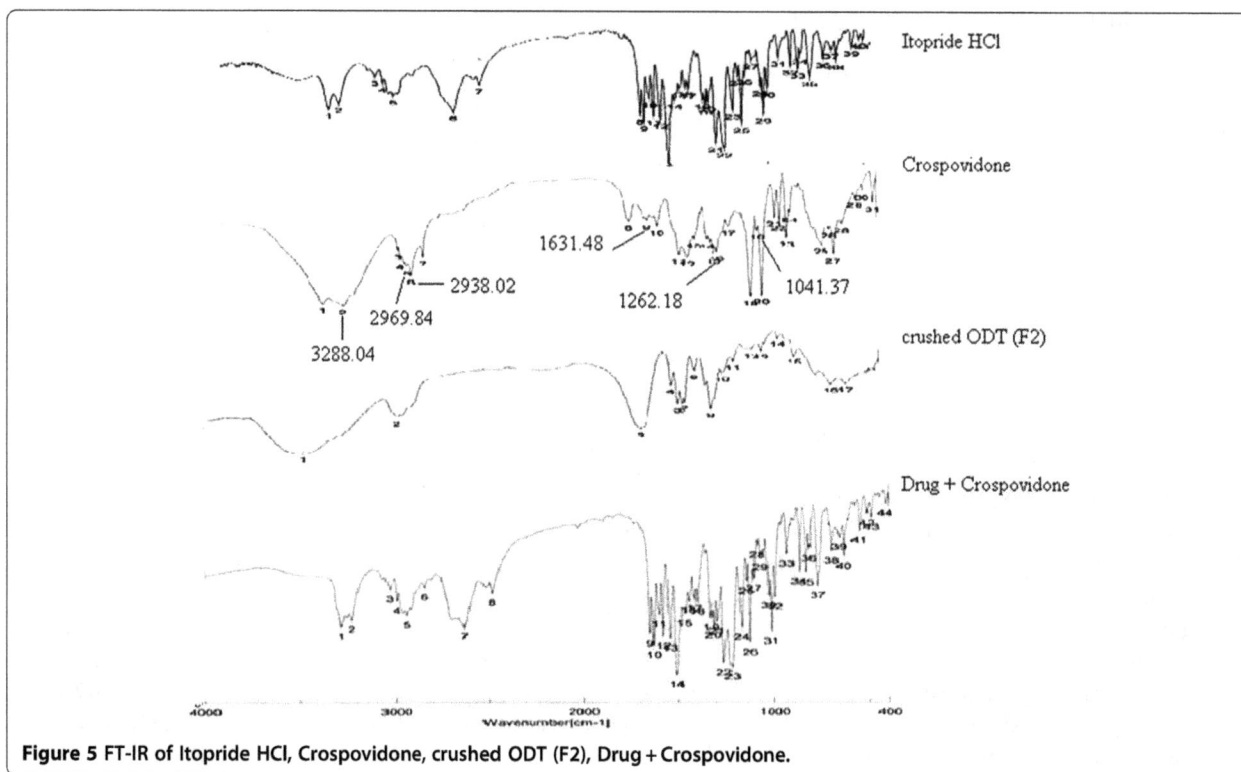

Figure 5 FT-IR of Itopride HCl, Crospovidone, crushed ODT (F2), Drug + Crospovidone.

In order to check chemical interaction between drug and polymer, thermal analysis was carried out by using DSC. The melting point of drug was confirmed from the endothermic peak of Itopride at 197°C in DSC analysis. DSC thermograms of Itopride HCl, Eudragit EPO and drug-loaded microspheres (E3) showed that there were no changes in the endotherms (Figure 4). The drug exhibited a small melting endotherm in the drug-loaded microspheres (E3) formulation. These slight changes in the melting endotherm of the drug may be attributed to the mixing process, which lowers the purity of each component in the mixture, thus resulting in slightly

broader and lower melting points, but not truly representing any incompatibility [31].

During formulation of orodispersible tablets of taste masked microspheres, three formulations with varying concentration of superdisintegrant: crospovidone (5, 7 and 10%w/w) were chosen on the basis of disintegration time of tablets (Table 4). Increasing the amount of Crospovidone from 5 (F1) to 7%w/w (F2) resulted in a decrease in the disintegration time of the tablets from 36 sec to 18 sec. However, further increase in the concentration to 10%w/w (F3) led to increase in disintegration time to 24 sec probably due to higher water

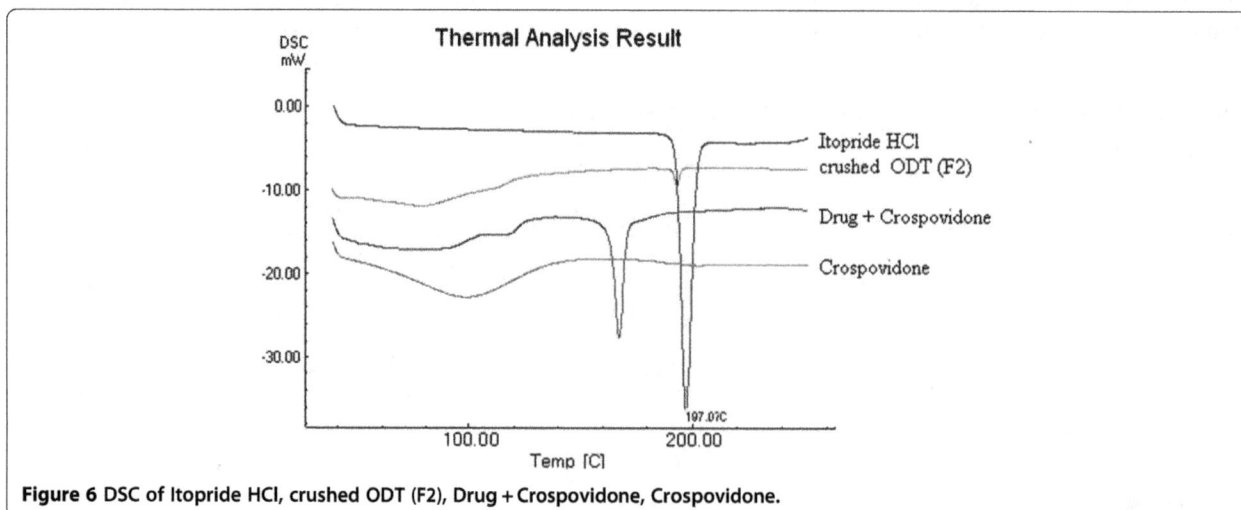

Figure 6 DSC of Itopride HCl, crushed ODT (F2), Drug + Crospovidone, Crospovidone.

Table 6 Dissolution profile of Orodispersible tablets (F2) and conventional tablet (Ganaton)*(Mean ± SD, n = 3)

Time (min)	Cumulative percentage drug release	
	ODT Batch (F2)	Conventional tablet (Ganaton)
0	0	0
2	73.6 ± 0.4	21.7 ± 0.9
5	84.6 ± 0.6	39.4 ± 0.2
10	98.5 ± 0.5	62.2 ± 0.9
15	100.5 ± 0.6	69.0 ± 0.2
30	100.7 ± 0.2	80.0 ± 0.4
45	100.7 ± 0.8	88.6 ± 0.9
60	101.3 ± 0.7	91.6 ± 0.4
90	101.4 ± 0.8	97.9 ± 0.3
120	101.1 ± 0.2	98.9 ± 0.8

requirement by a larger amount of Crospovidone, which consequently transformed into swelling force for rapid disintegration of the tablet. The obtained results were similar to the findings of Khan et al., 2007 [3] and Patel et al., 2004 [32]. Therefore, the suitable concentration of crospovidone was found to be 7%w/w for formulation of orodispersble tablet that showed minimal disintegration time of 18 seconds. Water insoluble diluents such as microcrystalline cellulose and dicalcium phosphate were not used in the study as they are expected to cause an unacceptable feeling of grittiness in the mouth. Among the soluble diluents, mannitol which is a hexahydric alcohol related to mannose was also used in the tablet formula as taste masking agent. Mannitol was also selected considering its advantages in terms of easy availability and negative heat of dissolution.

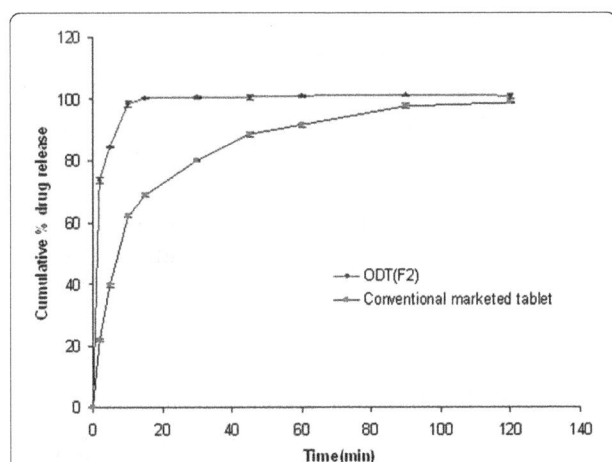

Figure 7 In-Vitro release profile of conventional marketed tablet (Ganaton) and formulation (F2) prepared using Crospovidone 7% and Itopride; Eudragit ratio of 1:2 in pH 1.2 HCl medium; errors bar indicate S.D, n = 3.

The tablets prepared by direct compression method were found to be free from capping, chipping and sticking. The prepared tablets were evaluated for various physical parametric tests (Table 5). The thickness of all the tablets was found in range of 4.18 to 4.24 mm and was within the prescribed limits of IP 1996 (±5%) [30]. Hardness of the all tablets was between 4.5–5.7 Kg/cm^2 during compression and was considered optimum for ODTs [32]. The average weights of tablets were found to be 399–401 mg. The acceptable weight range is ± 5% as per IP [22] for uniformity of weight thus indicating consistency in the preparation of the tablets and minimal batch to batch variation. The friability of all the formulations was found to be between 0.55 to 0.74%, which was found to be with in the pharmacopoeial requirement [33] (i.e. not more than 1%) indicating good mechanical resistance of tablet sufficient to withstand the rigors of transportation and handling. The drug content estimation data for all the batches were also found to be within the pharmacopoeial limit (i.e. 95.52 to 98.38%).

Wetting time is used as an indicator of the ease of the tablet disintegration in buccal cavity. It was observed that wetting time of tablets was in the range of 16 to 32 seconds which is desirable for ODT. Water absorption ratio, which is an important criteria for understanding the capacity of disintegrants to swell in presence of little amount of water, was calculated. It was found to be in the range of 74–84% which was considered to be optimum for an oro-dispersible tablet. Moisture uptake by tablets was found to be in the range of 0.71–0.82% and was considered satisfactory for an oro-dispersible tablet. All the formulations complied with the in vitro dispersion and disintegration time requirement of 60 sec for orodispersible tablets as per European Pharmacopoeia [34]. The formulation F2 containing crospovidone (7%w/w) had the least dispersion and disintegration time of 9 and 18 sec respectively.

Thus, formulation F2 possessed good disintegrating property among all formulations which was evaluated for in vitro disintegration, wetting time, in vitro dispersion time and in vivo studies.

Itopride HCl, crospovidone, crushed ODT (F2) and physical ad-mixture of drug plus Crospovidone was characterized by FTIR spectral analysis for any physical as well as chemical alteration of the drug characteristics (Figure 5). From the results, it was concluded that there was no interference in the functional groups as following principle peaks of the Itopride HCl such as at 3288.04 cm^{-1}, 2969.84 cm^{-1}, 2938.02 cm^{-1}, 1631.48 cm^{-1}, 1262.18 cm^{-1} and 1041.37 cm^{-1} were found in the spectra of the crushed ODT. All the peaks of Itopride HCl were found to be unaltered in the spectra of the drug-crospovidone physical admixture.

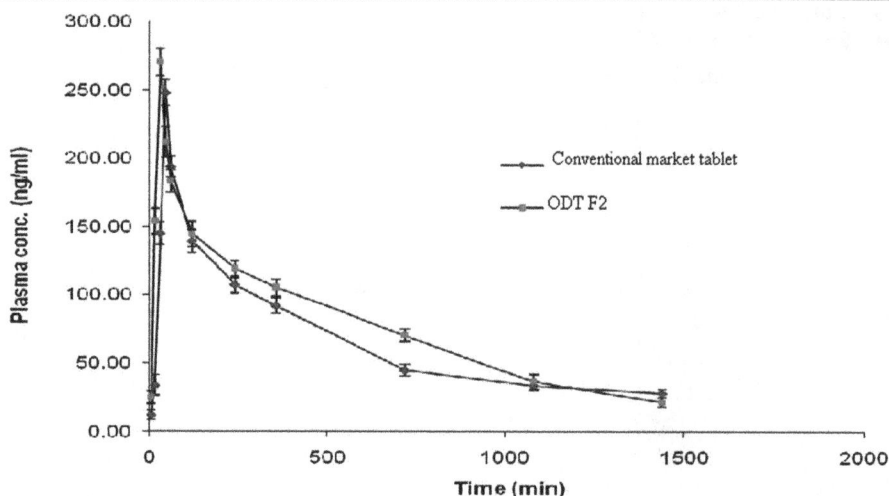

Figure 8 In vivo plasma profile comparison of GANATON and F2 prepared using crospovidone 7% and Itopride; Eudragit ratio of 1:2 in albino rabbits; errors bar indicate S.D, n = 3.

In DSC thermal analysis, Itopride HCl exhibited melting peak at 197.07°C, while in formulation F2 the drug exhibited a small melting peak at 195.80°C. These slight changes in the melting endotherm of the drug may be attributed to the mixing process, which lowers the purity of each component in the mixture, thus resulting in slightly broader and lower melting points, but not truly representing any incompatibility [31]. However, appearance of no new peak and only a slight shift in peak of drug + crospovidone, suggested absence of interaction between drug and other excipients (Figure 6).

From the cumulative percentage drug release of ODT formulation F2 and conventional tablet formulation (GANATON) available in the market, it was observed that in the first 2 min, only 21.7% drug was released from GANATON tablet while it was 73.6% in case of ODT F2 (Table 6). At the end of 10 min, 98.5% drug was released from F2 as compared to conventional tablet formulation in which only 62.2% drug was released (Figure 7). Thus, the release rate of Itopride hydrochloride was enhanced by formulating ODTs by using crospovidone (7%w/w) as superdisintegrant. According to the FDA guidance, value of similiarity factor (f2) between 50 and 100 ensure sameness or equivalence of the two dissolution profiles. The vaue of similiarity factor was found

to be 52 which indicate comparative equivalence with reference formulation.

Further, the formulation F2 and GANATON were subjected to in vivo pharmacokinetic studies to assess the bioequivalence. The mean plasma concentration as assessed by HPTLC as a function of time after oral administration of single animal dose of Itopride HCl immediate release tablets (GANATON) and oral disintegrating tablet (F2) is shown in Figure 8. The pharmacokinetic parameters as assessed by HPTLC for both formulations are illustrated in Table 7. The absorption from oral disintegrating tablet (F2) was faster compared to GANATON both showing T_{max} of 30 and 45 min respectively. The corresponding drug plasma concentration in rabbits after administration of F2 and Marketed tablet was 270 ng/ml and 248 ng/ml respectively.

The preliminary results of stability studies carried out on formulation (F2) at 40°C/75% RH for a specific time period upto 30 days are given in Table 8. The dispersion time after 1, 2, 3 and 4 weeks of storage were found to be within USFDA limits [35]. Also, no significant loss in the drug content was found at the end of one month. Hardness and friability values were also found to be within the pharmacopoeial range after 1 month storage at 40°C.

Conclusions

This study demonstrated that the prepared Itopride HCl oral disintegrating tablets possess short in vitro disintegration time and improved dissolution patterns as well as pharmacokinetic behavior in rabbits compared to the conventional product available in market. Therefore, it can be concluded that taste masking and rapid disintegration of tablets formulated in this investigation may

Table 7 Pharmacokinetic parameters of Orodispersible tablet (F2) and conventional tablet (Ganaton) in albino rabbits* (Mean ± SD, n = 3)

Parameter	Formulation F2	Ganaton tablet
Cmax (ng/ml)	270 ± 4.5	248 ± 5.6
Tmax (min)	30	45
AUC$_{0-t}$ (ng.h/ml)	123.98 ± 6.3	107.78 ± 5.3

Table 8 Stability studies of Orodispersible tablets ((Mean ± SD, n = 6)

Time	Evaluation parameters (F2)			
	Hardness (kg/cm^2)	Drug content %	Friability (%)	In-vitro Dispersion time (sec)
After 1 week	4.2 ±0.7	97.65 ± 0.04	0.50 ± 0.09	9 ± 1
After 2 week	4.1 ±0.9	95.99 ±0.04	0.47 ± 0.05	8 ± 0.5
After 3 week	4.0 ±0.6	95.47 ± 0.08	0.45 ± 0.01	8 ± 1
After 4 week	3.9 ±0.5	94.80 ± 0.02	0.42 ± 0.03	7 ± 0.9

possibly help in administration of Itopride HCl in a more palatable form without water during emesis. Thus, the present drug delivery technology could be expected to have higher patient compliance over conventional tablets thereby necessitating the extension of this technology to development of other potential drug candidates.

Competing interests

The authors declare that they have no competing interests.

Authors' contribution

SS, SM, SSA read and approved the final manuscript.

References

1. Kuchekar BS, Badhan AC, Mahajan HS: Mouth dissolving tablets of salbutamol sulphate: a novel drug delivery system. *Indian Drugs* 2004, 41:592–598.
2. Hoogstrate AJ, Verhoef JC, Tuk B, Pijpers A: In-vivo buccal delivery of fluorescin isothiocyanate-dextran 4400 with glycodeoxycholate as an absorption enhancer in pig. *J Pharm Sci* 1996, 85:457–460.
3. USFDA, "Inactive Ingredient Search for Approved Drug Products," Food and Drug Administration, Centre for Drug Evaluation and Research (CDER), Rockville, MD. 2009. http://www.accessdata.fda.gov/scripts/cder/iig/index. cfm.
4. Roy GM: Taste masking in oral pharmaceuticals. *Pharm. Tech* 1994, 18:85–91.
5. Nanda A, Kandarapu R, Garg S: An update on oral taste masking technologies for oral pharmaceuticals. *Indian J. Pharm. Sci* 2002, 64:10–17.
6. Anand V, Raghupathi K, Garg S: Ion-Exchange resins: carrying drug delivery forward. *Drug Discovery Today* 2001, 6:905–914.
7. Bodmeier R, Chen H, Tyle P, Jarosz P: Pseudoephedrine HCl microspheres formulated into an oral suspension dosage form. *J. Control. Release* 1991, 8:65–77.
8. Bogataj M, Mrhar A, Kristl A, Kozjek F: Eudragit E microspheres containing bacampicillin: preparation by solvent removal methods. *J Microencapsul* 1991, 8:401–406.
9. Goto S, Kawata M, Nakamura M, Maekawa K, Aoyoma T: Eudragit RS and RL (acrylic resins) microcapsules as pH insensitive and sustained release preparations of ketoprofen. *J Microencapsul* 1986, 3:293–304.
10. Lorenzo-Lamosa ML, Cuna M, Vila-Jato JL, Torres D, Alonso MJ: Development of a microencapsulated form of cefuroxime axetil using pH-sensitive acrylic polymers. *J Microencapsul* 1997, 14:607–616.
11. Pignatello R, Consoli P, Puglisi G: In vitro release kinetics of Tolmetin from tabletted Eudragit microparticles. *J Microencapsul* 2000, 17:373–383.
12. Bogataj M, Mrhar A, Kristl A, Kozjek F: Preparation and evaluation of Eudragit E microspheres containing bacampicillin. *Drug Dev. Ind. Pharm* 1991, 15:2295–2313.
13. Gupta S, Kapoor V, Kapoor B: Itopride a novel prokinetic agent. *J?K Science Drug Review* 2004, 6(2):106–108.
14. United States Pharmacopeia XXXII. Rockville (MD): National Formulary XXVII, USP Convention; 2009.
15. Lachman L, Liberman HA, Kanig JL: The theory and practice of industrial pharmacy. 3rd edition. Mumbai: Varghese Publishing House; 1991:209–303.
16. Lachman L, Liberman HA, Kanig JL: The theory and practice of industrial Pharmacy. 3rd edition. Mumbai: Varghese publishing house; 1987:184.
17. Levis SR, Deasy PB: Pharmaceutical applications of size reduced grades of surfactant co-processed micro crystalline cellulose. *Int J Pharm* 2001, 230:25–33.
18. SIEVE_CONVERSION_CHART.pdf. Accessed on; 2011. http://www. qclabequipment.com/.
19. Gao Y, Cui FD, Guan Y, Yang L, Wang YS, Zhang LN: Preparation of roxithromycin-polymeric microspheres by the emulsion solvent diffusion method for taste masking. *Int J Pharm* 2006, 318:62–69.
20. Ringard J: Guyot-Hermann AM. Calculation of disintegrant critical concentration in order to optimize tablets disintegration. *Drug Dev. Ind. Pharm* 1988, 14(15–17):1321–2339.
21. Marshall K, Lachman L, Lieberman HA, Kanig JL (Eds): The theory and practice of industrial Pharmacy. 3rd edition. Mumbai: Varghese publishing house; 1987.
22. Indian Pharmacopoeia. VIth edth edition. Delhi: Government of India, Ministry of Health and Family Welfare; 2010:1681–1683.
23. Zhao N: Augsburger LL. Functionality comparison of three classes of super-disintegrants in promoting aspirin tablets disintegration and dissolution. *AAPS PharmSci. Tech* 2005, 6(4):E634–40.
24. Bi Y: Preparation and evaluation of a compressed tablet rapidly disintegrating in the oral cavity. *Chem Pharm Bull* 1996, 44:2121–2127.
25. Amin AF, Shah TJ, Bhadani MN, Patel MM: Emerging trends in the development of orally disintegrating tablet technology; 2011. http://www. pharmainfo.net Accessed 6 April 2011.
26. Swamy PV, Shahidulla SM, Shirsand SB, Hiremath SN, Ali MY: Orodispersible tablets of carbmszepine prepared by direct compression method using 3^2 full factorial designs. *J Pharm Sci* 2008, 7:1–5.
27. Klancke J: Dissolution testing of orally disintegrating tablets. *Dissolution Technologies* 2003, 6:6–8.
28. Kulkarni GT, Subburaju T: Stability testing of pharmaceutical products: An over- View. *Ind. J. Pharm. Educ* 2004, 38(4):24–30.
29. Xu J, Bovet LL, Zhao K: In situ gelling hydrogels for pharmaceutical and biomedical application. *Int J Pharm* 2008, 359:63–69.
30. Hunter E, Fell JT, Sharma H: The gastric emptying of pellets contained in hard gelatin capsules. *Drug Dev. Ind. Pharm* 1982, 8:751–757.
31. Dooran AAV: Design of drug excipient interaction study. *Drug Dev. Ind. Pharm* 1983, 9:43–45.
32. Patel DM, Patel NM, Shah RR, Jogani PL, Balapatel AI: Studies in formulation of orodispersible tablets of rofecoxib. *Indian J. Pharm. Sci* 2004, 66:621–625.
33. Kaushik D, Dureja H, Saini TR: Formulation and evaluation of Olanzapine mouth dissolving tablets by effervescent formulation approach. *Indian Drugs* 2004, 41(7):410–2.
34. European Pharmacopoeia. 5, Vol Ith edition. Great Britain: Directorate of Medicine and Health; 2005, 628–629.
35. Khan S, Kataria P, Nakhat P, Yeole P: Taste Masking of Ondansetron Hydrochloride by Polymer Carrier System and Formulation of Rapid-Disintegrating Tablets. *AAPS PharmSci. Tech* 2007, 8:E1–E7.

Anticancer activity of *Pupalia lappacea* on chronic myeloid leukemia K562 cells

Alvala Ravi[1*], Mallika Alvala[2], Venkatesh Sama[1], Arunasree M Kalle[3], Vamshi K Irlapati[4] and B Madhava Reddy[1]

Abstract

Background: Cancer is one of the most prominent human diseases which has enthused scientific and commercial interest in the discovery of newer anticancer agents from natural sources. Here we demonstrated the anticancer activity of ethanolic extract of aerial parts of *Pupalia lappacea* (L) Juss (Amaranthaceae) (EAPL) on Chronic Myeloid Leukemia K562 cells.

Methods: Antiproliferative activity of EAPL was determined by MTT assay using carvacrol as a positive control. Induction of apoptosis was studied by annexin V, mitochondrial membrane potential, caspase activation and cell cycle analysis using flow cytometer and modulation in protein levels of p53, PCNA, Bax and Bcl2 ratio, cytochrome *c* and cleavage of PARP were studied by Western blot analysis. The standardization of the extract was performed through reverse phase-HPLC using Rutin as biomarker.

Results: The results showed dose dependent decrease in growth of K562 cells with an IC_{50} of 40 ± 0.01 μg/ml by EAPL. Induction of apoptosis by EAPL was dose dependent with the activation of p53, inhibition of PCNA, decrease in Bcl2/Bax ratio, decrease in the mitochondrial membrane potential resulting in release of cytochrome *c*, activation of multicaspase and cleavage of PARP. Further HPLC standardization of EAPL showed presence 0.024% of Rutin.

Conclusion: Present study significantly demonstrates anticancer activity of EAPL on Chronic Myeloid Leukemia (K562) cells which can lead to potential therapeutic agent in treating cancer. Rutin, a known anti cancer compound is being reported and quantified for the first time from EAPL.

Keywords: Pupalia lappacea, Anticancer activity, Chronic myeloid leukemia (K562) cells, Cytochrome *c*, p53, Multicaspase, PCNA

Background

Plant derived natural products gaining importance to cure various disease conditions. Side effects of several allopathic drugs and development of resistance to currently used drugs have led to increased emphasis on the use of plant materials as a source of medicines for a wide variety of human ailments. Incidentally plants and herbs are persistently being studied for the identification of novel therapeutic agents. Among the 2, 50,000 higher plant species on earth, more than 80,000 plants have medicinal values. India is one of the biodiversity centers with the presence of over 45,000 different plant species. Of these, about ~20,000 plants have good medicinal value. However, only ~7500 species are used for their medicinal values by traditional communities. It is well established that plants have always been useful source, for occurrence of anticancer compounds [1-3]. Approximately 60% of currently used anticancer chemotherapeutic drugs (vinblastin, vincristine) are derived from plant resource [4,5]. Moreover, traditionally, plants passed empirical testing against specific diseases and demonstrated that they are well tolerated in humans. Even though quite a few medicinal plants are applied against a wide variety of conditions, there are still numerous plants that have not been cross-tested in diseases apart from the traditional applications; one of such plant is *Pupalia lappacea*.

Pupalia lappacea (L) Juss. (Amaranthaceae) is an erect or straggling under shrub found in the hedges of fields and waste places from Kashmir to Kanyakumari and commonly known as forest Burr or creeping cock's

* Correspondence: ravi_alvala@yahoo.co.in
[1]G.Pulla Reddy College of Pharmacy, Mehdipatnam, Hyderabad 500 028, AP, India
Full list of author information is available at the end of the article

comb. In folklore medicine, the leaf paste of *Pupalia lappaceae* with edible oil is used to treat bone fractures and inflammatory conditions [6]. The fruit juice is applied locally for cuts, mixed with palm oil to treat boils and the fruit soup is used for cough and fever. In Africa, fruit is used as an ingredient in enema preparation; mixed with palm oil, it is applied as a dressing for boils and also applied to leprosy sores after making them bleed. Burnt plant is mixed with water to treat flatulence. Traditionally it is also used to treat jaundice, abdominal colics, cephalgias, diarrheas, paralysis, erectile dysfunction, vomiting and malaria [7]. Chemical investigations of *P. lappacea* revealed that foliage of this plant consists of 8 compounds, namely 1-docosanol, stearic acid, stigmasterol, sitosterol, N-benzoyl-L-Phenyl alaninol acetate, setosterol-3-O-D-glucopyranoside, stigmasterol-3-O-D-glucopyranoside and 20- hydroxyl ecdysone[8] The seeds are reported to consist of glycosides, saponins, steroids and alkaloids [9]. Aladedunye et al., reported the antioxidant activity of hexane and dichloromethane extract of *P. lappacea* foliage [8]. Sowemimo et al., in his preliminary studies reported the cytotoxic activity of whole plant of *P. lappacea* on HeLa cells [10]. Many of the natural antioxidants like curcumin, quercetin, resveratrol, berberine etc., are reported for potent anticancer activity in-vitro and in-vivo. Because of ethical considerations and the substantial time and expense required when using animal models, human cancer cell lines are preferred for most preliminary anticancer screening studies. The ability to inhibit cancer cell proliferation is considered as an indicator of anticancer potential, because the balance of tumor cell proliferation over cell death has been proposed to be one of the key factors in cancer evolution and progression. The present study was aimed to investigate *in vitro* anti proliferative activity of EAPL on K562 cells which is a proposed model for study of most of the cytotoxicity studies [11].

Methods
Plant material
The whole plant of *P. lappacea* was collected during flowering season from the Osmania University campus, Hyderabad, Andhra Pradesh, India, in the month of October 2010. Identification of plant was done by Dr. G. Bhagyanarayana, Taxonomist, Department of Botany, Osmania University, Hyderabad, India. The aerial parts (without flowers) were separated, cleaned, air dried and grounded to powder. The voucher specimen (PUL-203-07) is being maintained in department of Pharmacognosy, G. Pulla Reddy College of Pharmacy, Hyderabad, India.

Preparation of plant extract
The dried powder of aerial parts (1000 g) was extracted with 80% aqueous ethyl alcohol (5 liters) at room temperature by maceration for 7 days. The extract was filtered and concentrated under reduced pressure in rotary flash evaporator. The concentrated organic extract was lyophilized to remove the moisture and traces of solvent. The final yield of aerial part was 1.85% (18.5 g). The lyophilized product was qualitatively tested for the presence of phytoconstituents by TLC and test tube reactions [12,13].

Chemicals
3- (4, 5-dimethylthiazole-2-yl)-2, 5-diphenyl tetrazolium bromide (MTT), carvacrol were purchased from Sigma–Aldrich (Bangalore, India), Phosphate-buffered saline (PBS), RPMI medium, fetal bovine serum (FBS) were purchased from Gibco BRL (CA, USA). ECL reagent kit was purchased from GE Amersham whereas Nitrocellulose membrane from Millipore (Bangalore, India). Mouse monoclonal antibody against cytochrome *c* was from ChemiCon (CA, USA). Monoclonal antibodies of PARP (Poly (ADP-ribose) polymerase), BCl_2 ((B-cell lymphoma 2) and Bax were procured from Upstate (Charlottesville, VA, and USA). All the other chemicals and reagents used were of analytical and molecular biology grade.

Determination of effect of EAPL on cell proliferation by MTT assay
Cell culture
Human chronic myeloid leukemia K562 cells, Human embryonic kidney HEK-293 cells were procured from National Center for Cell Sciences, Pune, India. Cells were grown in RPMI media supplemented with 10% heat inactivated fetal bovine serum (FBS), 100 IU/ml penicillin, 100 mg/ml streptomycin and 2 mM-Glutamine. Cultures were maintained in a humidified atmosphere with 5% CO_2 at 37°C. The cells were subcultured twice a week, seeding at a density of about $2*10^3$ cells/ml. cell viability was determined by the trypan blue dye exclusion method.

Cell proliferation assay
Cell viability was determined by MTT assay. 5×10^3 cells/well (K562 and HEK-293) were seeded to 96-well culture plate and cultured with or without extract (10, 20, 30, 40, 50, 60, 70, 80, 90 & 100 µg/ml) or carvacrol (0, 0.5, 1, 10, 50,100 and 150 µg/ml) for 24 h in a final volume of 200 µl. After treatment, the medium was removed and 20 µl of MTT (5 mg/ml in PBS) was added to the fresh medium. After 3 h incubation at 37°C, cells were suspended in 100 µl of DMSO and plates were agitated for 1 min. Absorbance at 570 nm was recorded in a multi-well plate reader (Victor3 TM, Perkin Elmer, USA). Percent inhibition of proliferation was calculated as a fraction of control (without extract).

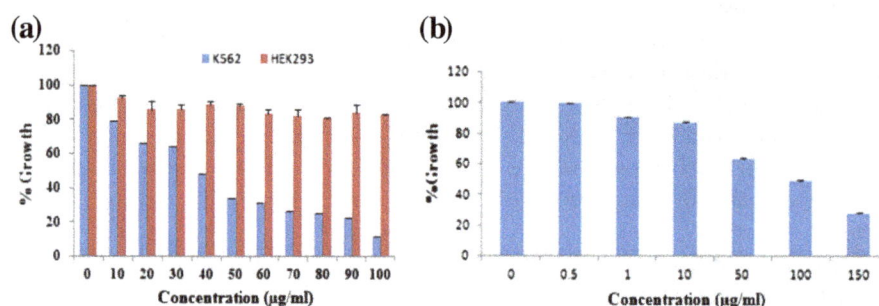

Figure 1 MTT assay: Cells treated with EAPL (a), Carvacrol for 24 h in K562 cell lines (b). Values were expressed as mean ± SEM (P < 0.05).

FACS analysis

Cell culture

$1*10^4$ cells/well were seeded in 96 well plates and incubated for 2–3 hrs at 37°C in humidified 5% CO_2 environment. Cells were treated with different concentrations (0, 25, 50, 100 μg/ml) of EAPL for 24 hrs, then harvested, stained and analyzed by Guava EasyCyte system for following experiments.

Annexin V assay

The Guava Nexin assay was conducted according to the manufacturer's protocol. Briefly, cells after harvesting, resuspended in 50 μl complete RPMI medium. A volume of 150 μl staining solution (135 μl 1X apoptosis buffer, 10 μl Annexin V-PE, and 5 μl of 7-AAD) was then added to each well, incubated in the dark at room temperature for 20 min and acquired by using Guava EasyCyte system ($5*10^3$ cells counted/sample, flow rate setting medium). The Nexin intensity gates were set to position the live population in the lower left corner of the dot plot. The angles of the gates were then positioned to divide the dot plot into four quadrants. Each quadrant of the dot plot contains a distinct population of cells that is dependent on the presence and intensity of cellular stains per cell.

Cell cycle analysis

Cell cycle analysis was conducted following the manufacturer's instructions. After harvesting, cells were washed with 1X PBS twice, and then fixed overnight at −20°C in 70% ethanol. After fixing, stained for DNA content with propidium iodide, and acquired by using Guava EasyCyte system ($5*10^3$ cells counted/sample, flow rate setting medium). The cell cycle gates were set to a position in dot plot which corresponds to four markers showing marker 1: G1 phase, marker 2: S phase, marker 3: G2/M phase and marker 4: sub-G0/G1 cells in histogram.

Mitochondrial membrane potential analysis

The Guava MitoPotential assay was conducted according to manufacturer's instructions. Briefly after harvesting, cells were resuspended in 200 μl of medium. A volume of 2 μl 100X JC-1 solution and 2 μl of 7-AAD was then added to each well. Plates were incubated for 30 minutes at 37°C in a 5% CO_2 incubator and acquired on a Guava EasyCyte system ($5*10^3$ cells counted/sample, flow rate setting medium). The membrane mitopotential intensity gates were set to position the live population in the lower left corner of the dot plot. The angles of the gates were then positioned to divide the dot plot into four

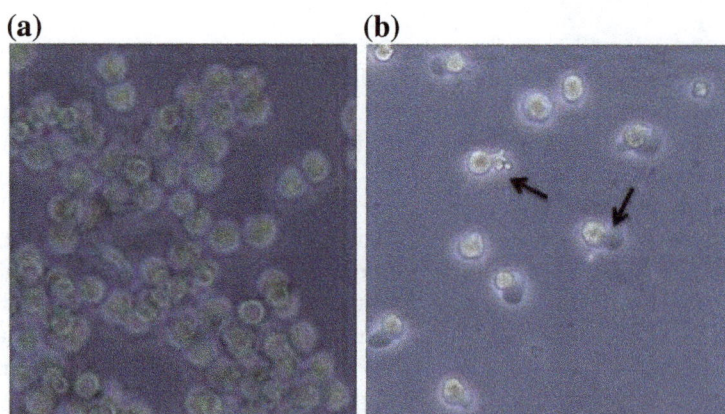

Figure 2 Microscopic photographs: untreated (a), treated (100 μg/ml) (b) cells. Arrows indicate apoptotic cells.

quadrants. Each quadrant of the dot plot contains a distinct population of cells that is dependent on the presences and intensity of cellular stains per cell. Finally percentage of apoptotic/dead cells corresponding to live cells was shown in dot plot.

Multicaspase activity analysis
Activation of multicaspase by EAPL was performed on Guava Easy Cyte Flow cytometer. Cells treated with EAPL were harvested, washed with PBS, stained with SR-VAD-FMK, 7-AAD and analyzed by flow cytometry according to manufacturer's protocol ($5*10^3$ cells counted/sample, flow rate setting medium). The activation of multicaspase intensity gates were set to position the live population in

the lower left corner of the dot plot. The angles of the gates were then positioned to divide the dot plot into four quadrants. Each quadrant of the dot plot contains a distinct population of cells that is dependent on the presence and intensity of cellular stains per cell.

Western blot analysis
Western blot analysis was performed as previously described [14]. Briefly, cells were lysed in a lysis buffer and centrifuged ($10,000 \times g$) for 10 min. The protein content of the supernatant was determined according to the Bradford method [15] and used as the whole-cell extracts. Proteins (100 μg) were separated on 8–12% sodium dodecyl sulphate - polyacrylamide gels (SDS-PAGE) along with

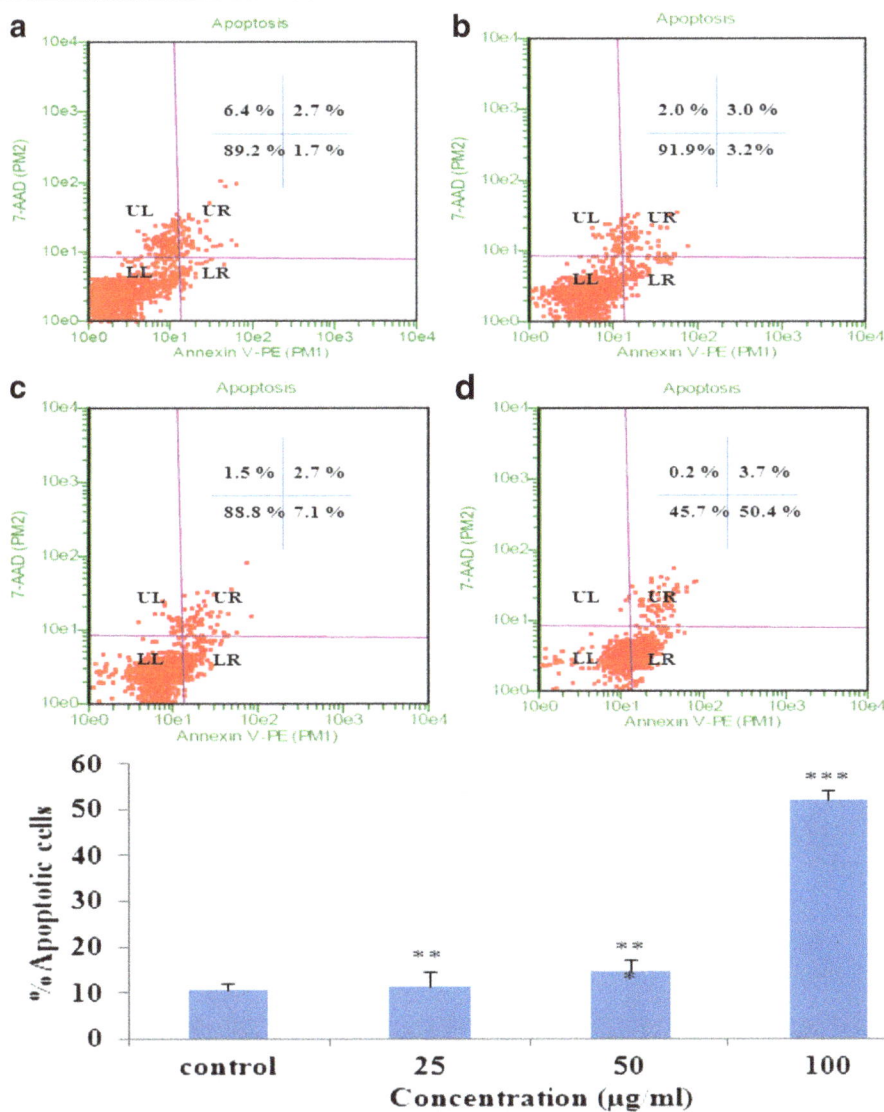

Figure 3 Annexin V assay: 5 x 10³ cells were treated with EAPL at different concentrations for 24 h analyzed by flow cytometer. (**a**) Control (**b**) 25 μg/ml (**c**) 50 μg/ml (**d**) 100 μg/ml. UL-Dead cells. UR-Late apoptotic cells. LR-Early apoptotic cells LL-live cells. Bar graph represents the % apoptotic cells (mean ± SEM).

protein molecular weight standards and electrophoretic-ally transferred to nitrocellulose membrane (Bio-Rad Laboratories, Hercules, CA). Non specific binding sites on the membranes were blocked with 5% (w/v) nonfat dry milk after checking the transfer using 0.5% Ponceau S in 1% acetic acid and then probed with a relevant antibody (Bax, Bcl2, PARP at 1:1000 dilution) for 8–12 h at 4°C followed by detection using peroxidase-conjugated secondary antibodies and Super Signal West Pico Chemiluminescence Substrate (Thermofisher scientific, USA). Equal protein loading was detected by probing the membrane with β-actin antibodies.

Release of cytochrome c from mitochondria was measured by immunoblot assay as previously described [16] with some modifications. Briefly, cells were washed once with ice-cold PBS and gently lysed for 30 s in 80 μl ice-cold lysis buffer (250 mM sucrose, 1 mM EDTA (ethylene diamine tetra acetic acid), 0.05% digitonin, 25 mM Tris, pH 6.8, 1 mM dithiothrietol, 1 mg/ml aprotinin, 1 mg/ml pepstatin, 1 mg/ml leupeptin, 1 mM PMSF (phenyl methane sulfonyl fluoride) and 1 mM benzamidine). Lysates were centrifuged at 12,000 × g at 4°C for 5 min to obtain the extracts (cytosolic extracts free of mitochondria). Supernatants were electrophoresed on 8-

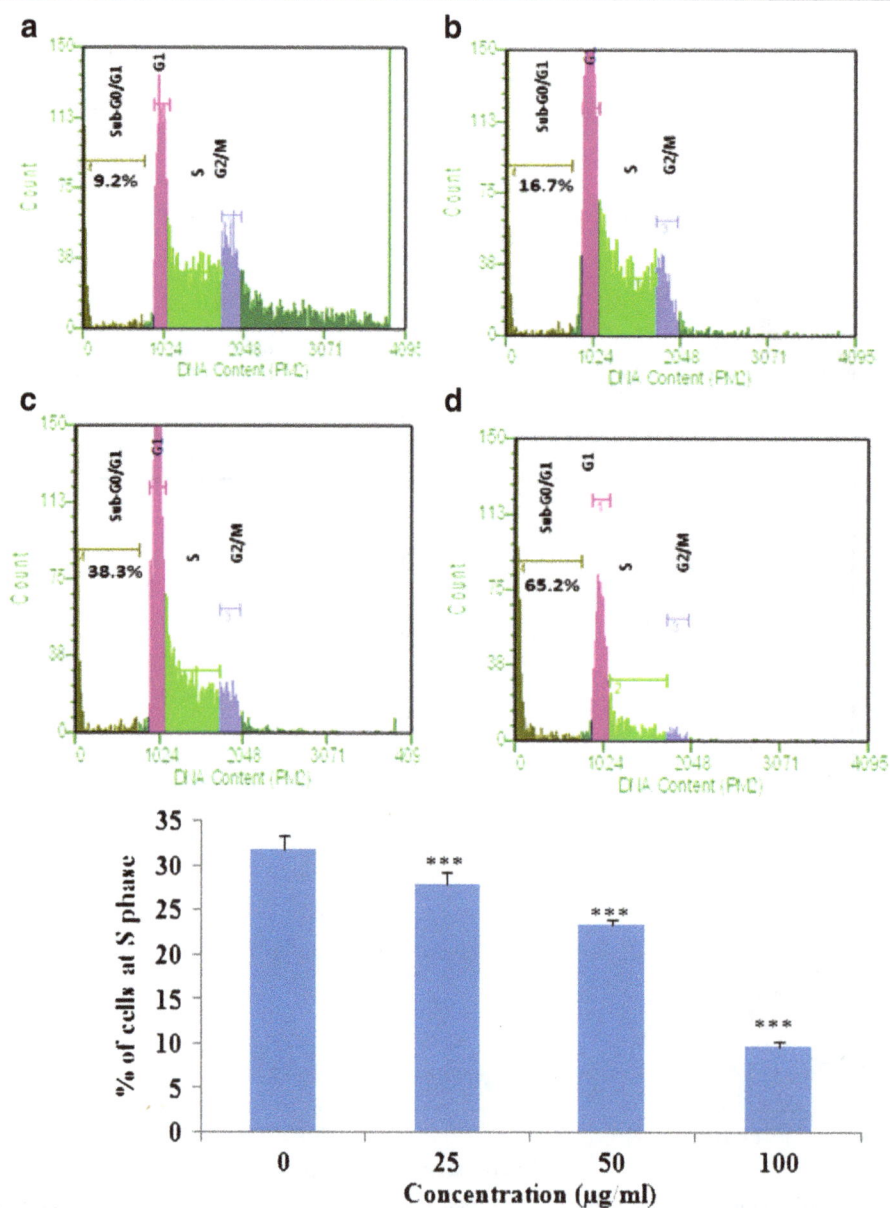

Figure 4 Cell cycle analysis: Cells exposed to different concentrations of EAPL (25, 50 and 100 μg/ml) for 24 h. (a) Control (b) 25 μg/ml (c) 50 μg/ml (d) 100 μg/ml. Bar graph represents the % cells at S phase (mean ± SEM).

15% SDS polyacrylamide gel and then analyzed by Western blot using cytochrome c antibody.

HPLC standardization

The sample was analyzed by reverse phase-high performance liquid chromatography using Shimadzu class LC-20 AD HPLC system, composed by a binary pump, 100 μl injection loop, Photo Diode Array (PDA) detector set at 250–350 nm under room temperature with a flow rate of 0.9 ml/min. Phenomenex Luna 5_ C-18 (2) (150 mm × 4.6 mm) was used as stationary phase. The mobile phase constituted 0.5% formic acid and acetonitrile (70:30, v/v). A serial dilution of standard rutin resulting to 15 ppm, 25 ppm, 50 ppm, 75 ppm and 100 ppm solutions were used for preparing calibration curve (Concentration Vs Area Under Curve). The amount of rutin present in EAPL was quantified from the standard graph.

Statistical analysis

All experiments were carried out in triplicate. Data were expressed as means ± SEM. Differences were evaluated by one-way analysis of variance (ANOVA) test completed by Dennett's test. * denotes $p < 0.05$, ** denotes $p < 0.01$ and *** denotes $p < 0.001$. The 50% inhibitory concentration (IC_{50}) was calculated by nonlinear regression curve with the use of Graphpad Prism version 5.0 for Windows (Graphpad Prism Software, San Diego, CA, USA).

Results and discussion

Phytochemical analysis

The aqueous ethanolic extract was found to contain steroids, terpenoids, flavonoids and/or their glycosides, tannins and carbohydrates. The alkaloids, coumarins, cardiac glycosides were absent.

The determination of IC_{50} by MTT assay

In an effort to gain mechanistic insights of EAPL-induced apoptosis on K562 cells, the anti-proliferative activity was evaluated by MTT assay along with normal (HEK 293) cells. As shown in Figure 1a, a dose-dependent decrease in the growth of cells was observed with increasing concentrations of EAPL and no significant difference was observed in the growth of normal cells. IC_{50} value of EAPL on K562 cells was calculated to be 40 ± 0.01 μg/ml (mean ± SEM) at 24 h by using Graphpad Prism. As a positive control, carvacrol was included in the study and the IC_{50} was determined to be was 110 μg/ml (Figure 1b) as reported earlier [17]. The assay suggests that EAPL is more specific towards cancer cells and ~3 fold more effective compare to carvacrol.

Morphological observations

In order to evaluate the cause of growth inhibition of K562 cells by EAPL, characteristic features of apoptosis

were studied. Apoptosis or programmed cell death is recognized by characteristic pattern of morphological, biochemical, and molecular changes occurring in a cell [18]. EAPL treated (100 μg/ml) cells for 24 h showed prominent morphological changes resembling cell shrinkage with rounding of cells and formation of membrane blebs (Figure 2b) compare to control (Figure 2a) cells which is a characteristic feature of apoptosis as evidenced by microscopic studies.

Annexin V assay

Redistribution of phosphatidylserine to the external side of the cell membrane occurs due to perturbation in the cellular membrane, is one of the biochemical features of apoptosis [19]. Annexin V, a recombinant phosphatidylserine-binding protein, interacts strongly and specifically with phosphatidylserine residues and is used for the detection of apoptosis [20]. Staining of cells with 7-AAD discriminate early apoptotic and dead cells. From Figure 3, the vast majority of K562 cells in the untreated (3a) were healthy and thus unstained for annexin V and 7-AAD. Whereas cells treatment with EAPL resulted in dose dependent increase in the Annexin V and 7-AAD positive cells (3b, 3c, 3d) demonstrating induction of apoptosis.

Cell cycle analysis

Loss of DNA content is a typical characteristic feature of apoptosis. Staining of cells with propidium iodide (PI) and analyzing by flow cytometer would helps in evaluating the cells at different (subG0/G1, G1, S, G2/M) phases of cell cycle. K562 cells were exposed with different concentrations (25, 50, 100 μg/ml) of EAPL for 24 h, washed and harvested and then analyzed in flow

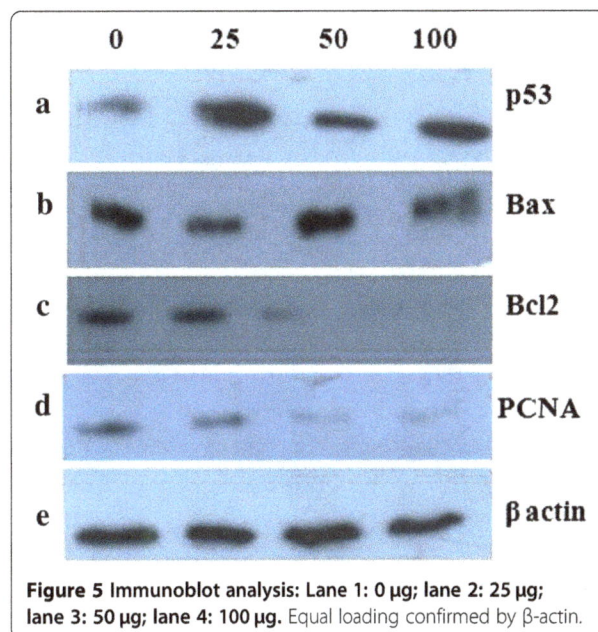

Figure 5 Immunoblot analysis: Lane 1: 0 μg; lane 2: 25 μg; lane 3: 50 μg; lane 4: 100 μg. Equal loading confirmed by β-actin.

cytometry (FACS). The percentage of cells in each phase of the cell cycle was calculated and shown in Figure 4. A dose dependent increase of sub G0/G1 phase (apoptotic peak) and decrease of S phase was observed, indicating the induction of apoptosis and inhibition of DNA synthesis in S phase. These results are in accordance with the previous results [14].

p53 mediated apoptosis

Further to understand the underlying molecular mechanism of apoptosis induced by EAPL, activation of the p53-mediated signaling network was evaluated. Modulation of p53 levels was evaluated by Western blot analysis using p53 antibody in K562 cells treated with different concentrations (25, 50, 100 μg/ml). The results showed an increase in p53 levels in a dose dependent manner

(Figure 5a). Bax homodimers are inducers of apoptosis whereas Bax-Bcl2 heterodimer formation results in cell survival. Both Bax and Bcl2 are transcriptional targets of p53 [21,22]. The levels of the pro-apoptotic protein Bax and anti-apoptotic protein Bcl2 were measured using Western blot. There is a significant decrease in the levels of Bcl2 (Figure 5c) with a little or no alteration in Bax protein, indicating the formation of Bax homodimers (Figure 5b). These changes resulted in increase within the Bax/Bcl2 ratio thereby pushing the cellular balance in the direction of apoptosis. Subsequently, proliferating cell nuclear antigen (PCNA), the marker of dividing cells, specifically inhibited by p53 [23,24] was also studied. The results illustrate a dose-dependent decrease in the expression of PCNA, suggesting induction of apoptosis (Figure 5d).

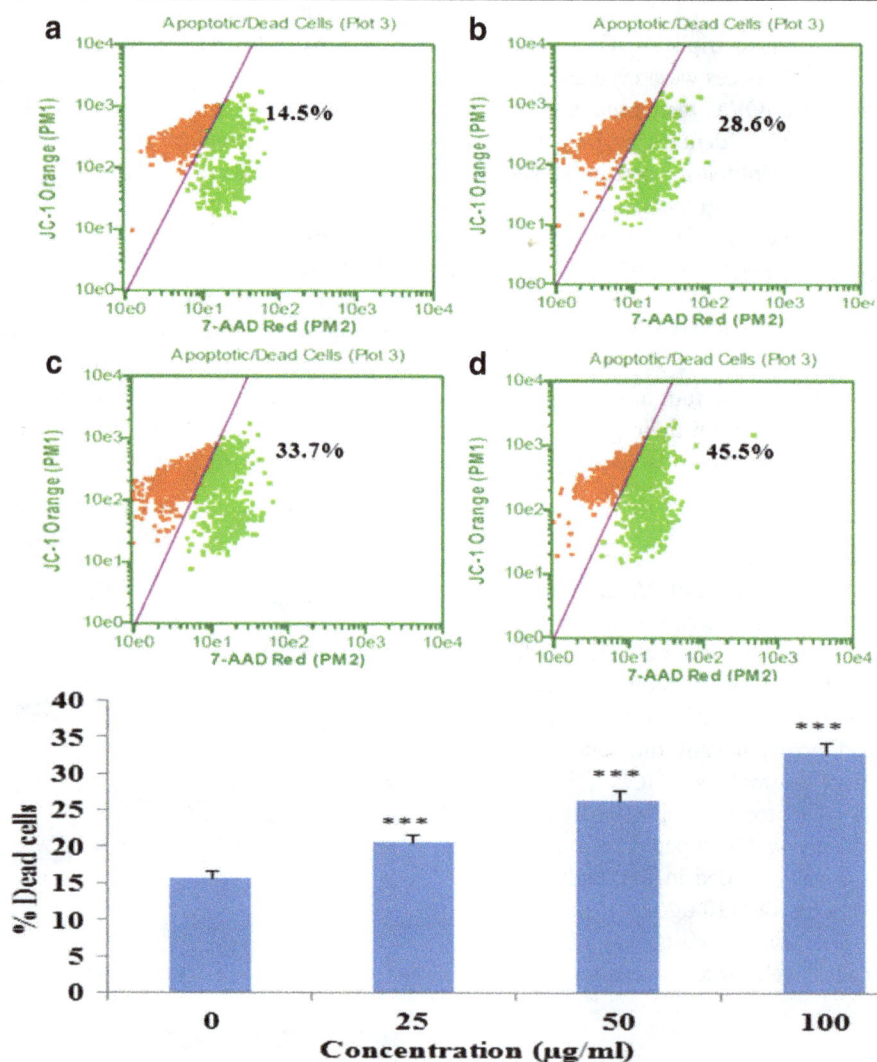

Figure 6 MitoPotential analysis. K562 cells treated with (25, 50, and 100 μg/ml) or without EAPL for 24 h and analyzed by flow cytometer. D-Dead cells. (**a**) Control (**b**) 25 μg/ml (**c**) 50 μg/ml (**d**) 100 μg/ml. Bar graph represents the % dead/apoptotic cells (mean ± SEM).

MitoPotential and multicaspase activation assay

Loss of mitochondrial inner transmembrane potential ($\Delta\Psi$m) is often [25-28], but not always [29,30] observed to be associated with the early stages of apoptosis. Collapse of this potential is believed to coincide with the opening of the mitochondrial permeability transition pores, leading to the release of cytochrome c into the cytosol. In cytoplasm, cytochrome c combines with caspase-9, Apaf-1 and dATP to form the apoptosome complex [31] which in turn activates caspase- 9, -3 and −7. The alteration in membrane mitopotential of the apoptotic cells was determined by flow cytometry and the results showed a dose dependent decrease in the membrane potential (Figure 6). Further the release of cytochrome c from mitochondria into cytosol was analyzed by Western blot analysis in cytosolic fractions of EAPL treated cells. There is a dose dependent increase in the levels of cytochrome c in the cytoplasm indicating

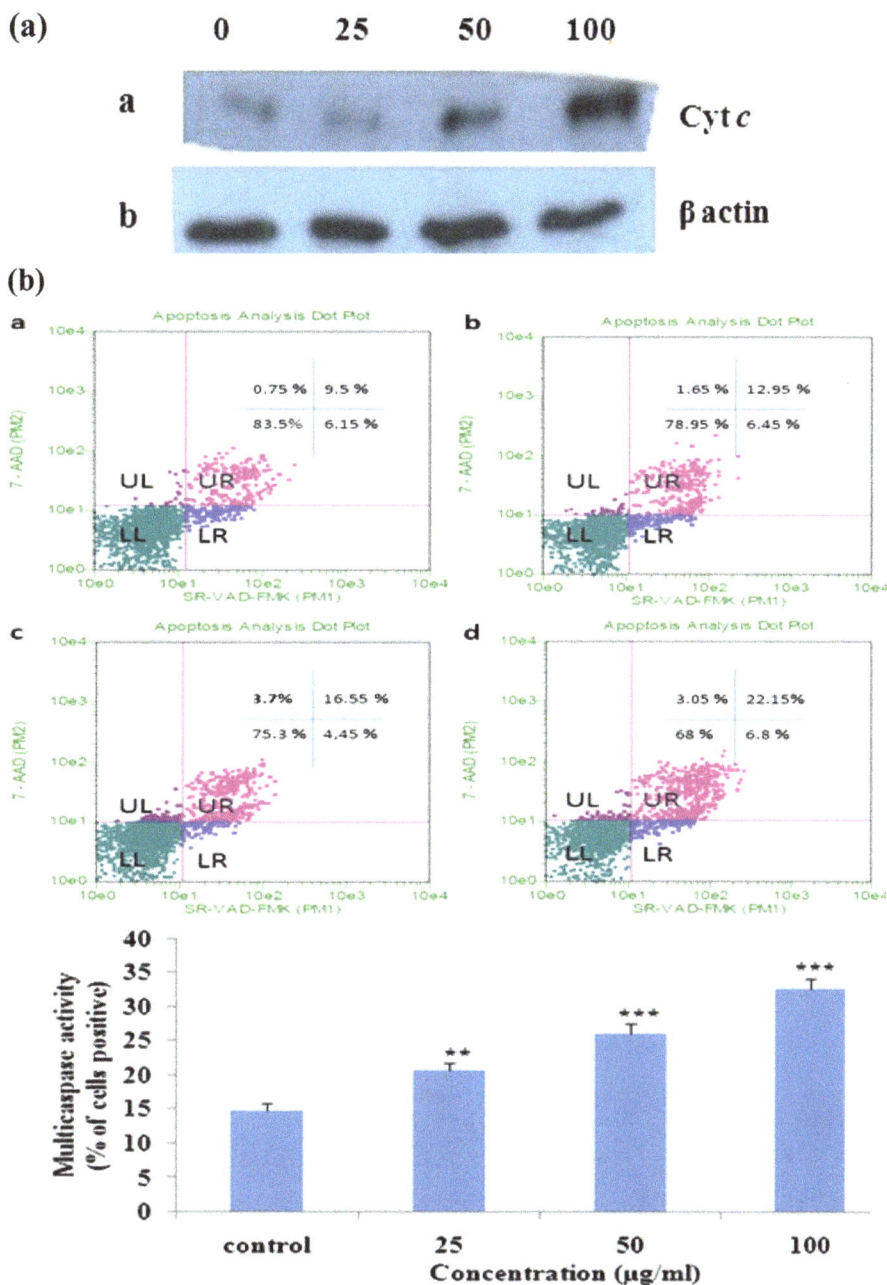

Figure 7 (a) Immunoblot analysis of Cyt c expression in EAPL treated (25, 50, 100 µg/ml) K562 cells. Equal loading confirmed by β-actin. (b) Multicaspase analysis. K562 cells treated with (25, 50, and 100 µg/ml) or without EAPL for 24 h and analyzed by flow cytometer. (a) Control (b) 25 µg/ml (c) 50 µg/ml (d) 100 µg/ml. Bar graph represents the % of caspase active cells (mean ± SEM).

the execution of apoptosis (Figure 7a). In addition activation of multicaspases was determined by FACS analysis and the results clearly demonstrated an increase in multicaspases activation with increase in concentration of EAPL (Figure 7b).

Cleavage of PARP

PARP (poly (ADP-ribose) polymerase) catalyzes the poly ADP-ribosylation of a variety of nuclear proteins with NAD as substrate. Upon DNA damage, PARP gets activated and depletes NAD as well as ATP in an attempt to repair the broken DNA. During apoptosis, caspase-3 inactivates PARP by cleaving it into 83 and 24 kDa fragments and thereby preserves ATP resources of the cell for apoptosis [32,33]. Results from immunoblot analysis using antibody that recognizes uncleaved (116 kDa) and cleaved (83 kDa) fragments of PARP, clearly demonstrate dose dependent inactivation of PARP in EAPL treated cells (Figure 8). The above mentioned studies clearly demonstrate that EAPL induces apoptosis in K562 cells by intrinsic death pathway.

HPLC standardization

Under the set of given analytical conditions, the retention time of standard rutin was observed as 3.8 min (see Additional file 1: Figure S1). The retention time of Rutin present in the sample was found to be identical (see Additional file 1: Figure S1) and the amount of Rutin in EAPL was calculated to be 0.024 % (w/w).

Conclusion

In conclusion, the current work demonstrates the antiproliferative effect of EAPL to induce programmed cell death in chronic myeloid leukemia (K562) cells with an IC_{50} of 40 ± 0.01 µg/ml, showing its anticancer property. It also explains the underlying molecular proceedings occurring in the presence of EAPL. Together, morphological changes such as cell shrinkage, rounding of cells, membrane blebbing, activation of p53, cell cycle arrest at S phase, increase in annexin V positive cells, increase in Bax/Bcl2 ratio, decrease in mitochondrial membrane potential and increase in cytochrome c release from

mitochondria, increase in caspase activity, cleavage of PARP and inhibition of PCNA demonstrate the molecular mechanism of programmed cell death by EAPL. Many of the natural antioxidants have been reported for anti cancer activity by the mechanism not yet clear but one example is curcumin induces apoptosis via a ROS-associated mechanism that converges on JNK activation, and to a lesser extent via a parallel ceramide-associated pathway [34]. Thus, the current work clearly reveals that EAPL could be a potent anti-cancer agent against chronic myeloid leukemia. Study of individual phytoconstituents of the EAPL extract may form the basis for future studies.

The use of natural drugs or food products rich in antioxidant property has been drawn great attention by many scientists for chemotherapeutic purposes, in part because these foods are generally recognized as safe. But natural drugs and food components showing strong antioxidant potential cannot always result in anticancer activities since the biological process of cancer development may be affected by phytochemicals via different mechanisms in addition to antioxidant effects. Many cell-culture based studies have been performed in an attempt to elucidate the relationship between antioxidant activities and anticancer properties of some plant-based drugs. To this end, conflicting findings were observed. Even though mechanism of antitumor activity of most of the plant based drugs has been established, still it is unclear with respect to mechanism of cancer cell death based on antioxidant property [35]. Many studies propose that there are additional functions accountable for the antitumor activity produced by these plant-based drugs that go beyond their antioxidant ability. Extensive molecular and metabolic studies are required to discover these other pathways [36]. Beside the use of cell-culture models, animal experiments and human clinical trials should be employed to explore the possible applications of phytochemical antioxidant rich drugs. These studies will provide more physiological insight into whether antioxidant capacities of plant base drugs are directly linked to their anticancer activities.

Additional file

Additional file 1: Figure S1A: HPLC chromatogram of standard Rutin (15, 25, 50, 75 and 100 ppm) and sample (EAPL). **Figure S1B:** HPLC chromatogram of ethanolic extract of aerial parts of Pupalia lappacea.

Competing interests

The authors declare that there is no conflict of interest that could influence the impartiality of the research reported. This article is original and has been written by the stated authors who are all aware of its content and approve its submission. It has not been published previously or under consideration for publication elsewhere, no conflict of interest exists. If accepted, the article will not be published elsewhere in the same form, in any language, without the written consent of the publisher.

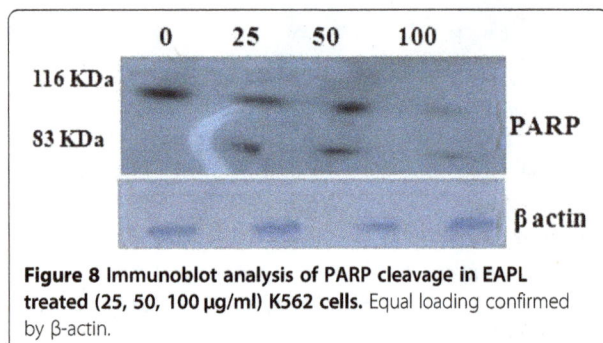

Figure 8 Immunoblot analysis of PARP cleavage in EAPL treated (25, 50, 100 µg/ml) K562 cells. Equal loading confirmed by β-actin.

Authors' contributions

AR, AM participated in the design of the study, performed most of the experimental work and drafted the manuscript. VS performed extraction and phytochemical analysis, selection of the journal. AMK, VKI, AR, AM performed western blot analysis. BMR involved in review of the paper. All authors read and approved the final version of the manuscript.

Author details

[1]G.Pulla Reddy College of Pharmacy, Mehdipatnam, Hyderabad 500 028, AP, India. [2]Birla Institute of Technology and Science, Pilani-Hyderabad Campus, Hyderabad 500 078, AP, India. [3]Department of Animal Sciences, School of Life Sciences, University of Hyderabad, Hyderabad 500046, India. [4]Institute of Life Sciences, University of Hyderabad Campus, Hyderabad, AP 500 046, India.

References

1. Stankovic MS, Curcic MG, Zizic JB, Topuzovic MD, Solujic SR, Markovic SD: Teucrium plant species as natural sources of novel anticancer compounds: antiproliferative, proapoptotic and antioxidant properties. *Int J Mol Sci* 2011, **12:**4190–4205.
2. Reddy L, Odhav B, Bhoola KD: **Natural products for cancer prevention: a global perspective.** *Pharmacol Ther* 2003, **99:**1–13.
3. Guo X, Zhu K, Zhang H, Yao H: **Anti-tumor activity of a novel protein obtained from tartary buckwheat.** *Int J Mol Sci* 2010, **11:**5201–5211.
4. Cragg GM, Newman DJ: **Plants as a source of anti-cancer agents.** *J Ethnopharmacol* 2005, **100:**72–79.
5. Tan G, Gyllenhaal C, Soejarto DD: **Biodiversity as a source of anticancer drugs.** *Curr Drug Targets* 2006, **7:**265–277.
6. Jalalpure SSAN, Patil MB, Chimkode R, Tripathi A: **Antimicrobial and wound healing activities of leaves of Alternanthera sessilis Linn.** *Int J Green Pharm* 2008, **3:**145–148.
7. Bero J, Ganfon H, Jonville MC, Frederich M, Gbaguidi F, DeMol P, Moudachirou M, Quetin-Leclercq J: **In vitro antiplasmodial activity of plants used in Benin in traditional medicine to treat malaria.** *J Ethnopharmacol* 2009, **122:**439–444.
8. Aladedunye Felix OD: **Antioxidant Activity and Chemical Constituents of Pupalia lappacea (L.).** *Juss. Res J Bio Sci* 2008, **3:**783–785.
9. Madhavachetty K (Ed): *Flowering plants of Chittoor District.* Andhra Pradesh, India: Students Offset printers; 2008.
10. Sowemimo A, van de Venter M, Baatjies L, Koekemoer T: **Cytotoxic activity of selected Nigerian plants.** *Afr J Tradit Complement Altern Med* 2009, **6:**526–528.
11. Shetab-Boushehri SV, Abdollahi M: **Current Concerns on the Validity of *in vitro* Models that use Transformed Neoplastic Cells in Pharmacology and Toxicology.** *Int J Pharmacol* 2012, **8:**594–595.
12. Trease E: *Text Book of Pharmacognosy.* New Delhi: India. Elsevier Publishers; 1983.
13. Kokate C: *Practical Pharmacognosy.* Nirali Prakashan: India; 1994.
14. Ravi A, Mallika A, Sama V, Begum AS, Khan RS, Reddy BM: **Antiproliferative activity and standardization of Tecomella undulata bark extract on K562 cells.** *J Ethnopharmacol* 2011, **137:**1353–1359.
15. Bradford MM: **A rapid and sensitive method for the quantitation of microgram quantities of protein utilizing the principle of protein-dye binding.** *Anal Biochem* 1976, **72:**248–254.
16. Chandra J, Niemer I, Gilbreath J, Kliche KO, Andreeff M, Freireich EJ, Keating M, McConkey DJ: **Proteasome inhibitors induce apoptosis in glucocorticoid-resistant chronic lymphocytic leukemic lymphocytes.** *Blood* 1998, **92:**4220–4229.
17. Abdeslam M: **Prenatal Immune Stress in Rats Dampens Fever during Adulthood.** *Dev Neurosci* 2012, **34:**318–326.
18. Elmore S: **Apoptosis: a review of programmed cell death.** *Toxicol Pathol* 2007, **35:**495–516.
19. Bratton DL, Fadok VA, Richter DA, Kailey JM, Guthrie LA, Henson PM: **Appearance of phosphatidylserine on apoptotic cells requires calcium-mediated nonspecific flip-flop and is enhanced by loss of the aminophospholipid translocase.** *J Biol Chem* 1997, **272:**26159–26165.
20. Arur S, Uche UE, Rezaul K, Fong M, Scranton V, Cowan AE, Mohler W, Han DK: **Annexin I is an endogenous ligand that mediates apoptotic cell engulfment.** *Dev Cell* 2003, **4:**587–598.
21. Chipuk JE, Green DR: **Cytoplasmic p53: bax and forward.** *Cell Cycle* 2004, **3:**429–431.
22. Green DR, Chipuk JE: **Apoptosis: Stabbed in the BAX.** *Nature* 2008, **455:**1047–1049.
23. Mercer WE, Shields MT, Lin D, Appella E, Ullrich SJ: **Growth suppression induced by wild-type p53 protein is accompanied by selective down-regulation of proliferating-cell nuclear antigen expression.** *Proc Natl Acad Sci USA* 1991, **88:**1958–1962.
24. Jackson P, Ridgway P, Rayner J, Noble J, Braithwaite A: **Transcriptional regulation of the PCNA promoter by p53.** *Biochem Biophys Res Commun* 1994, **203:**133–140.
25. Hearps AC, Burrows J, Connor CE, Woods GM, Lowenthal RM, Ragg SJ: **Mitochondrial cytochrome c release precedes transmembrane depolarisation and caspase-3 activation during ceramide-induced apoptosis of Jurkat T cells.** *Apoptosis* 2002, **7:**387–394.
26. Krysko DV, Roels F, Leybaert L, D'Herde K: **Mitochondrial transmembrane potential changes support the concept of mitochondrial heterogeneity during apoptosis.** *J Histochem Cytochem* 2001, **49:**1277–1284.
27. Ly JD, Grubb DR, Lawen A: **The mitochondrial membrane potential (delta psi(m)) in apoptosis; an update.** *Apoptosis* 2003, **8:**115–128.
28. Zamzami N, Susin SA, Marchetti P, Hirsch T, Gomez-Monterrey I, Castedo M, Kroemer G: **Mitochondrial control of nuclear apoptosis.** *J Exp Med* 1996, **183:**1533–1544.
29. Friedrich MJ: **Scientists probe roles of mitochondria in neurological disease and injury.** *JAMA* 2004, **291:**679–681.
30. Gollapudi S, McCormick MJ, Gupta S: **Changes in mitochondrial membrane potential and mitochondrial mass occur independent of the activation of caspase-8 and caspase-3 during CD95-mediated apoptosis in peripheral blood T cells.** *Int J Oncol* 2003, **22:**597–600.
31. Chinnaiyan AM: **The apoptosome: heart and soul of the cell death machine.** *Neoplasia* 1999, **1:**5–15.
32. Saraste A, Pulkki K: **Morphologic and biochemical hallmarks of apoptosis.** *Cardiovasc Res* 2000, **45:**528–537.
33. Soldani C, Scovassi AI: **Poly(ADP-ribose) polymerase-1 cleavage during apoptosis: an update.** *Apoptosis* 2002, **7:**321–328.
34. Moussavi M, Assi K, Gomez-Munoz A, Salh B: **Curcumin mediates ceramide generation via the de novo pathway in colon cancer cells.** *Carcinogenesis* 2006, **27:**1636–1644.
35. Abdollahi M, Shetab-Boushehri SV: **Is it right to look for anti-cancer drugs amongst compounds having antioxidant effect?** *DARU* 2012, **20:**61.
36. Wang S, Meckling KA, Marcone MF, Kakuda Y, Tsao R: **Can phytochemical antioxidant rich foods act as anti-cancer agents?** *Food Res Int* 2011, **44:**2545–2554.

Modified Gadonanotubes as a promising novel MRI contrasting agent

Rouzbeh Jahanbakhsh[1], Fatemeh Atyabi[1,2*], Saeed Shanehsazzadeh[3], Zahra Sobhani[1], Mohsen Adeli[4,5] and Rassoul Dinarvand[1,2]

Abstract

Background and purpose of the study: Carbon nanotubes (CNTs) are emerging drug and imaging carrier systems which show significant versatility. One of the extraordinary characteristics of CNTs as Magnetic Resonance Imaging (MRI) contrasting agent is the extremely large proton relaxivities when loaded with gadolinium ion (Gd_n^{3+}) clusters.

Methods: In this study equated Gd_n^{3+} clusters were loaded in the sidewall defects of oxidized multiwalled (MW) CNTs. The amount of loaded gadolinium ion into the MWCNTs was quantified by inductively coupled plasma (ICP) method. To improve water solubility and biocompatibility of the system, the complexes were functionalized using diamine-terminated oligomeric poly (ethylene glycol) via a thermal reaction method.

Results: Gd_n^{3+} loaded PEGylated oxidized CNTs (Gd_n^{3+}@CNTs-PEG) is freely soluble in water and stable in phosphate buffer saline having particle size of about 200 nm. Transmission electron microscopy (TEM) images clearly showed formation of PEGylated CNTs. MRI analysis showed that the prepared solution represents 10% more signal intensity even in half concentration of Gd^{3+} in comparison with commerciality available contrasting agent Magnevist®. In addition hydrophilic layer of PEG at the surface of CNTs could prepare stealth nanoparticles to escape RES.

Conclusion: It was shown that Gd_n^{3+}@CNTs-PEG was capable to accumulate in tumors through enhanced permeability and retention effect. Moreover this system has a potential for early detection of diseases or tumors at the initial stages.

Keywords: Carbon nanotubes, Contrast agent, MRI, Functionalization, Gadolinium, Pegylation

Introduction

Carbon nanotubes (CNTs) have unique physicochemical properties in biomedical and biological applications; hence have attracted attentions in different fields of nanotechnology [1-3]. Large specific surface area, efficient thermal and electrical conductivities, high mechanical strength, heat release in a radiofrequency field and capability of carrying therapeutics and imaging agents are some of these multifunctional features [4,5]. One of the extraordinary characteristics of CNTs loaded with gadolinium is their extremely large proton relaxivities which potentially could be used as magnetic resonance imaging (MRI) contrast agents (CA).

MRI is a powerful noninvasive imaging technique based on the differences between proton relaxation rates of water [6]. To enhance the contrast between different tissues and to detect disease states, using MRI CAs is inevitable [7,8]. Gadolinium (Gd^{3+}) with seven unpaired electrons and large magnetic moment is a suitable agent for this purpose. Although the equated Gd^{3+} ion is toxic, the most contrast enhancements are based on Gd^{3+}. Chelation or encapsulation of Gd^{3+}, decreases the toxicity of this ion for medical applications [7,9]. One of the most commercially used CA is gadolinium-diethylene triamine penta acetic acid, (Gd^{3+}-DTPA) commercially available as Magnevist®. Due to lack of specificity and sensitivity, this product is not very effective in early detection of the disease, so it has been classified as a traditional CAs [8].

Sitharaman et al. developed the first CNT-based contrast agent. They demonstrated that Gd@Ultra-short single-walled carbon nanotubes (gadonanotubes) drastically

* Correspondence: atyabifa@tums.ac.ir
[1]Department of Pharmaceutics, Faculty of Pharmacy, Tehran University of Medical Sciences, Tehran 14174, Iran
[2]Nanotechnology Research Centre, Faculty of Pharmacy, Tehran University of Medical Sciences, Tehran 14174, Iran
Full list of author information is available at the end of the article

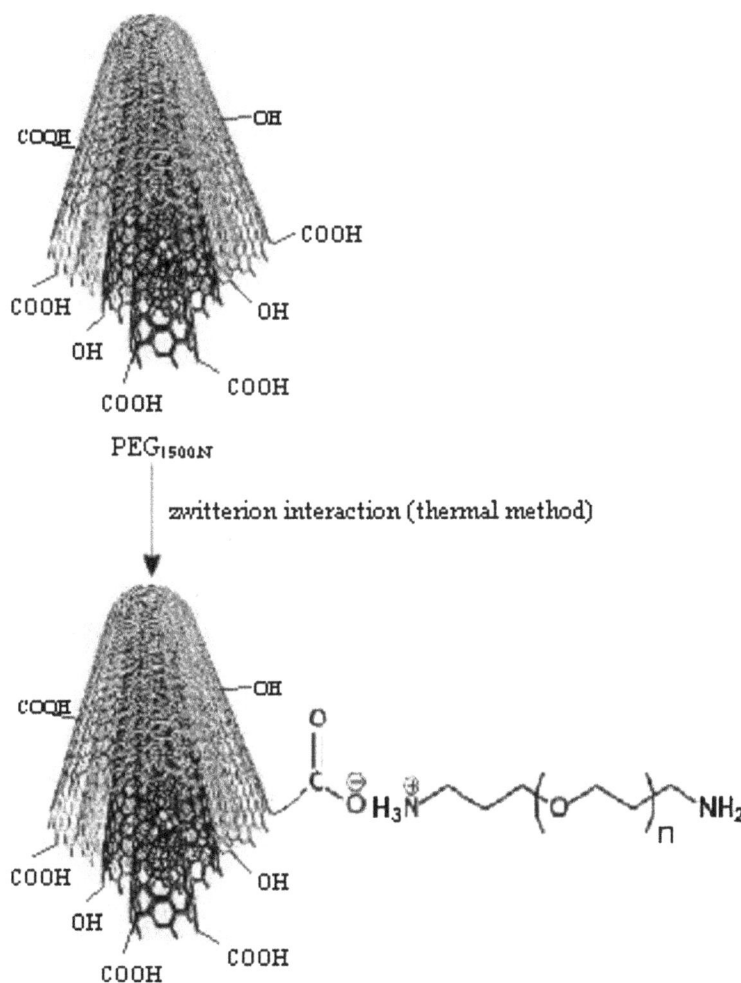

Figure 1 Schematic diagram of functionalization of oxidized CNTs loaded with Gd^{3+} (Gd_n^{3+}@CNTs) with diamine-terminated PEG via zwitterion interactions.

increase MRI efficacy compared to the traditional CAs [9]. However, the most challenging part of using CNTs in biological system is lack of solubility and hence its toxicity. Even though oxidation of CNTs improve their dispersibility, but it`s still not enough to call them as a suitable carriers.

Wrapping biocompatible and biodegradable polyethylene glycol (PEG) onto the CNTs makes them soluble and helping them to escape reticuloendothelial system (RES) uptake. This modification causes longer blood circulation of CNTs and facilitates the passive targeting to the cancer cells

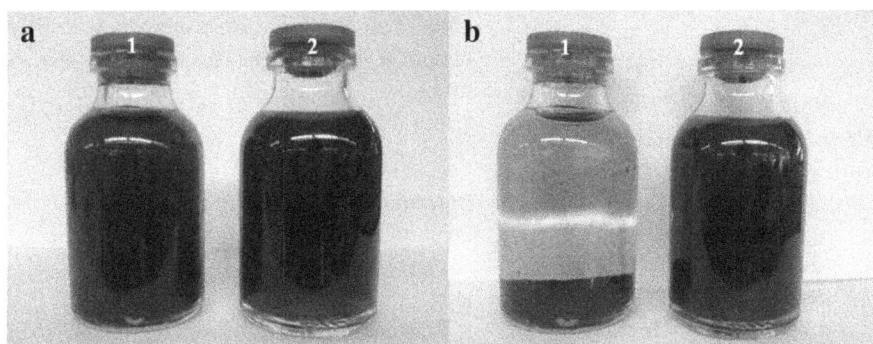

Figure 2 Dispersion of Gd_n^{3+}@CNTs (1) and Gd_n^{3+}@CNTs-PEG (2) immediately after sonication in PBS (a) and 2 months later (b).

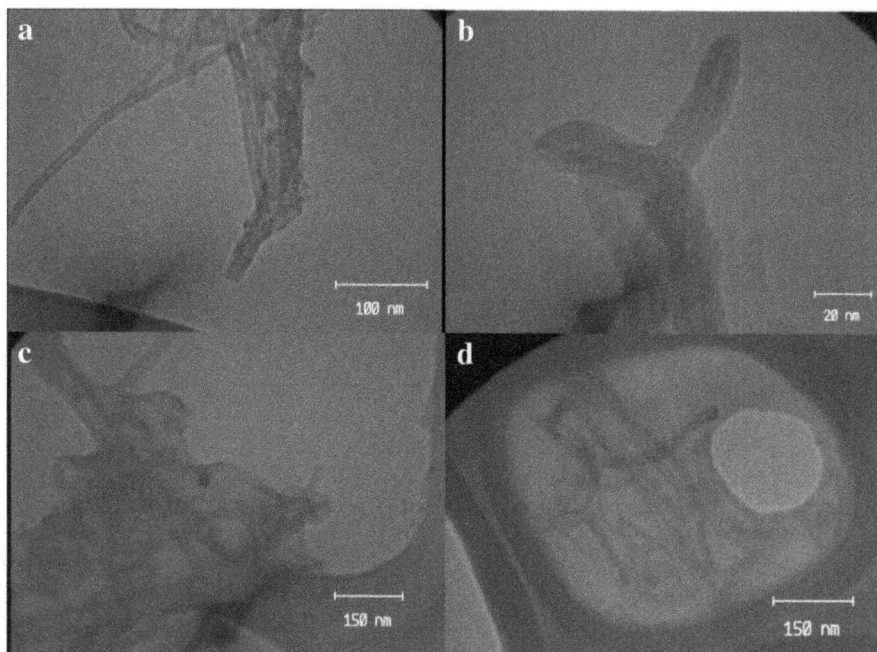

Figure 3 TEM images of Gd_n^{3+}@CNTs (a-b) and Gd_n^{3+}@CNTs-PEG (c-d).

through the enhanced permeability and retention (EPR) effect of tumor blood vessels [10-12]. Accordingly these particles can be applied for detection of tumors at the early stages.

In this work multi walled CNTs were functionalized by PEGylation and loaded with Gd_n^{3+} enhance contrast effect of commercial Gd. T_1/T_2 measurements revealed that signal intensity of Gd_n^{3+}@CNTs-PEG was more than commercial Magnevist®.

Methods and materials
Oxidation of MWCNTs
MWCNTs (number of walls 3–15, outer diameter 5–20 nm, and length 1–10 μm) were purchased from Plasmachem (GmbH, Berlin, Germany). CNTs were oxidized according to the procedure reported before [13]. Briefly, 20 ml of sulfuric acid and nitric acid mixture (3:1 v/v) were added to 1 g of MWCNTs in a reaction flask and the mixture was sonicated for 30 min. Reaction medium was refluxed for 21 h at 120°C. The mixture was cooled and diluted with 1 L of distilled water, filtered, and washed with deionized water to adjust pH to ≈ 6. The product was dried by vacuum oven.

Loading of GdCl₃ (H₂O)₆ into the oxidized MWCNTs
100 mg of oxidized MWCNTs (O-MWCNTs) and 100 mg of $GdCl_3.6H_2O$ (REacton®, 99.9%) were stirred together in 100 ml deionized water and sonicated in a bath sonicator for 60 min. The solution was left undisturbed overnight whereupon the Gd^{3+}-loaded oxidized CNTs (Gd_n^{3+}@CNTs)

flocculated from the solution. The supernatant was then decanted off. To remove any unabsorbed $GdCl_3$, remained sediment was dispersed in 25 ml of fresh deionized water with batch sonication and again, the Gd_n^{3+}@CNTs flocculated from solution was collected by decantation. This procedure was repeated 3 times. The final product was dried by vacuum oven.

Functionalization of Gd_n^{3+}@CNTs with PEG₁₅₀₀N
28 mg of Gd_n^{3+}@CNTs was mixed with 474 mg Poly (ethylene glycol) bis (3-aminopropyl) terminated (M_n~1,500, Aldrich) and the mixture was stirred at ≈ 120°C under nitrogen atmosphere for 6 days. Upon the addition of deionized water to the mixture, the suspension was placed in a membrane tube (molecular weight cutoff ~12000) for dialysis against fresh deionized water for 3 days to remove free PEG. Dialysis phases were also collected for the confirmation of absence of free Gd^{3+} ion by ICP. To removing large nanotube bundles the suspension was centrifuged three times at 13000 rpm for 15 min and the supernatant was freeze-dried.

Determination of size and morphology
Dynamic light scattering (DLS) (Malvern Zetasizer ZS, Malvern UK) was used to determine the dynamic diameter and size distributions of Gd_n^{3+}@CNTs-PEG.

Transmission electron microscopy (TEM) and Thermal gravimetric analyses (TGA) (Shimadzu, Japan) was applied for characterization of preparation.

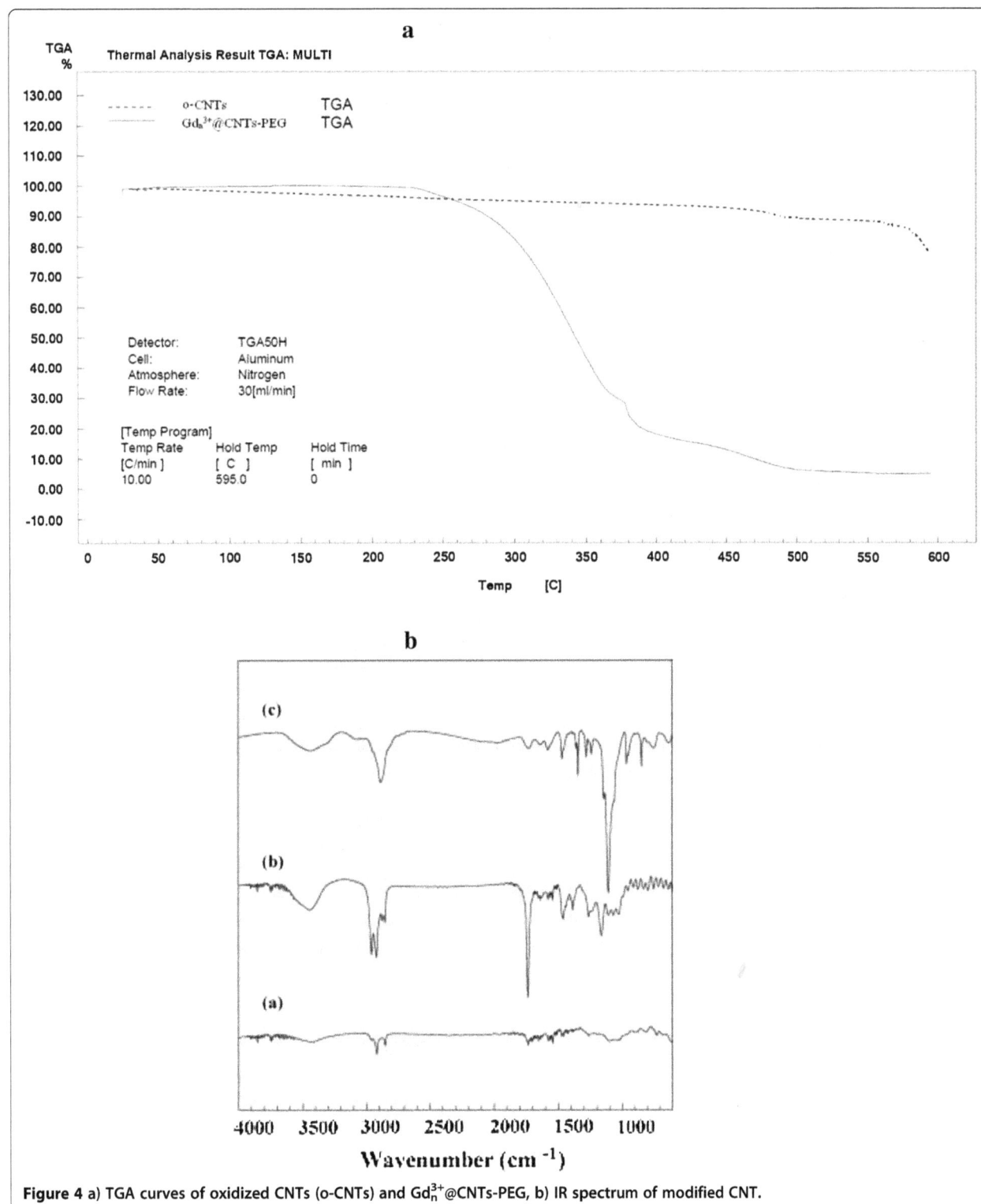

Figure 4 a) TGA curves of oxidized CNTs (o-CNTs) and Gd$_n^{3+}$@CNTs-PEG, b) IR spectrum of modified CNT.

ICP sample preparation

For ICP (Inductively Coupled Plasma) analysis, samples should digest with strong oxidizing agents like HNO3 or concentrated H2O2. As this harsh condition is not enough for digesting MWCNTs, in this study the nanotubes were first heated in oven at 650°C for 5 h. Fallowing cooling the sample, the solid residue was dissolved in the solution of $HNO_3(2\%)$ and the Gd content was

Table 1 T1 values (msec) derived from equations 1 and 2 for Gdn3+@CNTs-PEG with different Gd3+ concentration and Magnevist®

	Concentration of Gd mM/mL					Magnevist®	Water
TR (Sec)	**0.1818**	**0.1**	**0.05**	**0.025**	**0.0125**	**0.1818**	
T1	190.69	328.95	572.74	926.78	1385.23	405.35	3076.92
1/T1	0.005244	0.00304	0.001746	0.001079	0.0007219	0.002467	0.000325
R^2 value	**0.98**	**0.99**	**0.99**	**0.99**	**0.99**	**0.99**	**0.99**

determined by ICP-Optical Emission Spectrometer (Varian 720-ES).

In vitro T1/T2 measurement

The T1- and T2-weighted spin echo images at 1.5 Tesla (repetition time/echo time 250/16 msec and repetition time/echo time 4000/64 msec) were analyzed qualitatively. The signal intensities of vials with contrast medium in solution and contrast medium in cells with the corresponding Gd concentrations were visually compared.

For quantitative data analysis, the obtained MR images were transferred as digital imaging and communication in medicine (DICOM) images to a Dicom Works version 1.3.5 (DicomWorks, Lyon, France) [14,15]). For each concentration, three samplings and the maximum regions of interest were considered. Five concentrations of the carbon nanotubes (0.1818, 0.1, 0.05, 0.025 mM Gd or 0.1818, 0.1, 0.05, 0.025, 0.0125 mM/mL Gd) were prepared in sodium chloride 0.9%.

The imaging parameters were as follows: Standard Spin Echo, # of Echoes =1, TE=15 ms, TR=100, 200, 400, 600,1000, 2000 ms, Matrix=512*384, Slice Thickness=4 mm ,FOV=25 cm, NEX=3, Pixel Band width: 130 for T1 measurements and Standard Spin Echo, # of Echoes =4, TE=15/30/45/60 ms, TR=3000 ms, Matrix=512*384, Slice Thickness=4 mm, FOV=25 cm, NEX=3, Pixel Band width: 130 for T2 measurements.

T1 and T2 maps were calculated assuming mono exponential signal decay. T1 maps were calculated from four SE images with a fixed TE of 11 ms at 1.5T and variable TR values of 100, 200, 400, 600, 1000 and 2000 ms using a nonlinear function least-square curve fitting on a pixel-by-pixel basis. The signal intensity for each pixel as a function of time was expressed as follows (Equation 1) [16]:

$$Signal_{SE1}(TR, T_1) = S_{01}\left(1 - e^{-\frac{TR}{T_1}}\right)$$

T2 maps were calculated accordingly from four SE images with a fixed TR of 3000 ms and TE values of 15, 30, 45, and 60 ms on the 1.5T MR scanner. The signal intensity for each pixel as a function of time was expressed as follows (Equation 2):

$$Signal_{SE4}(TE, T_2) = S_0 e^{-\frac{TE}{T_2}} \Rightarrow ln(Signal_{SE4})$$
$$= ln(S_0) - \frac{TE}{T_2}$$

Care was taken to analyze only data points with signal intensities significantly above the noise level.

Statistical analysis

One-way analysis of variance was used for comparison of the results. P values of 0.05 or less were considered as significant.

Results and discussion
Loading of Gd_n^{3+} into the CNTs

In the presence study, MWCNTs were oxidized with harsh acid condition and then loaded with Gd_n^{3+}. Oxidizing occurred with the mixture of sulfuric and nitric acid (3:1). This procedure removes metal catalysts impurity and creates an open end termini in the structure and also sidewall defects that are stabilized by –COOH and –OH groups [12,17-19]. These hydrophilic holes are the very well place for accumulation of hydrophilic metal ions (e.g. Gd^{3+}) on the surface or inside of the interior of a CNT [18,20]. Besides the –COOH group could be coupled to different chemical or biochemical groups [18-21].

Table 2 T2 values (msec) derived from equations 1 and 2 for Gd_n^{3+}@CNTs-PEG with different Gd^{3+} concentration and Magnevist®

	Concentration of Gd mM/mL					Magnevist®	
TE (Sec)	**0.1818**	**0.1**	**0.05**	**0.025**	**0.0125**	**0.1818**	**Water**
1/T2	19.95	15.29	12.36	10.90	9.85	6.42	8.80
T2	0.0501	0.0654	0.0809	0.0917	0.1015	0.1558	0.1136
R^2 value	0.99	0.99	0.99	0.98	0.97	0.99	96

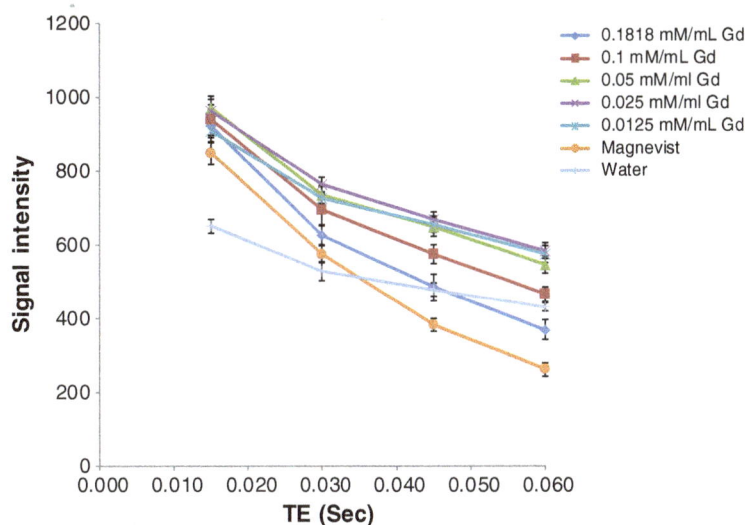

Figure 5 Signal changes based on echo time variation.

The oxidized MWCNTs were loaded by soaking and sonicating them in double distilled water containing aqueous $GdCl_3$. After sedimentation and dialysis to remove unloaded Gd^{3+} into the oxidized MWCNTs, $Gd_n^{3+}@CNTs$ was functionalized with PEG. ICP analysis showed the Gd_n^{3+} content of $Gd_n^{3+}@CNTs$ and $Gd_n^{3+}@CNTs$-PEG to be 4.328% and 0.02% (w/w) respectively. The absence of free Gd^{3+} ion in the sample was confirmed by analysis the final dialysis medium through ICP, no detectable Gd^{3+} was shown.

Solubilization and stabilization of $Gd_n^{3+}@CNTs$ with PEG

Carbon nanotubes have a rigid structure and presence in bundles, so they are essentially insoluble in any

solvents. As a result, solubilization of CNTs via chemical functionalization has been attracted much recent attentions [1,5,10,17,18]. Among the possible hydrophilic polymers, with regard to biocompatibility, PEG is attractive for use with CNTs because of being nontoxic, properly stable and having a low immunogenicity [1,10,11,21]. $Gd_n^{3+}@CNTs$ was functionalized with PEG_{1500N} ($Gd_n^{3+}@CNTs$-PEG). As reported by other researches, the attachment of diamine-terminated poly(ethylene glycol) with $Gd_n^{3+}@CNTs$ were done via thermal reaction and zwitterion interaction between terminated amines of PEG and carboxylic groups of oxidized CNTs as shown in Figure 1 [21].

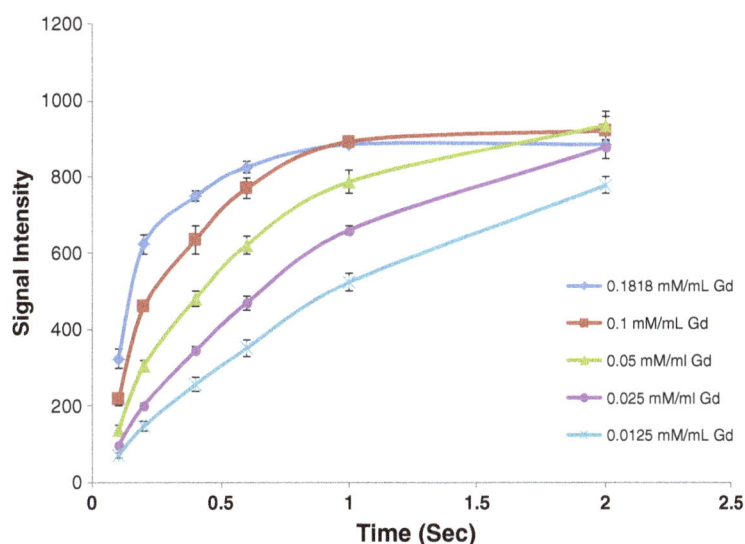

Figure 6 Signal changes based on repetition time variation.

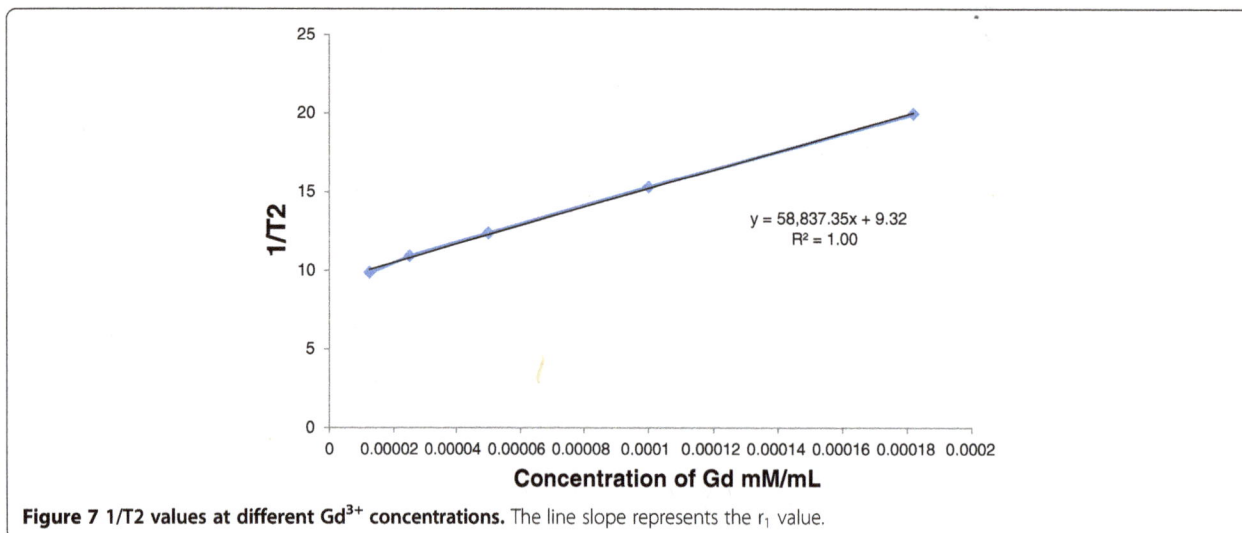

Figure 7 1/T2 values at different Gd^{3+} concentrations. The line slope represents the r$_1$ value.

As expected, the solution of the Gd$_n^{3+}$@CNTs-PEG was more stable than Gd$_n^{3+}$@CNTs in PBS. The Gd$_n^{3+}$@CNTs-PEG remained homogeneous over 2 months of observation time whereas in the Gd$_n^{3+}$@CNTs black precipitation appeared after a few days (Figure 2).

Characterization of Gd$_n^{3+}$@CNTs-PEG

The particle size of Gd$_n^{3+}$@CNTs-PEG in water evaluated by Dynamic Light Scattering technique was about 200 nm with narrow poly dispersity index (PDI : 0.361). This particle size is appropriate for IV administration of solubilized gadonanotubes as a contrasting agent.

Typical transmission electron microscopy (TEM) images of the functionalized MWCNTs loaded Gd^{3+} ions are shown in Figure 3. In the Gd$_n^{3+}$@CNTs-PEG image, wrapping PEG is can be clearly found around the nanotubes and the outer layer of polymer phase is discontinuous. Additionally nanotubes are dispersed either individually or in small bundles whereas in the image of Gd$_n^{3+}$@CNTs, tight bundles of nanotubes can be seen.

Thermo gravimetric analysis (TGA) and IR spectroscopy was employed to determine either the tube is wrapped by polymer chains. Thermograms and IR spectrum of Gd$_n^{3+}$@CNTs-PEG and oxidized MWCNTs are shown in Figure 4. Wrapped PEG started to thermally degrade in the temperature range of 312°C. When the temperature reached to 450°C, PEG had essentially decomposed completely. According to the weight loss of PEG in Gd$_n^{3+}$@CNTs-PEG (about 95%), content of MWCNT in this compound is low. TEM images and ICP results also confirmed this low content of MWCNT in the Gd$_n^{3+}$@CNTs-PEG.

For oxidized MWCNTs, a weight loss was detected at 470°C, which can be attributed to the thermally unstable functional groups, e.g. −COOH and −OH on MWCNTs, formed during oxidation. These results indicate that PEG chains have successfully wrapped onto the MWCNT surfaces.

T1/T2 measurement

T1/T2 measurements were performed in vitro, using magnetic resonance imaging apparatus. The analysis investigated that Gd$_n^{3+}$@CNTs-PEG solution in almost same and half concentration of Gd^{3+} compare to Magnevist® showed 29% and 9% more signal intensity respectively.

The results of T1/T2 relaxation time (derived from equations 1 and 2) are shown in Tables 1 and 2 and Figures 5 and 6.

Gd$_n^{3+}$@CNTs-PEG clearly caused a significant decrease in both T1 and T2 relaxation time compared with Magnevist®. As shown in Table 1, the T1 values at the same concentration of Gd^{3+} in the Gd$_n^{3+}$@CNTs-PEG and Magnevist® were 190.7 msec and 405.4 msec, respectively. If we depicted the 1/T1 value at different Gd^{3+} concentration the r$_1$ value will be obtained 26.6 (mMol^{-1}.sec^{-1}) as shown in Figure 7, while other studies show that the r$_1$ value for Magnevist® was only 13.4 (mMol^{-1}.sec^{-1}) [22].

Table 2 shows the T2 values for Gd$_n^{3+}$@CNTs-PEG at different Gd^{3+} concentrations. The r$_2$ value for Gd$_n^{3+}$@CNTs-PEG was 58.8 (mMol^{-1}.sec^{-1}) which was greater than Magnevist®. Data in tables and T1/T2 weighted images (Figure 8) showed that the signal increments of Gd$_n^{3+}$@CNTs-PEG were much higher even with half

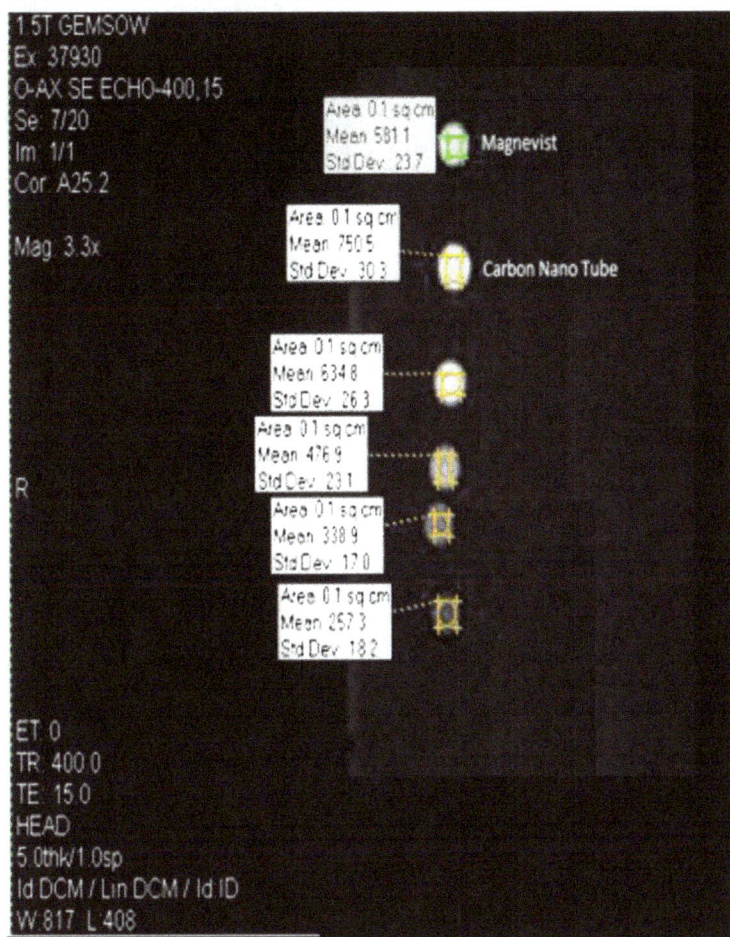

Figure 8 The discrepancies among different concentrations of Gd^{3+} in the Gd$_n^{3+}$@CNTs-PEG and Magnevist$^®$ at T1 weighted image. Five concentrations of the Gd$_n^{3+}$@CNTs-PEG (0.1818, 0.1, 0.05, 0.025 mMolarGd) were sorted, respectively from top to bottom by diluting with sodium chloride 0.9%.

concentration of Gd^{3+} compare with the conventional contrast agent Magnevist$^®$.

MR imaging of the samples (in test tubes) was performed using a 1.5T MR scanner (Signa, GE Medical Systems, Milwaukee, WI, USA) and a standard circularly polarized head coil (Clinical MR Solutions, Brookfield, WI, USA). All probes were placed in a water-containing plastic container (as shown in Figure 8) at room temperature (25°C) to avoid susceptibility artifacts from the surrounding air in the scans.

As shown in Figure 8 the signal intensity of Magnevist$^®$ and Gd$_n^{3+}$@CNTs-PEG at the same image condition, same protocol, same region of interest (ROI) area, and same Gd^{3+} concentration was 581.1 and 750.5, respectively. Therefore the signal intensity of Gd$_n^{3+}$@CNTs-PEG PEG was 29% and 9% more than Magnevist$^®$, at equal or half of Gd^{3+} concentration, respectively.

Conclusions

In order to increase proton relaxivity characteristics of gadolinium ion (Gd$_n^{3+}$ -ion) clusters, carbon nanotubes have been proven to be a good candidate. Addition of polyethylene glycol to this complex could improve the expected properties of the preparation as far as its solubility, stability and more over MRI contrasting ability of them. This could be the basis for further study to reach ideal goal which is detection of any abnormal tissues or tumors at the early stages.

Competing interest
The authors declare that they have no competing interests regarding present work.

Authors' contributions
RJ conducted the experimental work and help in drafting the manuscript, FA conceived the study supervised the work and is the corresponding author of the work, SS performed the MRI experiments and ZS helped with the interpretation of the data analysis, MA helped with synthesis part of the work, RD reviewed and edited the manuscript. All authors read and approved the final manuscript.

Acknowledgments

The author would like to thanks the kind help of Dr. Keith B Hartman for his useful suggestions.

Author details

[1]Department of Pharmaceutics, Faculty of Pharmacy, Tehran University of Medical Sciences, Tehran 14174, Iran. [2]Nanotechnology Research Centre, Faculty of Pharmacy, Tehran University of Medical Sciences, Tehran 14174, Iran. [3]Department of Biomedical Physics and Engineering, School of Medicine, Tehran University of Medical Sciences, Tehran, Iran. [4]Department of Chemistry, Sharif University of Technology, Tehran, Iran. [5]Department of Chemistry, Faculty of Science, Lorestan University, Khoramabad, Iran.

References

1. Liu Z, Tabakman S, Welsher K, Dai H: **Carbon nanotubes in biology and medicine: In vitro and in vivo detection, imaging and drug delivery.** *Nano Research* 2009, **2**:85–120.
2. Hartman KB, Wilson LJ, Rosenblum MG: **Detecting and Treating Cancer with Nanotechnology.** *Mol Diag Ther* 2008, **12**:1–14.
3. Sobhani Z, Dinarvand R, Atyabi F, Ghahremani M, Adeli M: **Increased paclitaxel cytotoxicity against cancer cell lines using a novel functionalized carbon nanotube.** *Int J Nanomedicine* 2011, **6**:705–719.
4. Gannon CJ, Cherukuri P, Yakobson BI, Cognet L, Kanzius JS, Kittrell C, Weisman RB, Pasquali M, Schmidt HK, Smalley RE, Curley SA: **Carbon nanotube-enhanced thermal destruction of cancer cells in a noninvasive radiofrequency field.** *Cancer* 2007, **110**:2654–2665.
5. Kam NWS, O'Connell M, Wisdom JA, Dai HJ: **Carbon nanotubes as multifunctional biological transporters and near-infrared agents for selective cancer cell destruction.** *P Natl Acad Sci USA* 2005, **102**:11600–11605.
6. Geraldes CF, Laurent S: **Classification and basic properties of contrast agents for magnetic resonance imaging.** *Contrast Media Mol Imaging* 2009, **4**:1–23.
7. Sitharaman B, Wilson LJ: **Gadofullerenes and gadonanotubes: A new paradigm for high-performance magnetic resonance imaging contrast agent probes.** *J Biomed Nanotechnol* 2007, **3**:342–352.
8. Mody W, Nounou MI, Bikram M: **Novel nanomedicine-based MRI contrast agents for gynecological malignancies.** *Adv Drug Deliv Rev* 2009, **61**:795–807.
9. Sitharaman B, Kissell KR, Hartman KB, Tran LA, Baikalov A, Rusakova I, Sun Y, Khant HA, Ludtke SJ, Chiu W: **Superparamagnetic gadonanotubes are high-performance MRI contrast agents.** *Chem Commun* 2005, **31**:3915–3917.
10. Foldvari M, Bagonluri M: **Carbon nanotubes as functional excipients for nanomedicines: II. Drug delivery and biocompatibility issues.** *Nanomedicine: Nanotechnology, Biology, and Medicine* 2008, **4**:183–200.
11. Yang ST, Fernando KA, Liu JH, Wang J, Sun HF, Liu Y, Chen M, Huang Y, Wang X, Wang H, Sun YP: **Covalently PEGylated carbon nanotubes with stealth character in vivo.** *Small* 2008, **4**:940–944.
12. Firme CP III, Bandaru PR: **Toxicity issues in the application of carbon nanotubes to biological systems.** *Nanomedicine: Nanotechnology, Biology and Medicine* 2010, **6**:245–256.
13. Tsang SC, Chen YK, Harris PJF, Green MLH: **A Simple Chemical Method of Opening and Filling Carbon Nanotubes.** *Nature* 1994, **372**:159–162.
14. Puech PA, Boussel L, Belfkih S, Lemaitre L, Douek P, Beuscart R: **DicomWorks: software for reviewing DICOM studies and promoting low-cost teleradiology.** *J Digit Imaging* 2007, **20**:122–130.
15. Jabr-Milane LS, van Vlerken LE, Yadav S, Amiji MM: **Multi-functional nanocarriers to overcome tumor drug resistance.** *Cancer Treat Rev* 2008, **34**:592–602.
16. Engström M, Klasson A, Pedersen H, Vahlberg C, Käll PO, Uvdal K: **High proton relaxivity for gadolinium oxide nanoparticles.** *Magnetic Resonance Materials in Physics, Biology and Medicine* 2006, **19**:180–186.
17. Klumpp C, Kostarelos K, Prato M, Bianco A: **Functionalized carbon nanotubes as emerging nanovectors for the delivery of therapeutics.** *Biochim Biophys Acta* 2006, **1758**:404–412.
18. Prato M, Kostarelos K, Bianco A: **Functionalized carbon nanotubes in drug design and discovery.** *Accounts of chemical research* 2007, **41**:60–68.
19. Cai SY, Kong JL: **Advance in Research on Carbon Nanotubes as Diagnostic and Therapeutic Agents for Tumor.** *Chin J Anal Chem* 2009, **37**:1240–1246.
20. Hashimoto A, Yorimitsu H, Ajima K, Suenaga K, Isobe H, Miyawaki J, Yudasaka M, Iijima S, Nakamura E: **Selective deposition of a gadolinium(III) cluster in a hole opening of single-wall carbon nanohorn.** *Proc Natl Acad Sci USA* 2004, **101**:8527–8530.
21. Huang W, Fernando S, Allard LF, Sun YP: **Solubilization of single-walled carbon nanotubes with diamine-terminated oligomeric poly (ethylene glycol) in different functionalization reactions.** *Nano Lett* 2003, **3**:565–568.
22. Svenson S, Prud'homme RK: **Polymer modified nanoparticles as targeted MR imaging agents.** In *Multifunctional nanoparticles for drug delivery applications: imaging, targeting, and delivery.* New York: Springer; 2012:186.

19

Design and characterization of diclofenac diethylamine transdermal patch using silicone and acrylic adhesives combination

Dandigi M Panchaxari[1], Sowjanya Pampana[1*], Tapas Pal[2], Bhavana Devabhaktuni[2] and Anil Kumar Aravapalli[1]

Abstract

Background and purpose of the study: The objective of the study was to develop and characterize Diclofenac Diethylamine (DDEA) transdermal patch using Silicone and acrylic adhesives combination.

Methods: Modified solvent evaporation method was employed for casting of film over Fluoropolymer coated polyester release liner. Initial studies included solubilization of drug in the polymers using solubilizers. The formulations with combination of adhesives were attempted to combine the desirable features of both the adhesives. The effect of the permeation enhancers on the drug permeation were studied using pig ear skin. All the optimized patches were subjected to adhesion, dissolution and stability studies. A 7-day skin irritancy test on albino rabbits and an in vivo anti-inflammatory study on wistar rats by carrageenan induced paw edema method were also performed.

Results: The results indicated the high percent drug permeation (% CDP-23.582) and low solubility nature (1%) of Silicone adhesive and high solubility (20%) and low% CDP (10.72%) of acrylic adhesive. The combination of adhesives showed desirable characteristics for DDEA permeation with adequate % CDP and sufficient solubility. Release profiles were found to be dependent on proportion of polymer and type of permeation enhancer. The anti-inflammatory study revealed the sustaining effect and high percentage inhibition of edema of C4/OLA (99.68%). The acute skin irritancy studies advocated the non-irritant nature of the adhesives used.

Conclusion: It was concluded that an ideal of combination of adhesives would serve as the best choice, for fabrication of DDEA patches, for sustained effect of DDEA with better enhancement in permeation characteristics and robustness.

Keywords: Transdermal drug delivery system, Silicone adhesive, Acrylic adhesive, Permeation study, Dissolution, Skin irritancy and anti-inflammatory

Introduction

Drugs can be delivered across the skin to have an effect on the tissues adjacent to the site of application (topical delivery) or to have an effect after distribution through the circulatory system (systemic delivery). While there are many advantages for delivering drugs through the skin the barrier properties of the skin provide a significant challenge. By understanding the mechanisms by which compounds cross the skin it will be possible to devise means for improving drug delivery [1]. In the last decades, transdermal dosage forms have been introduced for providing a controlled delivery via the skin into the circulation system.

A transdermal patch or skin patch is a medicated adhesive patch that is placed on the skin to deliver a specific dose of medication through the skin and into the blood stream. Drug-in-adhesive-type patches have been gaining increasing popularity as effective transdermal delivery systems during the last two decades [2] due to various advantages over other systems namely, they are easy to construct, less chances of dose dumping and patches with less thicknesses can be prepared.

Diclofenac is a well-established non-steroidal anti-inflammatory agent, widely used in musculoskeletal

* Correspondence: soujanya.pampana@gmail.com
[1]Department of Pharmaceutics, KLEU's college of Pharmacy, Nehru Nagar, Belgaum, Karnataka 590010, India
Full list of author information is available at the end of the article

disorders, arthritis, toothache, dysmenorrhea, etc., for symptomatic relief of pain and inflammation [3]. Diethylammonium salt of Diclofenac (Diclofenac Diethylamine) is reportedly used for topical applications. Diclofenac Diethylamine (DDEA) gel (1.16%; Voltaren® Emulgel®, Novartis, Nyon, Switzerland) has been used extensively in Europe since 1985 to relieve the symptoms of OA of the knee, as well as other painful, inflammatory tendon, ligament, muscle, and joint conditions [4]. However, all NSAIDs include a boxed warning highlighting the potential for increased risk of cardiovascular events as well as serious potential life-threatening gastrointestinal bleeding. The drug undergoes substantial hepatic first-pass metabolism and thus only about 50% of the administered dose reaches systemic circulation [3,5]. This originates the need of an alternative route of administration, which can bypass the hepatic first-pass metabolism. Transdermal route is an alternative choice of route of administration for such drugs. The drug, Diclofenac Diethylamine also possesses the ideal characteristics, such as poor bioavailability (40 to 60%), short biological half-life (2 to 3 h), smaller dose (25 to 50 mg), etc., to be formulated into a transdermal patch. Transdermal patches offer added advantages, such as maintenance of constant and prolonged drug level, reduced frequency of dosing, minimization of inter and intra patient variability, self-administration and easy termination of medication, leading to patient compliance [6].

It has been postulated that Diclofenac transdermal exerts its pharmacological effects through localized accumulation at the site of application rather than from the systemic absorption. The bioavailability of Diclofenac transdermal is approximately 1% that of oral Diclofenac, with an elimination half-life of 12 h compared with 1.2 to 2 h with oral Diclofenac [7].

The present study aimed at developing TDDS drug-in-adhesive patches of DDEA using Silicone adhesives, Acrylic adhesives and blend of Silicone and Acrylic adhesives.

Material and methods
Materials
The Silicone polymers (S_1 to S_6) were purchased from Dow Corning Corporation, (midland, MIA, USA), Acrylic polymer (A) was purchased from National Starch and Chemical company (Bridge Water, NJ, USA). Fluoropolymer coated polyester release liner and Polyester Backing laminate was purchased from 3 M Scotchpak (st. paul, USA). The drug Diclofenac Diethylamine B.P (DDEA) was obtained from Sparsha Pharma International Pvt Ltd (Hyd, India). Methanol and Acetonnitrile were of HPLC grade and purchased from Sigma-Aldrich corporation, India. All other reagents used were of highest reagent grade available.

Preparation of patches containing silicone adhesives
Preparation of placebo silicone patches
Transdermal patches were prepared by modified solvent evaporation method. It is similar to conventional method except, that the drug-polymeric solution was spread over the release liner with the help of manual coater over release liner. Transdermal patches using different silicone polymers (Table 1) without drug were prepared. For preparing transdermal patches, an adequate amount of polymeric solution was taken and then spread over the release liner with the help of a manual coater. The polymeric solution coated liner was dried at 80°C in an oven for 10 min. The patches were then finally laminated with polyester backing membrane. The obtained sheets were punched using suitable dyes (3, 10 and 50 cm²) to get patches of appropriate sizes, packed in aluminum foil and stored in a desiccator for further studies. Patches were prepared using different grades of silicone adhesives.

Physical evaluation of placebo patches
The tack of the patches – ball tack test
Tack is the ability of a pressure-sensitive adhesive to bond under conditions of light contact pressure and a

Table 1 Details of silicone and acrylic polymers used in the study

Code	Functional group	Solvent	Solid content (%)	Viscosity (Mpa.s)
Silicone Polymer				
S1	Amine compatible	Ethyl acetate	60	350
S2	Amine compatible	Ethyl acetate	60	800
S3	Amine compatible	Ethyl acetate	60	1200
S4	-	Ethyl acetate	60	650
S5	-	Ethyl acetate	65	2500
S6	-	Ethyl acetate	60	2600
Acrylic polymer				
A, Polyacrylate	COOH	Ethylacetae and Hexane	43.2	7000-19000

short contact time. The tack of the skin contact adhesive was measured by the rolling ball tack test using primary adhesive tester (Labthink Instruments Co. Ltd., China). The patch with a size of 50 cm^2 was fixed on a plate. Different diameter steel balls were released from the top of the inclined plate (angle 45°C). The number of the largest ball (0 – 9) which did not roll down was reported as the tack value [8].

Peel strength of patches

Peel strength measures the force required to peel away a pressure-sensitive adhesive once it has been attached to a surface. The test was performed with a Digital Peel tester with a load capacity up to 5 kg (Make: International Equipments, Model: CO). A piece of the patch which has a width of 10 mm and length of 25 mm was prepared, applied quickly to the end of the stainless steel plate and left the apparatus for 10 min.

The cello tape was affixed on the product. The free end of this tape was bending back 180° and it was attached firmly to the upper part of a peel testing machine with a clamp. The instrument was started with a speed of 300 mm/min and the values were recorded. Five patches form each batch were used measuring strength and their values were averaged [8].

Preparation of drug loaded silicone patches
Solubility of drug in adhesives

The solubility of drug in adhesive was tested in silicone adhesives (S_3 and S_6). Different concentrations of drug (5% w/w, 3% w/w, 2% w/w and 1% w/w of final patch formulation) were added to the adhesives under constant stirring with the help of magnetic stirrer. The stirring was continued for a period of 4 h in order to ensure complete mixing. The solution was kept aside overnight for visual observation. The solutions that showed turbidity were discarded and solutions that remained clear were coated over release liner and finally laminated with backing layer as described in the section 2.2.1.

Solubility enhancement techniques

Various solubility enhancements used to increase the solubility of Diclofenac Diethylamine in silicone adhesives include

Addition of solubilizers
Polyethylene glycol – 400 (PEG 400) and Propylene glycol (PG) in different concentrations (% w/w of final patch formulation) were used [9]. The adhesive polymeric solution, drug and solubilizer in required quantities were weighed and mixed with the aid of magnetic stirrer for a period of about 4–5 h. The solutions were monitored visually for appearance of turbidity/sedimentation. The formulations that showed

clear solution after 24 h were coated over release liner and laminated with polyester backing laminate. The patches were packed in aluminum foil, kept aside for 10 days for appearence of crystals visually and microscopically. The patches which did not show crystals after 10 days were selected for further study.

Addition of oils
Four oils were slected based on preliminary study to improve the solubility of Diclofenac Diethylamine [10]. The oils, Oleic acid (OLA), Iso stearic acid (ISA), Pharamasolve (PS) and Iso propyl myristate (IPM) in different ratios of drug: solubilizer were mixed with polymeric solution and then monitored visually for turbidity. The clear solutions were used for preparation of patches which were kept aside for 10 days for appearance of crystals.

Ex vivo skin permeation studies
Preparation of skin barrier

Fresh full-thickness (75–80 mm) pig ear skin was used for the study. The experiment was carried out according to the guidelines of the Committee for the Purpose of Control and Supervision of Experiments on Animals and approved by Animal Ethical Committee of Department of Genetics, Osmania University, Hyderabad, India (approval no.380/01/a/CPCSEA). Fresh pig ears were obtained from a local abattoir; to ensure integrity of the skin barrier, ears were removed post-sacrifice. The skin was dermatomed (Zimmer electric Dermatome Handset) to remove dermis [11,12]. The isolated epidermis (100 μm) was rapidly rinsed with hexane to remove surface lipids and then rinsed with water and used immediately.

The *ex vivo* skin permeation from the prepared drug polymeric patches across the porcine ear skin barrier was studied using Franz diffusion cell (Orchid Scientifics & Innovative India Pvt Ltd.), [13,14]. Twenty - five milliliters of phosphate buffer of pH 7.4 was used as an elution medium. The diameter of the donor compartment cell provided an effective constant area of 3.4 cm^2. The dermatomed pig ear skin was mounted between the two compartments of Franz diffusion cell with stratum corneum facing towards the donor compartment. A 3 cm^2 patch was used for the study. The release liner was removed. The patches to be studied were placed in between the donor and the receptor compartment in such a way that the drug releasing surface faced toward the receptor compartment. After securely clamping the donor and receptor compartments together, the elution medium was magnetically stirred for uniform drug distribution at a speed of 60 rpm. The temperature of the whole assembly was maintained at 32 ± 0.5°C by thermostatic arrangements. An aliquot of 0.5 mL was withdrawn at preset time intervals for a period of 24 h and an equivalent volume of fresh buffer was replaced. The samples removed were analysed by HPLC described below.

Preparation of patches containing acrylic adhesive

The formulations containing different concentrations of drug with acrylic adhesive were prepared by the method described under section 2.2. The patches prepared were monitered for appearance of crystals visually for 10 days. The properties of acrylic adhesive were mentioned in the Table 1. The patches which showed stability were subjected to peel test, ball test (described under 2.2) and permeation study (described in section 2.3).

Preparation of patches containing combination of silicone and arylic adhesives

Placebo patches containing combination of silicone and acrylate adhesives in different ratios and drug containing combinational patches were prepared by the following method:

In First step, required amount of drug (% w/w of final patch formulation) was made to dissolve completely in appropriate amount of acrylate adhesive by continuous stirring. Second step involves addition of silicone polymeric solution to clear solution formed in step 1 and then continuing mixing for a period of 12 h. The formulations that showed drug solubility after 24 h were laminated into patches. The patches which showed stability were subjected to peel test, ball test (described under 2.2) and permeation study (described in section 2.3).

Effect of permeation enhancers on drug loaded combinational patches

The incorporation of a permeation enhancer is indispensable for achieving the desired permeation rate for almost all drugs with the limited size of the patch. The permeation enhancers Oleic acid (OLA), Iso Stearic acid (ISA) and Isopropyl Myristate (IPM) at concentraions of 5% each were chosen to study their effect on permeation of Diclofenac Diethylamine across the skin. The solubilized combinational patches (C_4 and C_5) along with different permeation enhancers (5% concentration) were formulated and subjected for permeation study as described under 2.3.

Characterization of optimized patches

Various physicochemical tests employed for optimized transdermal patches were as shown

Thickness

Patch thickness was measured using digital micrometer screw gauge (Mitutoyo, Japan) at five different places. The average and standard deviation of five readings were calculated for each batch of the drug-loaded films.

Table 2 Draize evaluation of dermal reaction

Scoring	Reaction	
	Erythema	Edema
0	No erythema	No edema
1	Very slight erythema	Very slight edema
2	Well-defined erythema	Slight edema
3	Moderate to severe erythema	Moderate edema
4	Severe erythema	Severe edema

Weight uniformity

Five different films from individual batches were weighed individuall, and the average weight was calculated the individual weight should not deviate significantly from the weight was calculated, the individual weight should not deviate significantly from the average weight, so the standard deviation was calculated [15].

Drug content

Assay of Diclofenac Diethylamine was done with the help of HPLC. All the solvents used were of HPLC grade [16].

Sample solution

For determination of drug content one patch of 50 cm^2 was taken, dissolved in HPLC grade methanol and sonicated for 15 min. From above solution 1 mL was taken into a 50 mL volumetric flask, diluted up to the mark with methanol, filtered through Nylon membrane filters of 0.45 μ size (Pall Pharmalab Filtration Pvt. Ltd.) and injected (20 mL) into the HPLC column.

Standard solution

For preparing standard solution, 50 mg of Diclofenac Diethylamine was dissolved in 50 mL methanol (HPLC grade). From the above solution, 1 mL was taken and diluted to 50 mL with methanol which was finally filtered through a Nylon membrane filters of 0.45 μ size (Whatman GF/C) and injected (20 mL) into the HPLC column.

HPLC conditions

The HPLC system consisted of L-7110 pump (Shimadzu Corporation, Japan) with L-7420 variable-wavelength ultraviolet absorbance detector (Shimadzu Corporation, Japan) set at 274 nm. Analysis was performed on a reversed-phase column made of silica

Table 3 Adhesive mass values, ball test and peel test values for placebo silicone patches

Parameter and thickness	Polymer type				
	S_2	S_3	S_4	S_5	S_6
Ball tack test [a]	4	8	0	5	8
Peel test (Kg/cm) [b]	0.384	0.646	0.0938	0.495	0.645

(S_2, S_3, S_4, S_5 and S_6 represents different Silicone polymers used; a = 3 and b = 5).

Table 4 Solubilization summary of drug loaded silicone polymers

Formulation code	Drug concentration	Solubilizer concentration	Observation
DS_3	5%	-	Clear solution was not formed.
DS_3	3%	-	Clear solution was not formed.
DS_3	2%	-	Clear solution was not formed.
DS_3	1%	-	Clear solution indicating solubilization of drug
DS_3	0.5%	-	Clear solution indicating solubilization of drug.
DS_6	1%	-	Clear solution was not formed.
DS_3E_1	5%	5% PEG-400	Clear solution was not formed.
DS_3E_2	3%	5% PEG-400	Clear solution was not formed.
DS_3E_3	2%	3% PEG-400	Clear solution was formed.
DS_6E_4	1%	3% PEG-400	Clear solution was formed.
DS_6E_5	2%	3% PEG-400	Clear solution was not formed.
DS_3G_1	5%	5% PG	Clear solution was not formed.
DS_3G_2	2%	5% PG	Clear solution was formed.
DS_3G_3	1%	2% PG	Clear solution was formed.
DS_3O_1	3%	2% OLA	Clear solution was not formed
DS_3O_2	2%	2% OLA	Clear solution was not formed
DS_3O_3	1%	2% OLA	Clear solution was formed
DS_3I_1	4%	2% ISA	Clear solution was not formed
DS_3I_2	3%	2% ISA	Clear solution was not formed
DS_3I_3	1%	2% ISA	Clear solution was formed
DS_3M_1	1%	2% IPM	Clear solution was not formed
DS_3P_1	1%	2% Pharmasolve	Clear solution was not formed
$DS_3O_4I_4$	3%	5% OLA & 5% ISA	Clear solution was formed.

DS: drug with silicone polymer; S_3: Silicone polymer grade, S_3; S_6: Silicone polymer grade S_6; OLA: oleic acid; ISA: Iso stearic acid; IPM: Isopalmitic acid; PEG 400: Polyethylene glycol –400; PG: Propylene glycol.

(150 mm × 4.6 mm i.d., 5 μm, Chemsil BDS C18, Beijing China), operated at 40°C. The mobile phase consisted of 45: 55 ratio of 0.5% Glacial acetic acid in water and Acetonitrile. HPLC grade water was used for the preparation of 0.5% Glacial acetic acid solution. The flow rate of mobile phase was set at 0.8 mL/min, was used. The injection volume is 20 μL.

In vitro release – dissolution studies

The release-rate determination is one of the most important studies to be conducted for all controlled release delivery systems. The dissolution studies of patches are very crucial, because one needs to maintain the drug concentration on the surface of stratum corneum consistently and substantially greater than the drug concentration in the body, to achieve a constant rate of drug permeation [17].

A Paddle over disc assembly (USP 23, Apparatus 5) was used for the assessment of release of DDEA. The TDDS patch was mounted on the disc and placed at the bottom of the dissolution vessel. The dissolution medium, 900 ml degassed distilled water at pH 7.0. The apparatus was equilibrated to 32 ± 0.5°C and operated at 50 rpm [18] during the entire study period (24 h). The dissolution medium was degassed by a combination of heating up to 45°C and vacuum filtration followed by vigorous stirring of media under vacuum.

Stability study

The optimized formulations were subjected to stability study by storing patches at 40 ± 2°C and 75% RH in stability chamber for three months. Two parameters namely, peel strength and drug content were analyzed.

Surface morphology

The surface morphology of formulated transdermal patches (both stable and unstable) were investigated by using Scanning electron microscope (model: SEM JSM-6610) at 15 kV under different magnifications (950x, 1000x and 1500x). In order to make the samples electrically conductive the samples were gold coated prior to the study.

Acute skin irritancy test

The study was conducted on the basis of the approval of institutional animal ethical committee. Albino rabbits of either sex, each weighing 1.5 to 2.0 kg, divided into two groups, were used in this study (n = 4 in each group) [14]. They were housed in cages in the animal house under controlled temperature and light conditions. They were fed a standard laboratory diet and had access to water *ad libitum*. The dorsal surface of the rabbits was cleared and the hair was removed by shaving. The skin was cleared with rectified spirit. The experimental patch

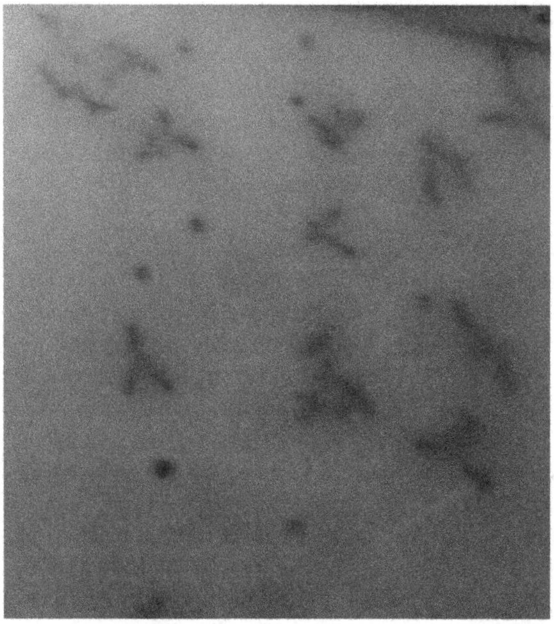

Figure 1 Photograph of Silicone patch, DS_3O_1, showing crystal formation.

(A1, group II), one patch per day, were applied to the shaved skin of rabbits and secured using USP adhesive tape (Johnson & Johnson limited, Mumbai). A 0.8% (v/v) aqueous solution of formaldehyde was applied as a standard irritant (group I). Its effect was compared with the test [19]. The animals were observed for any sign of erythema and edema for a period of 7 days and scored as reported by Draize et al. (1944) [20]. The Draize method of scoring was shown in Table 2.

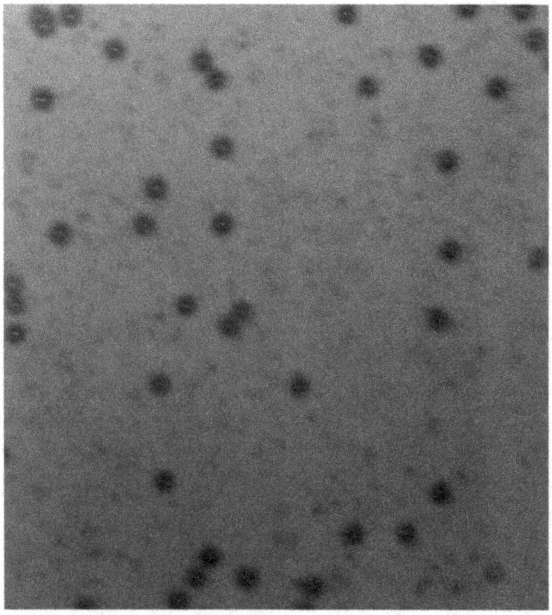

Figure 2 Photograph of Silicone patch, DS_3I_3, showing crystal formation.

Anti-inflammatory study

The study was conducted in accordance with the Ethical Guide- lines for Investigations in Laboratory Animals and was approved by the Ethics Review Committee for Animal Experimentation of Osmania University. The anti-inflammatory activity and sustaining action of the drug-loaded drug in adhesive patches were evaluated using "carrageenan-induced hind paw edema" method developed by Winter et al. (1965) [21]. Wistar rats were used after being allowed to acclimatize for 1 week. Before the day of administration, rats were fasted overnight but were allowed access to water ad libitum. Eight rats weighing 180–220 g (6–8 weeks old) divided into two groups were used for the study. The backsides of rats were shaved 12 h before starting the experiments.

Group – I (Control group): Paw edema was induced by injecting 0.1 mL of a 1% w/v homogeneous suspension of carrageenan in double-distilled water [21] The volume of injected paw was measured immediately (0 h) and at 0.5, 0.75, 1, 2, 3, 4, 5, 6, 8, 10, 12, 16 and 24 h after injection using a IMCORP plethysmometer [22]. The amount of paw swelling with respect to initial volume was determined time to time. It is obtained by subtracting volume of injected paw at time '0' from volume of injected paw at time 't' divided by volume of injected paw at time '0'.

Group – II (Test): Treated similar to control group except that patches were applied half an hour before sub-plantar injection of carrageenan. Percent (%) inhibition of edema produced by each patch- treated group was calculated against the respective control group using the following formula

$$\%\ Inhibition = \%\ edema(control) - \%\ edema(drug) / \%\ edema(control) \times 100 \tag{1}$$

Results and discussion

Evaluation of placebo silicone patches

The placebo patches using six grades of silicone polymer were prepared. The patches were smooth, flexible and uniform. The S_1 patches were ruled out because during preparation of patches after drying the polymer completely lost its adhesive property.

An ideal adhesive polymer for drug-in-adhesive system is one that exhibit greater adhesion value. The initial screening of the silicone adhesives was done by ball tack test and peel strength of patches. The peel test, ball test and adhesive mass test values of all placebo silicone

Table 5 Crystallization summary of drug loaded silicone patches with or without solubilizers

Formulation code	Drug concentration	Solubilizers concentration	Patch Observation after 10 days	Solution observation after 10 days
DS_3	0.5%	-	No sign of crystallization	Same as first day
DS_3	1%	-	No sign of crystallization	Same as first day
DS_3E_3	2%	3% PEG-400	No sign of crystallization	Oil globules were formed and the solution turned oily
DS_6E_4	1%	3% PEG-400	No sign of crystallization	Oil globules were formed and the solution turned oily
DS_3G_2	2%	5% PG	No sign of crystallization.	Oil globules were formed and the solution turned oily
DS_3G_3	1%	2% PG	No sign of crystallization.	Oil globules were formed and the solution turned oily
DS_3O_3	1%	2% OLA	Crystallization was seen.	Same as first day
DS_3I_3	1%	2% ISA	Crystallization was seen.	Same as first day
$DS_3O_4I_4$	3%	5% OLA & 5% ISA	Crystallization was seen.	Same as first day

patches of different thicknesses were as shown in Table 3. The ball test and peel test values for different formulations of thickness 200 μm were in the following order: S3 > S6 > S5 > S2 > S4. Hence, S_6 and S_3 polymers showed better peel adhesion and ball test values hence, selected for further study.

Evaluation of drug loaded silicone patches
Solubility of drug in pure silicone adhesives
The solubility of Diclofenac Diethylamine in S_3 and S_6 was tested. The solutions that remained clear after 24 h were coated over the release liner. Results were shown in (Table 4). The Polymeric adhesive S_3 only showed clear solution with 1% drug concentration. The results indicated low solubility of Diclofenac Diethylamine in Silicone adhesives and stresses on the need for the solubilizers for solubilization of drug.

Solubility enhancement techniques
Solubility of Drug in Silicone adhesives in the presence of solubilizers
Two solubilizers namely PEG - 400 and PG were tested to increase the solubility of Diclofenac Diethylamine in

Silicone adhesives. Though PEG - 400 and PG increased Diclofenac Diethylamine solubility in water [9], their role to solubilize the drug in Silicone adhesive was abortive. Table 4 shows the drug concentration and solubilizer concentration used. Except few, all the solutions showed turbidity. In case of DS_3E_3 a clear solution was formed with 2% drug and 3% PEG - 400 while, in formulations containing S_6 polymer (DS_6E_5) a clear solution was not formed with 2% drug and 3% PEG - 400. Similar to PEG - 400, PG showed slight improvement in solubility of drug in S_3 polymer.

From solubility studies, it can be concluded that compared to S_6, S_3 polymer showed solubilization of DDEA to some extent. So, S_3 polymer was chosen for further study.

Solubility of Drug in Silicone adhesives in the presence of oils
As formulations with PEG - 400 and PG showed little/no improvement in solubility, various oils namely oleic acid (OLA), IsoStearic acid (ISA), Pharmsolve® and Isopropyl Myristate (IPM) were tested for their ability to improve solubility of drug using the method described in experimental section. The formulations which remained clear after 24 h were coated over release liner. Among various oils tested, OLA and ISA were promising. However, only

Table 6 Permeation study of formulation DS_3 and DA

S. No	TIME (h)	DS_3		DA	
		CDP (μg/cm²)	% CDP	CDP (μg/cm²)	% CDP
1.	0	0	0	0	0
2.	2	1.185	1.405138	5.934	0.84051
3.	4	2.6843	3.182964	12.847	1.819688
4.	6	4.2813	5.07664	19.131	2.709773
5.	8	5.9842	7.095889	25.819	3.657082
6.	10	7.7583	9.199565	31.824	4.507649
7.	12	9.3142	11.04451	38.119	5.399292
8.	14	11.042	13.09328	45.248	6.409065
9.	24	19.573	23.20909	75.692	10.72125

CDP: Cumulative drug permeated; % CDP: percent cumulative drug permeated; DA: drug with Acrylic polymer alone.

Table 7 Solubilization summary, peel test, ball test and adhesive mass value for acrylic adhesive patches

Polymer	Drug concentration	Observation
A	10%	Clear solution formed
A	15%	Clear solution formed
A	20%	Clear solution formed
A	25%	Clear solution was not formed
Parameter evaluated		**DA**
Peel test (Kg/cm)		0.9306
Ball test		8

(n is equal to 5 and 3 for Peel test and Ball test respectively).

Table 8 Solubility of drug in combinational patches

Formulation code	Ratio of Silicone: Acrylic	Targeted drug concentration	Solubility observation
C_1	10:90	10%	YES
C_2	20:80	10%	YES
C_3	30:70	10%	YES
C_4	40:60	10%	YES
C_5	50:50	10%	YES
C_6	60:40	10%	NO
C_7	70:30	10%	NO
C_8	80:20	10%	NO
C_9	90:10	10%	NO

C: combination patches with Acrylic and Silicone adhesives.

1% drug was solubilized in both the cases (DS_3O_3 and DS_3I_3) While, IPM and Pharmsolve® did not even solubilize 1% drug. Combination of solubilizers was also tested but, only 3% drug solubilization was achieved in S_3 polymeric adhesive at 10% solubilizer concentration (OLA and ISA, 5% each).

The prepared patches (DS_3 with 1% drug, DS_3E_3, DS_6E_4, DS_3G_2, DS_3G_3, DS_3O_3, DS_3I_3 and $DS_3O_4I_4$) were uniform. However, after 10 days patches with additives OLA and ISA (DS_3O_3, DS_3I_3 and $DS_3O_4I_4$) ended up with formation of crystal growth. Figure 1 and Figure 2 shows crystallization in patches DS_3O_3 and DS_3I_3, respectively.

In case of formulations containing PEG - 400 and PG as additives, though the patches showed no crystallization, the solutions after 10 days took oil like consistency due to formation of oil globules in the solution resulting in loss of adhesion (Table 5).

The patches which did not contain any additives remained clear even after 10 days hence considered stable. Among various formulations prepared, DS_3 containing 1% drug was chosen for further study.

Ex vivo skin permeation study

The DS_3 patch containing 1% drug was chosen for conducting permeation study. The cumulative amount of drug permeated (CPD) at the end of 24 h was found to be 19.573 mcg/cm^2 (Table 6). Though the amount of drug permeated was low, the percentage cumulative amount of drug permeated was 23.209%. The low CPD value might be due to less amount of drug (1%) in the patch.

Evaluation of drug loaded acrylic patches

The extensive solubilization study conducted revealed that the silicone polymer is unsuitable for achieving very high concentrations of DDEA. Hence, solubility of drug in acrylic adhesive was tested by method described under experimental section I of IIIA. It was noticed that drug concentrations up to 20% was solubilized without use of any additives. The prepared patches were also stable after 10 days and did not showed crystal formation. While 25% of drug polymeric solution resulted in turbidity (Table 7). This might be because of drug loading greater than the saturation solubility of the drug in the adhesive used. However, the concentration of drug was fixed at 10% for further study since the formulation being studied is intended for topical use. The Ball test and peel strength values for DA were shown in Table 7.

Ex vivo skin permeation study

Skin permeation of Diclofenac Diethylamine was studied using DA patch containing 10% drug. Study was conducted for 24 h without using permeation enhancer. The cumulative amount of drug permeated into the receptor compartment was 75.692 mcg/cm^2 after 24 h (Table 6) that represents 10.72% of the total drug placed in the donor compartment.

Though the CDP of DA was significantly greater than CDP of DS_3 the percent drug permeated was high in case of DS_3 (23.209%). The CDP of DA was found to be

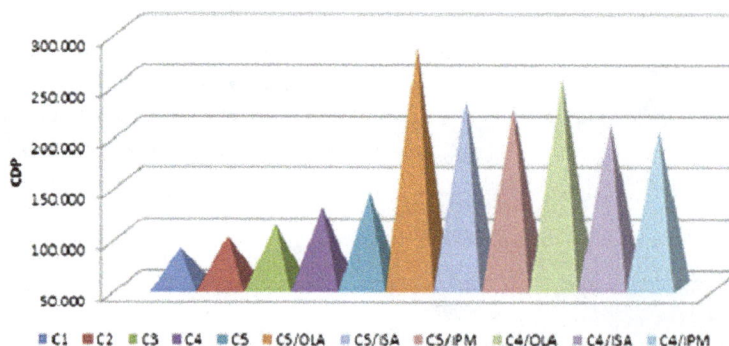

Figure 3 Graph showing cumulative amount of drug permeated (CDP) at the end of 24 h with and without permeation enhancers for combinational patches (C_4/OLA, C_4/ISA and C_4/IPM reprsents C_4 patch with oleic acid (OLA), Isostearic acid and Isopalmitic Myristate as permeation enhancers, respectively. Similar in case of C_5 combinational patches).

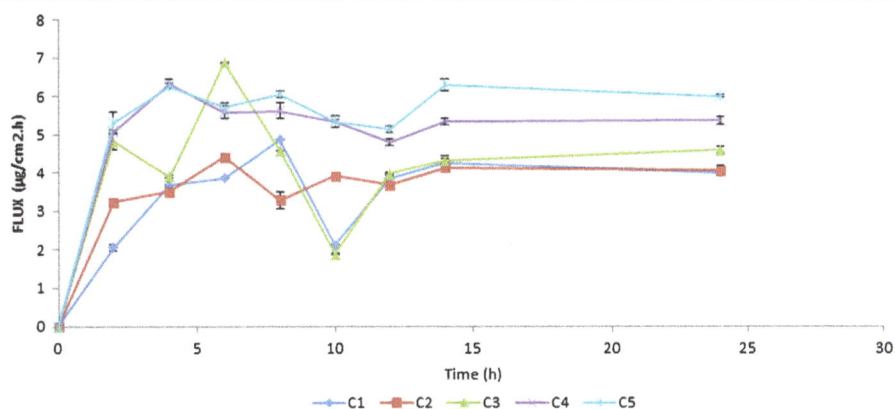

Figure 4 Graph showing the plot between Flux ($\mu g/cm^2.h$) and time (h) for C_1, C_2, C_3, C_4 and C_5 patches (data represented as mean ± S.D).

significantly high because the drug concentration in DA was 10 times greater than that of DS_3.

Evaluation of drug loaded combinational patches

Studies on Silicone adhesives revealed poor solubilization capacity and high percent cumulative drug permeation (%CDP) value whereas; acrylic polymers solubilized higher concentrations of drug but exhibited less%CDP. Hence an attempt was made to combine high%CDP property of Silicone and greater drug solubilization property of acrylic polymer by fabricating a drug formulation with combination of adhesives.

The placebo solutions containing different proportions of Silicone and Acrylic adhesives were prepared and used as reference for checking the solubility of drug in combination of adhesives. The combinations from C_1 to C_5 showed similar consistency as compared to respective

placebo patches after addition of drug. Table 8 shows the Solubility data of different combinations of Silicone and acrylic with 10% drug. The results indicated that minimum 50% acrylic polymer is required in the formulation to achieve 10% drug solubility (As acrylic polymer alone can solubilize 20% drug without any solubilizer as mentioned earlier, it is evident that 50% acrylic polymer is sufficient to solubilize 10% drug). Hence, formulations C_1, C_2, C_3, C_4 and C_5 were used for further study.

Ex vivo skin permeation experiment

In all the combinational patches, the CDP of combinational patches was higher than that DA patches which contains Acrylic polymer alone. Figure 3 shows the amount of drug permeated at the end of 24 h with and without combinational patches. The CDP of different combinational patches were in the following order:

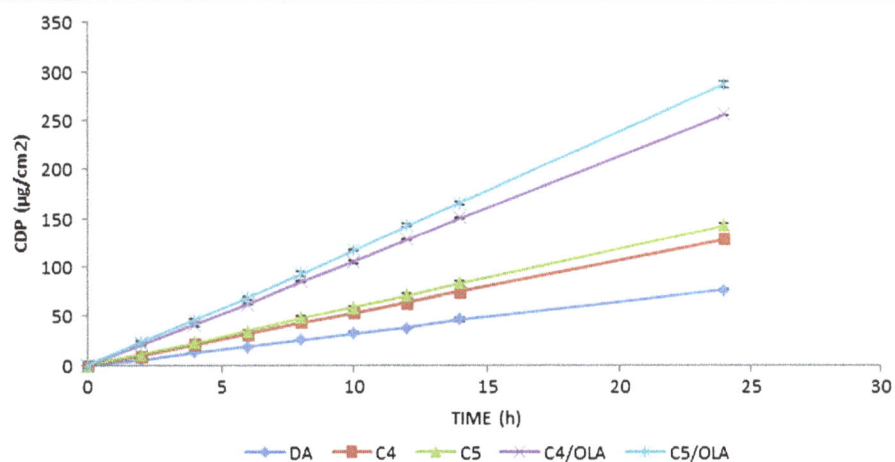

Figure 5 Graph showing the plot between cumulative amount of drug permeated (CDP, $\mu g/cm^2$) and time (h) for DA, C_4, C_5, C_5/OLA and C_4/OLA (data represented as mean ± S.D).

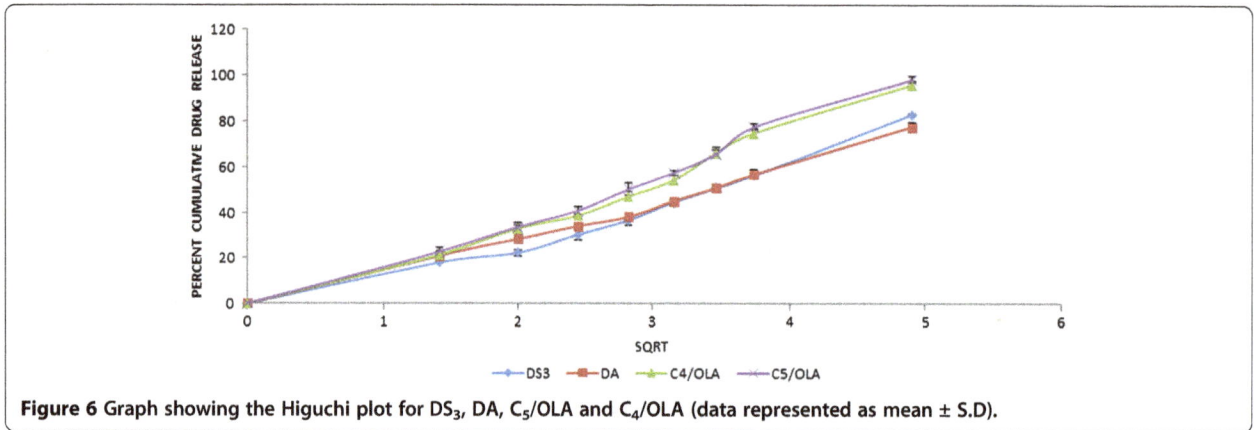

Figure 6 Graph showing the Higuchi plot for DS_3, DA, C_5/OLA and C_4/OLA (data represented as mean ± S.D).

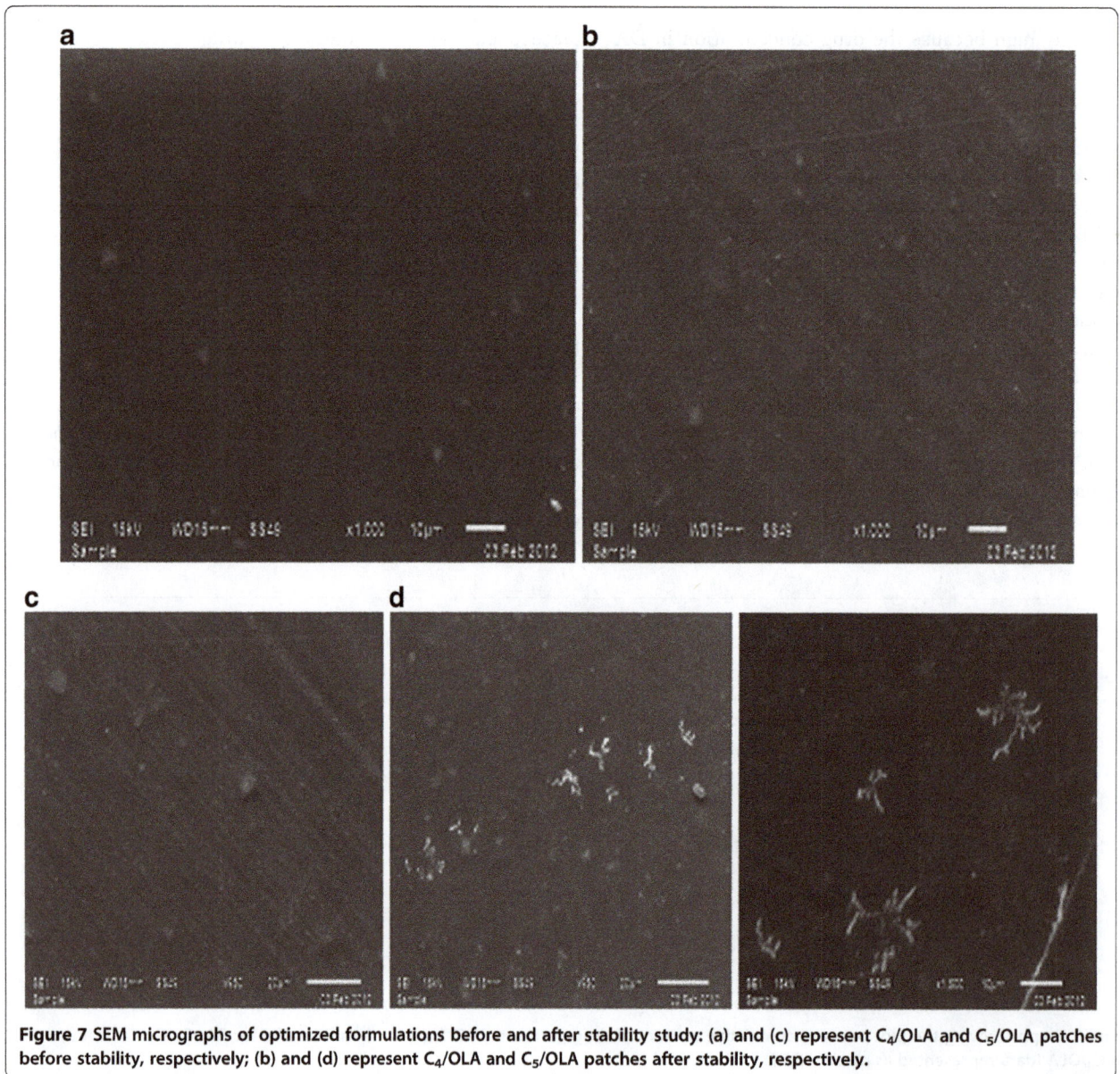

Figure 7 SEM micrographs of optimized formulations before and after stability study: (a) and (c) represent C_4/OLA and C_5/OLA patches before stability, respectively; (b) and (d) represent C_4/OLA and C_5/OLA patches after stability, respectively.

Table 9 Stability data for formulation C_4/OLA and C_5/OLA

Tested parameters	0 days	45 days	90 days
C_4/OLA			
Peel Strength (Kg/cm)	0.663	0.646	0.659
Drug content (%)	104.6	103.6	104.1
C_5/OLA			
Peel Strength (Kg/cm)	0.654	0.649	0.652
Drug content (%)	101.64	98.86	94.38

(C_4/OLA: C_4 combination patch with oleic acid, OLA, as permeation enhancer; C_5/OLA: C_5 combination patch with oleic acid, OLA, as permeation enhancer; n=3 for Drug content and n=5 for Peel strength).

$$C_5 > C_4 > C_3 > C_2 > C_1.$$

The above order once again reflected the previous results i.e. with increase in amount of Silicone polymer the amount of CDP increased. Among all five formulations C_5 displayed high CDP value due to its high Silicone content (50% of the total polymer).

Figure 4 shows plot between flux and time for all the five combinations. The graph showed little/less variation in the flux between different time intervals for C_4 and C_5. Moreover, the CDP was found to be relatively high for these two formulations. Hence, the formulations C_4 and C_5 were chosen for further study.

Effect of permeation enhancers on the permeation of DDEA

Three permeation enhancers namely, OLA, ISA and IPM were used at 5% concentration. The cumulative amount of drug permeated at the end of 24 h was represented in Figure 3. The permeation data revealed greater penetration enhancing capability of OLA than ISA and IPM. This is in line with the result reported where OLA increased the permeation of DDEA by 7–9 folds (Hussain Shah et al. 2012) [10]. Thus, it can be concluded that vehicles used here were predominantly influencing the partition of the drug into the skin. Hence, C_4/OLA and C_5/OLA which exhibited greater CDP among all were chosen as optimized formulations.

Figure 5 shows the plot between CDP and time for different formulations. From the graph, it can be predicted

Figure 8 Photograph of the patches C_4/OLA after stability.

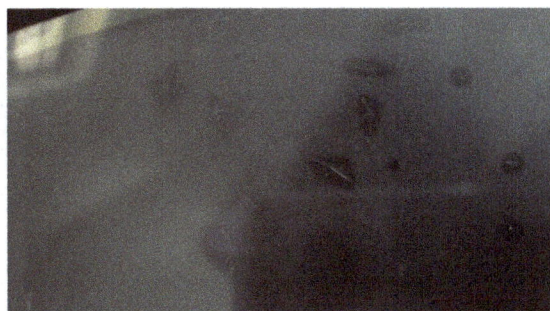

Figure 9 Photograph of the patches C_5/OLA after stability.

that C_4 and C_5 showed high CDP compared to DA indicating more drug permeation capacity compared to individual Acrylic formulations. OLA application as a permeation enhancer was well justified as significant increase in CDP value was observed compared to patches without enhancers.

Dissolution study of patches

In vitro release profile is an important tool that predicts in advance how the drug will behave in vivo. Thus, we can eliminate the risk of hazards during experimentation in living system. Five patches, DS_3, DA, C_4/OLA and C_5/OLA were studied for drug release. The study was conducted for a period of 24 h. The percent drug release (Figure 6) was found to be in the following order:

$$C_5/OLA > C_4/OLA > DS_3 > DA$$

The dissolution values revealed that formulations containing OLA exhibited greater percent cumulative drug release (%CDR) than DS_3 and DA. This might be due to increased solubility of poorly soluble drug, DDEA, in water due to OLA. Among C_5/OLA and C_4/OLA the formulation containing greater portion of silicone polymer, C_5/OLA, showed greater%CDR.

Release kinetics

The dissolution data of C_4/OLA and C_5/OLA was put forth for release kinetic studies. Based on high R^2 value it was shown that drug release from the formulations followed Higuchi pattern of drug release, with R^2 value 0.978 for C_4/OLA and 0.981 for C_5/OLA, (Figure 6) where drug diffusion through the polymeric system was the main mechanism. The 'n' value from the korsemeyer-peppas plot revealed non-fickian/anomalous diffusion pattern (n>0.5).

Stability study

The formulations C_5/OLA and C_4/OLA were kept for 3 month stability study. During stability study in case of

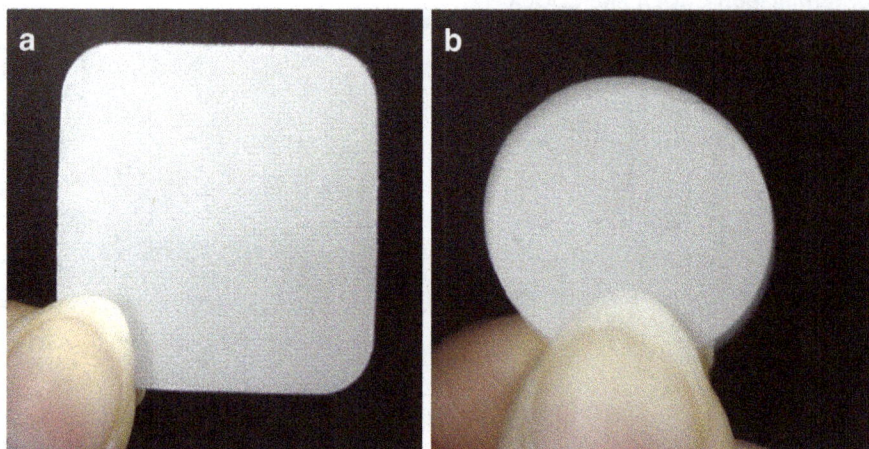

Figure 10 Photograph of optimized C_4/OLA patches both 10 cm² (a) and 3 cm² (b) patches.

C_5/OLA, crystallization (Figure 7) was observed which might be due to saturation of drug solubility which resulted in slow precipitation of drug. This is also reflected in its drug content shown in Table 9 where the percent drug content of the formulation kept on decreasing. Such a saturated matrix is unstable and the drug will recrystallize in such systems over time [23-25]. Recrystallization may however not be apparent immediately after manufacture because of the relatively low diffusion coefficients of drug in such highly viscous systems and the requirement of nucleation for the initiation of crystallization. Figure 8 shows the photograph of the C_4/OLA after stability with no crystals and Figure 9 shows photograph of the C_5/OLA after stability with crystal formation.

The peel test of both the formulations showed no significant change during stability study indicating the sustainability of adhesive property of the polymeric combination.

However, in case of C_4/OLA crystallization was not found and moreover the drug content remained stable representing robustness of the formulation during 3 month stability. Hence, the formulation C_4/OLA was found to be the optimized formulation.

Physical evaluation of optimized patches

Figure 10(a) and 10(b) shows the original patch C_4/OLA of sizes 10 cm² and 3 cm², respectively. The optimized formulation C_4/OLA was tested for various physical parameters. The thickness (n = 5) of C_4/OLA patches was found to be 181.63 ± 0.03 μm. Good weight uniformity among the batches was observed for all formulations and ranged from 214.33 – 216.35 mg. The results indicate that the process which was employed to prepare patches in this study was capable to produce patches with uniform drug content and minimal patch variability.

Acute skin irritancy study

The 7 day skin irritancy study revealed that the test formulation showed a skin irritation score (erythema and edema) of less than 1 (Table 10 & Figure 11). From the Draize method of scoring, the control animals showed severe erythema and moderate to slight edema whereas the test animals showed only very slight erythema and no edema on the site of application. According to Draize et al. (1944) [20] compounds producing scores of 2 or less are considered non-irritant [14]. Hence from the study, we can conclude that formulations are non-irritable to skin and safer for therapeutic use.

In vivo anti-inflammatory studies

The result of carrageenan induced paw edema test was shown in the Table 11. The table shows the data for the percent increase in edema with respect to initial volume and percentage inhibition of edema with respect to control during 24 h study for the test formulation. As shown in the table in case of control group animals, the mean percent increase in edema with respect to initial volume (Group –I) was 114.3 ± 15.0 at the end of 24 h which is because of swelling nature of carrageenan. While in case of test group animals the value is 0.37 ± 0.54 at the end of 24 h indicating that test patches, C_4/OLA, are

Table 10 Acute skin irritancy data for C_5/OLA (n = 4)

Day	Parameter	Standard				Test			
		1	2	3	4	1	2	3	4
Day 0	Erythema	0	0	0	0	0	0	0	0
	Edema	0	0	0	0	0	0	0	0
Day 7	Erythema	4	4	3	4	0	1	1	1
	Edema	3	2	2	3	0	0	0	0

(C_4/OLA: C_4 combination patch with oleic acid, OLA, as permeation enhancer).

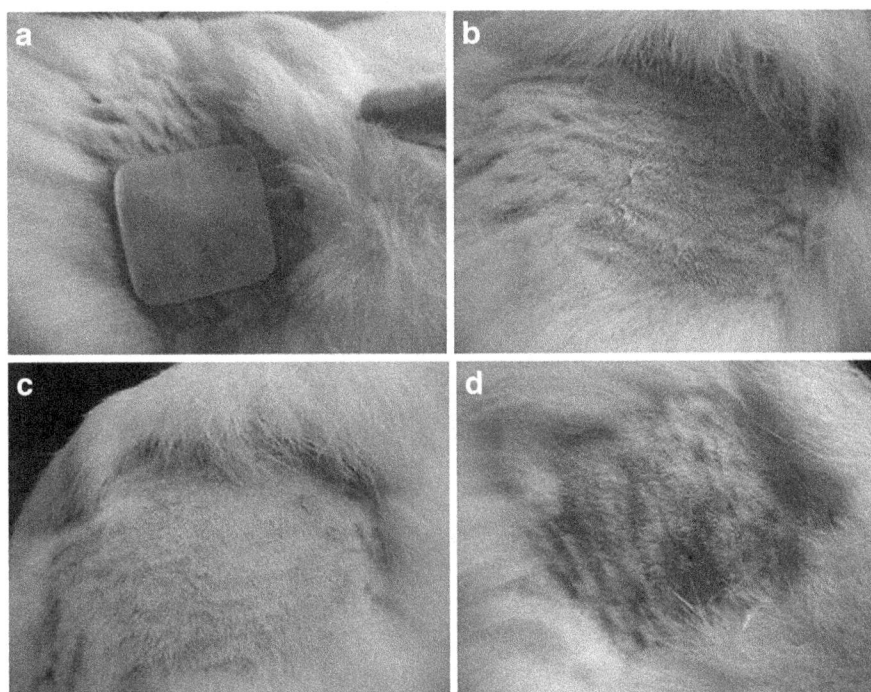

Figure 11 Images of skin irritancy study: (a) patch application to shaved area; (b) skin of rabbit at 0 day; (c) skin of test group rabbit after 7 days of patch application; (d) skin of standard group rabbit after 7 days.

effective in inhibiting carrageenan induced inflammation. Moreover, the test group animals showed 99.68% inhibition of edema with respect to control after 24 h indicating the efficacy of the formulation during the period. The initial percent increase in edema with respect to initial volume in case of test group half an hour after the carrageenan induction was 0.4 ± 0.54 as opposed to Control group (3.57 ±1.08) indicating that the test patch, C_4/OLA showed action from the first hour without any appreciable lag time. Throughout the study the percent increase in edema value with respect to initial volume for test group remained well below than the control group indicating the sustaining effect of the drug against carrageenan challenge.

Conclusion

The extensive solubilization study conducted on Silicone adhesive polymers revealed their unsuitability in fabrication of DDEA transdermal patches alone as not more than 1% drug was solubilized even with high concentration of solubilizer. On the other hand, Acrylic polymer showed high drug loading and greater control releasing capacity hence, alone can be used for fabricating transdermal patches of DDEA. However, use of Acrylic alone requires greater amount of drug incorporation due to its low value of percent cumulative drug permitted (10.72%). Hence, the combinations of adhesives were tested with the objective combining the greater permeation capacity of Silicone polymer and greater drug loading capacity of

Table 11 Paw edema data obtained on carrageenan induced rats half an hour after the patch application (data represented as mean ± S.D, n = 4)

	Time (h)													
	0.5	0.75	1	2	3	4	5	6	7	8	10	12	16	24
	% Edema with respect to initial volume													
Control	3.57 ±1.08	14.28 ± 2.05	35.71 ± 7.06	42.8 ±9.64	50.0 ± 12.95	60.7 ± 20.82	71.5 ± 19.72	83.0 ± 21.85	92.8 ± 11.05	100.0 ± 15.1	111.1 ± 18.6	121.4 ± 11.76	121.4 ±15.9	114.3 ± 15.0
Test (C_4/OLA)	0.4 ± 0.54	5.6 ± 2.91	11.3 ± 5.83	18.5 ± 0.97	39.4 ± 4.16	54.1 ± 0.31	62.6 ± 1.44	52.7 ± 9.29	42.6 ± 0.39	36.2 ± 4.39	21.2 ± 2.68	15.6 ± 0.82	2.5 ± 2.49	0.37 ± 0.54
	% inhibition of Edema with respect to control													
Test (C_4/OLA)	88.80	60.78	68.36	56.78	21.20	10.87	12.45	36.51	54.09	63.80	80.92	87.15	97.94	99.68

(C_4/OLA: C_4 combination patch with oleic acid, OLA, as permeation enhancer).

Acrylic polymer. The combinational patches incorporating the both the desired properties were successfully prepared. Among various permeation enhancers tested OLA proved to be a good permeation enhancer as compared to ISA and IPM for DDEA. C_4/OLA was found to be optimized formulation displaying robustness in stability. The skin irritancy study revealed the non-irritant nature of the C_4/OLA patches and sustaining action of the patches were confirmed by anti-inflammatory test by carrageenan induced paw edema model. Thus, it can be concluded that an ideal of combination of adhesives would serve as the best choice, for fabrication of DDEA patches, for sustained effect of DDEA with better enhancement in permeation characteristics and robustness.

Competing interests

The manuscript has no conflict of interest and there are no financial sources for many organizations and the work is purely part of student thesis work.

Authors' contributions

The author DPM helped in conceptual design of entire work, the author SP was responsible for the entire practical work, TP contributed to the interpretation of data obtained at various steps, the author BD helped in carrying out the studies involving animals and AKA helped in the calculation part and in preparation and follow up of the manuscript. All authors read and approved the final manuscript.

Acknowledgement

The authors are grateful to Sparsha Pharma International Pvt. Ltd., Hyderabad, India for extending their timely help and full co-operation for carrying out the entire research work under their guidance.

Author details

[1]Department of Pharmaceutics, KLEU's college of Pharmacy, Nehru Nagar, Belgaum, Karnataka 590010, India. [2]Research Scientist, R&D divison, Sparsha Pharma International Pvt. Ltd., Hyderabad, India.

References

1. Debjit B, Chiranjib, Chandira M, Jayakar B, Sampath KP: **Recent advances in transdermal drug delivery system.** *Int. J Pharm Tech Res* 2010, **2**(1):68–77.
2. Jain P, Banga AK: **Inhibition of crystallization in drug-in-adheisve-type transdermal therapeutic patches.** *Int J Pharm* 2010, **394**:68–74.
3. John VA: **The pharmacokinetics and metabolism of diclofenac sodium (Voltarol™) in animals and man.** *Rheumatol Rehabil* 1979, **Suppl 2**:22–37.
4. Fritz UN, Morris SG, Gail SS, Jiun-min L, Markus U, Helmut HA, Francois E: **Efficacy of topical diclofenac diethylamine gel in osteoarthritis of the knee.** *J Rheumatol* 2005, **32**:2384–2392.
5. Keith AD: **Polymer matrix consideration for transdermal devices.** *Drug Dev Ind Pharm* 1983, **9**:605–621.
6. Nauman Rahim K, Gul Majid K, Abdur Rahim K, Abdul W, Muhammad Junaid A, Muhammad A, Abid H: **Formulation, physical,** *in vitro* **and** *ex vivo* **evaluation ofdiclofenac diethylamine matrix patches containing turpentine oil as penetration enhancer.** *Afr J Pharm Pharmaco* 2012, **6**(6):434–439.
7. Haroutinaian S, Drennan DA, Lipman AG: **Topical NSAID therapy for musculoskeletal pain.** *Pain Med* 2010, **11**(4):535–549.
8. Changshun R, Liang F, Lei L, Qiang W, Sihai L, LiGang Z, Zhonggui H: **Design and evaluation of Indipamide transdermal patch.** *Int J Pharm* 2009, **370**(1–2):129–135.
9. Khalil E, Najjar S, Sallam A: **Aqueous solubility of diclofenac diethylamine in the presence of pharmaceutical additives: a comparative study with diclofenac sodium.** *Drug Dev Ind Pharm* 2000, **26**(4):375–381.
10. Hussain Shah SN, Salman M, Ahmad M, Rabbani M, Badshah A: **Effect of oleic acid on the permeation kinetics of Diclofenac Diethylamine.** *J Chem Soc Pak* 2012, **34**(1):1–8.
11. Atrux-Tallau N, Pirot F, Falson F, Roberts MS, Maibach HI: **Qualitative and quantitative comparison of heat separated epidermis and dermatomed skin in percutaneous absorption studies.** *Arch Dermatol Res* 2007, **299**(10):507–511.
12. Kaidi Z, Singh J: *In vitro* **percutaneous absorption enhancement of propranolol hydrochloride through porcine epidermis by terpenes/ethanol.** *J Control Rel* 1999, **62**(3):359–366.
13. Bonferoni M, Rossi S, Ferrari F, caramella C: **A modified Franz diffusion cell for simultaneous assessment of drug release and washability of mucoadhesive gels.** *Pharm Dev Technol* 1999, **4**(1):45–53.
14. Mamatha T, venkateswara rao J, Mukkanti K, Ramesh G: **Development of matrix type transdermal patches of lercanidipine hydrochloride: physicochemical and in-vitro characterization.** *DARU* 2010, **18**(1):9–16.
15. Verma PR, Iyer SS: **Transdermal delivery of propranolol using mixed grades of Eudragit: design and in-vitro and in-vivo evaluation.** *Drug Dev Ind Pharm* 2000, **26**(4):471–476.
16. Vijaya Bhanu P, Shanmugam V, Lakshmi PK: **Development and evaluation of Diclofenac Emulgel for topical drug delivery.** *Pharmacie Globale IJCP* 2011, **9**(10):1–4.
17. Sood A, Panchagnula R: **Role of dissolution studies in controlled release drug delivery system.** *STP Pharma Sci* 1999, **9**:157–168.
18. Mohamed A, Yamin S, Asgar A: **Matrix type transdermal drug delivery systems of metoprolol tartrate: in vitro characterization.** *Acta Pharm* 2003, **53**(2):119–125.
19. Shinde AJ, Shinde AL, More HN: **Design and evaluation transdermal drug delivery system of gliclazide.** *Asian J Pharm* 2010, **4**(2):121–129.
20. Draize JH, Woodword G, Calvery HO: **Methods for the study of irritation and toxicity of substances applied topically to the skin and mucous membranes.** *J Pharmacol Exp Ther* 1944, **8**:377–379.
21. Winter CA: **Antiinflammatory testing methods: Comparative evaluation of indomethacin and other agents.** In *Nonsteroidal antiinflammatory drugs.* Edited by Garattini S, Dukes MNG. Amsterdam: Excerpta Medica Foundation; 1965:190–202. series no. 82.
22. Priyanka A, Biswajit M: **Design, development, physicochemical, and in vitro and** *In Vivo* **evaluation of transdermal patches containing diclofenac diethylammonium salt.** *J Pharm Sci* 2002, **91**(9):2076–2089.
23. Hadgraft J: **Passive enhancement strategies in topical and transdermal drug delivery.** *Int J Pharm* 1999, **184**(1):1–6.
24. Latsch S, Selzer T, Fink L, Kreuter J: **Determination of the physical state of norethindrone acetate containing transdermal drug delivery systems by isothermal microcalorimetry, X-ray diffraction, and optical microscopy.** *Eur J Pharm Biopharm* 2004, **57**(2):383–395.
25. Cilurzo F, Minghetti P, Casiraghi A, Tosi L, Pagani S, Montanari L: **Polymethacrylates as crystallization inhibitors in monolayer transdermal patches containing ibuprofen.** *Eur J Pharm Biopharm* 2005, **60**(1):61–66.

20

Metformin loaded non-ionic surfactant vesicles: optimization of formulation, effect of process variables and characterization

Anchal Sankhyan and Pravin K Pawar[*]

Abstract

Background: Metformin an oral hypoglycemic has been widely used as a fist line of treatment of Type II Diabetes but in a very high dose 2–3 times a day and moreover suffers from a number of side effects like lactic acidosis, gastric discomfort, chest pain, allergic reactions being some of them. The present work was conducted with the aim of sustaining the release of metformin so as to decrease its side effects and also reduce its dosing frequency using a novel delivery system niosomes (non-ionic surfactant vesicles). Non-ionic surfactant vesicles of different surfactants were prepared using thin film hydration technique and were investigated for morphology, entrapment, in-vitro release, TEM (transmission electron microscopy) and physical stability. Optimized formulation was further studied for the effect of Surfactant concentration, DCP (Dicetyl phosphate), Surfactant: cholesterol ratio and volume of hydration. The release studies data was subjected to release kinetics models.

Results: The prepared vesicles were uniform and spherical in size. Optimized formulation MN3 entrapped the drug with 84.50±0.184 efficiency in the vesicles of the size 487.60±2.646 and showed the most sustained release of 73.89±0.126. Also it was resulted that 100 molar concentration of cholesterol and surfactant, Presence of DCP, equimolar ratio of span 60: cholesterol and 15 ml of volume of hydration were found to be optimum for miosome preparation.

Conclusions: The present work concluded metformin loaded niosomes to be effective in sustaining the drug release leading to decreased side effects and increased patient compliance.

Keywords: Anti-diabetic, Niosomes, Metformin, Dicetyl phosphate, Sustained release

Background

With the advent of therapeutics, oral delivery is the most widely used and the most convenient route of drug delivery. Despite of phenomenal advances in other dosage routes viz. injectable, inhalable, transdermal, nasal, oral delivery still remain well ahead of the pack as the preferred delivery route. Higher concentration is focused in making the oral formulations viable if it is not immediately viable, than in plumping for an alternative delivery method. The top 50 drugs selling in the world have 84% oral delivery [1]. Variety of approaches have been tried to enhance the oral bioavailability of poorly soluble drugs using the excipients with approved or GRAS (generally regarded as safe) status. Micronization by spray-drying, freeze-drying, crystallization and milling; nanosizing into nanoparticles by various techniques with high-pressure homogenization being one of most efficient; crystal engineering of polymorphs, hydrates, solvates, co-crystals, supercritical fluid and sonocrystallization; solid dispersions developed by melt-mixing, solvent evaporation, supercritical fluid and melt extrusion; solubilizing ability of cyclodextrins; solid lipid nanoparticles prepared by high-pressure homogenization and microemulsion technology and other colloidal drug delivery systems including emulsions, microemulsions, self-emulsified and self-microemulsified drug delivery systems, liposomes etc. have been widely researched for enhancement of oral bioavailability [2]. Other attempts of enhancing oral bioavailability include Solid lipid nanoparticles, mucoadhesive delivery system, lipid digestion models, Supersaturatable Formulations, nanoemulsion, nanocapsules, fast-dispersing dosage forms and pH-sensitive supramolecular assemblies [3-10].

* Correspondence: pkpawar80@yahoo.com
Chitkara College of Pharmacy, Chitkara University, Chandigarh-Patiala Highway, Rajpura, Patiala, Punjab 140401, India

Diabetes is a group of chronic carbohydrate metabolism disorders resulting from diminished or absent action of insulin by altered secretion, decreased insulin efficacy or combination of both the factors leading to hyperglycemia. Type II diabetes is the most common type counting about 90-95% of the diagnosed cases, characterized with normal or even excess of insulin levels with insulin resistance being the major cause of increased glucose levels [11]. Metformin a biguanide enhances insulin sensitivity, found to be effective in impaired glucose tolerance, obese patients and patients with cardiovascular diseases and is used as first line of drug in treatment of Type II diabetes [12].

The oral bioavailability of Metformin is 50-60% as it is BCS (Biopharmaceutical Classification System) class III drug and has site-specific absorption in the GI tract [13]. The drug has negligible plasma protein binding, relatively short half life of 1.5-4.5 hours and requires administration of 500 mg dose two or three times a day [14]. Moreover the drug suffers from serious but rare side effects of lactic acidosis with 50% mortality, chest pain, allergic reactions accompanied by high incidences of concomitant gastrointestinal symptoms such as diarrhea, abdominal discomfort, vomiting, stomachache, headache and lethargy [15]. Researchers endeavored for years to enhance the oral bioavailability, sustain the drug release for better patient compliance and reduced side effects of the most widely used oral hypoglycemic Metformin. The conventional dosage form of Metformin i.e. tablet has been modified by various approaches to get the desired results. Matrix tablets with sustained release have been prepared using hydroxypropyl methyl cellulose as a hydrophilic polymer, hydrophilic synthetic polymers and hydrophobic natural polymers and by incorporation of lipophillic waxes by melt granulation [14,16]. With the view to enhance patient compliance taste masked tablets and oro-dispersible tablets have also been formulated, also the FDA (Food and Drug Administration) has approved metformin-glipizide tablets for oral suspension, metformin-glyburide oral solution and linagliptin-metformin hydrochloride tablets [17-19]. Niosomes are non ionic surfactant vesicles having lamellar structure formed by self assembly of surfactant molecules. To improve the oral bioavailability of poorly water soluble drug like griseofulvin, the noisome (vesicular) system was developed [20]. In another report, the polysaccharide coated noisomes of propranolol HCl was developed for the oral drug delivery and studied the effect of polysaccharide cap using hydrophobic anchors on the non ionic surfactant vesicles [21]. The only novel delivery system so far utilized for the delivery of metformin is mucoadhesive ispaghula-sodium alginate beads [22]. Niosomes have been used to deliver a number of drugs and have shown pronounced benefits of enhanced

bioavailability, sustained release, targeted delivery, decreased side effects, high stability, easy modification, and so on [23]. In the present investigation niosomes have been prepared to enhance oral bioavailability of class III antidiabetic drug. The nonionic surfactant vesicles have been prepared and evaluated for entrapment efficiency, in vitro drug release, particle size, zeta potential, TEM. Also the effect of various parameters viz. molar concentration and molar ratio of cholesterol and surfactant, presence of DCP and volume of hydration was studied on the various evaluated parameters. The studied system is developed for efficient treatment of Type II diabetes.

Methods

Metformin was a kind gift sample from Matrix Laboratories (Hyderabad, India). Cholesterol was supplied by Fisher Scientific (Mumbai, India). The non-ionic surfactants viz. Span 20, Span 40, Span 60, Span 80, Tween 20, Tween 80 and Brij 30 were purchased from Loba Chemie Pvt. Ltd. (Mumbai, India). Tween 60 was procured from Sisco Research Laboratories Pvt. Ltd. (Mumbai, India) and HPLC chloroform was provided by Merck Specialities Pvt. Ltd. (Mumbai, India). All the ingredients used in the procedures were of analytical grade.

Preparation of niosomes

The nano sized vesicles were prepared using Thin Film Hydration Method. The specified quantities of cholesterol, non-ionic surfactant and Dicetyl Phosphate (DCP) were completely dissolved in 10 ml HPLC chloroform contained in a clean and dry Round Bottom Flask (Table 1). The transparent solution was reduced to a thin dry film using Rotary Vaccum Evaporator (Perfit, India) at 50.00±2.00°C. Metformin was dissolved in phosphate buffer pH 6.8 and the thin dry film was hydrated using this buffered drug solution. The film is allowed to hydrate for about 1 hour for the formation of niosomes [22]. Milky dispersion is prepared which is kept at 4°C for 24 hours for maturation of the formed vesicles.

Entrapment efficiency

The entrapment efficiency of the matured niosomes was determined using centrifugation method. The measured volume 5 ml of the prepared dispersion was centrifuged using cooling centrifuge (RIS-24BL, REMI India) at 6°C for 1 hour to separate the free drug from niosomes. The niosomes formed a cake floating at the top of tube and clear solvent containing the unentrapped drug remained at the bottom. The cake was resuspended in 5 ml phosphate buffer pH 6.8 and the process was repeated twice by centrifugation for 30 minutes to ensure complete removal of free drug. After suitable dilution with

Table 1 Composition (molar ratio), entrapment efficiency and particle size of metformin niosomes

Formulation code	Cholesterol	Surfactant	Dicetyl phosphate (mg)	Entrapment* efficiency (%)	Particle size* (nm)
MN1	250	Span 60 (250)	5	85.16±0.12	574.33±2.08
MN2	250	Span 60 (250)	-	87.12±0.05	636.00±2.65
MN3	100	Span 60 (100)	5	84.50±0.18	487.60±2.65
MN4	100	Span 60 (100)	-	86.51±0.15	504.66±2.52
MN5	75	Span 60 (75)	5	83.66±0.08	388.0±3.61
MN6	75	Span 60 (75)	-	84.71±0.05	496.66±3.51
MN7	250	Span 40 (250)	5	83.91±0.01	565.33±2.52
MN8	250	Span 40 (250)	-	85.07±0.08	624.67±2.08
MN9	100	Span 40 (100)	5	83.71±0.12	462.33±2.08
MN10	100	Span 40 (100)	-	84.88±0.11	496.33±1.53
MN11	75	Span 40 (75)	5	84.56±0.08	378.67±1.53
MN12	75	Span 40 (75)	-	86.63±0.02	484.67±1.53

*Mean ± SD, n = 3.

Phosphate buffer pH6.8 the clear fraction was used for the determination of free drug spectrophotometrically by UV-visible Spectrophotometer (AU-2701, Systronics, Mumbai, India) [24]. The entrapment efficiency was calculated using the formula

$$PercentEntrapmentEfficiency = \frac{InitialDrug(D_i) - Unentrappeddrug(D_u)}{InitialDrug(D_i)} X100$$

In-vitro drug release
The in-vitro drug release pattern was studied using modified USP dissolution apparatus I. Samples were placed on the dialysis membrane previously soaked overnight in phosphate buffer pH 6.8 and attached to lower end of a glass tube. The tubes were immersed in dissolution vessel containing phosphate buffer pH 6.8 maintained at 37±0.5°C. Samples were withdrawn at regular interval of time and replaced with equal amount of buffer to maintain sink condition [25]. The samples were analyzed by UV/Visible spectrophotometer (AU-2701, Systronics, Mumbai, India) for the drug release pattern. The study was continued upto 8 hours.

Particle size and zeta potential
The particle size of the non-ionic surfactant vesicles was determined by dynamic light scattering technique also known as photon correlation spectroscopy using Zetasizer Nano ZS-90 (Malvern Instruments Ltd., UK) [26]. The samples diluted suitably by filtered water (0.5 micrometer filter- Himedia) were placed in the cuvettes and the procedure was carried out at 90° angle and temperature 25°C to determine the size of the particles in the range of 0.6nm to 3 microns. The zeta potential was determined using combination of laser Doppler

velocimetry and phase analysis light scattering by Zetasizer Nano ZS-90 (Malvern Instruments Ltd.; UK). The diluted niosome dispersions were located in zeta meter cell for determination of electrophoretic mobility [27]. All the experiments were performed in triplicate.

Transmission electron microscopy
The morphology of the vesicles was examined by transmission electron microscopy (TEM). A drop of niosomal dispersion was diluted 10 times and was stratified onto a carbon-coated copper grid for 1 minute and excess was removed by filter paper. A drop of 2% phosphotungstic acid solution was stratified to stain the vesicles; excess was removed by a tip of filter paper and left to air dry. The grid was observed by transmission electron microscopy (Hitachi, H-7500) and by using imaging viewer software the images were analyzed and captured [28].

Drug release kinetic data analysis
The release data obtained from various formulations was studied further for fitness of data in different kinetic models like Zero order, First order, Higuchi and Korsmeyer-Peppas release models [29].

Physical stability testing
Physical stability of the niosomes was studied by leaching of the drug from the vesicles in the native prepared form i.e. dispersion stored under refrigeration. The optimized dispersion with the composition of cholesterol and span in 100:100 molar ratio with DCP was sealed in glass vials and stored under refrigeration temperature (2-8°C) for a period of 90 days. Samples were withdrawn at definite intervals of time and the amount of drug remaining was calculated by the method employed for entrapment efficiency determination [30].

Results

Span 20, Span 80, Tween 20, Tween 60, Tween 80 and Brij 30 did not formed thin and dry film at the round bottom flask so were not used further in the study. Thereby Span 40 and Span 60 were used for the preparation and evaluation in the study.

Morphology

The prepared niosomal solution was a homogeneous dispersion and after maturation of 24 hours was studied under the microscope for morphological evaluation. The vesicles were uniform, spherical in shape with traces of aggregation. The formulations prepared with inclusion of DCP were found to be free from aggregation.

Entrapment efficiency

The amount of drug loaded in the vesicles was determined by centrifugation method which separates the entrapped and the unentrapped drug. The percent entrapment efficiency was calculated and was found to be in the range of 83.66 ± 0.08-87.12 ± 0.05 (Table 1).

In-vitro release

The release pattern of the drug from the niosomes was studied using modified USP dissolution apparatus I. The formulations presented sustained release upto 8 hours with MN3 having the most sustained release of 73.89 ± 0.13 at the end of 8 hours. On the basis of most sustained release and sufficient entrapment of 84.50 ± 0.18 MN3 was selected as the optimized formulation (Figure 1) (Figure 2).

Particle size and zeta potential

The average vesicular size of niosomes of all the batches was measured in the range of 388.0 ± 3.61-644.67 ± 2.08 (Table 1). Also the surface charge was studied by zeta potential measurement. The niosomes were found to be

stabilized by large negative values of zeta potential and the polydispersity index (PDI) was 0.123.

Transmission electron microscopy

The TEM photomicrographs clearly indicate that vesicles were uniform, unilamellar and spherical in shape. Also the positive staining showed the drug to be concentrated in the core of the vesicles with drug free bilayer (Figure 3).

Release kinetics

The study of drug release kinetics showed that in all the formulations the best fit model was found to be Korsmeyer-Peppas with 'n' smaller than 0.45 suggesting the Fickian diffusion release mechanism for the drug. Formulation MN3 showed the lowest release of 73.89 ± 0.13 in 8 hours and had correlation coefficient (r =0.996) (Table 2).

Physical stability

The formulation investigated for physical stability studies showed the residual drug content in the niosomes to be 77.61 ± 0.22 at the end of three months. The results concluded that almost 99% of the drug was retained upto 1 month and at the end of the study 91.84% drug was retained by the formulation (Table 3).

Discussion
Effect of type of surfactants

The effect of non-ionic surfactant was studied on the entrapment efficiency, particle size and in-vitro release of the prepared niosomes. Span 60 and Span 40 were the two surfactants used in the study and the formulations were prepared by varying their concentrations to the same extent. Span 60 preceded Span 40 in terms of in-vitro release and entrapment efficiency by presenting the most sustained release in all the prepared batches and

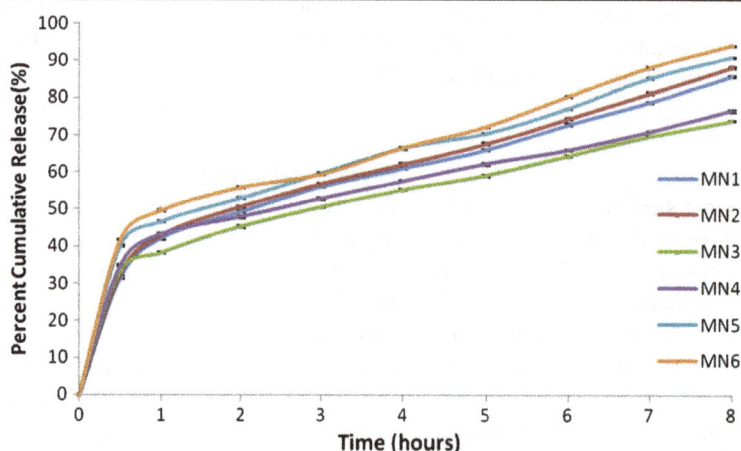

Figure 1 In vitro drug release pattern of metformin niosomes using Span 60.

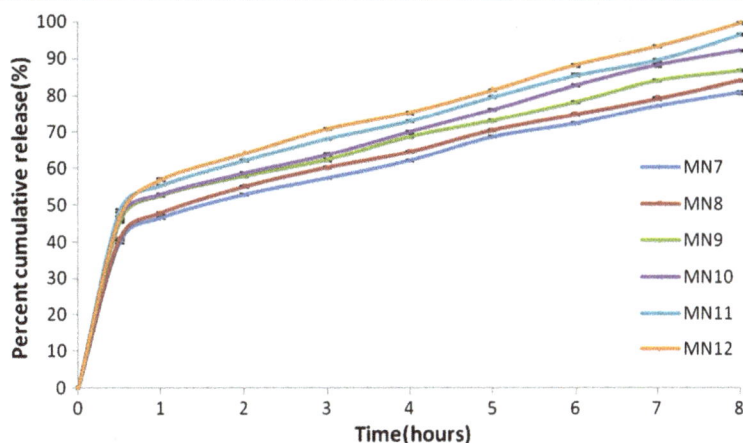

Figure 2 In vitro drug release pattern of metformin niosomes using Span 40.

higher entrapment efficiencies when compared to corresponding formulations (Figure 1) (Figure 2). Span 60 and Span 40 has the same head group and differs in the chain length of the alkyl chain which determines their performance. Span 60 having longer chain length provide more stable vesicles contributing to the higher entrapment and delayed release. Also the ordered gel state and higher phase transition temperature offered by Span 60 plays a significant role in the observed outcomes [31,32]. The size of the vesicles was slightly high in

formulations prepared by Span 60 at the same molar concentration of Span 40. This may be the repercussion of the longer alkyl chain and its stronger interactions with cholesterol molecules which resulted larger core space providing larger entrapment [33]. Decreased molar concentrations of surfactant and cholesterol reduced the entrapment of the drug and the size which may be the aftermath of the insufficient bilayer material to form a strong membrane and to encapsulate the drug efficiently. The case was not similar for the drug release an

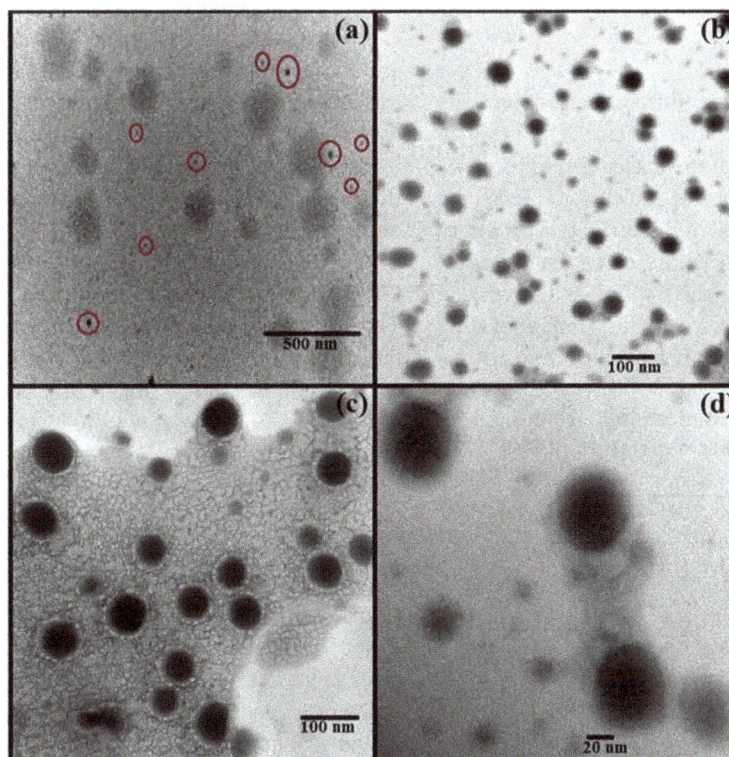

Figure 3 TEM images (a) Uniform distribution; (b) Uniform spherical shape & size; (c) Visible membrane & dark core; (d) Uniform shape.

Table 2 Drug release kinetics profile of metformin niosomes

S. NO	Formulation code	Zero order		First order		Higuchi		Korsemeyer - Peppas		
		r^2	K	r^2	K	r^2	K	r^2	K	n
1	MN1	0.851	24.00	0.566	0.137	0.973	7.98	0.993	1.620	0.267
2	MN2	0.855	24.35	0.564	0.139	0.973	7.97	0.995	1.629	0.264
3	MN3	0.809	23.66	0.541	0.135	0.953	9.75	0.996	1.580	0.261
4	MN4	0.779	25.86	0.506	0.142	0.937	11.51	0.968	1.629	0.204
5	MN5	0.824	27.81	0.511	0.150	0.954	11.07	0.975	1.660	0.252
6	MN6	0.821	28.82	0.500	0.153	0.946	11.76	0.968	1.601	0.336
7	MN7	0.760	28.96	0.474	0.151	0.927	13.51	0.992	1.664	0.203
8	MN8	0.759	29.94	0.469	0.153	0.928	13.90	0.998	1.676	0.216
9	MN9	0.734	32.70	0.440	0.160	0.909	16.13	0.960	1.714	0.184
10	MN10	0.767	32.54	0.454	0.161	0.925	15.19	0.969	1.717	0.195
11	MN11	0.754	34.53	0.440	0.165	0.920	16.47	0.991	1.739	0.198
12	MN12	0.769	34.65	0.450	0.165	0.932	15.79	0.992	1.751	0.202
13	MN13	0.812	30.27	0.487	0.156	0.943	12.70	0.957	1.692	0.214
14	MN14	0.814	23.35	0.538	0.135	0.939	9.86	0.959	1.589	0.203
15	MN15	0.793	25.36	0.509	0.141	0.929	11.30	0.952	1.624	0.190
16	MN16	0.702	37.27	0.405	0.170	0.883	19.50	0.963	1.766	0.156
17	MN17	0.820	23.06	0.546	0.134	0.948	9.46	0.988	1.579	0.223
18	MN18	0.820	24.69	0.535	0.139	0.954	9.91	0.976	1.606	0.235

*r^2=regression coefficient, K= release rate constant, n=diffusional exponent.

optimized amount was required for the controlled effect and increase or decrease in the amount of surfactant lead to early drug loss (Table 1).

Effect of DCP

Charge inducer used was also scrutinized to corroborate its effects on the characteristics of the vesicles. The negative charge induced by DCP resulted in smaller size of the vesicles leading to lower entrapment efficiency (Table 1). Charge on the surface of the bilayer cause repulsive forces which compel the vesicles to be more curved and smaller in sizes. Smaller the size smaller will be the volume enclosed in the core and smaller will be the amount of drug entrapped. DCP was also found to have an advantageous

Table 3 Stability of optimized metformin niosome formulation under refrigeration temperature (2-8°C) storage condition

Time (days)	Entrapment efficiency* (%)	Drug remaining* (%)
0	84.50±0.19	100.00±0.00
7	84.36±0.10	99.83±0.12
15	84.24±0.13	99.68±0.15
30	83.91±0.08	99.30±0.09
45	83.39±0.10	98.69±0.12
60	81.55±0.21	96.50±0.25
90	77.61±0.22	91.84±0.26

*Mean ± SD, n = 3.

impact in retarding the drug release rate which may be attributed to the stability provided by it to the membrane [34] (Figure 1) (Figure 2). DCP has reported effects of providing integrity and uniformity and preventing aggregation and fusion which have been established in the study by the maintenance of sustained release and evident reduction of aggregation in photomicrographs and visual observations [35]. Aggregation has also been lowered by sonication of the prepared dispersion clearly visible in photomicrographs of the vesicles.

Effect of surfactant: cholesterol ratio

The surfactant: cholesterol ratio used, plays a decisive determinant of the properties and the behavior of the bilayer of the niosomes. So to predict the consequences, different molar ratios of surfactants were incorporated into different batches and were investigated for the parameters of particle size, entrapment and in-vitro release. The evaluation proposed equimolar ratio to be the most apt for development of a superior delivery system providing all the required features. Surfactant is the core material for bilayer formation, but the bilayer of just the non-ionic surfactant is not strong enough to serve as host for the drug. So cholesterol having a steroidal rigid structure provides the required strength to the bilayer, despite of the fact that cholesterol itself is incapable of layer formation [36]. When the molar ratio of the surfactant was increased from 75:100 to 125:100 in context with cholesterol the entrapment enhanced to an optimum level and then declined, here the optimized ratio was equimolar i.e. 100:100. The excess of cholesterol at lower ratio tend to disrupt the regular bilayer structure leading to lower entrapment and higher drug release caused by leakage. Irregularities in the membrane structure added by the excess of cholesterol may have lead to increase in the vesicular size. With the increased ratio of the surfactant the entrapment has also improved to an optimized level as the excess of cholesterol is compensated by the added surfactant. At the molar ratio of 100:100 the surfactant and the cholesterol have the best fit arrangement in the bilayer serving to be efficient drug carrier. As the cholesterol acts as the rigidizing agent having the ability to cement the leakages, its deficiency upon increasing the ratio of the surfactant after the optimized ratio lead to the formation of leakage points resulting in lower entrapment and increased drug release [37]. The particle size has decreased with the increasing concentration of surfactant, may be due to bilayer formation with decreased cholesterol content. MN14 being the optimized formulation has highest entrapment of 84.14±0.07, with the most sustained release of 74.37±0.22 after 8 hours and the smallest particle size of all 481.33±3.06 nm (Table 4).

Effect of volume of hydration

Hydration of the thin dry film by the aqueous media is a critical step and the volume used determines the resulting features of the niosomes. The drug used being hydrophilic in nature was dissolved in the buffer and this solution was used for hydration. So the volume also altered the concentration obtained. The results showed no specific pattern of relationship between volume and the evaluated parameters. MN17 prepared using 15 ml of hydrating media served to be best fit formulation with highest entrapment and most retarded release. Any increase or decrease in volume hampered the entrapment and subsequently the release (Table 4). The possible reason for such a behavior could be stated as 15 ml providing ample space for vesicle formation. The lower volume may have lead to incomplete or distorted formation of bilayer due to excess of material and less of space. Whereas in the case of larger volume, the material have

been dispersed in large volume with large interacting area. This may have caused formation of smaller vesicles with decreased entrapment efficiency.

The in vitro release revealed prolonged delivery of the drug for about 8 hours which suffice the daily requirement in Type II diabetes treatment. The sustained release is also proven to decrease the side effects resulting from higher drug concentrations or presence of drug at the areas other than the target site [38]. Also the patient compliance is enhanced by use of niosomes with the possibility of once daily dose as compared to 2–3 doses per day. The negative zeta potential exhibit the negative charge developed on the surface causing the repulsive forces preserving the formulation from aggregation and fusion of vesicles thereby maintaining their integrity and uniformity [35]. The stability testing imply minimal drug lose from the vesicles upto 3 months at refrigeration temperature. In the light of above facts niosomes have been found to meet the requirements for successful delivery of the drug. Furthermore successful encapsulation of the drug in niosomes has also opened the doors for exploitation of other benefits presented by this novel delivery system viz. enhanced penetration, targeted delivery, reduced dose, protection from harsh environment etc.

Conclusions

The investigation conclusively supported niosomes to be an advantageous drug delivery system with high degree of entrapment and sustained release of the drug over extended period of time. The results also concluded that the studied variables have a significant impact on the entrapment and release of drug from the niosomes. Also the Molar concentration and molar ratio of cholesterol and surfactant, the charge inducer DCP and the volume of hydration used should be in optimized value and greatly influence the entrapment of drug in the vesicles and also alters the performance of niosomes. The optimized formulation (cholesterol: surfactant, 100:100 molar concentration) with DCP (5 mg) and 15 ml volume of hydration showed the most sustained release of drug and was found to be the best formulation. The careful control of all the above factors allow the production of a dosage form with sustained release capable of

Table 4 Effect of surfactant: cholesterol ratio on entrapment efficiency, particle size and in vitro drug release

Formulation code	Cholesterol:surfactant (Span 60)	Volume of hydration (ml)	Entrapment efficiency* (%)	Particle size* (nm)	In vitro drug release* (%)
MN13	100:75	15	78.84±0.09	524.33±3.06	94.18±0.50
MN14	100:100	15	84.14±0.07	481.33±3.06	74.37±0.22
MN15	100:125	15	79.27±0.04	445.33±2.08	79.03±0.10
MN16	100:100	10	66.92±0.33	490.67±2.52	94.03±0.14
MN17	100:100	15	83.37±0.09	477.33±2.08	74.60±0.33
MN18	100:100	20	79.36±0.10	455.0±2.64	78.31±0.20

*Mean ± SD, n = 3.

combating the side effects and also reducing the dosing frequency with the greater patient compliance. Suggesting metformin loaded niosomes to be an efficient drug carrier system in treatment of Type II Diabetes.

Abbreviations
DCP: Dicetyl Phosphate; TEM: Transmission Electron Microscopy.

Competing interests
The author(s) declare that they have no competing interests.

Authors' contributions
All authors have read and approved the final manuscript.

Acknowledgements
The authors are thankful to Matrix Laboratories, Hyderabad, India, for providing metformin as a kind gift sample. Authors are grateful to Dr. Madhu Chitkara, Vice chancellor, Chitkara University, Rajpura, Punjab for financial and infrastructure support for the project.

References
1. Furness G: *OnDrugDelivery*. [http://www.ondrugdelivery.com/publications/Oral_Drug_Delivery_07.pdf].
2. Krishnaiah YSR: **Pharmaceutical technologies for enhancing oral bioavailability of poorly soluble drugs.** *J Bioequiv Availab* 2010, **2**:28–36.
3. Luo YF, Chen DW, Ren LX, Zhao XL, Qin J: **Solid lipid nanoparticles for enhancing vinpocetine's oral bioavailability.** *J Control Release* 2006, **114**:53–59.
4. Schnürch AB, Guggib D, Pinter Y: **Thiolated chitosans: development and in vitro evaluation of a mucoadhesive, permeation enhancing oral drug delivery system.** *J Control Release* 2004, **94**:177–186.
5. Fatouros DG, Mullertz A: **In vitro lipid digestion models in design of drug delivery systems for enhancing oral bioavailability.** *Expert Opin Drug Metab Toxicol* 2008, **4**:65–76.
6. Gao P, Guyton ME, Huang T, Bauer JM, Stefanski KJ, Lu Q: **Enhanced oral bioavailability of a poorly water soluble drug PNU91325 by supersaturatable formulations.** *Drug Dev Ind Pharm* 2004, **30**:221–229.
7. Vyas TK, Shahiwala A, Amiji MM: **Improved oralbioavailability and brain transport of Saquinavir upon administration in novel nanoemulsion formulations.** *Int J Pharm* 2008, **347**:93–101.
8. Nassara T, Roma A, Nyskab A, Benita S: **Novel double coated nanocapsules for intestinal delivery and enhanced oral bioavailability of tacrolimus, a P-gp substrate drug.** *J Control Release* 2009, **133**:77–84.
9. Sastry SV, Nyshadham JR, Fix JA: **Recent technological advances in oral drug delivery – a review.** *Pharm Sci Technol To* 2000, **3**:138–145.
10. Sant VP, Smith D, Lerouxa JC: **Novel pH-sensitive supramolecular assemblies for oral delivery of poorly water soluble drugs: preparation and characterization.** *J Control Release* 2004, **97**:301–312.
11. Deshpande AD, Hayes MH, Schootman M: **Epidemiology of Diabetes and Diabetes-Related Complications.** *Phys Ther* 2008, **88**:1254–1264.
12. Slama G: **The potential of metformin for diabetes prevention.** *Diabetes Metab* 2003, **29**:104–111.
13. Tajiri S, Kanamaru T, Yoshida K, Hosoi Y, Konno T, Yada S, Nakagami H: **The Relationship between the Drug Concentration Profiles in Plasma and the Drug Doses in the Colon.** *Chem Pharm Bull* 2010, **58**:1295–1300.
14. Mandal U, Gowda V, Ghosh A, Selvan S, Solomon S, Pal TK: **Formulation and Optimization of Sustained release matrix tablet of Metformin HCl 500mg using response surface methodology.** *Yakugaku Zasshi* 2007, **127**:1281–1290.
15. Brown JB, Pedula K, Barzilay J, Herson MK, Latare P: **Lactic Acidosis Rates in Type 2 Diabetes.** *Diabetes Care* 1998, **21**:1659–1663.
16. Wadher KJ, Kakde RB, Umekar MJ: **Formulation and Evaluation of Sustained-Release Tablets of Metformin Hydrochloride Using Hydrophilic Synthetic and Hydrophobic Natural Polymers. Indian.** *J Pharm Sci* 2011, **73**:208–215.
17. The Weinberg Group Inc.: FDA: [http://www.fda.gov/ohrms/dockets/dailys/04/may04/050404/04p-0208-cp00001-03-Attachment-02-vol1.pdf?

utm_campaign=Google2&utm_source=fdaSearch&utm_medium=website&utm_term=metformin-glipizide%20tablets%20for%20oral%20suspension&utm_content=1].
18. Lachman Consultant Services Inc.: FDA: [http://www.fda.gov/ohrms/dockets/dailys/03/Nov03/112193/03p-0534-cp00001-03-attachment-2-vol1.pdf?utm_campaign=Google2&utm_source=fdaSearch&utm_medium=website&utm_term=metformin-glyburide%20oral%20solution&utm_content=1].
19. Boehringer Ingelheim: FDA;; [http://www.accessdata.fda.gov/scripts/cder/drugsatfda/index.cfm?fuseaction=Search.DrugDetails].
20. Jadon PS, Gajbhiye V, Jadon RS, Gajbhiye KR, Ganesh N: **Enhanced Oral Bioavailability of Griseofulvin via Niosomes.** *AAPS PharmSciTech* 2009, **10**:1186–1192.
21. Sihorkar V, Vyas SP: **Polysaccharide coated niosomes for oral drug delivery: formulation and in vitro stability studies.** *Pharmazie* 2000, **55**:107–13.
22. Patel FM, Patel AN, Rathore KS: **Release of metformin hydrochloride from ispaghula sodium alginate beads adhered cock intestinal mucosa.** *Int J Curr Pharmaceut Res* 2011, **3**:52–55.
23. Kumar GP, Rajeshwarrao P: **Nonionic surfactant vesicular systems for effective drug delivery—an overview.** *Acta Pharmaceutica Sinica B* 2011, **1**:208–219.
24. Chengjiu H, David Rhodes G: **Proniosomes: A Novel Drug Carrier Preparation.** *Int J Pharm* 1999, **185**:23–35.
25. Abdel-Mottaleb MMA, Lamprecht A: **Standardized in vitro drug release test for colloidal drug carriers using modified USP dissolution apparatus.** *Drug Dev Ind Pharm* 2011, **37**:178–184.
26. Junyaprasert VB, Teeranachaideekul V, Supaperm T: **Effect of Charged and Non-ionic Membrane Additives on Physicochemical Properties and Stability of Niosomes.** *AAPS PharmSciTech* 2008, **9**:851–859.
27. Singh G, Dwivedi H, Saraf SK, Saraf SA: **Niosomal Delivery of Isoniazid - Development and Characterization.** *Trop J Pharm Res* 2011, **10**:203–210.
28. Muzzalupo R, Tavano L, Trombino S, Cassano R, Picci N, Mesa CL: **Niosomes from α, ω-trioxyethylene-bis(sodium2-dodecyloxy-propylenesulfonate): Preparation and characterization.** *Colloids Surf B Biointerfaces* 2008, **64**:200–207.
29. Srinivas S, Kumar YA, Hemanth A, Anitha M: **Preparation and evaluation of niosomes containing Aceclofenac.** *Dig J Nanomater Bios* 2010, **5**:249–254.
30. Shahiwala A, Misra A: **Studies in topical application of niosomally entrapped nimuslide.** *J Pharm Pharm Sci* 2002, **5**:220–225.
31. Attia IA, El-Gizawy SA, Fouda MA, Donia AM: **Influence of a Niosomal Formulation on the Oral Bioavailability of Acyclovir in Rabbits.** *AAPS PharmSciTech* 2007, **8**:E1–E7.
32. Hao YM, Li K: **Entrapment and release difference resulting from hydrogen bonding interactions in niosome.** *Int J Pharm* 2011, **403**:245–253.
33. Manconi M, Sinico C, Valenti D, Loy G, Fadda AM: **Niosomes as carriers for tretinoin. I. Preparation and properties.** *Int J Pharm* 2002, **234**:237–248.
34. Namdeo A, Jain NK: **Niosomal delivery of 5-Fluorouracil.** *J Microencapsul* 1999, **16**:731–740.
35. Kandasamy R, Veintramuthu S: **Formulation and Optimization of Zidovudine Niosomes.** *AAPS PharmSciTech* 2010, **11**:1119–1127.
36. Korchowiec B, Paluch M, Corvis Y, Rogalska E: **A Langmuir film approach to elucidating interactions in lipid membranes: 1,2-dipalmitoyl-sn-glycero-3- phosphoethanolamine/ cholesterol/ metal cation systems.** *Chem Phys Lipids* 2006, **144**:127–136.
37. Guinedi AS, Mortada ND, Mansour S, Hathout RM: **Preparation and evaluation of reverse-phase evaporation and multilamellar niosomes as ophthalmic carriers of acetazolamide.** *Int J Pharm* 2005, **306**:71–82.
38. Bayindir ZS, Yuksel N: **Characterization of niosomes prepared with various nonionic surfactants for paclitaxel oral delivery.** *J Pharm Sci* 2010, **99**:2049–2060.

Design and evaluation of Lumefantrine – Oleic acid self nanoemulsifying ionic complex for enhanced dissolution

Ketan Patel, Vidur Sarma and Pradeep Vavia[*]

Abstract

Background: Lumefantrine, an antimalarial molecule has very low and variable bioavailability owing to its extremely poor solubility in water. It is recommended to be taken with milk to enhance its solubility and bioavailability. The aim of present study was to develop a Self Nanoemulsifying Delivery system (SNEDs) of lumefantrine (LF) to achieve rapid and complete dissolution independent of food-fat and surfactant in dissolution media.

Methods: Solubility of LF in oil, co-solvent/co-surfactant and surfactant solution and emulsification efficiency of surfactant were analyzed to optimize the LF loaded self nanoemulsifying preconcentrate. Effect of LF-oleic acid complexation on emulsification, droplet size, zeta potential and dissolution were investigated. Effect of milk concentration and fat content on saturation solubility and dissolution of LF was investigated. Dissolution of marketed formulation and LF-SNEDs was carried out in pH 1.2 and pH 6.8 phosphate buffer.

Results: LF exhibited very high solubility in oleic acid owing to complexation between tertiary amine of LF and carboxyl group of oleic acid (OA). Cremophore EL and medium chain monoglyceride were selected surfactant and co-surfactant, respectively. Significantly smaller droplet size (37 nm), shift in zeta potential from negative to positive value, very high drug loading in lipid based system (> 10%), no precipitation after dissolution are the major distinguish characteristics contributed by LF-OA complex in the SNED system. Saturation solubility and dissolution study in milk containing media pointed the significant increment in solubility of LF in the presence of milk-food fat. LF-SNEDs showed > 90% LF release within 30 min in pH 1.2 while marketed tablet showed almost 0% drug release.

Conclusion: Self nanoemulsification promoting ionic complexation between basic drug and oleic acid hold great promise in enhancing solubility of hydrophobic drugs.

Introduction

Poor aqueous solubility of the existing and New Chemical Entities adversely affects the oral bioavailability. Failure to mimic in vivo performance compare to in vitro potential, variable absorption and so the plasma concentration, requirement of higher dose than actually needed for desired pharmacological activity are some of the major problems associated with poor solubility of drugs. Further, molecules having very poor aqueous solubility with poor oil solubility impose greater formulation challenges for pharmaceutical scientists. Self emulsifying drug delivery system is one the promising strategy to overcome the solubility barrier of drugs, with commercial products in market e.g. Cyclosporin A, Ritonavir, Lopinavir, Fenofibrate etc. Although a versatile approach, it is not suitable for inherently poor oil soluble molecules e.g. Itraconazole, Carbamazepine, Lumefantrine etc. [1-3].

Lumefantrine (LF) is a highly lipophilic flourene derivative and a Biopharmaceutical Classification System (BCS) Class II drug which is an important agent in the treatment of falciparum malaria. Plasmodium Falciparum is an insidious malarial parasite that fatally threatens a major segment of the Sub-Saharan population in Africa. Thus far, existing therapies for treatment of this form of malaria

* Correspondence: vaviapr@yahoo.com
Center for Novel Drug Delivery Systems, Department of Pharmaceutical Sciences and Technology, Institute of Chemical Technology, University under Section 3 of UGC Act – 1956, Elite Status and Center of Excellence – Govt. of Maharashtra, TEQIP Phase II Funded, N. P. Marg, Matunga (E), Mumbai 400 019, India

have been futile due to irregular dosage regimen and insufficient bioavailability afforded by drugs of the quinine class. Lumefantrine is a blood schizonticide, acts by inhibiting detoxification of haem, this toxic haem and free radicals induce parasite death [4,5].

Although a very efficacious molecule, its activity is limited by extremely poor aqueous solubility. Its solubility is far below the critical solubility requirement and so the reported bioavailability is 4–11%. Such vast variability in bioavailability is contributed by the effect of food-fat consumption. Low intrinsic clearance and erratic oral variability and therapeutic levels are more reliably achieved by co-administration with a fatty meal. The oral bioavailability of lumefantrine is highly dependent on food and is consequently poor in acute malaria, showing high degree of variation in different subjects [6]. Poor solubilization leads to incomplete absorption and so inadequate plasma concentrations for antimalarial activity. Due to this chances of treatment failure are higher, which is again associated with increased morbidity, transmissibility and development of resistance. Lumefantrine is an extremely well-tolerated drug, so it is essential to ensure its maximum absorption [6]. Generally milk is recommended to be taken with lumefantrine but availability of milk and its fat content might vary region to region and the variation in antimalarial response to it. This inter-subject variability may gradually induce resistance to artemisinin-based combination therapy, thus making it crucial to increase the dosage regimen. There is only one report on enhancement of dissolution of LF by wet milling technique. However, Nano milling is very high energy consuming process; moreover paper states that nanopowder lumefantrine also requires benzalkonium chloride (BKC) in dissolution media for solubilization [7]. So far there is no report on solubility enhancement of LF by Self nanoemulsifying system. Self nanoemulsifying systems are very well reported in literature for enhancement in solubility of lipophilic drugs. Self emulsifying preconcentrate is made of oil, surfactant, co-surfactant and drug. On dispersion in water it forms < 100 nm sized droplets. Based on oil characteristic it is directly disseminate to systemic circulation or absorb via lymphatic pathway. Oil-surfactant-cosurfactant driven very high solubility, nano-size and permeability results in significantly rise in bioavailability. The spontaneous formation of nanosized emulsion droplets in stomach generates enormously high surface area for drug to diffuse in lumen and absorb rapidly [3,8].

Poor oil solubility of LF has restricted development of lipid based system. In view of this inadequacy, the current study aims at improving the solubility of lumefantrine, especially to eliminate the co administration of milk or any other fatty meal. Considering the basic nature of LF, we have planned to form LF-oleic acid ionic complex and to prepare self emulsifying system of complex by addition

of appropriate surfactant. Such a self emulsifying hydrophobic complex enable rapid dissolution of LF, without need of BKC in dissolution media, hence provide better correlation to in vivo condition. Till date, there is no report on preparation of self emulsification system with drug – oil ionic complex. The main objective of the study was to develop a self nanoemulsifying delivery system of lumefantrine to increase its solubility, which otherwise is dependent on food.

Materials and methods
Materials
Lumefantrine was procured from Mangalam Laboratories Pvt Ltd (India). The following materials were procured from gattefosse India and were used as received: Labrafac CM10 (C 8 -C 10 polyglycolized glycerides), Maisine 35–1 (glyceryl monolinoleate), Lauroglycol FCC (propylene glycol laurate), Labrafil 1944 CS (apricot kernel oil polyethylene glycol [PEG] 6 esters) and Labrafac PG (propylene glycol caprylate/caprate). Cremophor RH 40 (polyoxyl 40 hydrogenated castor oil), Cremophor EL (polyethoxylated castor oil and Solutol HS 15 (polyoxyethylene esters of 12-hydroxystearic acid) were obtained from BASF India Ltd. Gelucire 44/14 (PEG-32 glyceryl laurate) and 50/13 (PEG-32 glyceryl palmistearate) were received from Colorcon Asia (India). Oleic acid, Tween 80 (polyoxyethylene sorbitan monooleate) and PEG 400 were purchased from Merck (India). Deionized water was prepared by a Milli-Q purifi cation system from Millipore (France). Acetonitrile and methanol used in the present study were of high performance liquid chromatography (HPLC) grade. All other chemicals were reagent grade. Empty HPMC capsule shells were procured from ACG Capsules (Mumbai). Milk of different fat content was purchased from Aarey dairy (1.5% fat content) and Gokul dairy (3% fat content) India.

Analytical method
A simple HPLC method was developed for quantitative analysis of lumefantrine in the formulation. The HPLC system was equipped with Jasco PU2080 plus pumps with PDA detector and auto sampler unit. The drug was analyzed using Hypersil C18 column (250 mm × 4.6 mm, 5 μm) with mobile phase composition Methanol – 0.1% TFA in water in the ratio of 80:20 v/v, with 1.5 ml/min flow rate and detector wavelength set to 336 nm.

Methods
Screening of oil
Saturation solubility of Lumefantrine in oil was chosen as the criteria of selection. The solubility of the drug was determined in various natural and derived oils. 1 ml of each of the selected vehicles was added to each cap vial containing an excess of LF. Mixing of the systems was

performed using a vortex mixer. Formed suspensions were then shaken with a shaker at 37°C for 48 hours. After reaching equilibrium, each vial was centrifuged at 15,000 rpm for 5 minutes. The solubility of lumefantrine in oil was then quantified by HPLC method.

Screening of surfactant and co-surfactant

Screening of surfactant was done on the basis of (i) Solubility of LF in surfactant solution and (ii) its emulsification efficiency for LF-oil mixture.

Saturation solubility of the drug was determined in various surfactant solution (1% w/v solutions in water) and co-surfactant. An excess amount of LF was added to 5 ml of the surfactant solution and co-surfactant/co-solvent. Samples were placed in a water shaker bath for 48 hrs. The sample was then centrifuged (15,000) for 10 min followed by analysis of supernatant by HPLC. Oleic acid was selected as oil for lumefantrine solubilization. Various Surfactants, co surfactant and combination thereof were mixed with oleic acid and LF-oleic acid solution in various ratios. The co-solvent/co-surfactant were screened on the basis of emulsification time, droplet size, appearance of final system and its reports on compatibility with capsule shell. 500 mg of each mixture (oleic acid-surfactant or LF-oleic acid-surfactant) was added to 250 ml of water (37°C) with mild stirring (100 rpm on magnetic stirrer). The compositions were evaluated for their emulsifying efficiency for oleic acid and LF-oleic acid mixture. Emulsification time, appearance and type of emulsion, LF precipitation and stability for 24 h etc. parameters were considered to evaluate the emulsification efficiency of surfactant.

LF-SNEDs (Lumefantrine-Self Nanoemulsifying Delivery System) was prepared by dissolving LF in oleic acid (minimal amount require for LF solubilization). Optimized mixture of Surfactant and co-surfacacant were added to LF-oleic acid mixture. Fixed weight of Lumefantrine: Oleic acid (100 mg:325 mg) was mixed with various ratios of Cremophore EL and different co-solvents and co-surfactants. Droplet size and emulsification time was evaluated in order to optimize the quantity of surfactant and co solvent/co surfactant. The prepared LF-SNEDs preconcentrate was filled into HPMC capsules.

Droplet size and zeta potential measurement

One hundred microliters of each LF-SNEDs preconcentrate was added to 100 ml of miliQ water, and gently mixed using a glass rod. The resultant emulsion was analyzed for droplet size (z average diameter) by Dynamic Light Scattering (DLS) using Malvern Zetasizer, USA. The same procedure of dilution used to measure zeta potential by laser dopper microelectrophoresis using same instrument.

Saturation solubility of lumefantrine in milk containing media

Eventhough LF is recommended to be taken with milk, there has been no literature report hitherto on the effect of milk on the solubility of lumefantrine. In an attempt to check the solubility of lumefantrine in milk containing varying amounts of fat, the following two types of milk were chosen: milk containing 1.5% fat (a) and 3.1% fat (b).

Milk of types a and b were added to different test tubes containing water at pH 1.2 buffer USP (Hydrochloric acid) and pH 6.8 phosphate buffer USP at a concentration of 20% v/v under the assumption that an average person consumes 200 ml of milk in a day. Excess amount of drug was added to each test tube and it was kept in a water shaker bath for 24 hours. Thereafter solutions were filtered through 0.45 μm filter to remove the insoluble drugs. Filtrate was diluted suitably distilled water followed by extracted by chloroform. After evaporating chloroform and reconstituting with mobile phase LF was quantified using HPLC. The saturation solubility of lumefantrine with increasing concentrations of milk at different pH was calculated.

In vitro dissolution study

Dissolution of Marketed Formulation was carried out in surfactant free dissolution media with and without milk. Instead of using Fed state dissolution media, a real time method to account for variability in ingested food was used by adding 100 mL and 200 mL of low-fat milk (a) to each dissolution flask respectively. The composition of dissolution media for marketed formulation is mentioned in Table 1. Dissolution of marketed preparation was carried out using USP XXIII apparatus I at 37 ± 0.50°C with a rotating speed of 100 rpm. Samples were taken at every 15 min from each of the flasks and the percentage cumulative release was calculated.

LF-SNEDs preconcentrate was filled in size '0' HPMC capsules. Dissolution Test of LF-SNEDs was carried out in similar dissolution media using sinker. The composition of milk containing dissolution media showed in Table 1.

Table 1 Preparation of dissolution media

Dissolution media	Deionised water	Milk
pH 1.2 buffer USP (HCl)	900	0
	800	100
	700	200
pH 6.8 phosphate buffer USP	900	0
	800	100
	700	200

Results

Screening of oil

The core part of SNEDs is composed of oil, in which drug is solubilized. Hence, it is very much essential to choose the oil having higher solubility for drug. Various types of oil have been screened including fatty acids, medium chain mono/di/tri glycerides, propylene mono/di glycerides and long chain triglycerides. Castor oil and GMO showed minimal solubility of LF while Medium chain triglycerides, Isopropyl myristate, rice germ oil etc. showed moderate solubility of LF (Table 2). The higher solubility in rice germ oil may be attributed to its high oleic acid content and γ-orizynol [9]. Oleic acid showed significantly higher solubility of lumefantrine – 157 mg of LF/gm of oleic acid. Such a higher solubility is not merely expected form hydrophobic interaction between LF and oleic acid. There must be ionic interaction attributes to this solubility enhancement.

Screening of surfactant

Selection of suitable surfactant is very crucial part for self emulsifying system especially when a fine translucent nanosized emulsion is required. Surfactant was selected on the basis of two criterions: saturation solubility of lumefantrine in 1% w/v surfactant solution (Table 3) and its emulsification efficiency for LF-oleic acid (Table 4).

Table 2 Saturation solubilities of drug in vehicles

Vehicle	Solubility (mg/gm) ± SD (n=3)
Oil	
Castor Oil	5.91± 0.21
Glyceryl Monooleate	7.79 ± 0.29
Sunflower oil	10.57 ± 0.42
Olive oil	11.67 ± 0.37
Acconon CO7	13.22 ± 0.24
Groundnut Oil	14.16 ± 0.43
Corn Oil	19.34 ± 0.61
Captex 300	29.62 ± 0.72
Till oil	33.40 ± 0.8
Isopropyl Myristate	40.85 ± 0.74
Rice germ Oil	59.92 ± 1.19
Oleic Acid	157.20 ± 1.38
Co-surfactant	
Capmul MCM C8	14.99 ± 0.48
Capmul PG8	18.13 ± 0.49
Co-solvent	
Propylene Glycol	0.432 ± 0.11
Ethanol	2.831 ± 0.29
PEG 400	2.852 ± 0.18
Transcutol P	19.267 ± 0.58
Benzyl alcohol	78.024 ± 1.41

Table 3 Saturation solubility of LF in surfactant solution

Surfactant solution (1%)	Solubility (µg/ml) (Mean± SD) (n=3)
Acconon MC8	0.26 ± 0.14
Sodium Deoxytaurocholate	1.33 ± 0.09
Sodium taurocholate	1.42 ± 0.14
Tween 20	9.18 ± 0.13
SLS	10.75 ± 0.28
Lutrol	13.01 ± 0.15
Acconon S 35	13.05 ± 0.17
Gelusire	15.18 ± 0.17
Solutol HS 15	22.49 ± 0.21
TPGS	27.18 ± 0.28
Cremophore EL	44.52 ± 0.29
Cremophore RH40	46.94 ± 0.25
Tween 80	101.63 ± 0.37

Surfactants of chemical diversity – ionic (cholate, SLS) and non ionic (PEG fatty acid esters, PEO-PPO-PEO block co polymers, PEG vitamin E esters etc.) have been screened for solubility of lumefantrine. LF was almost negligible soluble in PEG-medium chain fatty acid ester (Acconon MC8), marginal solubility in ionic surfactant, with highest solubility in Tween 80 (100 ppm). Tween 80 was selected as the surfactant in trials with different co-surfactants to assess the ability of the co-surfactants to improve the clarity of the system. However, Tween 80 does not show good emulsification as the final system remained hazy. Eventhough LF exhibited highest solubility in Tween 80, it was rejected bacause its poor emulsification property for LF-oleic acid (Table 4).

LF-oleic acid-cremophore EL preconcentrate was self nanoemulsify to 50–100 nm sized droplet depending on the amount of cremophore EL (Table 5). However, in all the bathces have shown longer self emulsification time (~ 7 min) on additon into water (Table 6). Reduction in self emulsification time is necessary to release LF immidiately. In order to reduce the emulsification time, addition of co-solvent or co-surfactant facilitating the emulsification process was added. Various co-solvent/co-surfactant were screened for this purpose. Solubility of LF in Co co-solvent/co-surfactant was not considered as an important criteria for its selection because of very poor solubility of LF in Medium chain monoglycerides, ethanol, PEG and transcutol P. solubiliy of LF was found to be higher in benzyle alcohol compare to other solvents but was rejected in formualtion due to its lower acceptibilty limit and volatile nature.

The emulsification time and appearance of the formulation with different co-surfactants with Cremophore EL were shown in Table 6. Further, droplet size and polydispersity index of various batches of LF-oleic acid mixture with in different ratio of cremophore EL with

Table 4 Emulsification behavior of Oil and Surfactant mixture

Composition	Surfactant	Observation	Emulsification
Oleic Acid	Gelusire 44/14, Tween 80, Solutol HS 15, TPGS, Lutrol F68	Turbid	Poor
LF-Oleic Acid	Gelusire 44/14, Tween 80, Solutol HS 15, TPGS	Turbid	Poor
Oleic Acid	Cremophor RH40	Translucent milky solution	Satisfactory
LF-Oleic acid	Cremophor RH40	Translucent	Good
Oleic Acid	Cremophore EL	Translucent	Good
LF-Oleic Acid	Cremophore EL	Clear and translucent	Excellent

various Co-surfactant/Co-solvent has mentioned in Table 5.

It was found that a oil:surfactant ratio of 1:1.2 yielded the smallest droplet size and a clear translucent system, however, in an attempt to reduce the amount of surfactant in the system the droplet size was compromised slightly and the surfactant concentration was reduced. Thus, a system with an oil:surfactant ratio of 1:1 was chosen. Although transcutol acts as an effective co-solvent in terms of emulsification capacity, it slows down the emulsification time for the system. PEG-400, inspite of being a good candidate for a co-solvent was not chosen due to its hygroscopic tendencies in soft and hard gelatin capsules. Ethanol was not considered as a co-solvent in the final formulation due to its tendency to diffuse out of the shell and it threatens the integrity of the capsule. Capmul MCM-C8, a medium chain monoglyceride was selected as co-surfactant in finally optimized system (LF-SNEDs) since it has given minimal droplet size of 37 nm (Table 5) with comparatively rapid emulification (Table 6). Moreover there is no report on its any chemical or physical interaction with capsule shell.

Zeta potential

In this study, to account for the electrostatic effects of the drug-lipid interaction, the zeta potential values of self-emulsified formulation were measured at the same drug to lipid ratios as optimized in the above experiments. Zeta potential of SNEDs with and without drug was evaluated to understand effect of LF-oleic acid complex on surface charge. The Zeta Potential of oleic acid self emulsifying system was found to be – 6.73 mv while LF loaded SNEDs exhibited + 4.4 mv zeta potential. The graphical presentation of droplet size, zeta potential and possible orientation of surfactant in LF-SNEDs showed in Figure 1. This indicates the blank formulation has negative zeta potential while addition of drug lead to shift in zeta potential to positive side. The results are in agreement with a study by Nagarsenker et al., suggesting that addition of a basic drug lead to shift in zeta potential from negative to positive [10]. The final composition of LF-SNEDs is mentioned in Table 7.

Saturation solubility of lumefantrine in milk containing media

The saturation solubility of lumefantrine in milk containing media at gastric and intestinal pH was analyzed (Figure 2). Saturation solubility of LF was found to be significantly influenced by pH and presence milk. However, in absence of milk LF showed almost negligible solubility in both pH 1.2 and pH 6.8 buffers. As expected LF has higher solubility at lower pH due to its

Table 5 Particle size analysis of various formulations

Formulation	Co-solvent/Co- surfactant (mg)	Cremophore EL (mg)	Particle size (nm)	PDI
F1	0	250	94.51 ± 7.67	0.329
F2	0	325	65.43 ± 5.49	0.229
F3	0	400	48.4 ± 5.3	0.25
F4	Transcutol P (25)	250	72.25 ± 6.7	0.235
F5	Transcutol P (25)	325	60.5 ± 5.3	0.21
F6	Transcutol P (25)	400	50.25 ± 6.2	0.227
F7	Capmul MCM (25)	250	80.39 ± 8.7	0.254
LF-SNEDs	Capmul MCM (25)	325	37.96 ± 4.1	0.184
F9	Capmul MCM (25)	400	53.78 ± 4.81	0.211
F10	Capmul MCM (50)	325	39.49 ± 4.4	0.119
F11	PEG 400 (25)	325	52.98 ± 4.7	0.123
F12	Ethanol (25)	325	41.59 ± 3.5	0.139
F13	Capmul PG8	325	51.71 ± 3.9	0.122

Table 6 Effect of different co-surfactants on emulsification time

Co-surfactant	Emulsification time (min)	Observations
Transcutol P	6.17	Long time to disperse but final system is clear
PEG-400	4.30	Clear system
Capmul PG8	4.70	Translucent nanoemulsion
Capmul MCM-C8	3.16	Translucent nanoemulsion
Without any co-solvent	7.0	Highly viscous clumps take a long time to disperse

basic nature. Saturation solubility of LF increase with increase the fat content of milk, with maximum solubility of 24 ppm was observed in media containing 20% v/v high fat milk at pH 1.2 (Figure 2). Further increase in fat content or milk concentration is expected to proportionally enhance the solubility of LF.

Dissolution profile of marketed formulation in milk containing media

Dissolution profile clearly states that release of LF is highly depend on concenration of milk in dissolution media (Figure 3). The results of dissolution sutdies are complemetaty to saturation solubility study of LF in milk containing media. The dissolution medium without milk showed negligible release and hence it can be predicted that without fat containig food suppliment, bioavailbility and therefore therapeutic response may be very poor. Milk containing dissolution media showed marginal improvement in dissolution of LF. Dissolution of LF is higher at pH 1.2 media compare to pH 6.8, irrespective of milk content. Higher dissolution at pH 1.2 is due to its higher solubility at lower pH. The cumulative

release increases to maximum 12% upon the ingestion of 200 ml of milk in gastric pH.

Dissolution test of lumefantrine self nanoemulsifying system

Comparable dissoluiton profile of marketed formulation and LF-SNEDs at pH 1.2 and pH 6.8 shown in Figure 4. Marketed formulation showed almost negligible release over the period of 60 min, which is by virtue of extemley poor solubility of lumefantrine in aqeous media. LF-SNEDs exhibited significantly enhancement in dissolution compare to marketed preparation. At pH 1.2, more than 90% of LF was found to release within 30 min account of rapid formation of nanoemulasion in contact with aqeuous medium.

Discussion

Oleic acid showed highest solubilizaion capacity of LF owing to complexation between tertiary amine of LF and oleic acid. Complexation of LF and oleic acid was indirectly confirmed by addition of stronger base than lumefantrine. It was assumed that addition of stronger

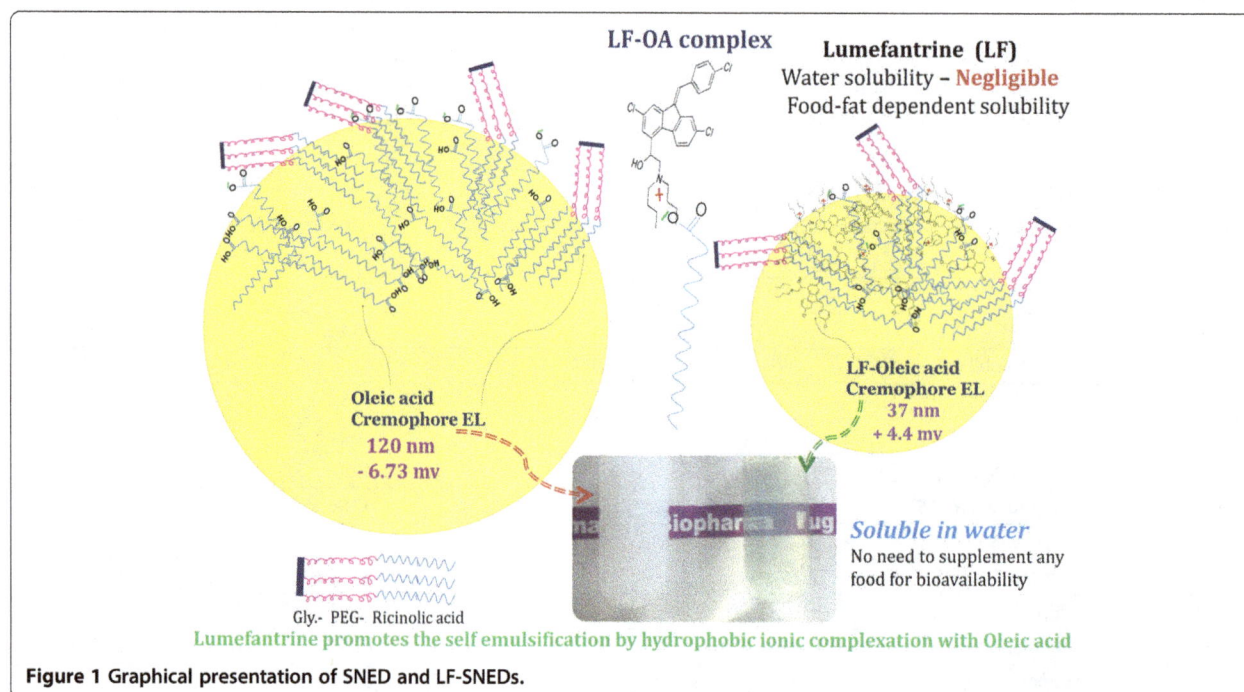

Figure 1 Graphical presentation of SNED and LF-SNEDs.

Table 7 Composition of LF-SNEDs

Lumefantrine	100 mg
Oleic acid	325 mg
Cremophore EL	325 mg
Capmul MCM	25 mg
Total	775 mg

amine containing group in oleic acid will interfere in complexation of amine group of LF with carboxylic acid of oleic acid. The reported pKa value of halofantrine (a similar class of drug) is in the range of 8.2 [11]. So on the basis of structural similarity we assumed that lumefantrine has similar pKa. The pKa of Triethylamine (TEA) is 10.5, which depicts that it is stronger base than lumefantrine. LF was found to be insoluble in oleic acid in the presence of TEA. On this basis it was confirmed that ionic complexation is responsible for significant higher solubility of LF in oleic acid.

Further experimentation on self emulsification property of oleic acid and LF-oleic acid suggested the proof of concept of ionic complexation between LF and oleic acid promote self emulsification (see graphical abstract). It was discovered that a system consisting of only oleic acid (no drug), surfactant and co-solvent is self nanoemulsifying to 120 ± 12 nm while system containing LF-oleic acid, surfactant and consurfactant easily emulsify to nano size translucent dispersion of 37.96 ± 4.1 nm. Addition of LF showed 4 times reduction in droplet size. It means that LF-oleic acid complex is itself promoting the self emulsification, which is otherwise difficult to emulsify oleic acid. We can attribute this to the fact that oleic acid interacts with the amine drug and forms a hydrophobic ion-pairing complex with its carboxylic group. Thus, the functional

group of oleic acid which might br interfering in self emulsification, on complexation with drug to it promote the self-emulsifying property. Based on the above results, Oleic acid was selected as the oil. The interaction was reflected in zeta potential study. Shift in Zeta potential of plain oleic acid nanoemulsion – 6.73 mv to + 4.4 mv with LF-oleic acid nanoemulsion also support the ionic interaction between amine of LF and carboxylic acid group of oleic acid. The blank formulation has a negative charge due to the predominance of the anionic oleic acid. The negative charge of blank system is due to presence of carboxylic acid group on surface. Very marginal negative potential of the system is due to poor ionization of oleic acid (pKa – 9.85). Moreover, dense network of PEG of cremophore EL on surface mask zeta potential of the ionized species on surface. Zeta potential of LF-SNEDs was found to be slightly positive, clearly indicating the ionic interaction of LF-oleic acid. The positive charge, in LF-SNEDs can be attributed to masking of anionic charge of oleic acid by complexation with LF and surface orientation of amine group of LF in nanoglobules. This interaction results in significantly higher solubility of LF in oleic acid, further LF-oleic acid complex is expected to be more soluble in oleic acid than lumefantrine itself.

Tween and cremphore both are PEG fatty acid esters but their chemical structures have vast diffence. Cremphore surfactants are more bulky and having higher molecular weight compare to Tween surfactants. Tween 80 has single chian of oleic acid as lipophilic part while cremophore surfactants have three fatty acid chain attahced to PEG-glycerol. This bulkier lipophilic part of cremophore may contributed to better emulsification property of cremophore EL and cremophore RH 40. Hence, further formulations were tested with Cremophore

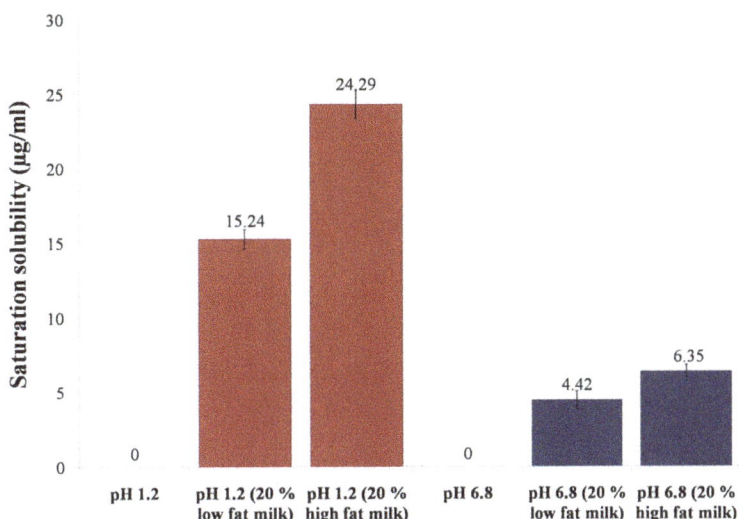

Figure 2 Saturation solubility of lumefantrine in different types of milk at different pH.

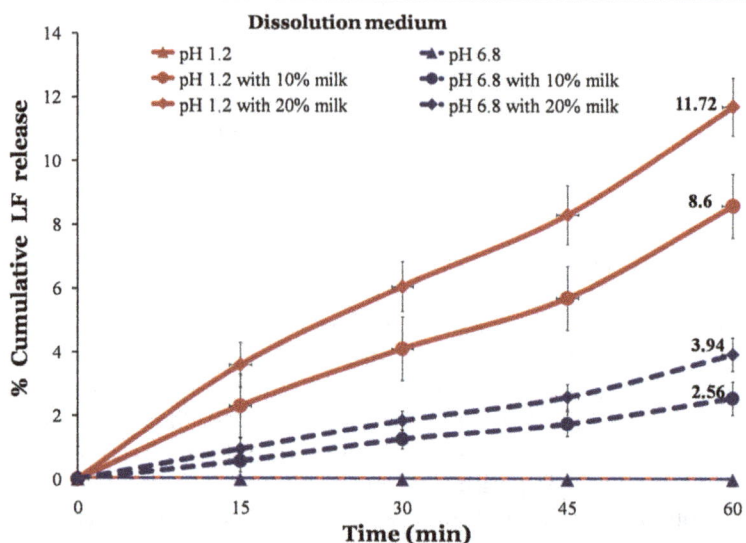

Figure 3 Dissolution profile of marketed formulation in milk containing dissolution media.

EL and Cremophore RH 40. We have observed that free fatty acid e.g. oleic acid is difficult to emulsify in comparision to its glyceryl esters. Though Cremophore RH 40 showed a slightly better solubilising capacity, it was dismissed in favour of Cremophore EL as the latter portrayed a clearer and more transparent emulsion on redispersion. Also, Cremophor RH40 (polyoxyl 40 hydrogenated castor oil) appeared to be less readily digested than Cremophor EL (polyoxyl 35 castor oil). An explanation for differences in the digestability of the structurally similar Cremophor surfactants is not very clear in literature but may reflect differences in the reactivity of the saturated (hydrogenated) castor oil glyceride backbone in Cremophor RH40 leading to the generation of slightly different reaction products with polyethylene oxide, when compared with Cremophor EL (which is generated by polyethoxylation of unsaturated castor oil) [12]. Alternatively the slightly larger polyethylene oxide content of Cremophor RH 40 may have more effectively masked the approach and binding of pancreatic enzymes (and therefore hydrolysis) when compared with Cremophor EL. Cremophore EL has an IIG limit of 599 mg making it a feasible and non-toxic component in the system.

Self-emulsification of oil-surfacatant preconcentrate proceeds through formation of Liquid Crystalline phase (LC) at oil–water interface. The rate and extent of water penetration into LC phase determines the rate of emulsification. Rapidity of self emulsification is governed by weakness and viscosity of intermediate LC [13,14]. Medium chain monoglyceride (MCM) has ability to

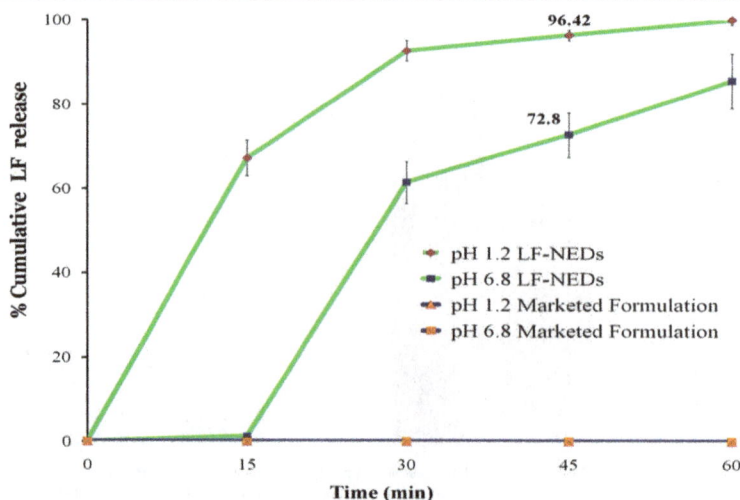

Figure 4 Dissolution profile of marketed formulation and LF-SNEDs.

form such LC phase especially when mixed with hydrophilic surfactant [14].

It was observed that increasing concentrations of fat in milk brought about an increase in saturation solubility of lumefantrine whereas no solubility was observed at the gastric and intestinal pH in the absence of milk. Triglycerides are the major component of milk fat. These medium to long chain triglycerides of milk contributing to marginal solubility of lumefantrine in milk. Higher the fat content of milk, higher will be the solubility of LF in it.

This indicates the extreme necessity of fat containing diet for its solublilization and therefore absoption. Possibility of failure in therapetic response can not be denied with such a poorly soluble drug as discussed in introduction part.

Increase in solubility with increase in milk content is prime reason for enhacement in bioavailability of LF when given with milk. The results are in agreement with a bioavailability study carried out on healthy human volunteer to evaluate the effect of food/fat on bioavailability of LF. Bindschedle et al. have reported 16 fold enhancement in bioavailability in the presence of food [15]. Ashley et al. have reported 90% of maximum AUC was achieved with 36 ml of soya milk [6]. Ensuring that volunteer receives milk or fat with given medicine is feasible under study conditions but difficult to guarantee during routine treatment in malaria patients. However, the availability of milk, composition of fat and the amount of milk consumed varies from person to person and thus there is no conclusive prediction of the bioavailability in the LF.

LF-oleic acid ionic hydrophobic complex emulsify to nanosize by cremophore EL, generating an enormously high surface area. Accroding to noyes-whitney equation reduction in droplet size lead to significant enhancement in dissolution while Prandlt equation suggests the significant reduction in diffusion layer thickness with nanosizing of particle [16].

One more important thing to take into consideration is dissolution media does not contain any surfactant. Generally, in dissolutin studies of hydrophobic drug, surfactant is added to maintain sink condition and to prevent precipitaion of drug-in dissolution media. USP recommonds use of 1% w/v Benzalkonium chloride (BKC) in dissoultion media. The saturation solubilty of LF in 0.1 M HCl with 1% w/v BKC is 119 ± 3 ppm, sufficient to solubilize 120 mg of LF in dissolution media [16]. The most important advantage of LF-SNEDs system is complete dissolution of LF without use of such surfactant in dissoltion media. Both the dissolution media pH 1.2 and pH 6.8, do not contain BKC or other surfactant, still LF-SNEDs capable enough to solubilize drug without precipiatation. Amount of cremophore EL in dosage form is just 325 mg, leading to 0.36% w/v in

900 ml of dissolution media. This concentration is much below to maitain sink condition for LF in dissolution media (Table 3). Hence, we can predict that LF remains in solubilized state in dissolution media because of its comlexation with oleic acid. The complex formation promote the faster self emulsification and dissolution and further inhibit the precipitaion of drug once solubilized. In phosphate buffer 6.8, slow dissolution of capsule shell resulted in 10 min lag period for solubilitzation. After opening of capsule dissolution profile is similar to that of pH 1.2.

Conclusion

Hydrophobic ionic complexation based self nanoemulsifying delivery system of LF showed remarkabley higher dissolution profile, eliminating the requirement of food/fat for LF solubilization. Lumefantrine has very high solubility in oleic acid due to complexation between tertiary amine of LF and oleic acid. Higher the solubiilty of drug in oil, higher the drug loading capacity of formulation. For drug having higher dose, ionic complexation with oleic acid would be effective strategy to enhance solibilty by self nanoemulisfying formulation. Selection of an ideal surfactant and co-surfactant is very much essential to emulsify the complex to nano sized globule within short period of time. Spontaneous formation of nanoemulsion lead to rapid dissolution of a hydrophobic drug, which may offer food/fat independent bioavailability. Ionic complexation with self emulsifying delivery offer an easy, cost effective and industry feasible approach for solubilization of basic hydrophobic drugs.

Competing interest
The authors declare that they have no competing interest.

Authors' contributions
KP and VS have carried out studies mentioned in article. PV has guided this project and made substantial contributions for data interpretation and involved in drafting the manuscript and revising it critically. All authors read and approved the final manuscript.

Acknowledgment
Authors are thankful to University Grant Commission, Govt. of India for research fellowship awarded and All India Council for Technical Education (AICTE-NAFETIC) for research facilities provided.

References
1. Thomas VH, Bhattachar S, Hitchingham L, Zocharski P, Naath M, Surendran N: The road map to oral bioavailability: an industrial perspective. Expert Opin Drug Metab Toxicol 2006, 2:591–608.
2. Stegemann S, Leveiller F, Franchi D, de Jong H, Lindén H: When poor solubility becomes an issue: from early stage to proof of concept. Eur J Pharma Sci 2007, 31:249–61. Patel AR, Vavia PR: Preparation and in vivo evaluation of SMEDDS (self-microemulsifying drug delivery system) containing fenofibrate. AAPS J 2007, 9:E344–E345.
3. Singh SP, Raju KSR, Nafis A, Puri SK, Jain GK: Intravenous pharmacokinetics, oral bioavailability, dose proportionality and in situ permeability of anti-malarial lumefantrine in rats. Malar J 2011, 10:293.

4.   Ezzet F, Mull R, Karbwang J: **The population pharmacokinetics of CGP 56697 and its effects on the therapeutic response in malaria patients.** *Br J Clin Pharmacol* 1998, **46:**553–561.

5.   Ashley EA, Annerberg A, Kham A, Brockman A, Singhasivanon P, White NJ: **How much fat is necessary to optimize lumefantrine oral bioavailability?** *Trop Med Int Health* 2007, **12:**195–200.

6.   Gahoi S, Jain GK, Tripathi R, Pandey SK, Anwar M, Warsi MH: **Enhanced antimalarialactivity of lumefantrine nanopowder prepared by wet-milling DYNO MILL technique.** *Colloids Surf B: Biointerf* 2012, **95:**16–22.

7.   Date AA, Nagarsenker MS: **Design and evaluation of self-nanoemulsifying drug delivery systems (SNEDDS) for cefpodoxime proxetil.** *Int J Pharm* 2007, **329:**166–172.

8.   Pawar SK, Vavia PR: **Rice Germ Oil as Multifunctional Excipient in Preparation of Self- Microemulsifying Drug Delivery System (SMEDDS) of Tacrolimus.** *AAPS PharmSciTech* 2012, **13:**254–261.

9.   Patel KD, Padhye SG, Nagarsenker MS: **Duloxetine HCl lipid nanoparticles: preparation, characterization, and dosage form design.** *AAPS Pharm Sci Tech* 2012, **13:**125–133.

10. Babalola CP, Adegoke AO, Ogunjinmi MA, Osimosu MO: **Determination of physicochemical properties of halofantrine.** *Afr J Med Med Sci* 2003, **32:**357–359.

11. Cuiné JF, McEvoy CL, Charman WN, Pouton CW, Edwards GA, Benameur H, Porter CJ: **Evaluation of the impact of surfactant digestion on the bioavailability of danazol after oral administration of lipidic self-emulsifying formulations to dogs.** *J Pharm Sci* 2008, **97:**995–1012.

12. Lopez-Montilla JC, Herrera-Morales PE, Pandey S, Shah D: **Spontaneous emulsification:mechanisms, physicochemical aspects, modeling and applications.** *J Disp Sci Techn* 2002, **23:**219–268.

13. Biradar SV, Dhumal RS, Paradkar AR: **Rheological investigation of self-emulsification process: effect of co-surfactant.** *J Pharm Pharm Sci* 2009, **12:**164–174.

14. Bindschedler M, Degen P, Lu ZL, Jiao XQ, Liu GY, Fan F: **Comparative biovailability of benflumetol after administration of single oral doses of co-artemether under fed and fasted conditions to healthy subjects (abstract P-01-96).** *Proceedings of the XIvth International Congress for Tropical Medicine and Malaria, Nagasaki, Japan* 1996:17–22.

15. Müller RH, Jacobs C, Kayser O: **Nanosuspensions as particulate drug formulations in therapy.** *Rationale for development and what we can expect for the future. Adv drug deliv rev* 2001, **23:**3–19.

16. Umapathi P, Ayyappan J, Quine SD: **Development and Validation of a Dissolution Test Method for Artemether and Lumefantrine in Tablets.** *Trop J Pharm Res* 2011, **10:**643–653.

Isolation and characterization of exopolysaccharide with immunomodulatory activity from fermentation broth of *Morchella conica*

Chao-an Su[1], Xiao-yan Xu[2], De-yun Liu[1], Ming Wu[2], Fan-qing Zeng[1], Meng-yao Zeng[2], Wei Wei[2], Nan Jiang[2] and Xia Luo[2*]

Abstract

Background and the purpose of this study: Mushroom polysaccharides have traditionally been used for the prevention and treatment of a multitude of disorders like infectious illnesses, cancers and various autoimmune diseases. *In vitro and in vivo* studies suggest that certain polysaccharides affect immune system function. *Morchella conica (M. conica)* is a species of rare edible mushroom whose multiple medicinal functions have been proven. Thus, the objective of this study is to isolate and characterize of exopolysaccharide from submerged mycelial culture of *M. conica,* and to evaluate its immunomodulatory activity.

Methods: A water-soluble *Morchella conica* Polysaccharides (MCP) were extracted and isolated from the fermentation broth of *M. conica* through a combination of DEAE-cellulose and Sephacryl S-300 HR chromatograph. NMR and IR spectroscopy has played a developing role in identification of polysaccharide with different structure and composition from fungal and plant sources, as well as complex glycosaminoglycans of animal origin. Thus, NMR and IR spectroscopy were used to analyze the chemical structure and composition of the isolated polysaccharide. Moreover, the polysaccharide was tested for its immunomodulatory activity at different concentrations using *in vitro* model.

Results: The results showed that MCP may significantly modulate nitric oxide production in macrophages, and promote splenocytes proliferation. Analysis from HPLC, infrared spectra and nuclear magnetic resonance spectroscopy showed that MCP was a homogeneous mannan with an average molecular weight of approximately 81.2 kDa. The glycosidic bond links is →6)-α-D-Man *p*-(1→.

Conclusion: The results suggested that the extracted MCP may modulate nitric oxide production in macrophages and promote splenocytes proliferation, and it may act as a potent immunomodulatory agent.

Keywords: Morchella conica, Exopolysaccharides, Submerged liquid culture, Immunomodulatory activity

Introduction

Medicinal mushrooms have become an attractive option for functional food or as a source for the development of pharmaceuticals and nutraceuticals. The medicinal properties are due to various cellular components and secondary metabolites, which have been isolated and identified from the fruiting-body, cultured mycelium and cultured broth of mushrooms [1]. Exopolysaccharides (EPS) are referred to secondary metabolite of microorganisms during the growth process, and secreted into the extracellular broth. Recently, many polysaccharides have been isolated from mushrooms [2]. They have emerged as an important class of bioactive natural products in the biochemical and medical areas due to their specific biological activities such as hepatoprotective, antioxidant activity, immunomodulatory property, inhibition early stages

---
* Correspondence: luox2009@163.com
[2]Laboratory of Cellular and Molecular Biology, Sichuan Academy of Chinese Medicine Science, Chengdu 610041, China
Full list of author information is available at the end of the article

of biofouling and gastroprotective effects [3]. The documented immune-active polysaccharides, isolated from *Opuntia polyacantha*, *Bupleurum smithii*, and *Sipunculus nudus*, exhibited innate immunomodulatory activities through enhancing phagocytosis of macrophages, increasing production of NO and secretion of cytokine [4-6]. Previous reports have demonstrated that EPS from *longan pulp*, and *Enteromorpha prolifera* may not only modulate macrophages activities, but also enhance the spleen lymphocyte proliferation and cytokine production [7,8]. These suggested that EPS represent a potential therapeutics with immunomodulatory action for their low toxicity and high potency.

Morchella conica, is an edible mushroom belonging to genus *Morchella*. It was used in Traditional Chinese Medicine to treat indigestion, excessive phlegm and shortness of breath. It has also been consumed as tasted food, health nutritional supplement for its high gastronomic quality, fatigue resistance and gastroprotective effects [9,10]. However, wild *Morchella conica* is difficult to culture, and its price is expensive price [11]. The fermentation broth of *M. conica* contains similar bioactive compounds and is rich in quantity compared with fermentation broth of *M. conica* and wild *M. conica*. Thus, bioactive compounds are obtained from fermentation broth of *M. conica*, and may serve as an ideal substitute for the wild *M. conica*, thereby resolving the problem of its limited production from wilds. To the best of our knowledge, there is no available report yet on the exopolysaccharides from fermentation broth of *Morchella conica*. In the present study, an immunomodulatory activity exopolysaccharide was isolated from submerged fermentation broth of *Morchella conica*. Beside, chemical structure of the isolated polysaccharide was also elucidated.

Material and method
Chemicals and materials
The strain of *Morchella conica* (labeled, No. 20110802) was obtained from the Sichuan Agricultural Academy of Sciences, Chengdu, China. DEAE-cellulose 52 and Sephacryl HR-300 were purchased from GE Healthcare Life Sciences (Uppsala, Sweden). Dextran T-2000, T-500, T-200 and T-70 were purchased from Pharmacia Co., Ltd. (Uppsala, Sweden). RAW264.7 cells were obtained from American Type Culture Collection (Manassass, VA, USA). Kunming mice (18~20 g) were obtained from the Animal Facility of the Institute of Chinese Traditional Medicine, Sichuan, China. The protocols of feeding were formed in accordance with the Guidelines of Institute of Chinese Traditional Medicine Animals Research Committee. All other reagents used were of analytical grade.

Extraction and isolation of exopolysaccharide
M. conica was cultured on synthetic potato dextrose agar (PDA) plates in a Petri dish at 25°C for 7 d. Then the seeds were grown in 250 ml Erlenmeyer flasks containing 100 ml liquid culture medium under agitation at 150 rev min^{-1} for 7 days at 25°C. 10% (v/v) of the seed culture was transferred into 20 L culture media (pH 6.4) on a rotary shaker incubator under agitation at 50 rev min^{-1} for 5 d at 28°C. The liquid culture medium used in this study is composed of 3 g/l glucose, 7 g/l sucrose, 3 g/l yeast extract, 5 g/l peptone, 0.1 g/l K_2HPO_4, 0.5 g/l KH_2PO_4, and 0.5 g/l $MgSO_4$. The fermentation broth was harvested and centrifuged at 3000 rpm for 20 min from the culture. After centrifuging, the supernatant was treated by the Sevag method to remove protein and lipid, etc. [12]. In brief, a mixed solution of chloroform: butanol = 4:1 was added in amount of 10% to the supernatant, which was stirred for 12 h. Then, this solution was subjected to centrifugal separation for 20 min at 10000 rpm to remove precipitation, and the supernatant was collected for next study. Next, after adding four-fold volume of 95% ethanol to this supernatant, the crude polysaccharide was obtained through precipitation. This agglutinant was filtered off to remove ethanol, and dialyzed for 12 h (MWCO 5000, Sigma) and lyophilized using Thermo Savant MODULYO freeze-dryer (EC Apparatus Corp., Holbrook, NY, USA) for further study. The sample was re-dissolved in 20 mM Tris–HCl (pH 8.0) and applied to DEAE-Cellulose 52 anion-exchange chromatography column (2.6 × 50 cm, Whatmann) equilibrated with 20 mM Tris–HCl (pH 8.0), and eluted with a linear gradient of NaCl from 0 mM to 500 mM in 20 mM Tris–HCl (pH 8.0) at a flow rate of 2 mL/min. The eluted samples were monitored by the phenol-sulfuric acid method [13], and the four yielded fractions were collected and combined. Subsequently, the samples were further subjected to Sephacryl S-300HR column (2.6 × 100 cm, Pharmacia Co.) and eluted with 10 mM NaCl at a flow rate of 1 mL/min. Fractions containing EPS were pooled and dialyzed. Then, the sample was subjected to lyophilized, and used directly for analysis or stored at -20°C for further study.

Innate and adaptive immunomodulatory activity of MCP
Measurement of NO production
RAW264.7 cells were plated in 24-well culture plates in RPMI 1640 at a density of 1×10^6 for 2 h. LPS (10 µg/ml), and different concentrations MCP (0, 50, 100, 200, 300, 400 and 500 µg/ml) were added, and the mixture was incubated for 48 h. Production of nitric oxide (NO) was measured according to the Griess method [14]. Briefly, supernatants were mixed with an equal volume of Griess reagent, which was prepared by mixing one part of 0.1% (w/v) N-(1-naphthyl) ethylenediamine with one part of 1% (w/v) sulfanilamide in 5% phosphoric acid. After 20 min,

absorbance was measured at 540 nm using a UV/vis spectrophotometer (TU-1901, Purkinje General, Beijing, China). The nitrite concentration was calculated using sodium nitrite as a standard.

Lymphocyte proliferation test in vitro

Spleen lymphocytes were prepared as reported previously with some modifications [15]. Briefly, mice were killed by cervical dislocation, and obtained spleen sterile. Medium containing spleen lymphocytes was collected, and added equal volume 0.83% Tris-NH$_4$Cl for lysis the red blood cells for 5 min. The suspended cells were centrifuged at 1500 rpm for 15 min, and resuspended with complete RPMI-1640. The resuspended cells were subsequently seeded onto culture plates for 1 h at 37°C and 5% CO$_2$ to remove the adherent cells. The non-adherent cells were designated as spleen lymphocytes. Cell viability was ≥95% in all experiments. The non-adherent cells, which were spleen lymphocytes, were plated in 96-well culture plates in RPMI 1640 at a density of 1×10^6. Different concentration MCP (0, 50, 100, 200, 300, 400 and 500 μg/ml) was added into 9-wells, and one of three wells added 5 μg/ml ConA, and the other three wells added 5 μg/ml LPS, the rest three wells was just MCP without ConA and LPS. The mixture was incubated for 72 h at 37°C and 5% CO$_2$. The splenocytes proliferation was assessed by using MTT-based colorimetric assay.

Measurement of homogeneity and molecular weight of MCP

The homogeneity and average molecular weight of MCP were measured and determined by the high performance gel permeation chromatography (HPGPC)method on a Waters 1525 HPLC system (Waters, Boston, US) equipped with a TSK gel 5000 PWXL column (7.8 × 300 mm, Tosoh Co., Tokyo, Japan) and a Alltech 2000ES (Alltech Associates, Inc., USA) Evaporative Light Scatttering Detector (ELSD). The molecular weight was estimated by reference to the calibration curve made under the conditions described above from Dextran T-series standards (T70, T200, T500 and T2000) of known molecular weight.

Monosaccharide composition analysis of MCP

The polysaccharide, MCP (~2 mg), was hydrolysed with 2 M trifluoroacetic acid (TFA) for 10 h at 110°C in a sealed glass tube. When the residual acid was removed using methyl alcohol, and the hydrolysate was analyzed by HPLC/ELSD system. The chromatograph was fitted with an Alltech Prevail carbohydrate column (Alltech Associates, Inc., USA). Results were compared with the following monosaccharide standards: D-glucose, L-rhamnose, D-xylose, D-galactose, D-mannose and L-arabinose.

Analysis of Infrared (IR) spectra and Nuclear magnetic resonance (NMR)

IR spectroscopy, and ^{1}H and ^{13}C NMR were used to analyze the structural features of MCP. IR spectrum of MCP were recorded on a Fourier transform infrared spectroscopy (Nicolet 170 SX, FTIR, US), and the test specimens of polysaccharide film were prepared by KBr-disk method. The ^{1}H and ^{13}C NMR measurements were carried out at 600 and 150 Hz, respectively, on a Bruke 600 Hz NMR instrument (Bruker Avance, Karlsruhe, Germany). All chemical shifts were in relative to Me$_4$Si.

Statistical analysis

Data were expressed as means ± SD. The significance of difference was evaluated with one-way ANOVA, followed by Student's t-test to statistically identify differences between the control and treated groups. Significant differences were set at $P < 0.05$ and $P < 0.01$.

Results and discussion
Isolation and purification of polysaccharide

During EPS isolation and purification, removing abundant protein, DNA and RNA contaminations in *Morchella conica* extract was an essential step when obtaining EPS. Different methods obtained from the literature were tested to efficiently isolate the soluble EPS fraction from harvested cells [1]. These contaminations were effectively removed by precipitating with 95% ethanol, dialyzed, DEAE-Cellulose 52 anion-exchange (Figure 1) and Sephacryl S-300HR chromatography (data not shown) during the purification procedure. Several sample fractions were taken after each treatment and the relative purification was determined using Nanodrop (DNA and

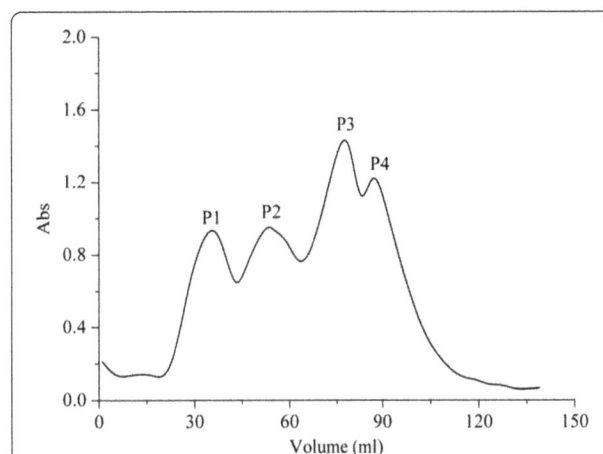

Figure 1 Elution pattern of the crude polysaccharide produced from submerged mycelial culture of *M. conica* on DEAE-Cellulose 52 anion-exchange chromatography column (2.6 × 50 cm, Whatmann). The four peaks of P1, P2, P3 and P4 were eluted with a linear gradient of NaCl from 0 mM to 500 mM in 20 mM Tris–HCl (pH 8.0), and the activity were also measured.

Table 1 Purification and production yields of Morchella conica polysaccharide

Steps	Volume (ml)	Concentration (mg/ml)	Total Polysaccharide (mg)	Yield (%)
Crude extract	1000	1.06	10600	100
Pre-treatment	150.3	45.9	6898.8	65.1
DEAE-cellulose	17.4	38.5	669.9	6.32
Sephacryl S-300	26.3	20.5	539.2	5.09

Total polysaccharide is equal to Volume × Concentration. Data represent mean values ± SD (n =3).

protein) quantification, protein assays and a total carbohydrate assay. As a result, a peak of P3 represents the purified EPS with the purity up to 95%, which designed as MCP. Thus, this process may isolate approximately 539.2 mg EPS from one liter fermentation broth of *M. conica* (Table 1).

Molecular weight and monosaccharide composition

Molecular weight has been recognized as a critical parameter in the antigenicity of polysaccharides. Most polysaccharides with medicinal properties are high molecules above 100 kDa of molecular weight. Moreover, some polysaccharides have low molecular weights, such as polysaccharide from *Ganoderma lucidum* (8 kDa, 22 kDa), *Euphorbia fischeriana* (49.5 kDa) *and Armillariella tabescens* (49.5 kDa), etc., which were found to exhibit bioactivity [14,16,17]. The molecular weight of purified MCP was about 81.2 kDa by HPLC analysis using dextrans as standards, which was in the range reported for other mushroom polysaccharides. According to HPLC equipped with a Alltech Prevail

carbohydrate column and ELSD analyzing, it was found that MCP was composed of only one monosaccharide, D-mannose (data not shown).

Structure elucidation of MCP

It well known that the configuration of polysaccharides was very important for the biological activity. Most of documented immuno-active polysaccharides from medicinal fungi are β-glycosidic linkage polysaccharides [4,16,18]. Recent reports suggested that polysaccharides with α-glycosidic linkage exhibit immune activity from *Ganoderma lucidum, Armillariella tabescens,* and *Cordyceps sinensis* [15,17,19]. As shown in Figure 2, the intensity of bands around 3424.93 cm^{-1} in the IR spectrum was due to the -OH stretching vibration of the polysaccharide and as expected they were broad. The bands in the region of 2887.40 cm^{-1} were due to C-H stretching vibration, and the bands in the region of 1635.29 cm^{-1} were due to associated water. Three strong absorption bands at 1060.87 cm^{-1}, 1101.31 cm^{-1} and 1149.31 cm^{-1} in the range of 1200-1000 cm^{-1} in the IR spectrum suggested that the monosaccharide in MCP had a pyranose-ring. The absorption at 842.77 cm^{-1} indicated that MCP had α-glucopyranose linkages. These findings suggested that the MCP have α-glycosidic linkage in the molecule configuration. As shown in Figure 3, the resonances in the region of 98-106 ppm in the ^{13}C NMR spectrum of MCP were attributed to the anomeric carbon atoms of mannopyranose (Man*p*), which was in good agreement with the monosaccharide composition [20]. Bases on the above results, it could be concluded that MCP was α-mannopyranose, composed of a repeating unit with the possible structure as [→6)-α-D-Man*p*-(1→6)-[α-D-Man*p*-(1→6)-]n-α-D-Man*p*-(1→.

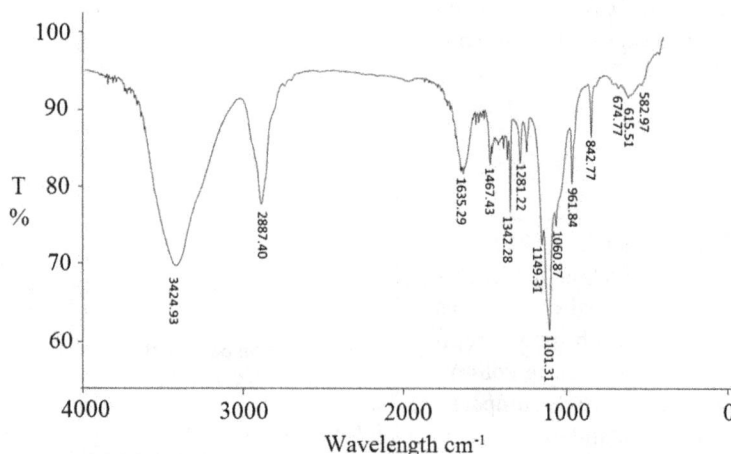

Figure 2 IR analysis of *M. conica* polysaccharides (MCP).

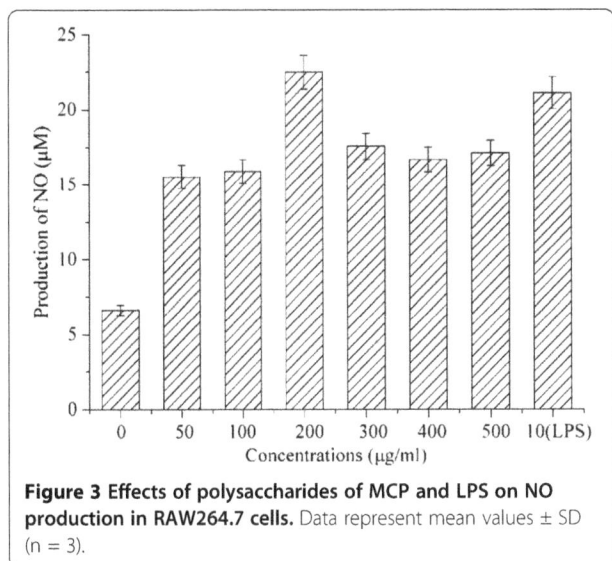

Figure 3 Effects of polysaccharides of MCP and LPS on NO production in RAW264.7 cells. Data represent mean values ± SD (n = 3).

Measurement of NO production in vitro

After RAW264.7 cells were incubated with different concentrations of polysaccharides (0, 50, 100, 200, 300, 400 and 500 μg/ml) or LPS (10 μg/ml) for 24 h, NO concentrations in culture supernatants were assessed by NO_2^- contents in the Griess reaction. As shown in Figure 3, 10 μg/ml LPS could significantly increase production of NO (p<0.01), and MCP may significantly induce the production of NO with a dose-dependent manner at 50-200 μg/ml. However, the stimulate roles showed decrease treads when the concentrations of EPS concentrations are higher than 200 μg/ml. Earlier studies showed that the mannose receptor (MR) was existed on the cell surface of macrophage, and involved in the process of production reactive oxidants, phagocytosis, and endocytosis [21]. The polysaccharides with mannose, trehalose and N-acetyl glucosamine residues may bind to MR, and then the complex may active macrophage *via* NF-κB pathway or other signaling pathways, which will enhance the secretion of cytokines, such as IL-1β, IL-6, and GM-CSF, etc. [22,23]. Thus, they play critical role in cell-mediated immunity and humoral immunity. In the present study, results showed that MCP may induce the production of NO, and modulate the innate immune response at the specific concentration ranges.

Lymphocyte proliferation in vitro

Lymphocyte proliferation is a crucial event in the activation cascade of both cellular and humoral immune responses [3,24]. To investigate the immunomodulatory effect of the polysaccharides, MTT assay was used to evaluate spleen lymphocyte proliferation (Figure 4). The results showed that MCP may promote lymphocyte proliferation in dose-dependent manner. These results are

similar with the additions of LPS and/or ConA on lymphocyte proliferation (p<0.05). At a lower concentration of 50 μg/ml, MCP could significantly enhance the proliferation of lymphocyte (P<0.05), and the MCP concentration of 500 μg/ml exhibited the highest co-mitogenic activities compared to those of the normal control groups. It is well known that lymphocyte proliferation effect were either directly activated or by the cytokines exopolysaccharide-induced by other cells secretion such as macrophages and natural killer (NK). Earlier reports suggested that polysaccharides from *Morchella esculenta* could directly activate T cells [24]. Moreover, ConA also can selectively promote the proliferation of T cells. Thus, the effects of MCP on lymphocyte proliferation may be an adaptive immune response *via* T cell-mediated. However, the mechanism of MCP is directly activated *via* T cells or by the cytokines need further study.

Conclusion

Culture of *M. conica* fruiting bodies usually takes at least three months; therefore compared with the extraction of polysaccharides from the fruiting bodies of *M. conica*, the production and purification of polysaccharides from fermentation broth can significantly shorten the culture period and provide a faster way of polysaccharide production. In the present study, we showed, for the first time that the polysaccharides isolated and characterized from fermentation broth of *M. conica*. In addition, it is important to note that MCP has immunomodulatory activity, and may be seen as a promising immunopotentiating agent in health-care food or the treatment of infectious diseases. Further in-depth study will focus on between the mechanism of immunomodulatory activity and structure-function relationship.

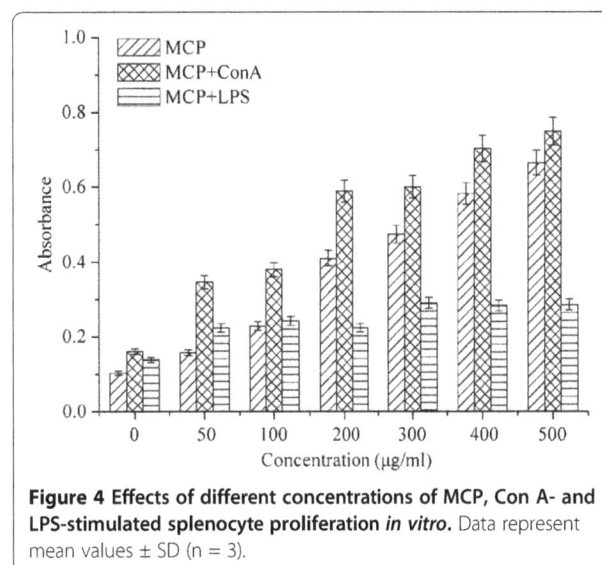

Figure 4 Effects of different concentrations of MCP, Con A- and LPS-stimulated splenocyte proliferation *in vitro*. Data represent mean values ± SD (n = 3).

Competing interests
The authors declare that they have no competing interests.

Authors' contribution
CS, Experiment operator; XX, data collection and analysis; DL, literature search; MW, Manuscript editing and review; FZ, Manuscript editing and review; MY, fermentation culture assistant; WW, fermentation culture assistant; NJ, figures preparation; LX, Experiment design and manuscript writing. All authors read and approved the final manuscript.

Acknowledgements
This work was supported by Fungus medicine research and development of Sichuan Provincial Science and Technology Innovation Team, Sichuan mushroom innovative team deep processing of post construction project (Chuan [2009] No. 75), Resource collection and breeding of medicinal fungi, and Sichuan Province Key Scientific and Technological Projects.

Author details
[1]Lishui Agricultural Academy of Sciences, Lishui, Zhejiang 32300, China. [2]Laboratory of Cellular and Molecular Biology, Sichuan Academy of Chinese Medicine Science, Chengdu 610041, China.

References
1. Wasser SP: Current findings, future trends, and unsolved problems in studies of medicinal mushrooms. *Appl Microbiol Biotechnol* 2011, **89**:1323–1332.
2. Stachowiak B, Reguła J: Health-promoting potential of edible macromycetes under special consideration of polysaccharides: a review. *Eur Food Res Technol* 2012, **234**:369–380.
3. Borchers AT, Krishnamurthy A, Keen CL, Meyers FJ, Gershwin ME: The immunobiology of mushrooms. *Exp Biol Med* 2008, **233**:259–276.
4. Schepetkin IA, Xie G, Kirpotina LN, Klein RA, Jutila MA, Quinn MT: Macrophage immunomodulatory activity of polysaccharides isolated from *Opuntia polyacantha. Int Immunopharmacol* 2008, **8**:1455–1466.
5. Cheng XQ, Li H, Yue XL, Xie JY, Zhang YY, Di HY, Chen DF: Macrophage immunomodulatory activity of the polysaccharides from the roots of Bupleurum smithii var. parvifolium. *Ethnopharmacol* 2010, **130**:363–368.
6. Zhang CX, Dai ZR: Immunomodulatory activities on macrophage of a polysaccharide from *Sipunculus nudus* L. *Food Chem Toxicol* 2011, **49**:2961–2967.
7. Kuang H, Xia Y, Yang B, Wang Q, Wang Y: Screening and comparison of the immunosuppressive activities of polysaccharides from the stems of *Ephedra sinica Stapf. Carbohydr Polymers* 2011, **83**:787–795.
8. Kim JK, Cho ML, Karnjanapratum S, Shin IS, You SG: *In vitro* and *in vivo* immunomodulatory activity of sulfated polysaccharides from *Enteromorpha prolifera. Int J Biol Macromol* 2011, **49**:1051–1058.
9. Gursoy N, Sarikurkcu C, Cengiz M, Solak MH: Antioxidant activities, metal contents, total phenolics and flavonoids of seven *Morchella* species. *Food Chem Toxicol* 2009, **47**:2381–2388.
10. Ismet O, Serkan S, Ugur S, Lutfiye E, Osman S: Bioactivity and mineral contents of wild-grown edible *Morchella conica* in the Mediterranean Region. *J Consumer Protection Food Safety* 2010, **5**:453–457.
11. Turkoglu A, Kivrak I, Mercan N, Duru ME, Gezer K, Turkoglu H: Antioxidant and antimicrobial activities of *Morchella conica Pers. Afr J Biotechnol* 2006, **5**:1146–1150.
12. Alum N, Gupta PC: Structure of a water-soluble polysaccharide from the seeds of *Cassia angustifolia. Planta Med* 1986, **50**:308–310.
13. Masuko T, Minami A, Iwasaki N, Majima T, Nishimura S, Lee YC: Carbohydrate analysis by a phenol-sulfuric acid method in microplate format. *Anal Biochem* 2005, **339**:69–72.
14. Schepetkin IA, Faulkner CL, Nelson-Overton LK, Wiley JA, Quinn MT: Macrophage immunomodulatory activity of polysaccharides isolated from *Juniperus scopolorum. Int Immunopharmacol* 2005, **5**:1783–1799.
15. Luo X, Xu XY, Yu MY, Yang ZR, Zheng LY: Characterisation and immunostimulatory activity of an [alpha]-(1->6)-d-glucan from the cultured Armillariella tabescens mycelia. *Food Chem* 2008, **111**:357–363.
16. Liu J, Sun Y, Yu C, Liu L: Chemical structure of one low molecular weight and water-soluble polysaccharide (EFP-W1) from the roots of *Euphorbia fischeriana. Food Chem* 2012, **87**:1236–1240.
17. Joseph S, Sabulal B, George V, Antony KR, Janardhanan KK: Antitumor and anti-inflammatory activities of polysaccharides isolated from *Ganoderma lucidum. Acta Pharm* 2011, **61**:335–342.
18. Jung YS, Yang BK, Jeong YT, Islam R, Kim SM, Song CH: Immunomodulating activities of water-soluble exopolysaccharides obtained from submerged culture of Lentinus lepideus. *J Microbiol Biotechnol* 2008, **18**:1431–1438.
19. Wang ZM, Peng X, Daniel Lee KL, Cheuk-on TJ, Chi-Keung Cheung P, Wu JY: Structural characterisation and immunomodulatory property of an acidic polysaccharide from mycelial culture of *Cordyceps sinensis* fungus Cs-HK1. *Food Chem* 2011, **125**:637–643.
20. Zhao GH, Kan JQ, Li ZX, Chen ZD: Structural features and immunological activity of a polysaccharide from *Dioscorea opposita Thunb* roots. *Carbohydr Polymers* 2005, **61**:125–131.
21. Schepetkin IA, Quinn MT: Botanical polysaccharides: macrophage immunomodulation and therapeutic potential. *Int Immunopharmacol* 2006, **6**:317–333.
22. Jiang Z, Hama Y, Yamaguchi K, Oda T: Inhibitory effect of sulphated polysaccharide porphyran on nitric oxide production in lipopolysaccharide-stimulated RAW264.7 macrophages. *J Biochem* 2012, **151**:65–74.
23. Monick MM, Hunninghake GW: Activation of second messenger pathways in alveolar macrophages by endotoxin. *Eur Respir J* 2002, **20**:210–222.
24. Lai CY, Hung JT, Lin HH, Yu AL, Chen SH, Tsai YC, Shao LE, Yang WB, Yu J: Immunomodulatory and adjuvant activities of a polysaccharide extract of *Ganoderma lucidum in vivo* and *in vitro. Vaccine* 2010, **28**:4945–4954.

Biological activity and microscopic characterization of *Lythrum salicaria* L

Azadeh Manayi[1], Mahnaz Khanavi[1,2], Soodabeh Saiednia[3], Ebrahim Azizi[4], Mohammad Reza Mahmoodpour[1], Fatemeh Vafi[1], Maryam Malmir[5], Farideh Siavashi[6] and Abbas Hadjiakhoondi[1,3*]

Abstract

Background: There are several plants have been used worldwide in the folk medicine with high incidence for treatment of human disorders, of which *Lythrum salicaria* belongs to the Lythraceae family has traditionally reputation for some medicinal usage and recently many biological and pharmacological activity of the plant have been studied.

Methods: In this study, microscopic characterizations of the aerial parts of the plant were determined. Moreover, the plant extract (aqueous methanol 80%) was subjected to an anti-diabetic activity test (in a rat model of streptozocin induced diabetes), anti-*Helicobacter pylori* (using disc diffusion method) along with antioxidant activity against DPPH (stable free radical) tests. Besides, total flavonoids, phenols, tannins, as well as polysaccharides contents have been assessed using spectroscopic methods.

Results: The microscopic properties of the plant fragments revealed anomocytic stomata, conical shape trichomes, and abundant spherical pollen grains as a characteristic pattern for the aerial parts of the plant. The extract of the plant at concentration of 15 g/kg showed mild lowering activity on blood glucose level to 12.6% and 7.3% after 2 and 3 h of administration. Additionally, clinically isolated *H. pylori* strain was inhibited with the plant extract at concentration of 500 mg/mL (zone of inhibition: 17 ± 0.08 mm). Moreover, IC_{50} values for DPPH inhibition of the plant extract, vitamin E, BHA were examined as 13.5, 14.2, and 7.8 µg/mL, respectively. Total flavonoids, phenols, tannin, and polysaccharides contents of the extract were successfully evaluated as 5.8 ± 0.4 µg QE/mg EXT, 331 ± 3.7 µg GAE/mg EXT, 340 ± 2.3 µg TAE/mg EXT, 21 ± 0.2 µg GE/mg EXT, respectively.

Conclusions: The results suggested that *L. salicaria* has low anti-diabetic and anti-*Helicobacter pylori* effects, but high antioxidant activity, just the same as positive standard (vitamin E), which might be attributed to the high content of phenolic compounds in the extract.

Keywords: *Lythrum salicaria*, Antioxidant, Diabetes, *H. pylori*, Microscopy characterization

Background

Plants have performed a substantial role in traditional treatment or prevention of the complexity of diseases. They reduce the risk of many chronic diseases including diabetes, cancer, cardiovascular disorders and other sicknesses [1]. Identification of the plants powders is a complex criterion for herbalist. Although recognition of plant materials is one of the main concerns in phytotherapy, microscopical examination has been accepted as a standard technique for determination of herbal drugs in a powdered mixture [2].

Lythrum salicaria is a perennial herbaceous plant belonging to the Lythraceae family, which consists of 30 species. Seven of the mentioned species are growing wildly in Iran. This plant distributed in the north and north-west of Iran in the wetlands near streams [3,4]. The plant is well- known as "Turbinkwash", "Yerpoose" and "Surmankhal" in Persian language [4]. Despite of the fact that this plant was considered as a wild invasive herb, its flowering aerial part has been used as a medicinal plant from ancient time. Aerial parts of the plant

* Correspondence: abbhadji@tums.ac.ir
[1]Department of Pharmacognosy, Faculty of Pharmacy, Tehran University of Medical Sciences, Tehran, Iran
[3]Medicinal Plants Research Center, Faculty of Pharmacy, Tehran University of Medical Sciences, Tehran, Iran
Full list of author information is available at the end of the article

have been traditionally employed for treatment of diarrhoea, dysentery, inflammation of intestine, haematuria, leucorrhoea, epitaxis and dysmenorrhoea. Additionally, the plant used externally for cleaning impetigo, eczema, lupus and inflammation of female genito-urinary system in the north-west of Iran [5]. Scientific investigations of *L. salicaria* recently demonstrated antibacterial, antifungal, antioxidant, anti-inflammatory, anti-nociceptive, and cytotoxicity effects [6-10]. The literatures revealed that *L. salicaria* extracts showed decreasing activity on blood glucose level in both normoglycemic and glucose induced hyperglycemic rats as well as rabbits through augmentation of insulin secretion, and also it could reduce the plasma level of triglycerides [11,12]. Betulinic acid and its derivatives, isolated from ethyl acetate extract of the plant, exhibited suppressive activity on human Acyl-CoA: cholesterol acyl transferase (hACAT), suggesting that the plant might be useful for the hypercholesterolemia and atherosclerosis treatment and prevention [13]. Lately, anti-tussive and bronchodilator activity of the plant was determined due to polysaccharide-polyphenolic conjugate in the guinea pig [14]. Moreover, the high mass molecules (polysaccharide-polyphenolic conjugate) showed controversial anticoagulant and procoagulant effects in the preceding experiments [15,16]. Phytochemical purification of the plant have been revealed the presence of various bioactive compounds such as tannins, flavonoids, phenolic acids, anthocyanins, alkaloids, sterols, and triterpens in preceding studies [6,17-19]. It is also explored that there are three forms of plant flowers varying in both size and type of stigma, which facilitate legitimate pollination [20].

In the present study, microscopic characterization of the aerial parts of the plant as well as anti-diabetic, anti-*Helicobacter pylori*, and antioxidant effects of the aqueous methanol extract (80%) of *L. salicaria* have been assessed along with phytochemical contents of the extract. This is the first report of the microscopic structural characterization and anti-*Helicobacter pylori* activity of the plant followed by polysaccharides content.

Methods
Plant material
Aerial parts of *L. salicaria* were collected in May 2011 from Lahidjan city, Guilan province in the north of Iran and has been deposited at the Herbarium of Institute of Medicinal Plants, Jahade-Daneshgahi (ACECR), Karaj, Iran (Ajani 313). The cleaned plant materials were dried in the shade at room temperature and extracted with aqueous methanol (80%) using percolation apparatus.

Powdered plant characterization
One gram of each tissue powder (flower, leave, and stem) of *L. salicaria* was heated in potassium hydroxide

solution (10%) in a backer on heater for 30 seconds (flower and leave) or 1 minute (stem) depending on the tissue hardness, and washed afterwards with distilled water three times. The treated powders were sequentially washed with sodium hypochlorite for whitening and then rinsing with distilled water. The preparation was mounted in aqueous glycerin [2]. Photomicrographs were taken using Zeiss microscope attached with a digital camera. Photomicrographs of sections were captured at various magnifications conditional upon the microscopic details to be observed.

Anti-diabetic test

Animals
Male Wistar rats weighing about 190–200 g body weight were housed at standard laboratory conditions and fed with rodent pellet diet and water *ad libitum*. The animals were kept at room temperature and a photoperiod of 12 h day/night cycle. They considered as fasted were deprived of food for 14 h but had free access to water. The rats were obtained from animal house of Faculty of Pharmacy, Tehran University of Medical Sciences. All ethical manners for use of animals in scientific research have been carefully considered.

Induction of diabetes
Streptozocin (STZ) was freshly prepared in normal saline (22 mg/mL). Type 2 diabetes mellitus (T2DM) was induced in overnight fasted rats by a single intraperitoneal injection of STZ (55 mg/kg). Hyperglycemia was confirmed polydipsia, polyuria and by the elevated glucose degree in plasma, calculated at 60 h after injection by glucometer. Rats with a blood glucose level above 250 mg/dL were choosing for the experiments.

In vivo determination of anti-diabetic activity (T2DM model)
The animals (n = 24) were divided into four groups of six animals. The extract of the plant dissolved in DMSO that orally administered to the experimental groups (15 and 12.5 g/kg body weight) and a control group were also fed with DMSO (10 mL/kg). Previous investigation demonstrated that LD$_{50}$ of DMSO (lethal dose, 50%) in rats is 20 mL/kg [21]. Glibenclamide (3 mg/kg) was administered to the diabetic rats as a positive control. Samples of blood were achieved from the tail at 1, 2 and 3 h after vehicle, samples and drug administration. Concentration of blood glucose was estimated by enzymatic glucose oxidase method using a commercial glucometer (Accucheck, Germany). The percentage variation of

glycemia for each group was calculated in relation to initial (0 h) level, according to:

$$\%\text{Variation of glycemia} = [(Gi\text{-}G0)/G0] \times 100$$

G0: initial glycemia values and Gi: glycemia values at 1, 2 and 3 h, respectively.

Assay of anti-*Helicobacter pylori* effect

Helicobacter pylori were isolated from patients with chronic gastritis who had been introduced to the Endoscopy Unit at Shariati Hospital, Tehran, Iran. The biopsies from patient with antrum gastritis or peptic ulcer and positive rapid urea breath test were cultured on selective brucella agar under microaerobic situation. Isolated *H. pylori* were characterized using Gram stains, exhibited Gram negative spiral forms, positive urease, oxidase and catalase tests. The surface of brucella agar plus 7-8% blood plates were inoculated with 100 μL of bacterial suspension (bacterial suspensions in normal saline with the turbidity of McFarland standard No. 2 equivalent to 6×10^8 cell/mL) and dried at room temperature for 10 min. Afterwards, the sterile blank disc (diameter: 6 mm) were impregnated in the plant extract (500 mg/mL) and placed on the plates, these plates were incubated at 37°C under microaerobic conditions and examined after 3–5 days [22]. Positive control plates included discs impregnated with amoxicillin (1 μg/mL) and the inhibition zone diameters (IZD) were recorded.

Free radical scavenging activity assay

Free stable radical, 2,2-Diphenyl-1-picryl-hydrazyl (DPPH), has been widely used to evaluate the free radical scavenging activity of natural products. The plant extract activity against free radical was examined by DPPH method which described previously [23]. The absorptions at 517 nm were measured after 30 min. Free radical 50% inhibition (IC_{50}) provided by extracts concentrations were calculated according to the plot of inhibition percentage against extracts concentration. Besides, vitamin E and BHA were used as positive standards.

Assay of total flavonoids

The flavonoids content were measured at 425 nm by creating a complex with $AlCl_3$ in a methanol-ethyl acetate-acetic acid medium [24]. The contents of total flavonoids, expressed as quercetin equivalent in the extract (μg QE/mg EXT), were calculated from following expression: $(A \times 0.875)/b$

A: the absorbance of the test solution at 425 nm
b: the mass of the powdered extract in grams

Assay of total phenols

Total phenolics content of the plant extract was examined and expressed as gallic acid equivalent (μg GAE/mg EXT) using Folin Ciocalteu method [23]. The sample absorbance was compared to gallic acid calibration curve.

Assay of total tannins

The method of total tannins could be coupled with the use of insoluble matrix, polyvinylpolypyrrolidone (PVPP) which binds with tannin-phenolics for measurement of tannins. The percentage of total tannins was calculated as tannic acid equivalent in dry extract (μg TAE/mg EXT) using tannic acid calibration curve (Y = 0.042X + 0.077, r^2 = 0.974) [25].

Determination of total polysaccharides

Total sugar (including polysaccharides) content or polysaccharides content was determined according to previous study [26]. In this method, all the glycosidic linkages in the presence of sulfuric acid are broken and a colored aromatic complex achieved between phenol and the carbohydrate, afterwards absorbance of this complex was measured. The samples absorptions were compared to calibration curve of different concentration of glucose (5–50 μg/mL) and the results reported as glucose equivalent in the extract (μg GE/mg EXT) using glucose calibration curve (Y = 0.014X + 0.024, R^2 = 0.998).

General

Substances (all by analytical grades) including solvents, glucose, gallic acid, Folin Ciocalteu, DMSO and brucella agar were purchased from Merck (Germany), along with Glibenclamide and STZ purchased from Tehran Chemistry (Iran) and Pharmacia and Upjohn (USA), respectively.

Statistical analysis

All values were expressed as mean ± SE. Statistical significance was estimated by analysis of variance (ANOVA) following by Tukey post hoc test for multiple comparisons, $p < 0.05$ implies significance.

Results and discussion
Microscopic characterization

Microscopic structures of *L. salicaria* aerial parts provide a useful and reliable criterion to the examination of powdered materials of the herb. The fragments of corolla were abundant in the powder of the plant aerial parts (Figure 1). The epidermal cells of corolla possessed thin, wavy walls with striated cuticle and also the calyx epidermis with anomocytic stomata and cicatrix were observed in the flower fragments. The fragments of the styles and stigmas were found in the powder, the structure of style was composed of thin-walled, longitudinally

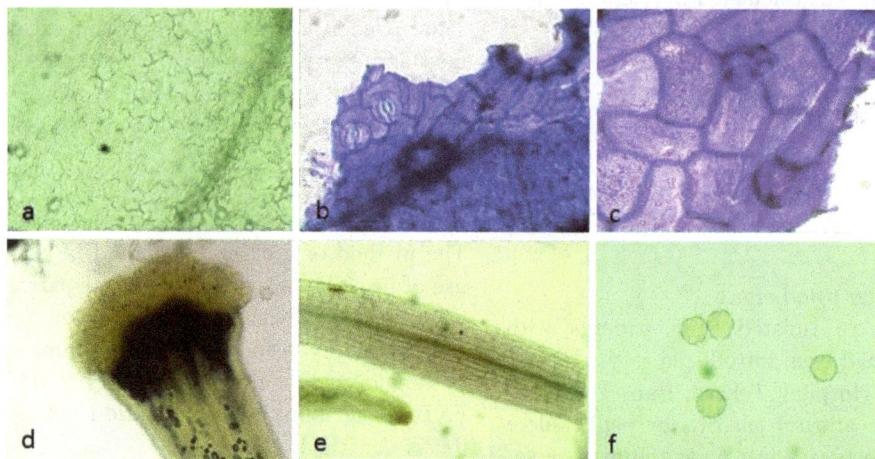

Figure 1 Microscopic characterization of *L. salicaria* flower, a: corolla epidermis cells, b: anomocytic stomata of calyx, c: cicatrix of calyx, d: papillae of stigma and style, e: anther in surface view, f: pollen grains.

elongated cells. The epidermal cells of the apices of the stigmas were extended to form elongated, finger like papillae. Moreover, the occasional fragments of the fibrous layer of the anthers were composed of fairly large cells, while the abundant small spherical pollen grains were discovered with some furrows and a finely pitted exine. The cells of upper epidermis of the leaf were larger than lower epidermis; both were thin-walled in surface view (Figure 2). The walls of the epidermis cells were sinuous or wavy shapes and almost anomocytic stomata observed on both surfaces. The palisade cells underlying the upper epidermis were large and closely packed. The spongy mesophyll was composed of thin-walled spherical cells, in which the clusters of calcium oxalate were found. Covering trichomes were found abundantly on both epidermises, mainly along the veins on the lower epidermis. They were all conical and taper abruptly to a point at the apex, composed of one or two cells with slightly thickened and warty walls. The fragments of the stems consisted of large annularly, spiral, and reticulate thickened vessels accompanied with fibrous layer in some cases (Figure 3). The anomocytic stomata with cicatrix and covering trichomes were also observed in the stem parts of the plant same as other segments.

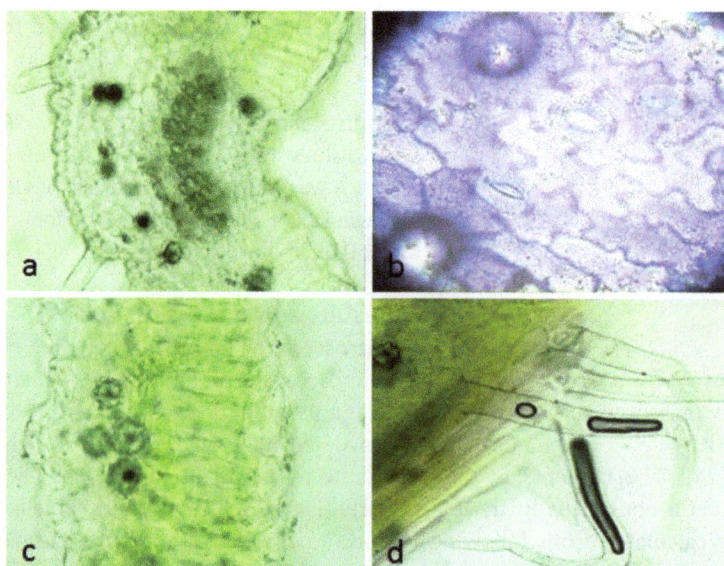

Figure 2 Microscopic characterization of *L. salicaria* leaf, a: leaf in the sectional view, b: epidermis with sinuous cell walls, anomocytic stomata and cicatrix, c: upper and lower epidermises, palisade cells and mesophylls containing calcium oxalate clusters, d: covering trichomes.

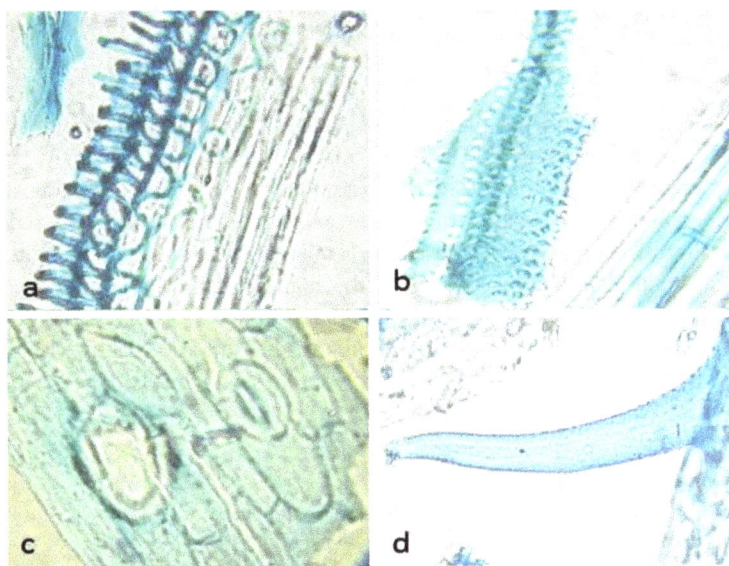

Figure 3 Microscopic characterization of *L. salicaria* stem, a: vessels of the stem with spiral thickening, b: vessels with reticulate thickening and fibrous layer, c: anomocytic stomata and cicatrix, d: covering trachoma attached to the stem.

Anti-diabetic activity

Anti-diabetic activity of the plant extract was tested using STZ-induced diabetic rats (Table 1). The results of this study revealed that the extract (15 g/kg) was significantly decreased blood glucose level. The plant extract (at dose of 15 g/kg) could reduce the blood glucose level by 12.6% and 7.3% during the second and third hours of administration, respectively. However, the rats treated with glibenclamide showed decreasing by 227% significantly after 2 h of administration. The plant extract with concentration of 12.5 g/kg was not effective to decrease the blood glucose level in the diabetic rats. The present results are in consistency with previous reports on hypoglycemic effect of *L. salicaria* extract suggesting augmentation of insulin secretion from langerhans cells [11,27]. Additionally, bioactive compounds of the plant

Table 1 Biological activity and phytochemical contents of *L. salicaria* extract

Various biological assays	Results (mean ± SE)
Anti-diabetic[1]	−12.6%[2]
Anti-helicobacter	17 ± 0.08 mm[3]
Antioxidant	13.52[4]
Total flavonoids	5.8 ± 0.4 µg QE/mg EXT[5]
Total phenols	331 ± 3.7 µg GAE/mg EXT[6]
Total tannins	340 ± 2.3 µg TAE/mg EXT[7]
Total polysaccharides	21 ± 0.21 µg GE/mg EXT[8]

1: The plant extract was tested using STZ-induced diabetic rats, 2: % variation of glycemia in the second hour, 3: inhibition zone diameter (IZD), 4: free radical 50% inhibition (IC_{50}), 5: quercetin equivalent in the extract (QE/EXT), 6: gallic acid equivalent in the extract (GAE/EXT), 7: tannic acid equivalent in the extract (TAE/EXT), 8: glucose equivalent in the extract (GE/EXT).

have been previously isolated and identified as ursolic acid and oleanolic acid [6]. The mentioned triterpenes, purified from the *L. salicaria* extract, possess pentacylic structure with carboxylic functional group at C28, which forms an extensive hydrogen bond network. Previous results revealed that oleanolic acid administration to STZ-induced diabetic rats can significantly reduce the blood glucose level [28]. Moreover, these triterpenic acids are reported to induce a significant inhibition on protein tyrosine phosphatase 1B (PTP-1B), as an important enzyme, to influence insulin sensitivity through enhancing insulin receptor phosphorylation and stimulating glucose uptake [29,30]. Oleanolic acid was also able to enhance insulin secretion just the same as sulfonylurea at both basal and glucose-stimulated conditions in cultured cell [31]. Generally, *L. salicaria* extract is weakly able to decrease the blood glucose level probably by two mechanisms including high insulin secretion and sensitivity attributed to its active components.

Anti-*Helicobacter pylori* activity

L. salicaria traditionally has been used for some intestinal disorders. Therefore, in the present study its anti-*Helicobacter* activity was assessed against clinically isolated strain. In the preliminary evaluation, the plant extract exhibited low inhibitory activity against *H. pylori* isolated from patient with gastric disorder using disc diffusion method (Table 1). The extract of the plant (500 mg/mL) and Amoxicillin (1 µg/mL) inhibited the growth of the strain with zone diameter of inhibition as 17 ± 0.08 and 30 ± 0.04 mm, respectively. In addition, blood hemolysis was observed in the culture medium of the bacterium treated with the plant extract.

Antioxidant activity

Value of IC_{50} for radical scavenging activity of the plant extract was also measured as 13.5 µg/mL using DPPH method (Table 1). Antioxidant activities of vitamin E and BHA were tested as positive controls and IC_{50} values of them evaluated as 14.2, and 7.8 (µg/mL), respectively. The plant extract showed higher free radical inhibition than vitamin E. Previous preliminary studies have also exhibited antioxidant effect of the polar extracts of *L. salicaria* corroborating the results of this study [8,32].

Phytochemical contents of the extract

The plant extract was subjected to chemical evaluation in the present study using different methods (Table 1). However, various genuine compounds (gallic acid, tannic acid and glucose) were employed to depict of standard curves in order to estimate the concentration of those components. Total contents of flavonoids, phenols, and tannins as well as polysaccharides were measured in the extract as 5.8 ± 0.4 µg QE/mg EXT, 331 ± 3.7 µg GAE/mg EXT, 340 ± 2.3 µg TA/mg EXT, and 21 ± 0.2 µg GE/mg EXT, respectively. Various extracts of the plant were previously subjected to evaluation of flavonoids, phenols, and tannins contents together with antioxidant activity [32,33]. The results indicate that the phytochemical contents are found here in less concentration than those reported in previous study. This condition could be attributed to different plants origins and also application of diverse extraction methods.

Conclusions

Taking together, microscopic structures of the plant powder, mentioned in this paper, could be an important identification method for determining the plant identity in the mixed herbal powders administered by traditional herbalist. The anomocytic stomata, conical trichomes with warty cell, and pollen grains were found as the main characteristics of the plant powder. Additionally, aqueous methanol extract (80%) of *L. salicaria* was found to exhibit low hypoglycemic effect in STZ-induced diabetic rats as well as anti-*Helicobacter pylori*. It seems that the triterpenic constituents, including oleanolic acid and ursolic acid, are responsible to induce sensitivity to the insulin [6,31]. Additionally, the results of preliminary studies revealed that the plant extract increased insulin secretion in the experimental animals [11,27]. Therefore, it could be concluded that the plant extract is able to decrease blood glucose level by two possible mechanisms: increasing insulin secretion and also augmenting of insulin sensitivity. In spite of the fact that, the lowering effect of blood glucose level due to the ingestion of plant extract is very light in comparison to the positive control, it might be important if the plant materials administrated with other anti-diabetic medicines. Although, the result of blood lowering effect of the plant extract is in consistency with previous studies, the mentioned effect of the plant is weaker than it consider as a blood glucose lowering agent. Moreover, the plant extract displayed excellent radical scavenging activity similar to vitamin E as a standard antioxidant, due to the high contents of phenolic compounds including tannins and flavonoids. The traditional use of this plant as an anti-inflammation factor could be attributed to the high content of its antioxidant chemicals.

Competing interests

The authors declare that they have no competing interests.

Authors' contributions

AM: extraction, manuscript drafting and interpreting of data, MK: proposing of the plant, SS: participating in manuscript drafting and interpreting of data, EA: designing antidiabetic test and interpreting its data, MRM: performing plant extraction and anti-diabetic test, FV: phytochemical contents test, MM: participating in microscopic characterization, FS: *Helicobacter* test, AH: proposing of the plant. All authors read and approved the final manuscript.

Author details

[1]Department of Pharmacognosy, Faculty of Pharmacy, Tehran University of Medical Sciences, Tehran, Iran. [2]Traditional Iranian Medicine and Pharmacy Research Center, Tehran University of Medical Sciences, Tehran, Iran. [3]Medicinal Plants Research Center, Faculty of Pharmacy, Tehran University of Medical Sciences, Tehran, Iran. [4]Department of Pharmacology and Toxicology, Faculty of Pharmacy, Tehran University of Medical Sciences, Tehran, Iran. [5]Med.UL, Faculty of Pharmacy, University of Lisbon, Lisbon, Portugal. [6]Microbiology Department, Faculty of Sciences, University of Tehran, Tehran, Iran.

References

1. Soumyanath A: *Traditional herbal medicines for modern times, anti-diabetic plants.* New York: Taylor and Francis; 2006.
2. Jackson B, Snowdown DW: *Atlas of microscopy of medicinal plants, culinary herbs and spices.* London: Belhaven Press; 1999.
3. Rechinger KH: *Lythracea L. In Flora Iranica.* Austria: Akademische Druck-u; 1968.
4. Soltani A: *Encyclopaedia of traditional medicine (dictionary of medicinal plants).* Tehran: Arjomand; 2011.
5. Miraldi E, Ferri S, Mostaghimi V: **Botanical drugs and preparations in the traditional medicine of West Azerbaijan (Iran).** *J Ethnopharmacol* 2001, **77:**77–87.
6. Becker H, Scher J, Speakman JB, Zapp J: **Bioactivity guided isolation of antimicrobial compounds from Lythrum salicaria.** *Fitoterapia* 2005, **76:**580–584.
7. Citoglu GS, Altanlar N: **Ankara Antimicrobial activity of some plants used in folk medicine.** *J Fac Pharm* 2003, **32:**159–163.
8. Coban T, Citoglu GS, Sever B, Iscan M: **Antioxidant activities of plants used in traditional medicine in Turkey.** *Pharm Biol* 2003, **41:**608–613.
9. Lopez V, Akerreta S, Casanova E, Garcia-Mina JM, Cavero RY, Calvo MI: **Screening of Spanish medicinal plants for antioxidant and antifungal activities.** *PharmBiol* 2008, **46:**602–609.
10. Khanavi M, Moshteh M, Manayi A, MR S a, Vazirian M, Ajani Y, Ostad SN: **Cytotoxic acivity of Lythrum salicaria L.** *Res J Biol Sci* 2011, **6:**55–57.
11. Lamela M, Cadavid I, Calleja JM: **Effects of Lythrum salicaria extracts on hyperglycemic rats and mice.** *J Ethnopharmacol* 1986, **15:**153–160.
12. Torres IC, Suarez JC: **A preliminary study of hypoglycemic activity of Lythrum salicaria.** *J Nat Prod* 1980, **43:**559–563.
13. Kim GS, Lee SE, Jeong TS, Park CG, Sung JS, Kim JB, Hong YP, Kim YC, Song KS: **Human Acyl-CoA: cholesterol acyltransferase (hACAT)-inhibiting triterpenes from Lythrum salicaria L.** *J Korean Soc Appl Biol Chem* 2011, **54:**628–632.

14. Sutovska M, Capek P, Franova S, Pawlaczyk I, Gancarz R: **Antitussive and bronchodilatory effects of** *Lythrum salicaria* **polysaccharide-polyphenolic conjugate.** *Inter J Biol Macromol* 2012, **51**:794–799.

15. Pawlaczyka I, Capek P, Czerchawsk L, Bijak J, Lewik Tsirigotisa M, Pliszczak-Krold A, Gancarz R: **An anticoagulant effect and chemical characterization of** *Lythrum salicaria* **L. glycoconjugates.** *Carbohyrd Polym* 2011, **86**:277–284.

16. Pawlaczyk I, Czerchawski L, Kanska J, Bijak J, Capek P, Pliszczak-Kropl A, Gancarz R: **An acidic glycoconjugate from** *Lythrum salicaria* **L. with controversial effects on haemostasis.** *J Ethnopharmacol* 2010, **131**:63–69.

17. Zhou J, Xie G, Yan Z: *Encyclopaedia of traditional Chinese medicines.* Berlin: Springer; 2011.

18. Rauha JP, Remes S, Heinonen M, Hopia A, Kahkonen M, Kujala T, Pihlaja K, Vuorela H, Vuorela P: **Antimicrobial effects of Finnish plant extracts containing flavonoids and other phenolic compounds.** *Inter J Food Microbiol* 2000, **56**:3–12.

19. Manayi A, Saeidnia S, Faramarzi MA, Samadi N, Jafari S, Vazirian M, Ghaderi A, Mirnezami T, Hadjiakhoondi A, Shams Ardekani MR, Khanavi M: **A comparative study of anti-Candida activity and phenolic contents of the calluses from** *Lythrum salicaria* **L. in different treatments.** *Appl Biochem Biotech* 2013, **170**:176–184.

20. Hermann BP, Mal TK, Williams RJ, Dollahon NR: **Quantitative evaluation of stigma polymorphism in a tristylous weed,** *Lythrum salicaria* **(Lythraceae).** *Amer J Bot* 1999, **86**:1121–1129.

21. Brown VK, Robinson J, Stevenson DE: **A note on the toxicity of solvent properties of dimethyl sulphoxide.** *J Pharm Pharmacol* 1963, **15**:688–692.

22. Shahani S, Monsef-Esfahani HR, Saeidnia S, Saniee P, Siavoshi F, Foroumadi A, Samadi N, Gohari AR: **Anti-***Helicobacter pylori* **activity of the methanolic extract of** *Geum iranicum* **and its main compounds.** *Z Naturforsch C* 2012, **67**:172–180.

23. Manayi A, Mirnezami T, Saeidnia S, Ajani Y: **Pharmacognostical evaluation, phytochemical analysis and antioxidant activity of the roots of** *Achillea tenuifolia* **LAM.** *Pharmacog J* 2012, **4**:14–19.

24. Tomczyk M, Pleszczynska M, Wiater A: **Variation in total polyphenolics contents of aerial parts of** *Potentilla* **species and their anticariogenic activity.** *Molecules* 2010, **15**:4639–4651.

25. Hagerman A, Muller-Harvey I, P.S. Makkar H: *FAO/IAEA division of nuclear techniques in food and agriculture, Quantification of tannins in tree foliage.* Vienna: IAEA; 2000.

26. Nakamura T, Nishi H, Kakehi K: **Investigation on the evaluation method of fungi polysaccharide marker substance for the identification by gel permeation chromatography.** *Chromatogra* 2009, **30**:25–35.

27. Lamela M, Cadavid I, Gato A, Calleja JM: **Effects of** *Lythrum salicaria* **in normoglycemic rats.** *J Ethnopharmacol* 1985, **14**:83–91.

28. Ramirez-Espinosa JJ, Yolanda Rios M, Lopez-Martinez S, Lopez-Vallejo F, Medina-Franco JL, Paoli P, Camici G, Navarrete-Vazquez G, Ortiz-Andrade R, Estrada-Soto S: **Antidiabetic activity of some pentacyclic acid triterpenoids, role of PTPe1B:** *In vitro*, **in silico, and** *in vivo* approaches. *Eur J Med Chem* 2011, **46**:2243–2251.

29. Zhang W, Hong D, Zhou Y, Zhang Y, Shen Q, Li JY, Hu LH, Li J: **Ursolic acid and its derivative inhibit protein tyrosine phosphatase 1B, enhancing insulin receptor phosphorylation and stimulating glucose uptake.** *Biochem Biophys Acta* 2006, **1760**:1505–1512.

30. Shi L, Zhang W, Zhou Y, Zhang YN, Li JY, Hu LH, Li J: **Corosolic acid stimulates glucose uptake via enhancing insulin receptor phosphorylation.** *Eur J Pharmacol* 2008, **584**:21–29.

31. Teodoroa T, Zhang L, Alexander T, Yue J, Vranic M, Volchuk A: **Oleanolic acid enhances insulin secretion in pancreatic b-cells.** *FEBS Let* 2008, **582**:1375–1380.

32. Tunalier Z, Kosar M, Kupeli E, Calis I, Can Baser KH: **Antioxidant, anti-inflammatory, anti-nociceptive activities and composition of** *Lythrum salicaria* **L. extracts.** *J Ethnopharmacol* 2007, **110**:539–547.

33. Humadi SS, Istudor V: *Lythrum salicaria* **(purple loosestrife) medicinal use, extraction andidentification of its total phenoliccompounds.** *Farmacia* 2009, **57**:192–199.

A cytotoxic hydroperoxy sterol from the brown alga, *Nizamuddinia zanardinii*

Maryam Hamzeloo Moghadam[1], Jamileh Firouzi[2], Soodabeh Saeidnia[3], Homa Hajimehdipoor[1], Shahla Jamili[4], Abdolhossein Rustaiyan[5] and Ahmad R Gohari[3*]

Abstract

Background: The marine environment is a unique source of bioactive natural products, of which *Nizamuddinia zanardinii* is an important brown algae distributed in Oman Sea. Literature revealed that there is no report on phytochemistry and pharmacology of this valuable algae.

Methods: Bioguided fractionation of the methanolic extract of *Nizamuddinia zanardinii*, collected from Oman Sea, led to the isolation of a hydroperoxy sterol. Its structure was determined by analysis of the spectroscopic data as 24-hydroperoxy-24-vinyl cholesterol (HVC). In vitro cytotoxic activity of this compound was evaluated against HT29, MCF7, A549, HepG2 and MDBK cell lines.

Results: Although 24(R)-hydroproxy-24-vinylcholesterol has been previously reported from *Sargassum* and *Padina* species, it is the first report on the presence of this compound from *N. zanardinii*. This compound exhibited cytotoxicity in all cell lines (IC_{50}, 3.62, 9.09, 17.96, 32.31 and 37.31 µg/mL respectively). HVC was also evaluated for apoptotic activity and demonstrated positive results in terminal deoxynucleotidyl transferase dUTP Nick End labeling (TUNEL) assay suggesting it a candidate for further apoptotic studies.

Conclusions: *Nizamuddinia zanardinii*, a remarkable brown algae of Oman Sea, is a good source of hydroproxy sterols with promising cytotoxic on various cell lines particularly human colon adenocarcinoma.

Keywords: *Nizamuddinia zanardinii*, Brown algae, Sterol, MTT assay, TUNEL, Apoptosis

Background

Cancer is the second leading cause of death in the world. Almost all synthetic agents currently being used in cancer therapy are known to be toxic with severe damage to normal cells [1]. Naturally occurring compounds found in food and medicinal plants could serve as alternatives to chemically designed anticancer agents [2] and those that restrain the proliferation of malignant cells by inducing apoptosis may represent a useful mechanistic approach to both cancer chemoprevention and chemotherapy. Thus, there is growing attention in the use of natural products for treatment of various cancers and development of safer and more effective therapeutic agents [1].

The marine environment is a unique source of bioactive natural products, many of which exhibit structural features not found in terrestrial natural products [3]. Marine algae are the important source of novel bioactive substances and the medicinal importance of seaweeds has been reported from various countries throughout the world. However, Brown algae (Phaeophyceae) have been the object of phytochemical investigations that resulted in the discovery of more than 500 new metabolites [4,5]. *Nizamuddinia zanardinii* (Schiffner) P.C. Silva is one of the brown algae distributed in Oman Sea (Qishn in Yemen, Chabahar and Tang in Iran) and there is no report on chemical compounds of this alga. In this article, we explained the cytotoxic evaluation of 24-Hydroperoxy-24-vinyl cholesterol (HVC) which was isolated and identified from methanolic extract of *N. zanardinii*, using MTT assay on different cell lines followed by TUNEL assay (apoptotic induction in MCF-7 cells).

* Correspondence: goharii_a@tums.ac.ir
[3]Medicinal Plants Research Center, Faculty of Pharmacy, Tehran University of Medical Sciences, Tehran, Iran
Full list of author information is available at the end of the article

Methods

General procedures

^{1}H and ^{13}C-NMR spectra were measured on a Bruker Avance TM 500 DRX (500 MHz for ^{1}H and 125 MHz for ^{13}C) spectrometer with tetramethylsilane as an internal standard and chemical shifts are given in δ (ppm). The MS data were recorded on an Agilent Technology (HP TM) instrument with 5973 Network Mass Selective Detector (MS model). The separation and purification of the compounds were carried out with silica gel 60 (Merck, 35–70 and 230–400 mesh). Silica gel 60 F-254 (Merck, Aluminum sheet) was used for TLC analyses. Spots were detected by spraying anisaldehyde-sulfuric acid reagent followed by heating (120°C for 5 min).

Chemicals and reagents

DMEM medium and FBS (Gibco), RPMI 1640 medium, penicillin-streptomycin (Sigma), MTT [3-(4, 5-dimethyl-thiazol-2-yl)-2, 4-diphenyltetrazolium bromide] (Sigma), DMSO (Merck) and in Situ Cell Death Detection Kit, POD (Roche) were used in cytotoxicity and apoptosis studies. Methanol and other solvents were analytical grade from Merck.

Algae material

The brown algae, Nizamuddinia zanardinii (Schiffner) P.C. Silva, was collected from Oman Sea (region of Chabahr) in November 2010 and identified by Mr. B. M. Gharanjik. A voucher specimen (No. 51-17P) was deposited at the Research Center of Persian Gulf Biotechnology (Qeshm Island, Iran).

Extraction and isolation

N. zanardinii were dried (700 g dried weight), reduced to small pieces and extracted with MeOH (3 times), for 48 - hours at room temperature. The extract was concentrated and dried with freeze dryer. The methalonic extract (150 g) was subjected to silica gel CC, eluting with CHCl$_3$: EtOAc (7:3, 0:10) and EtOAc:MeOH (5:5, 0:10) to give eight fractions (A-H). The fraction C (2.3 g) was submitted to silica gel CC, which was eluted with CHCl$_3$: EtOAc (9:1, 8:2, 5:5) to obtain six fractions (C$_1$-C$_6$). The fraction C$_3$ (910 mg) was subjected to silica gel CC, eluting with CHCl$_3$: EtOAc (8:2) to yield seven fractions (C$_{31}$-C$_{37}$). The fraction C$_{34}$ (27 mg) was purified as HVC.

Preparation of HVC for MTT assay

HVC was dissolved in DMSO (10 mg/mL of to make stock solution). Serial dilutions were prepared accordingly from the stock solution to reach the final concentrations (100 µg/mL, 50 µg/mL, 25 µg/mL, 12.5 µg/mL, 6.25 µg/mL and 3.125 µg/mL) with DMSO not exceeding 1%.

Cell lines

MCF7 (human breast adenocarcinoma), HepG2 (human Hepatocellular carcinoma), MDBK (bovine kidney cells), A549 (Non-small cell lung carcinoma) and HT29 (human colon adenocarcinoma) cells were obtained from Pasteur Institute, Tehran, Iran. MCF7 cells were maintained in DMEM medium with 5% FBS and HT29 cells were cultured in DMEM medium with 20% FBS while the other cell lines were maintained in RPMI 1640 medium with 10% FBS to maintain the desired growth. All cell lines were treated with 1% penicillin-streptomycin, in a humidified incubator at 37°C in an atmosphere of 5% CO$_2$. The growth curve of each cell line was assessed.

MTT assay

Cell viability was assessed in a micro culture tetrazolium/formazan assay (MTT assay) [6]. The cells were seeded in 96-well plates at 8×10^3 for MCF7, 15×10^3 for HepG2, 11×10^3 for MDBK, 8×10^3 for A549 and 5×10^3 for HT29 cells. They were then incubated at 37°C. After

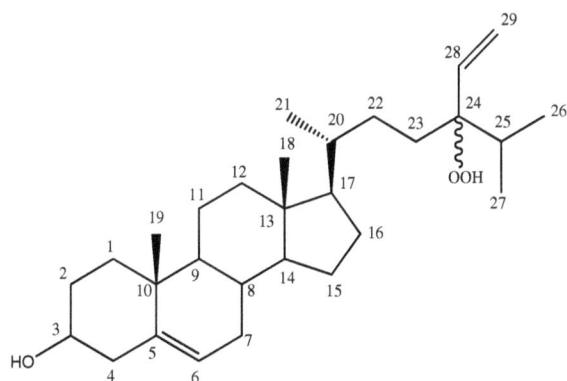

Figure 1 Structure of 24-hydroperoxy-24-vinyl cholesterol.

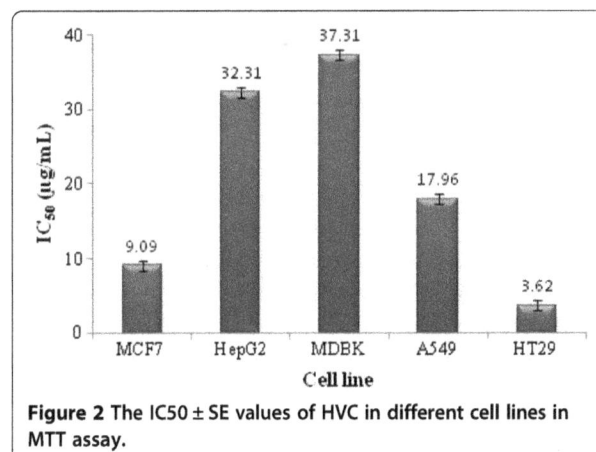

Figure 2 The IC50 ± SE values of HVC in different cell lines in MTT assay.

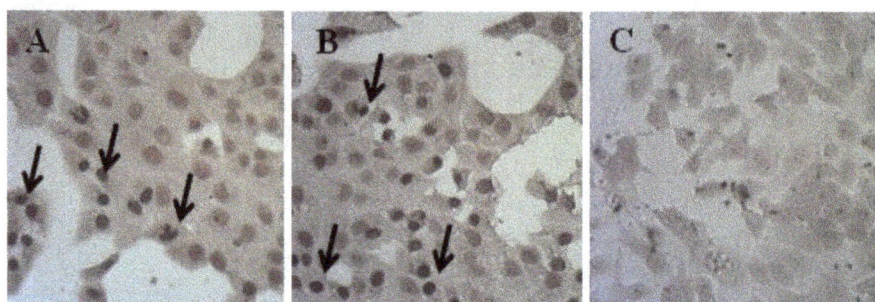

Figure 3 Results of TUNEL assay; A) HVC, B) positive control (tamoxifen), C) negative control; the arrows point to the condensed nuclei of MCF-7 cells treated with HVC or tamoxifen.

24 h the medium was replaced with fresh medium containing different concentrations of HVC. After 72 h exposure of cells at 37°C to HVC, the medium was replaced with fresh medium containing MTT with a final concentration of 0.5 mg/mL. The cells were incubated for another 4 h in a humidified atmosphere at 37°C, then the medium containing MTT was removed and the remaining MTT-formazan crystals were dissolved in DMSO. The absorbance was recorded at 570 nm with an ELISA reader (TECAN). Tamoxifen was used as positive control.

The relative cell viability (%) was calculated by $[A]_{samples}$ / $[A]_{control} \times 100$. Where $[A]_{samples}$ is the absorbance of wells with sample and $[A]_{control}$ is the absorbance of wells in absence of sample. To calculate IC_{50} dose–response curves were graphed by Microsoft Excel.

Assessments of apoptosis induction

Apoptosis induction was detected in MCF7 cells using terminal deoxynucleotidyl transferase (TdT) mediated deoxyuridine triphosphate (dUTP) Nick-End Labelling (TUNEL) system. MCF-7 cells cultured in 96 well plates were treated with HVC at 12.5 µg/mL and incubated for 24 h. The assay was conducted according to the manufacturer's instructions. Briefly, treated cells were blocked with 3% H_2O_2 followed by fixing with 4% *p*-formaldehyde, then washing with phosphate buffer saline (PBS). Cells were then, permeabilized using 0.1% triton X-100. Fluorescein-dUTP and TdT, were added to label the fragmented DNA at 37°C for one hour, next step was treating with anti-fluorescein antibody conjugated with horse-radish peroxidase (POD) at 37°C for half an hour, followed by adding DAB as substrate for the above enzyme (10 min at room temperature). The stained cells were then analyzed under light microscope. Untreated cells (cells, cell culture medium and DMSO 1%) were used as a negative control and tomaxifen was used as positive control as well.

Results and discussion

24-hydroperoxy-24-vinylcholesterol (HVC)

^{1}H-NMR (500 MHz, CDCl$_3$): δ 5.74 (1H,*d* , *J* =17.8, 11.4 Hz, H-28, epimer 24R), 5.73 (1H, *d*, *J* =17.8, 11.4 Hz, H-28, epimer 24S), 5.27 (1H,*dd*, *J* =11.3, 1.5 Hz, H-29a), 5.35 (1H, *d*, *J* =5.3 Hz, H-6), 5.15 (1H, *dd*, *J* =17.8, 1.5 Hz, H-29b), 3.53 (1H, *m* , H-3), 1.01 (3H, *s* , H-19),), 0.97 (3H, *d*, *J* =6.4 Hz, H-21), 0.68 (3H, *s* , H-18).

^{13}C-NMR (125 MHz, CDCl$_3$): 37.3 (C-1), 31.7 (C-2), 71.8 (C-3), 42.3 (C-4), 140.7 (C-5), 121.7 (C-6), 31.9 (C-7, C-8), 50.1 (C-9), 36.5 (C-10), 21.1 (C-11), 39.8 (C-12), 42.3 (C-13), 56.8 (C-14), 24.3 (C-15), 28.4 (C-16), 55.9 (C-17), 11.9 (C-18), 19.3 and 19.4 (C-19, epimer 24*R* and 24*S*), 35.9 (C-20), 18.8 (C-21), 28.8 (C-22), 28.3 (C-23), 89.1 and 89.2 (C-24), 30.5 (C-25), 16.7 (C-26), 17.7 (C-27), 137.1 and 137.2 (C-28), 116.3 and 116.4 (C-29).

The isolated compound (Figure 1) from the MeOH extract of *N. zanardinii* were identified as a mixture of two epimer, epimers 24(*S*) and 24(*R*)-hydroproxy-24-vinylcholesterol, by comparison of their ^{1}H and ^{13}C-NMR spectral data with those reported in the literature [7,8]. Although this compound has been previously reported from *Dictyopteris justii, Spatoglossum schroederi* [9], *Turbinaria ornate* [10], *Sargassum oligocystum* [8] and *Padina pavonica* [11], it is the first report of the presence of 24 (R)-hydroproxy-24-vinylcholesterol from *N. zanardinii*.

MTT assay determines cell viability through reduction of tetrazolium salts to formazan by cellular enzymes where MTT is reduced to the water insoluble purple formazan, depending on the viability of the cells. Results of MTT assay demonstrated cytotoxic activity of HVC with IC_{50} of 9.09, 32.31, 37.31, 17.96 and 3.62 µg/mL in MCF7, HepG2, MDBK, A549 and HT29 cells, respectively (Figure 2) which were obtained from dose–response curves of each cell line. IC_{50} of tamoxifen against the above-mentioned cell lines was found 3.69, 4.38, 6.35, 10.68 and 2.89 µg/mL, respectively.

In TUNEL assay, Treating MCF7 cells with 12.5 µg/mL of HVC resulted in observation of dark stained nuclei of cells which indicated DNA fragmentation and nuclear condensation (Figure 3A). It was also detectable in tamoxifen as positive control (Figure 3B). No alteration in nuclei was observed in negative control (Figure 3C).

The results also indicated that HVC was more cytotoxic to HT-29 and MCF-7 cells compared to the other three cell lines. In addition to the role of estrogen receptor (ER) in breast cancer, it has been found that estrogen and progesterone receptors (ER and PR, respectively) expression in colorectal cancerous tissues were higher than those in normal mucosa and there was positive correlation in expressing ER and PR in cancerous tissues [12]. Therefore, ERs are involved in both breast and colorectal tumors. According to the finding that estrogen receptors play an important role in regulating the growth and differentiation of normal, premalignant and malignant cell types [13], it seems that HVC with sterol structure might possibly represent its cytotoxic properties through estrogen receptors. Therefore, higher cytotoxic activity of the compound in MCF-7 and HT-29 cells could be partly related to its sterol structure. It should be mentioned that, not only the sterol structure but also the hydroperoxy functional group might play an important role in cytotoxicity of this compound, since a literature review revealed that compounds with peroxy groups have indicated cytotoxicity in several studies. For instance, hydroperoxy sterols isolated from the red alga Galaxaura marginata have demonstrated a significant cytotoxicity against several tumor cell lines [14] and it has also been found that hydroperoxy group could oxidate the glutathione pyruvic and alpha ketoglutaric acids in bacteria resulted in death of the bacteria [15]. TUNEL assay revealed apoptotic induction in MCF-7 cells exposed to 12.5 μg/mL HVC. Hence, the cytotoxic activity of HVC could be a result of the induction of cell death by apoptosis. In order to determine the precise mechanism of HVC, further comprehensive investigations are necessary.

Conclusions

N. zanardinii, a remarkable brown algae of Oman Sea, is a good source of hydroproxy sterols with promising cytotoxic on various cell lines particularly human colon adenocarcinoma.

Competing interest
The authors declare that they have no competing interest.

Authors' contributions
MHM: cytotoxic evaluation; JF: carried out the isolation and purification process; SS: carried out the interpretation of the NMR data and identification of the compounds; HH: TUNEL test; SJ: Alga material preparation; AR: advise the isolation process; ARG: participated in design of the study, helped in structured elucidation and final approved of the version to be published and participated in drafting the manuscript and helped in isolation of the compounds. All authors read and approved the final manuscript.

Acknowledgements
This research was supported by Tehran University of Medical Sciences and Health Services grant (No.16373).

Author details
[1]Traditional Medicine and Materia Medica Research Center and Department of Traditional Pharmacy, School of Traditional Medicine, Shahid Beheshti University of Medical Sciences, Tehran, Iran. [2]Department of Marine Science and Technology, Science and Research Branch, Isalmic Azad University, Tehran, Iran. [3]Medicinal Plants Research Center, Faculty of Pharmacy, Tehran University of Medical Sciences, Tehran, Iran. [4]Department of Marine Biology, Science and Research Branch, Isalmic Azad University, Tehran, Iran. [5]Department of Chemistry, Science and Research Branch, Isalmic Azad University, Tehran, Iran.

References
1. Mohan S, Bustamam A, Ibrahim S, Al-Zubairi AS, Aspollah M, Abdullah R, Elhassan MM: In vitro ultramorphological assessment of apoptosis on CEMss induced by linoleic acid-R fraction from typhonium flagelliforme tuber. *Evid Based Complement Alternat Med* 2011, **2011**:421894.
2. Rao YK, Geethangili M, Fang SH, Tzeng YM: Antioxidant and cytotoxic activities of naturally occurring phenolic and related compounds: a comparative study. *Food Chem Toxicol* 2007, **45**:1770–1776.
3. Cantillo-Ciau Z, Moo-Puc R, Quijano L, Freile-Pelegrín Y: The tropical brown alga lobophora variegata: A source of antiprotozoal compounds. *Mar Drugs* 2010, **8**:1292–1304.
4. Faulkner DJ: **Marine natural products.** *Nat Prod Rep* 2002, **19**:1–49.
5. Blunt JW, Copp BR, Munro MHG, Northcote PT, Prinsep MR: **Marine natural products.** *Nat Prod Rep* 2006, **23**:26–78.
6. Mosaddegh M, Hamzeloo Moghadam M, Ghafari S, Naghibi F, Ostad SN, Read RW: **Sesquiterpene lactones from** Inula oculus-christi. *Nat Prod Commun* 2010, **5**:511–514.
7. Lo JM, Wang WL, Chiang YM, Chen CM: **Ceramides from the red algae** Ceratodictyon spongiosum **and symbiotic spong** Sigmadocia symbiotica. *J Chinese Chem Soc* 2001, **48**:821–826.
8. Permeh P, Saeidnia S, Mashinchian-Moradi A, Gohari AR: **Sterols from** Sargassum oligocystum, a brown algae from the Persian Gulf, and their bioactivity. *Nat Prod Res* 2011, **26**:774–777.
9. Teixeira VL, Barbosa JP, Rocha FD, Kaplan MAC, Houghton PJ: **Hydroperoxysterols from** Dictyopteris justii **and** Spatoglossum schroederi. *Nat Prod Commun* 2006, **4**:293–297.
10. Sheu J, Wang G, Sung P, Chiu Y, Duh C: **Cytotoxic sterols from the formosan brown algae** Turbinaria ornata. *Planta Med* 1997, **63**:571–572.
11. Ktari L, Guyot M: **A cytotoxic oxysterol from the marine algae** Padina pavonica. *J Appl Phycol* 1999, **11**:511–513.
12. Zhou ZW, Wan DS, Wang GQ, Pan ZZ, Lu HP, Gao JH, *et al*: **Expression of estrogen receptor and progesterone receptor in colorectal cancer: a quantitative study.** *Ai Zheng* 2004, **23**:851–854.
13. Fang YJ, Wang GQ, Lu ZH, Zhang LY, Pan ZZ, Zhou ZW, *et al*: **Effects of tamoxifen on apoptosis and matrix metalloproteinase-7 expression in estrogen receptor β-positive colorectal cancer cell line.** *Chinese J Cancer* 2008, **27**:428–431.
14. Sheu JH, Huang SY, Wang GH, Duh CY: **Oxygenated clerosterols isolated from the marine algae** Codium arabicum. *J Nat Prod* 1995, **58**:1521–1526.
15. Mucchielli A, Saint-Lebe L: **The mechanism action of hydrogen peroxide on bacterial metabolism.** *CRC Acad Sci Hebd Seances Acad Sci D* 1976, **283**:435–438.

Anti-inflammatory effects of apo-9'-fucoxanthinone from the brown alga, *Sargassum muticum*

Eun-Jin Yang[1,2†], Young Min Ham[1†], Wook Jae Lee[1], Nam Ho Lee[2] and Chang-Gu Hyun[2,3*]

Abstract

Background: The marine environment is a unique source of bioactive natural products, of which *Sargassum muticum* (Yendo) Fensholt is an important brown algae distributed in Jeju Island, Korea. *S. muticum* is a traditional Korean food stuff and has pharmacological functions including anti-inflammatory effects. However, the active ingredients from *S. muticum* have not been characterized.

Methods: Bioguided fractionation of the ethanolic extract of *S. muticum*, collected from Jeju island, led to the isolation of a norisoprenoid. Its structure was determined by analysis of the spectroscopic data. In vitro anti-inflammatory activity and mechanisms of action of this compound were examined using lipopolysaccharide (LPS)-stimulated RAW 264.7 cells through ELISA assays and Western blot analysis.

Results: Apo-9'-fucoxanthinone, belonging to the norisoprenoid family were identified. Apo-9'-fucoxanthinone effectively suppressed LPS-induced nitric oxide (NO) and prostaglandin E_2 (PGE_2) production. This compound also exerted their anti-inflammatory actions by down-regulating of NF-κB activation via suppression of IκB-α in macrophages.

Conclusions: This is the first report describing effective anti-inflammatory activity for apo-9'-fucoxanthinone'-fucoxanthnone isolated from *S. muticum*. Apo-9'-fucoxanthinone may be a good candidate for delaying the progression of human inflammatory diseases and warrants further studies.

Keywords: Apo-9'-fucoxanthinone, Brown alga, *Sargassum muticum*, Inflammation

Background

Inflammation is the response of an organism to invasion by foreign pathogens such as parasites, bacteria and viruses. The inflammatory response is an important protective reaction to injury, irritation and infection and is characterised by redness, heat, swelling, loss of function and pain [1]. In the inflammatory state, activated immune cells, such as macrophages secrete large amounts of proinflammatory cytokines, nitric oxide (NO), and prostaglandin E_2 (PGE_2). However, high levels of NO and PGE_2 in a chronic inflammation state can result in various pathological conditions [1-4]. For this reason, regulation of the production of NO and PGE_2 in macrophages are current research topics for the development of new anti-inflammatory agents. There have been many attempts to derive new anti-inflammatory agents from natural compounds [5-7]. Traditional remedies derived from terrestrial plants and maritime plants such as seaweeds have been considered safe, less toxic, and readily available, even through their modes of action are yet infinite for the most part. Thus, uncovering the molecular mechanism underlying the biological function of natural products might be a good strategy for identifying new therapeutic agents [8,9].

Sargassum muticum (Yendo) Fensholt, a brown alga, is the most important economic seaweed, and widely distributed on the seashore of southern and eastern Korea. It is commonly consumed as a popular marine vegetable for more than 1000 years in Korea, particularly in Jeju Island. It has various biological activities, including antioxidant, anti-inflammatory, and antibacterial activities

* Correspondence: cghyun@jejunu.ac.kr
†Equal contributors
2Department of Chemistry, Cosmetic Science Center, Jeju National University, Jeju 690-756, Korea
3LINC Agency, Jeju National University, Ara-1-dong, Jeju 690-756, Korea
Full list of author information is available at the end of the article

[10,11]. Previously, our research group documented the anti-inflammatory properties of various seaweads [11-14]. During our on-going screening program designed to identify the anti-inflammatory potential of natural compounds, we have isolated apo-9'-fucoxanthinone from *S. muticum*, using activity-directed fractionation, and characterized apo-9'-fucoxanthinone's structural identity using spectroscopy (^{1}H and [13]NMR) in this study. Also, as a prelude to revealing the anti-inflammatory effects and its mechanisms of apo-9'-fucoxanthinone, the present study focused on whether apo-9'-fucoxanthinone inhibited the production of NO and PGE_2 and expression of inducible nitric oxide synthase (iNOS) and cyclooxygenase (COX)-2 in LPS-stimulated macrophages.

Methods

Extraction and isolation of apo-9'-fucoxanthinone

S. muticum was collected from the coasts of Jeju Island in March 2009, and verified by Dr. Wook Jae Lee at Jeju Technopark (JTP). A voucher specimen (CSC-002) was deposited at Department of Chemistry, Jeju National University, Jeju, Korea. *S. muticum* were washed 3 times with water to remove any salt, epiphytes, and sand attached to the surface. They were dried at 60°C for 24 h in an oven, and pulverized in a grinder prior to extraction. The dried powder (800 g) was extracted with 70% aqueous ethanol with stirring for 2 days at room temperature. The filtrate was concentrated under reduced pressure. The extract (105 g) was suspended in water (1.0 L), and successively partitioned into *n*-hexane, methylene chloride, ethyl acetate, and *n*-butanol fractions. The fraction of methylene chloride (7 g), being dissolved in solvent, mixed with celite, and evaporated using a rotary vacuum evaporator. After lyophilization, it was chromatographed and eluted by using the solvents 500 mL of into *n*-hexane, methylene chloride/ethyl acetate (10:1, 5:1, 2:1), methylene chloride, ethyl acetate, and methanol in order. The hexane fraction was chromatographed over a silica gel column using n-hexane:EtOAc (3:1) in order to obtain 10 subfractions (F-1 to F-10). All fractions containing the same constituent(s) identified on the TLC plates were combined and the solvents were evaporated using a rotary vacuum evaporator. Structures of fraction 10 of them (F10, 2.3 g) were determined using proton-nuclear magnetic resonance (^{1}H NMR) and ^{13}C NMR. The compound's structural identity was determined by one-and two-dimensional nuclear magnetic resonance (NMR) spectroscopic analysis (Additional file 1) and comparison to published values. Structures of these compounds are given in Figure 1.

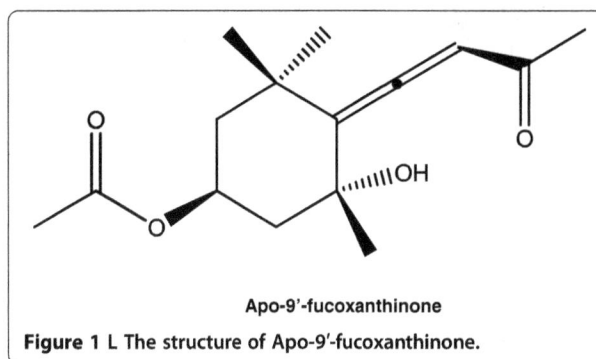

Figure 1 L The structure of Apo-9'-fucoxanthinone.

Chemicals and reagents

Dulbecco's modified Eagle's medium (DMEM) and foetal bovine serum (FBS) were obtained from Invitrogen-Gibco (Grand Island, NY, USA). Enzyme-linked immunosorbent assay (ELISA) kits for prostaglandin E_2 (PGE_2) was purchased from R&D Systems, Inc. (St. Louis, MO, USA). Anti-IκB-α, anti-phosphorylated IκB-α (anti-p-IκB-α) were purchased from Cell Signaling Technology (Beverly, MA, USA). Pyrollidine dithiocarbamate (PDTC, a specific inhibitor of NF-κB) was purchased from Calbiochem (San Diego, CA, USA). All other reagents were purchased from Sigma-Aldrich Chemical Co. (St Louis, MO, USA).

RAW 264.7 cell culture

RAW 264.7 cells were obtained from the Korean Cell Line Bank (KCLB; Seoul, Korea) and maintained at subconfluence in a 95% air, 5% CO_2 humidified atmosphere at 37°C as described previously [11-14]. Cells at passages 10–20 were used for the experiments and subcultured every 2–3 days. The medium for routine sub-cultivation was DMEM supplemented with FBS (10%), penicillin (100 units/mL), and streptomycin (100 µg/mL). Cells were counted with a haemocytometer, and the number of viable cells was assessed by trypan blue dye exclusion method.

MTT assay for cell viability

Cell viability was measured as described previously [11-14] with slight modification using MTT assay. RAW 264.7 cells were cultured in 96-well plates for 18 h, followed by treatment with LPS (1 µg/mL) in the presence of various concentrations of the sample. After a 24-h incubation, MTT was added to the medium for 4 h. Finally, the supernatant was removed and the formazan crystals were dissolved in DMSO. Absorbance was measured at 540 nm. The percentage of cells showing cytotoxicity relative to the control group was determined.

Nitric oxide determination

RAW 264.7 cells were plated at 1.5×10^5 cells/well in 24-well plates and then incubated with or without LPS (1 µg/mL) in the absence or presence of various concentrations (12.5,

25, 50, and 100 μg/mL) of apo-9-fucoxanthinone for 24 h. Nitrite levels in culture media were determined as described previously [11-14] with slight modification using the Griess reaction and presumed to reflect NO levels. Briefly, the culture supernatant (100 μL) was mixed with the same volume of Griess reagent (1% sulphanilamide and 0.1% N-[1-naphthyl]-ethylenediamine dihydrochloride in 5% phosphoric acid %) for 10 min. Absorbance was the measured at 540 nm using spectrophotometer. Fresh culture media were used as blanks in all experiments. NO levels in samples were read off a standard sodium nitrite curve.

Detection of PGE₂ in supernatant
Sandwich ELISA was used to determine the inhibitory effects of various concentrations (12.5, 25, 50, and 100 μg/mL) of apo-9-fucoxanthinone on the production of cytokines PGE_2 in LPS-treated RAW 264.7 cells. RAW 264.7 cells were stimulated for 24 h before the supernatant was harvested and assayed according to the manufacturer's protocol for the relevant ELISA kit. Results from 3 independent experiments were used for statistical analysis.

Western blot analysis
Western blotting was performed with a SDS-PAGE Electrophoresis System as described previously [11-14]. Briefly, the RAW 264.7 cells (5.0×10^5 cells/mL) were pre-incubated for 18 h and then treated with LPS (1 μg/mL) plus aliquots sample for 24 h. After incubation, the cells were washed twice with cold PBS. Whole-cell lysates (25 μg) were separated by 10% sodium dodecyl sulphate-polyacrylamide gel electrophoresis (SDS-PAGE) and electro-transferred to a polyvinylidene fluoride (PVDF) membrane (BIO-RAD, HC, USA). The membrane was incubated for 24 h with 5% skim milk and then incubated with iNOS (1:2500), COX-2 (1:2500), IκB-α (1:1000), phosphorylated IκB-α, antibodies (1:1000) at room temperature for 2 h. The membrane was washed 4 times with TTBS and incubated for 30 min with a peroxidase-conjugated secondary antibody (1:5000) at room temperature. Finally, The immunoactive proteins were detected using an enhanced chemiluminescence (ECL) Western blotting detection kit (Amersharm Pharmacia Biotech., NY, USA).

Statistical analysis
Results are presented as the means ± standard deviation of at least three replicates. The Student t-test was used for statistical analyses of the difference noted. P values of 0.05 or less were considered statistically significant.

Results and discussion
Brown algae have proven to be rich sources of structurally novel and biologically active natural compounds in recent study. These compounds have served as important chemical prototypes for the discovery of new drugs for use in the treatment of various human diseases [15]. Brown algae are also very popular sea vegetables, and many people consider this vegetable as a food of health benefit in East Asia such as Korea, China, and Japan. Jeju Island, the largest island in Korea, is located in the southwest of the Korean Strait, and is well known for its distinctive environment. In particular, the sea levels around this island are known to fluctuate rapidly as a result of global warming. Therefore, in response to this unusual environment, the brown algae that are present on Jeju Island may possess substantial endogenous protective mechanisms [12]. Some studies on brown algae-derived anti-inflammatory compounds have investigated potential inhibitory effects by using the LPS-stimulated murine macrophages [16-18]. Previously, we found that the a S. muticum extract displayed an appreciable anti-inflammatory effect in mouse macrophage RAW264.7 cells [11]. In the present study, we isolated the active substance, in an attempt to understand the possible anti-inflammatory mechanism of S. muticum. To identify its active components, the ethanol extract was suspended in H_2O and extracted successively with n-hexane, methylene chloride, ethyl acetate, and n-butanol. The methylene chloride fraction was subjected repeatedly to column chromatography over celite and silica gel in various solvent systems, to yield the active ingradent. It was identified as apo-9′fucoxanthinone (Figure 1) by comparison of physical and spectroscopic data with published values.

In murine macrophage RAW264.7 cells, LPS alone induces the transcription and protein synthesis of iNOS and COX-2, which produce large amounts of NO and PGE_2, respectively. Excess production of NO by iNOS has been implicated in a wide spectrum of diseases including septic shock, rheumatoid arthritis, cerebral ischemia, multiple sclerosis, and diabetes [19]. For this reason, NO production induced by LPS through iNOS can reflect the degree of inflammation, and a change in NO level through inhibition of iNOS enzyme activity or iNOS induction provides a means of assessing the effect of agents on the inflammatory process. Therefore, the modulation of macrophage-mediated inflammatory responses is emerging as a promising new therapeutic approach against inflammatory diseases [12-14,20,21]. In an effort to characterize the anti-inflammatory activities of apo-9′fucoxanthinone, we firstly assessed the effects of apo-9′fucoxanthinone on LPS induced NO production in RAW 264.7 cells. Since the half-life of NO is very short, we used nitrite production as an indicator of NO released by LPS-activated macrophages. As shown in Figure 2A, compared to in normal macrophages, NO production increased >15 fold in LPS-activated macrophages. apo-9′-fucoxanthinone reduced LPS-induced NO production

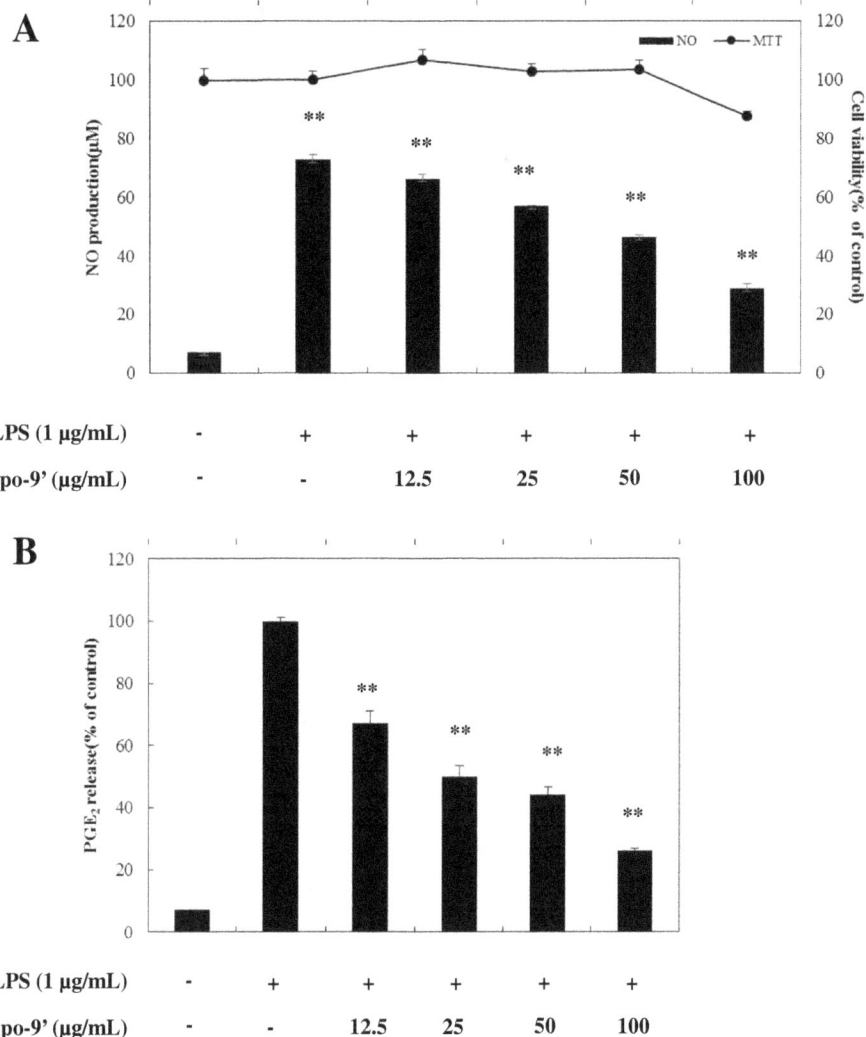

Figure 2 Effect of Apo-9′-fucoxanthinone on nitric oxide and PGE₂ production in LPS-stimulated RAW264.7 cells. The cells were stimulated with 1 μg/mL of LPS only or with LPS plus various concentrations (12.5, 25, 50, and 100 μg/mL) of Apo-9′ for 24 hr. Nitric oxide production was determined by the Griess reagent method. After a 24-h incubation, PGE₂ in the culture supernatants was measured by an enzyme-linked immunosorbent assay (ELISA) kit. Cell viability was determined from the 24 hr culture of cells stimulated with LPS (1 μg/mL) in the presence of Apo-9′. The data represent the mean ± SD of triplicate experiments.*$P < 0.05$, **$P < 0.01$ versus LPS alone.

in a dose-dependent manner: At apo-9′-fucoxanthinone concentrations of 12.5 μg/mL, 25 μg/mL, 50 μg/mL, and 100 μg/mL, the production of NO by LPS-treated macrophages decreased, as compared with LPS-treated macrophages not treated with apo-9′-fucoxanthinone (Figure 2A). DMSO, the vehicle control, had no effect on NO production (data not shown), reconfirming its immunological inertness. In parallel, the potential cyto-toxicity of apo-9′-fucoxanthinone was evaluated by an MTT assay after incubating cells for 24 h in the absence and presence of LPS. However, cell viability was negligibly affected at the concentrations used (12.5 μg/mL, 25 μg/mL, 50 μg/mL, and 100 μg/mL) to inhibit NO (Figure 2A). Thus, the inhibitory effects of apo-9′-fucoxanthinone were not attributable to cytotoxicity.

To further elucidate the mechanisms by which apo-9′-fucoxanthinone inhibited NO production in LPS-activated macrophages, we analyzed apo-9′-fucoxanthinone's effect on LPS-induced iNOS gene expression in macrophages. Under normal conditions, RAW 264.7 cells expressed non-detectable levels of iNOS mRNA, but iNOS mRNA levels increased markedly after 24 h of LPS stimulation (Figure 3A). With the addition of apo-9′-fucoxanthinone (12.5 μg/mL - 100 μg/mL), dose-dependent inhibition of iNOS expression was observed, indicating that apo-9′-fucoxanthinone modulates iNOS expression.

PGE₂ is an inflammatory mediator that is produced from the conversion of arachidonic acid by cyclooxygen-ase. In a variety of inflammatory cells, including macro-phages, COX-2 is induced by cytokines and other

A

| LPS (1 µg/mL) | - | + | + | + | + | + |
| Apo-9' (µg/mL) | - | - | 12.5 | 25 | 50 | 100 |

iNOS   130 kDa

β-actin   42 kDa

B

| LPS (1 µg/mL) | - | + | + | + | + | + |
| Apo-9 (µg/mL) | - | - | 12.5 | 25 | 50 | 100 |

COX-2   72 kDa

β-actin   42 kDa

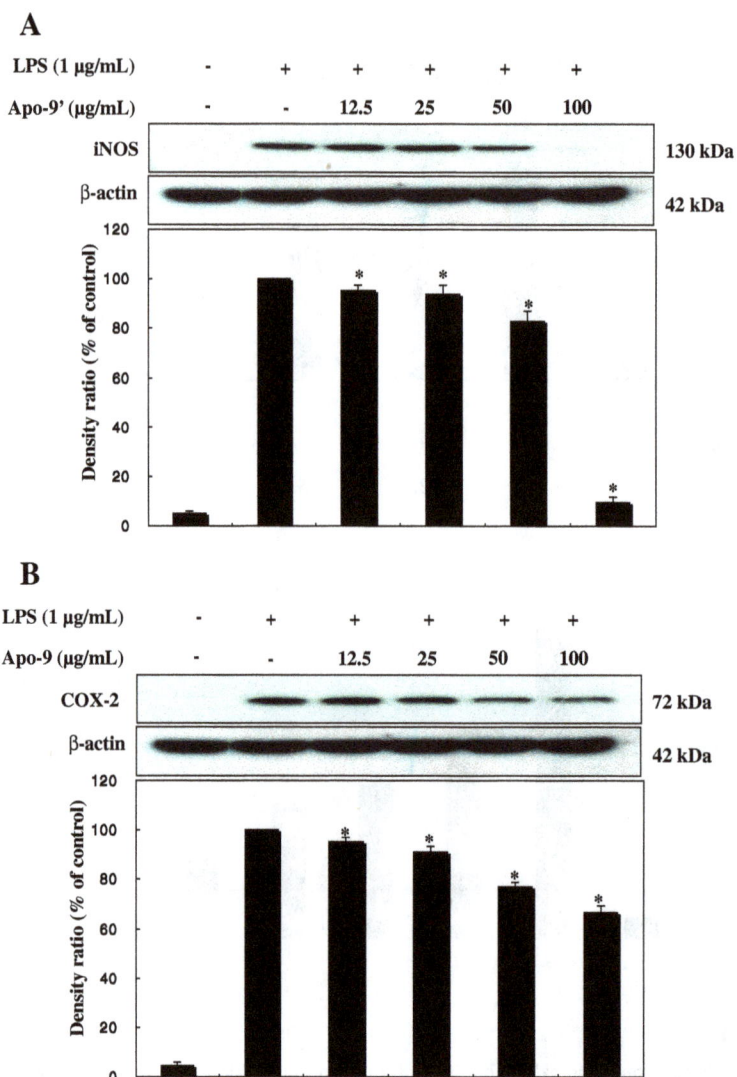

Figure 3 Effect of Apo-9'-fucoxanthinone on the activation of iNOS and COX-2 in LPS-stimulated RAW 264.7 cells. RAW 264.7 cells (5.0×10^5 cells/mL) were stimulated with LPS (1 µg/mL) in the Apo-9' (12.5, 25, 50, and 100 µg/mL) for 24 hr. Whole-cell lysate (25 µg) were prepared and the protein level was subjected to 10% SDS-PAGE, and expression of iNOS, COX-2, and β-actin were determined by Western blotting.

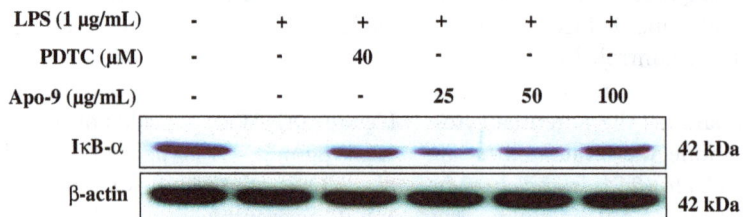

LPS (1 µg/mL)	-	+	+	+	+	+
PDTC (µM)	-	-	40	-	-	-
Apo-9 (µg/mL)	-	-	-	25	50	100

IκB-α   42 kDa

β-actin   42 kDa

Figure 4 Effects of Apo-9'-fucoxanthinone on the degradation of IκB-α in LPS stimulated RAW 264.7 cells. RAW 264.7 cells (1.0×10^6 cells/mL) were stimulated with LPS (1 µg/mL) in the presence of apo-9'-fucoxanthinone (12.5, 25, 50, and 100 µg/mL) or PDTC (40 µM) for 15 min. Whole cell lysates (30 ug) were prepared and the protein level was subjected to 12% SDS-PAGE, and expression of IκB-α and β-actin were determined by Western blotting. The β-actin antibody as a loading control.

activators, such as LPS, resulting in the release of a large amount of PGE_2 at inflammatory sites. Numerous studies have reported that prostaglandin $(PGE)_2$ participate in inflammatory and nociceptive events [22-24]. Therefore its ubiquitous role in the pathogenesis of inflammatory gene expression, PGE_2 is a current target for treating various diseases. For this reason, we next examined the effects of apo-9'-fucoxanthinone on PGE_2 production in LPS-stimulated RAW 264.7 macrophages. Cells were pre-incubated with apo-9'-fucoxanthinone for 1 h, following which they were stimulated with 1 μg/mL LPS for 24 h. As shown in Figure 2B, Compared to unstimulated macrophages, the PGE_2 level increased dramatically by 15-fold in LPS-stimulated macrophages. With the addition of apo-9'-fucoxanthinone (12.5 μg/mL, 25 μg/mL, 50 μg/mL, and 100 μg/mL) a dose-dependent reduction in PGE_2 was observed (Figure 2B). In order to determine the mechanism by which apo-9'-fucoxanthinone reduces LPS-induced PGE_2 production, we studied the ability of apo-9'-fucoxanthinone to influence the LPS-induced expression of COX-2. The addition of LPS resulted in a clearly defined increase in COX-2 expression that was markedly attenuated in a dose-dependent fashion when treated with apo-9'-fucoxanthinone (Figure 3B), corroborating that apo-9'-fucoxanthinone induces a decrease in COX-2, which translates into a dramatic decrease in PGE_2.

NF-κB activation, in response to pro-inflammatory stimuli, involves the rapid phosphorylation of IκBs by the IKK signalosome complex. Free NF-κB produced by this process translocates to the nucleus, where it binds to κB-binding sites in the promoter regions of target genes. It then induces the transcription of pro-inflammatory mediators such as iNOS and COX-2. Actually, several studies have shown that anti-inflammatory agents inhibit the activation of NF-κB by preventing IκB degradation [25-27]. Thus, we attempted in this study to determine whether or not apo-9'-fucoxanthinone inhibits the phosphorylation and degradation of IκB. Accordingly, RAW 264.7 cells were pretreated for 30 min with 9'fucoxanthinone, and IκB-α protein levels were determined after 15 min of further LPS exposure (1 μg/mL). As shown in Figure 4, apo-9'-fucoxanthinone was shown to significantly suppress the LPS-induced IκB-α degradation. As expected, the reference compounds 2-amino-4-methyl pyridine (iNOS inhibitor) also potently inhibited the LPS-induced IκB-α degradation at 40 μM. These results show that apo-9'-fucoxanthinone inhibits LPS induced NF-κB activation by preventing the IκB-α degradation.

Conclusions

The results of this study reveal, for the first time, that the apo-9'-fucoxanthinone isolated from *S. muticum* exhibit anti-inflammatory properties through suppressing NO and PGE_2 production in LPS-stimulated RAW 264.7 cells

by attenuation of NF-κB-mediated iNOS and COX-2 expression. It is proposed that that apo-9'-fucoxanthinone is a potential anti-inflammatory agent and may be used in the future to treat inflammation-associated human health. To our knowledge, this is the first report concerning the evaluation of the anti-inflammatory properties of apo-9'-fucoxanthinone.

Additional file

Additional file 1: Apo-9'-fucoxanthinone.

Competing interests
The authors declare that they have no competing interests.

Authors' contributions
EJY carried out the anti-inflammatory evaluation. YMH carried out the isolation and purification apo-9'-fucoxanthinone. WJL carried out the preparation and identification of alga material. NHL carried out the interpretation of the NMR data and identification of the compounds. CGH conceived of the study, and participated in its design and coordination and helped to draft the manuscript. All authors read and approved the final manuscript.

Acknowledgements
This research was supported financially by the Ministry of Trade, Industry & Energy, Korea Institute for Advancement of Technology through the Inter-ER Cooperation Projects (R0002016). We are grateful to Jeju Technopark for providing research facilities.

Author details
[1]Jeju Biodiversity Research Institute (JBRI), Jeju Technopark, Jeju 699-943, Korea. [2]Department of Chemistry, Cosmetic Science Center, Jeju National University, Jeju 690-756, Korea. [3]LINC Agency, Jeju National University, Ara-1-dong, Jeju 690-756, Korea.

References
1. Liu SX, Jin HZ, Shan L, Zeng HW, Chen BY, Sun QY, Zhang WD: **Inhibitory effect of 4,4'-dihydroxy-α-truxillic acid derivatives on NO production in lipopolysaccharide-induced RAW 264.7 macrophages and exploration of structure-activity relationships.** *Bioorg Med Chem Lett* 2013, **23:**2207–22311.
2. Medeiros A, Peres-Buzalaf C, Fortino Verdan F, Serezani CH: **Prostaglandin E₂ and the suppression of phagocyte innate immune responses in different organs.** *Mediators Inflamm* 2012, **2012:**327568.
3. Aoki T, Narumiya S: **Prostaglandins and chronic inflammation.** *Trends Pharmacol Sci* 2012, **33:**304–311.
4. Wang S, Xu Y, Jiang W, Zhang Y: **Isolation and identification of constituents with activity of inhibiting nitric oxide production in RAW 264.7 macrophages from *Gentiana triflora*.** *Planta Med* 2013, **79:**680–686.
5. Yan M, Zhu Y, Zhang HJ, Jiao WH, Han BN, Liu ZX, Qiu F, Chen WS, Lin HW: **Anti-inflammatory secondary metabolites from the leaves of *Rosa laevigata*.** *Bioorg Med Chem* 2013, **21:**3290–3297.
6. Lee J, Yang G, Lee K, Lee MH, Eom JW, Ham I, Choi HY: **Anti-inflammatory effect of *Prunus yedoensis* through inhibition of nuclear factor-kappaB in macrophages.** *BMC Complement Altern Med* 2013, **13:**92.
7. Chen TY, Sun HL, Yao HT, Lii CK, Chen HW, Chen PY, Li CC, Liu KL: **Suppressive effects of *Indigofera suffruticosa* Mill extracts on lipopolysaccharide-induced inflammatory responses in murine RAW 264.7 macrophages.** *Food Chem Toxicol* 2013, **55:**257–264.
8. Hwang PA, Chien SY, Chan YL, Lu MK, Wu CH, Kong ZL, Wu CJ: **Inhibition of lipopolysaccharide (LPS)-induced inflammatory responses by *Sargassum hemiphyllum* sulfated polysaccharide extract in RAW 264.7 macrophage cells.** *J Agric Food Chem* 2011, **59:**2062–2068.

9. Chen JH, Lim JD, Sohn EH, Choi YS, Han ET: Growth-inhibitory effect of a fucoidan from brown seaweed *Undaria pinnatifida* on *Plasmodium* parasites. *Parasitol Res* 2009, **104**:245–250.

10. Kim JY, Lee JA, Kim KN, Yoon WJ, Lee WJ, Park SY: Antioxidative and antimicrobial activities of *Sargassum muticum* extracts. *J Korean Soc Food Sci Nutr* 2007, **36**:663–669.

11. Yoon WJ, Ham YM, Lee WJ, Lee NH, Hyun CG: Brown alga *Sargassum muticum* inhibits proinflammatory cytokines, iNOS, and COX-2 expression in macrophage RAW 264.7 cells. *Turk J Biol* 2010, **34**:25–34.

12. Yang EJ, Moon JY, Kim MJ, Kim DS, Kim CS, Lee WJ, Lee NH, Hyun CG: Inhibitory effect of Jeju endemic seaweeds on the production of pro-inflammatory mediators in mouse macrophage cell line RAW 264.7. *J Zhejiang Univ Sci B* 2010, **11**:315–322.

13. Yang EJ, Moon JY, Kim MJ, Kim DS, Lee WJ, Lee NH, Hyun CG: Anti-inflammatory effect of *Petalonia binghamiae* in LPS-induced macrophages is mediated by suppression of iNOS and COX-2. *Int J Agri Biol* 2010, **12**:754–758.

14. Yang EJ, Ham YM, Kim DS, Kim JY, Hong JP, Kim MJ, Moon JY, Lee WJ, Lee NH, Hyun CG: *Ecklonia stolonifera* inhibits lipopolysaccharide-induced production of nitric oxide, prostaglandin E_2, and proinflammatory cytokines in RAW264.7 macrophages. *Biol* 2010, **65**:362–371.

15. Ham YM, Kim KN, Lee WJ, Lee NH, Hyun CG: Chemical constituents from *Sargassum micracanthum* and antioxidant activity. *Int J Pharmacol* 2010, **6**:147–151.

16. Yoon WJ, Heo SJ, Han SC, Lee HJ, Kang GJ, Kang HK, Hyun JW, Koh YS, Yoo ES: Anti-inflammatory effect of sargachromanol G isolated from *Sargassum siliquastrum* in RAW 264.7 cells. *Arch Pharm Res* 2012, **35**:1421–1430.

17. Heo SJ, Yoon WJ, Kim KN, Oh C, Choi YU, Yoon KT, Kang DH, Qian ZJ, Choi IW, Jung WK: Anti-inflammatory effect of fucoxanthin derivatives isolated from *Sargassum siliquastrum* in lipopolysaccharide-stimulated RAW 264.7 macrophage. *Food Chem Toxicol* 2012, **50**:3336–3342.

18. Dutot M, Fagon R, Hemon M, Rat P: Antioxidant, anti-inflammatory, and anti-senescence activities of a phlorotannin-rich natural extract from brown seaweed *Ascophyllum nodosum*. *Appl Biochem Biotechnol* 2012, **167**:2234–2240.

19. Galea E, Feinstein DL: Regulation of the expression of the inflammatory nitric oxide synthase (NOS2) by cyclic AMP. *FASEB J* 1999, **13**:2125–2137.

20. Kanwar JR, Kanwar RK, Burrow H, Baratchi S: Recent advances on the roles of NO in cancer and chronic inflammatory disorders. *Cur Med Chem* 2009, **16**:2373–2394.

21. Murakami A: Chemoprevention with phytochemicals targeting inducible nitric oxide synthase. *Forum Nutr* 2009, **61**:193–203.

22. Scher JU, Pillinger MH: The anti-inflammatory effects of prostaglandins. *J Invest Med* 2009, **57**:703–708.

23. Iyer JP, Srivastava PK, Dev R, Dastidar SG, Ray A: Prostaglandin E(2) synthase inhibition as a therapeutic target. *Expert Opin Ther Targets* 2009, **13**:849–865.

24. Rao P, Knaus EE: Evolution of nonsteroidal anti-inflammatory drugs (NSAIDs): cyclooxygenase (COX) inhibition and beyond. *J Pharm Pharmaceut Sci* 2008, **11**:81s–110s.

25. Kanarek N, Ben-Neriah Y: Regulation of NF-κB by ubiquitination and degradation of the IκBs. *Immunol Rev* 2012, **246**:77–94.

26. Kwak JH, Jung JK, Lee H: Nuclear factor-kappa B inhibitors; a patent review (2006–2010). *Expert Opin Ther Pat* 2011, **21**:1897–1910.

27. Skaug B, Jiang X, Chen ZJ: The role of ubiquitin in NF-kappaB regulatory pathways. *Annu Rev Biochem* 2009, **78**:769–796.

Statistical optimization of a novel excipient (CMEC) based gastro retentive floating tablets of propranolol HCl and it's *in vivo* buoyancy characterization in healthy human volunteers

Venkata Srikanth Meka[1*], Sreenivasa Rao Nali[2], Ambedkar Sunil Songa[2], Janaki Ram Battu[2] and Venkata Ramana Murthy Kolapalli[2]

Abstract

The objective of the present investigation is to formulate gastro retentive floating drug delivery systems (GRFDDS) of propranolol HCl by central composite design and to study the effect of formulation variables on floating lag time, D_{1hr} (% drug release at 1 hr) and t_{90} (time required to release 90% of the drug). 3 factor central composite design was employed for the development of GRFDDS containing novel semi synthetic polymer carboxymethyl ethyl cellulose (CMEC) as a release retarding polymer. CMEC, sodium bicarbonate and Povidone concentrations were included as independent variables. The tablets were prepared by direct compression method and were evaluated for *in vitro* buoyancy and dissolution studies. From the polynomial model fitting statistical analysis, it was confirmed that the response floating lag time and D_{1hr} is suggested to quadratic model and t_{90} is suggested to linear model. All the statistical formulations followed first order rate kinetics with non-Fickian diffusion mechanism. The desirability function was used to optimize the response variables, each having a different target, and the observed responses were highly agreed with experimental values. Statistically optimized formulation was characterized by FTIR and DSC studies and found no interactions between drug and polymer. The results demonstrate the feasibility of the model in the development of GRFDDS containing a propranolol HCl. Statistically optimized formulation was evaluated for *in vivo* buoyancy studies in healthy humans for both fed and fasted states. From the results, it was concluded that gastric residence time of the floating tablets were enhanced at fed stage but not in fasted state.

Keywords: Propranolol HCl, Gastro retentive, Floating, Central composite, Carboxymethyl ethyl cellulose

Introduction

Drug delivery systems (DDS) are used for maximizing the therapeutic index of the drug and also targeted for reduction in the side effects. All over delivery systems the oral drug delivery has become the mainstay of treatment due to higher patient compliance and reduced patient discomfort. Under certain circumstances prolonging the gastric retention of a DDS is desirable for achieving greater therapeutic benefit of the drug [1]. For example, drugs that are absorbed in the proximal part of the gastrointestinal tract (GIT), and the drugs that are less soluble or are degraded by the alkaline pH may benefit from prolong gastric retention. In addition, for local and sustained drug delivery to the stomach and the proximal small intestine to treat certain conditions, prolonging gastric retention of the therapeutic moiety may offer numerous advantages including improved bioavailability, therapeutic efficacy and possible reduction of the dose size [2-4]. All over the retentive systems gastric floating system for modulation of oral controlled drug delivery was found to be great importance. Hence in the present investigation effervescent floating systems were developed for prolonging the gastric retention.

* Correspondence: venkatasrikanthmeka@gmail.com
[1]School of Pharmacy, International Medical University, Kuala Lumpur 57000, Malaysia
Full list of author information is available at the end of the article

In the present investigation propranolol HCl was selected as a model drug for the development of gastro retentive floating drug delivery systems (GRFDDS). Propranolol is a nonselective beta-adrenergic receptor blocking agent possessing no other autonomic nervous system activity used for the treatment of hypertension [5]. It is highly lipophilic and almost completely absorbed after oral administration. However, it undergoes high first-pass metabolism by the liver and on average, only about 25% of propranolol reaches the systemic circulation [6]. Variability of propranolol bioavailability is depends upon the secretory transporter P-glycoprotein (P-gp) located on the epithelium cells. Although P-gp appears to be distributed throughout the GIT, its levels are higher in more distal regions (stomach < jejunum < colon). Absorption through P-gp prolongs the drug exposure to CYP3A4. The colocalization of P-gp and CYP3A4 in the mature enterocytes and their overlapping substrate specificity reasonably suggests that the function of these two proteins may be synergistic and appear to be coordinately regulated. Consequently, a greater proportion of drug will be metabolized since the repetitive two-way kinetics (drug excerption from the enterocytes into the lumen via P-gp and reabsorption back into enterocytes) will simply prolong the drug exposure to CYP3A4. This mechanism not only limits the absorption of a wide variety of drugs, including peptides, but also poses a threat for potential drug interactions [7,8].

Based on previously published literature, applications of gastro retentive drug delivery system (GRDDS) may be suitable for the drugs insoluble in intestinal fluids (acid soluble basic drugs), e.g., propranolol, metoprolol, diazepam [8]. As discussed earlier, propranolol has short half-life, high first-pass metabolism, presence of food increases the bioavailability, P-gp plays important role in the absorption, and the drug is acid-soluble basic drug which make it suitable for GRDDS. A novel semi synthetic polymer carboxy methyl ethyl cellulose (CMEC) was used as release retarding polymer in the present investigation. Till now there were no reports found on CMEC as a release retarding polymer.

In the normal conventional optimization process, a single independent variable is varied while all others are kept constant at a specific set of conditions. It's not possible to change more than one parameter at a time during the formulation development. This method may lead to unreliable results and improper conclusions besides wastage of excipients due to the requirement of large number of runs in achieving the desired goal. Response surface methodology (RSM) is an alternative to overcome this difficulty, which can be employed to optimize the formulations with suitable experimental design. RSM permits a deeper understanding of a process or product and has important applications like optimization and in establishing the robustness of that product. Central composite designs are a progression from the factorial designs which have been widely used in response-surface modeling and optimization [9].

The objective of the present investigation is to develop gastro retentive floating tablets (GRFT) of propranolol HCl using central composite design. In this study CMEC quantity, sodium bicarbonate concentration and Povidone concentration were selected as independent variables while floating lag time, D_{1hr} and t_{90} were selected as dependent variables. For this study Design Expert software was used which gives information regarding critical values for achieving the desired response and also the possible interaction effects of selected independent variables on dependent variable.

Experimental
Materials
Propranolol HCl was provided by Dr Reddy's Laboratories Ltd (Hyderabad, India). CMEC, sodium bicarbonate, Povidone K 30 and magnesium stearate were obtained as gift samples from Unichem Laboratories Ltd (Goa, India). All other reagents and chemicals were of analytical grade.

Experimental design
RSM is an experimental design technique by which the factors involved and their relative importance can be assessed. In the present study, a central composite design was employed containing 3 factors evaluated at 3 levels and experimental trials were performed at all 20 possible combinations. The levels of the 3 independent variables are shown in Table 1 and the formulation variables evaluated include:

X_1 = CMEC quantity in mg
X_2 = % w/w Sodium bicarbonate concentration (% w/w to the tablet weight)
X_3 = % w/w Povidone concentration (% w/w to the tablet weight)

The response variables include

Y_1 = Floating lag time (sec)
Y_2 = D_{1hr} (% drug released at 1 hr)
Y_3 = t_{90} (time required to release 90% of the drug)

Table 1 Experimental range and levels of the independent variables in CMEC based formulations

Variables	Range and levels		
	-1	0	+1
CMEC (mg) X_1	200	240	280
% w/w Sodium bicarbonate concentration X_2	5	10	15
% w/w povidone concentration X_3	2.5	5	7.5

Preparation of GRFT of propranolol HCl

All the ingredients sufficient for a batch of 100 tablets according to the formulae suggested by Design Expert software shown in Table 2 were accurately weighed and passed through the sieve 40. Propranolol HCl (80 mg) was geometrically mixed with CMEC until a homogeneous blend was achieved. Povidone and sodium bicarbonate was added to the above mixture and mixed for 5 min in a polybag. Blend was lubricated with presifted magnesium stearate (sieve 60) for 3 min in polybag. 1% w/w of magnesium stearate was used in all the formulations. The flow property of the final blend was found to be good so final blend was directly compressed into tablets on a 16-station rotary tablet punching machine (M/s. Cad mach Machinery Co. Pvt., Ltd., India) using 9 mm round plain punches.

Evaluation of GRFT
In vitro buoyancy studies

All the formulated floating tablets (n = 5) were subjected to in vitro buoyancy studies. The floating lag time was determined in one liter glass beaker containing 900 ml of 0.1 N HCl [10]. The time required for the tablet to rise to the surface and float was determined as floating lag time. Results are given in Table 2.

In vitro dissolution studies

In vitro release of propranolol hydrochloride from the prepared floating tablets was studied using USP XXIII dissolution test apparatus (LABINDIA, Disso 2000) employing the paddle stirrer (Apparatus-II). 900 ml of 0.1 N HCl was used as dissolution medium maintained at a temperature of 37 ± 0.5 °C and the paddle was rotated at 50 rpm [11]. Aliquots (5 ml each) were withdrawn at predetermined time intervals by means of a syringe fitted with 0.45 μm prefilter and immediately replaced with 5 ml of fresh medium maintained at 37 ± 0.5 °C. The filtered samples were suitably diluted with the dissolution medium wherever necessary and the absorbance of the samples was measured at 289 nm and results are given in Figure 1.

Release kinetics
Zero order release kinetics

Drug dissolution from dosage forms that do not disaggregate and release the drug slowly can be represented by the equation:

$$Q_t = Q_0 + K_0 t$$

Where Q_t is the amount of drug dissolved in time t, Q_0 is the initial amount of drug in the solution (most

Table 2 Formulations with the levels of independent variables and observed responses

Standard Order	CMEC quantity (mg) X_1	%w/w of Sodium bicarbonate X_2	%w/w of povidone X_3	Floating lag time (sec)	D_{1hr} (%)	t_{90} (hr)
PCMECR 01	200	5	2.5	650	40.22	6.6
PCMECR 02	280	5	2.5	550	31.11	8
PCMECR 03	200	15	2.5	720	36.58	8.2
PCMECR 04	280	15	2.5	510	18.99	10.8
PCMECR 05	200	5	7.5	300	32.12	8
PCMECR 06	280	5	7.5	600	23.45	9.9
PCMECR 07	200	15	7.5	495	22.12	9.9
PCMECR 08	280	15	7.5	670	13.84	12.2
PCMECR 09	172.73	10	5	570	27.23	9
PCMECR 10	307.27	10	5	369	18.12	11
PCMECR 11	240	1.59	5	450	28.15	8.85
PCMECR 12	240	18.41	5	300	18.99	12
PCMECR 13	240	10	0.80	310	34.59	9.8
PCMECR 14	240	10	9.20	280	26.68	11.15
PCMECR 15	240	10	5	312	19.12	10.3
PCMECR 16	240	10	5	369	18.99	10.4
PCMECR 17	240	10	5	435	19.89	10.25
PCMECR 18	240	10	5	401	19.99	10.2
PCMECR 19	240	10	5	467	19.01	10.15
PCMECR 20	240	10	5	420	18.78	10

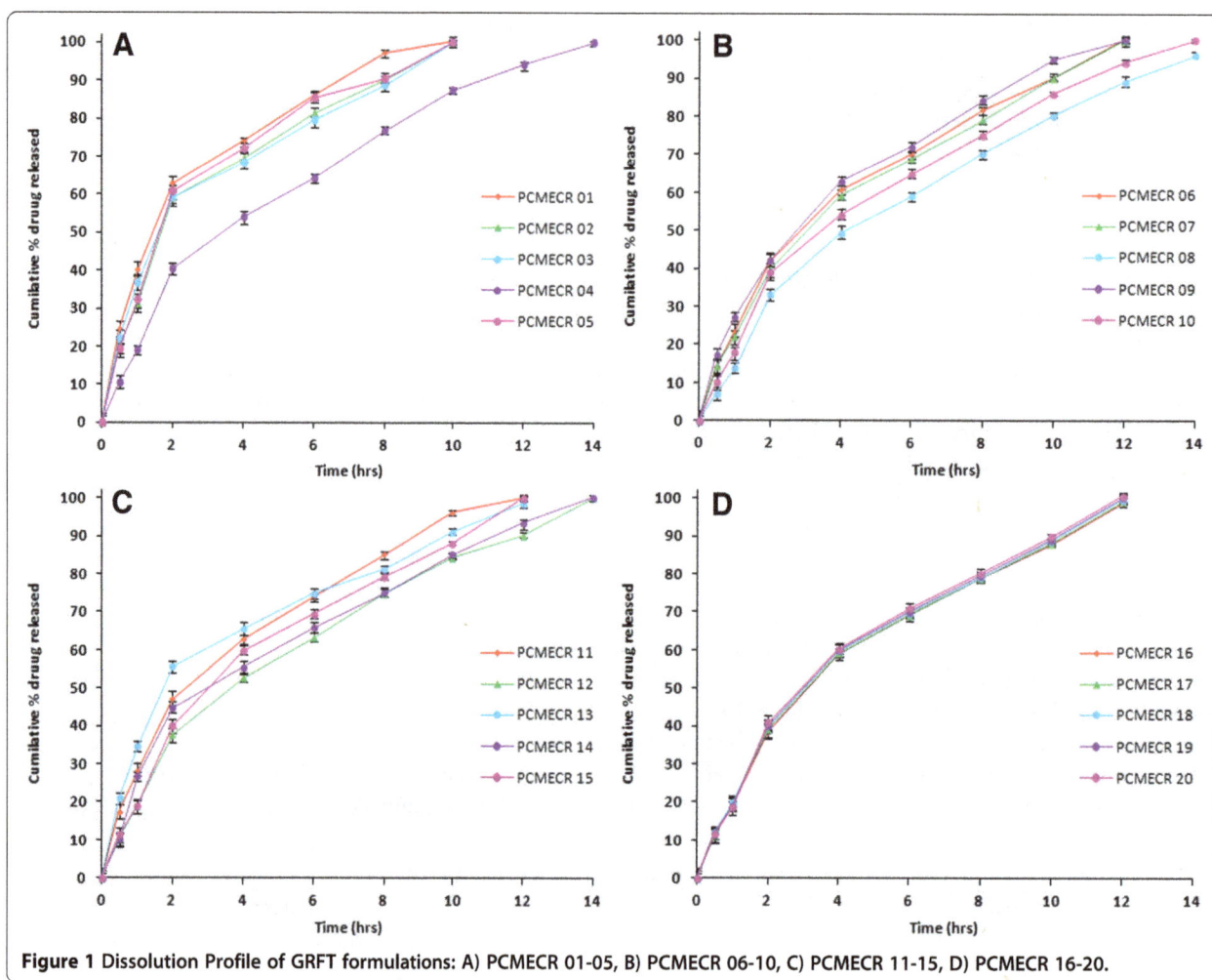

Figure 1 Dissolution Profile of GRFT formulations: A) PCMECR 01-05, B) PCMECR 06-10, C) PCMECR 11-15, D) PCMECR 16-20.

times, $Q_0 = 0$) and K_0 is the zero order release constant expressed in units of concentration/time [12].

First order release kinetics

The release of the drug which followed first order kinetics can be expressed by the equation [13]:

$$\frac{dC}{dt} = -Kc$$

Where K is first order rate constant expressed in units of time^{-1}.

This equation can be modified as

$$\log \quad C = \log C_0 - Kt/2.303$$

Where C_0 is the initial concentration of drug, k is the first order rate constant, and t is the time. The data obtained are plotted as log cumulative percentage of drug remaining vs. time which would yield a straight line with a slope of -K/2.303.

Higuchi equation

It defines a linear dependence of the active fraction released per unit of surface (Q) on the square root of time.

$$Q = k_2 t^{1/2}$$

Where, k_2 is the release rate constant.

A plot of the fraction of drug released against square root of time will be linear if the release obeys Higuchi equation. This equation describes drug release as a diffusion process based on the Fick's law, square root time dependent [14].

Korsmeyer-Peppas model

In order to define a model, which would represent a better fit for the formulation, dissolution data was further analyzed by Peppas and Korsmeyer equation (Power law).

$$M_t/M_\infty = k.t^n$$

Where, M_t is the amount of drug released at time t and M_∞ is the amount released at time ∞, thus the M_t/M_∞ is the fraction of drug released at time t, k is the kinetic constant and n is the diffusion exponent.

In this model, the value of *n* characterizes the release mechanism of drug. For the case of cylindrical tablets, 0.45 = n corresponds to a Fickian diffusion mechanism, 0.45 < n < 0.89 to non-Fickian transport, n = 0.89 to Case II (relaxation) transport, and n > 0.89 to super case II transport [15].

Hixson - Crowell model

Hixson and Crowell recognized that the particles regular area is proportional to the cube root of its volume. They derived the equation:

$$\left(W_0^{1/3} - W_t^{1/3}\right) = Kt$$

Where W_0 is the initial amount of drug in the pharmaceutical dosage form, W_t is the remaining amount of drug in the pharmaceutical dosage form at time t and K (kappa) is a constant incorporating the surface – volume relation [16]. The equation describes the release from systems where there is a change in surface area and diameter of particles or tablets.

Correlation coefficients and release rate kinetics are shown in the Table 3.

Statistical analysis of the data and optimization

Polynomial models including linear, interaction and quadratic terms were generated for all the response variables using Design Expert software. The best fitting model was selected based on the comparisons of several statically parameters including the coefficient of variation (CV), the coefficient of determination (R^2), adjusted coefficient of determination (adjusted R^2) and the predicted residual sum of square (PRESS) provided by Design Expert software. In addition, statistical analysis like analysis of variance (ANOVA) to identify significant effect of factors on response, regression coefficients, F test and P value were also calculated with the software. The results are given in Table 4-5.

The relationship between the dependent and independent variables was further elucidated by using response surface plots (Figure 2-3). These plots are useful in the study of the effects of factors on the response at one time and predict the responses of dependent variables at the intermediate levels of independent variables. Subsequently, a numerical optimization technique by the desirability approach (Figure 4) and graphical optimization technique by the overlay plot (Figure 4) were used to generate the new formulations with the desired responses.

Validation of the experimental design

To validate the chosen experimental design, the resultant experimental values of the responses were quantitatively compared with those of predicted values and % relative error was calculated by the following equation;

$$\% \text{ Relative error} = \frac{(\text{Predicted value} - \text{Experimant value})}{\text{Predicted value}} \times 100$$

Drug interaction studies
Fourier transformation-infrared spectroscopy (FTIR)

FTIR is used to identify the drug excipient interaction. FTIR studies were performed on drug, polymer and statistically optimized formulation. Samples were analyzed by potassium bromide pellet method in an IR spectrophotometer (Shimadzu, FTIR 8700) in the region between 3500-500 cm^{-1}.

Differential scanning calorimetry (DSC)

Differential Scanning Calorimetric analysis of drug, polymer and statistically optimized formulation were done using Differential Scanning Calorimeter (Mettler Toledo Star SW 8.10, Model no: DSC 822). In this process about 8-10 mg of the samples were weighed in aluminum pan and were heated under nitrogen atmosphere from 5 °C to 250 °C.

In vivo buoyancy studies

To confirm the spatial and temporary placement of floating drug delivery system, a variety of techniques have been used like string technique, endoscopy and gamma scintigraphy [17-20]. Of these techniques, X-ray technique was used to determine the gastric residence time of the tablets. In the present investigation X-ray studies were conducted for the evaluation of intragastric floating behavior of the statistically optimized GRFT of propranolol HCl both in fasted and fed states.

The *in vivo* X-ray evaluation of floating ability studies were carried out by administering GRFT of propranolol HCl containing barium sulfate ($BaSO_4$) in humans in fasted and fed state.

Two healthy male subjects of mean age 25 ± 2 yrs (ranging from 23 to 27), mean weight 68 ± 10 Kg (ranging from 58 to 78 kg) and a mean height of 170 ± 5 cm (ranging from 165 to 175 cm) participated in this study. The volunteers were judged healthy on the basis of their previous medical history, physical examination and routine laboratory tests. Both subjects were presented with full details of the investigation, verbally and in written form, prior to providing written informed consent and the study was conducted under the guidance of radiologist. The study was approved from an

Table 3 Correlation coefficient values and release kinetics of GRFT

Formulation	Zero order		First order		Higuchi	Hixson Crowell	Peppas	
	K_0	r	K_1	r	r	r	n	r
PCMECR 01	8.8464	0.9128	0.3922	0.9764	0.9856	0.9848	0.3821	0.9837
PCMECR 02	8.9460	0.9311	0.2738	0.9912	0.9889	0.9786	0.4640	0.9687
PCMECR 03	8.6046	0.9276	0.2519	0.9872	0.9893	0.9593	0.4007	0.9822
PCMECR 04	6.8619	0.9641	0.2158	0.9860	0.9955	0.9953	0.5905	0.9841
PCMECR 05	9.0042	0.9211	0.2886	0.9908	0.9835	0.9745	0.4530	0.9644
PCMECR 06	7.7720	0.9623	0.2174	0.9955	0.9969	0.9937	0.5565	0.9910
PCMECR 07	7.7709	0.9676	0.2119	0.9916	0.9972	0.9938	0.5791	0.9920
PCMECR 08	6.1913	0.9695	0.2027	0.9728	0.9950	0.9947	0.6678	0.9827
PCMECR 09	7.7972	0.9597	0.2660	0.9778	0.9981	0.9930	0.5213	0.9966
PCMECR 10	6.8746	0.9658	0.2119	0.9831	0.9957	0.9947	0.6067	0.9844
PCMECR 11	7.7522	0.9528	0.2840	0.9709	0.9968	0.9908	0.4961	0.9926
PCMECR 12	6.7415	0.9679	0.1835	0.9959	0.9965	0.9958	0.5917	0.9896
PCMECR 13	7.0102	0.9243	0.2830	0.9463	0.9881	0.9807	0.3870	0.9845
PCMECR 14	6.5653	0.9549	0.2004	0.9822	0.9942	0.9893	0.4732	0.9927
PCMECR 15	7.8594	0.9646	0.2036	0.9965	0.9943	0.9564	0.6207	0.9826
PCMECR 16	7.8342	0.9659	0.2929	0.9975	0.9942	0.9837	0.6264	0.9854
PCMECR 17	7.8163	0.9655	0.2022	0.9967	0.9950	0.9801	0.6101	0.9869
PCMECR 18	7.8216	0.9644	0.2063	0.9957	0.9951	0.9749	0.6073	0.9852
PCMECR 19	7.8945	0.9643	0.2096	0.9958	0.9944	0.9931	0.6246	0.9820
PCMECR 20	7.9658	0.9637	0.2169	0.9950	0.9941	0.9934	0.6288	0.9798

independent Institutional Ethics Committee of Andhra University, Visakhapatnam (India).

The statistically optimized GRFT of propranolol HCl was administered to the two volunteers, one under fasted and another one under fed states.

1. Fasted state: The subject was fasted overnight and then swallowed the gastric floating tablet with 200 ml of water. No food was allowed up to 3 hrs of dosing. Subject was not allowed to lay down for sleeping. Every one hour a glass of water (200 ml) was given.

Table 4 Summary of ANOVA results in analyzing lack of fit (LOF) and pure error

Parameters	Sum of squares	df	Mean Square	F value	p value Prob > F	Remark
			Floating lag time (Quadratic model)			
Model	171694	9	19077.11	1.122	0.4269	Not significant
Residual	170028	10	17002.78			
Lack of Fit	155211	5	31042.10	10.47	0.0111	significant
Pure Error	14817	5	2963.4667			
			D_{1hr} (Quadratic model)			
Model	942.28	9	104.6973	16.04	< 0.0001	significant
Residual	65.26	10	6.5265			
Lack of Fit	63.96	5	12.7915	48.93	0.0003	significant
Pure Error	1.31	5	0.2614			
			t_{90} (Linear model)			
Model	29.439	3	9.812	21.28	< 0.0001	significant
Residual	7.377	16	0.461			
Lack of Fit	7.2837	11	0.662	35.47	0.0005	significant
Pure Error	0.0933	5.0000	0.018			

Table 5 Statistical parameters

Parameters	Floating lag time	D_{1hr}	t_{90}
Std. Dev.	130.39	2.555	0.68
Mean	458.90	24.399	9.84
C.V. %	28.41	10.471	6.90
PRESS	1195095.90	502.960	12.95
R-Squared	0.5024	0.9352	0.7996
Adj R-Squared	0.0546	0.8769	0.7621
Pred R-Squared	-2.4973	0.5008	0.6484
Adeq Precision	3.4934	12.842	16.4605

2. Fed state: The subject was fasted overnight and in the morning given a high calorie-high fat breakfast with a total calorie value of approximately 900 Cal. The floating tablet was administered with 200 ml of water after half an hour of the breakfast. The subject was not allowed to eat anything up to 6 hrs but given a glass of water (200 ml) every hour.

Preparation of GRFT for in vivo studies

Optimized GRFT of propranolol HCl containing barium sulfate (PCMECRsoB) for *in vivo* X-ray evaluation were prepared by direct compression method. The amount of propranolol HCl was reduced to 40 mg for incorporating the barium sulfate (40 mg) as radio opaque substance to maintain the constant weight of the tablet. Propranolol HCl (40 mg) was geometrically mixed with CMEC until a homogeneous blend was achieved. Barium sulfate (40 mg), Povidone and sodium bicarbonate were added to the above blend, mixed and lubricated with magnesium stearate (1%w/w). Final blend was directly compressed into tablets on a 16-station rotary tablet punching machine (M/s. Cad mach Machinery Co Pvt Ltd. India) using 9 mm round plain punches at hardness of 4-6 kg/cm^2.

Results and discussion

All the floating tablets were passed physicochemical tests like weight variation, assay and friability. Floating lag times of all the formulations were within the range of 280 to 720 sec (Table 2). As the concentration of sodium bicarbonate increases, the floating lag time found to be decreased.

The cumulative percent drug releases from GRFDDS prepared by central composite design with CMEC are shown in the Figure 1. From the results, it was observed that as the concentration of polymer increased along with concentration of sodium bicarbonate the drug release was retarded. This may be due to increased intensity of air pockets surrounding the jellified surface of the tablet. Increase in the concentration of the sodium bicarbonate at constant polymer concentration also retarded the drug release due to high intensity of the carbon dioxide gas pockets. Drug retardation was directly proportional to the concentration of Povidone which may be due to the formation of strong compactness between the particles [21].

All CMEC based formulations followed first order rate constant with non Fickian diffusion mechanism. (Table 3).

The responses of the floating tablets were fitted to linear, interaction and quadratic model using Design Expert software. As suggested by the software the responses floating lag time, and D_{1hr} is suggested to quadratic model and t_{90} is suggested to linear model (Table 4).

Data analysis

By using semi synthetic polymer CMEC, 20 batches of formulations within the experimental design were prepared to obtain floating tablets which were evaluated for their floating lag time, D_{1hr} and t_{90}. From the ANOVA data, the F value for the floating lag time was found to be 1.12 which indicates that the model is non-significant, whereas for other responses D_{1hr} and t_{90} the F value was found to be 16.04 and 21.28 respectively which indicates that both models are significant. The values of Prob > F less than 0.05 for all the responses except floating lag time are indicating that the models are significant. The response floating lag time exhibited Prob > F value 0.4269, which indicating model was not significant (Table 4). In the response observation for D_{1hr} A, B, C, B^2 and C^2, for t_{90} A, B and C was found to be significant model terms. For floating lag time no significant model terms were found (A: CMEC, B: Sodium bicarbonate, C: Povidone). The lack

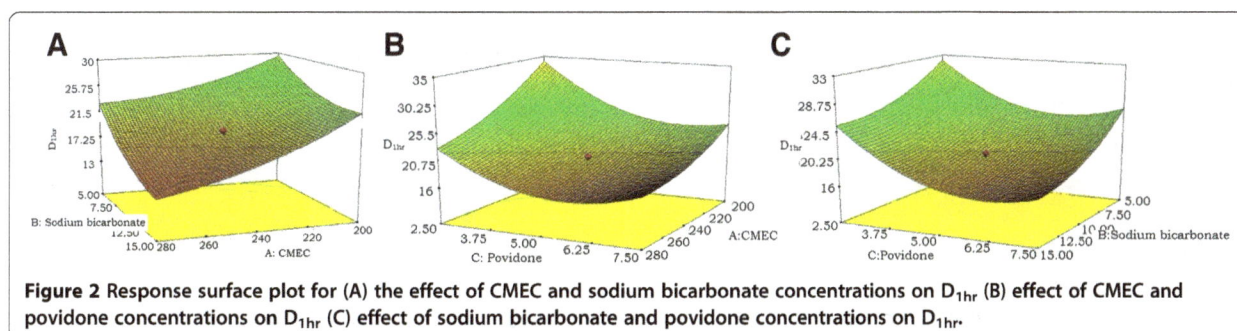

Figure 2 Response surface plot for (A) the effect of CMEC and sodium bicarbonate concentrations on D_{1hr} (B) effect of CMEC and povidone concentrations on D_{1hr} (C) effect of sodium bicarbonate and povidone concentrations on D_{1hr}.

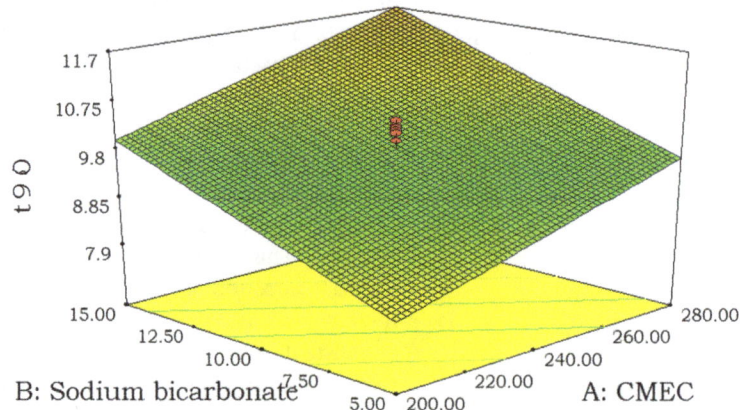

Figure 3 Response surface plot for (A) the effect of CMEC and sodium bicarbonate concentrations on t_{90}.

of fit F value for floating lag time, D_{1hr} and t_{90} was found to be 0.0111, 0.0003 and 0.0005 respectively implies that the lack of fit is significant. Similarly 'R- squared' value was also calculated for all responses. The ideal value is nearer to zero. 'R- Squared' value in the present model is near to zero which indicates towards a good model. In all the cases 'Pred R squared' values are in reasonable agreement with the 'Adj R squared' values except floating lag time (0.8769 & 0.5008 for D_{1hr} and 0.7621 & 0.6484 for t_{90}). A negative 'Pred R squared' was observed for the floating lag time response which implies that the overall mean is a better predictor of this response than current model. In all the case 'Adeq Precision' values are in the range of 12 – 17 except floating lag time which indicates an adequate signal and the model can be used to navigate the design space. For floating lag time 'Adeq Precision' was found to be 3.49 which indicates an inadequate signal and we should not used this model to navigate the design space (Table 5). Even though lack of fit was significant for all the variables, the model was preceded further because of the positive results obtained with other parameters such as F value, values of Prob > F, 'R- squared', 'Pred R squared' and 'Adj R

squared' for D_{1hr} and t_{90} responses. Hence in the present investigation only D_{1hr} and t_{90} responses were taken as dependent variables and optimization was proceeding with these parameters.

The application of response surface methodology yielded the following regression equations which are an empirical relationship between the logarithmic values of floating lag time, D_{1hr} and t_{90}. Test variables in coded units:

$$\text{Floating lag time} = 394.75 - 12.67 * A + 3.13 * B$$
$$- 30.42 * C - 29.37 * A * B$$
$$+ 98.13 * A * C + 29.38 * B * C$$
$$+ 63.02 * A^2 + 29.61 * B^2 + 1.32 * C^2$$

$$D_{1hr} = +19.25 - 4.32 * A - 3.72 * B - 3.56 * C$$
$$- 1.01 * A * B + 1.22 * A * C - 0.48 * B * C$$
$$+ 1.47 * A^2 + 1.78 * B^2 + 4.28 * C^2$$

$$t_{90} = 9.83 + 0.85 * A + 1.02 * B + 0.63 * C$$

The contour and response surface plots for the all responses of all the formulation factors are shown in

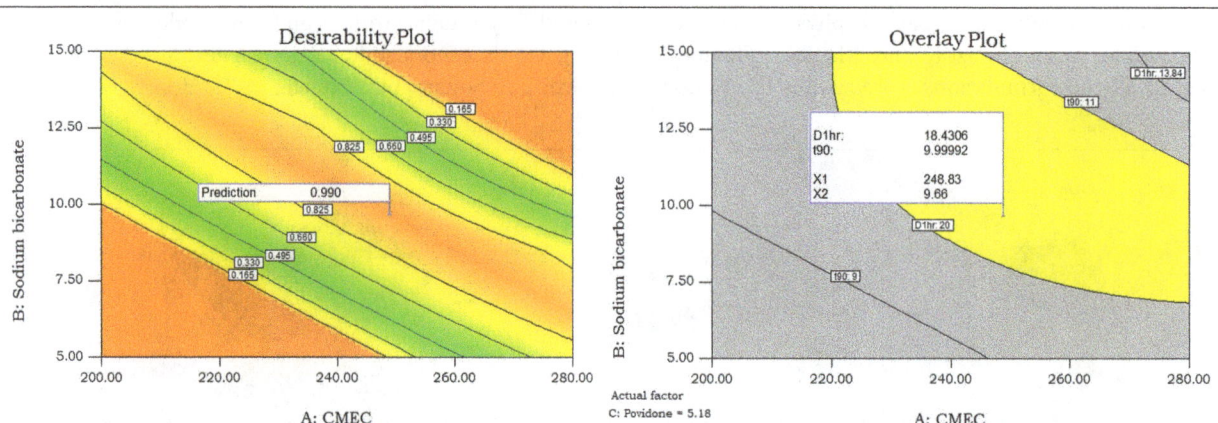

Figure 4 Desirability plot and Overlay plot for optimization of gastroretentive floating tablets of propranolol HCl.

Statistical optimization of a novel excipient (CMEC) based gastro retentive floating tablets of propranolol...

209

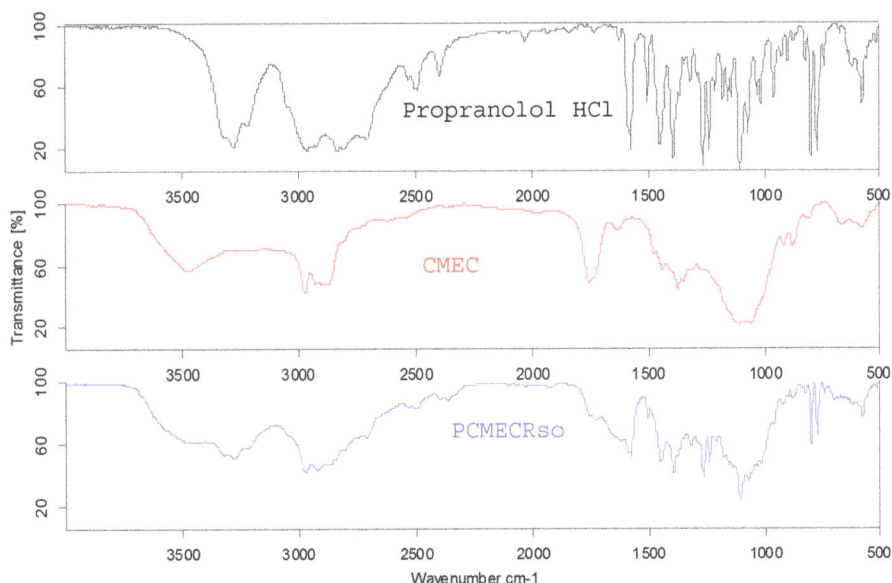

Figure 5 FTIR spectra of propranolol HCl, CMEC and PCMECRso.

Figure 2-3. Contour and response plots of the response surface as a function of two factors at a time, holding all other factors at fixed levels, are more helpful in understanding both the main and the interaction effects of these two factors.

Optimization

To optimize all the responses with different targets, a multi criteria decision approach like a numerical optimization technique by the desirability function and graphical optimization technique by the overlay plot were used (Figure 4). The optimized formulation was obtained by applying constraints on dependent variable responses and independent variables.

Optimized formulation was selected based on the criteria of less than 20% of the drug release at 1 hr (fixed by USP dissolution conditions [11]) and 90% of the drug released in between 10 to 11 hrs. Floating lag time was omitted in the optimization process as per the previous discussion. These constrains are common for all the formulations. The recommended concentrations of the independent variables were calculated by the Design Expert software from the above plots which has the highest desirability near to 1.0.

The optimum values of selected variables obtained by using Design Expert software was 248.88 mg of CMEC, 9.66% of sodium bicarbonate and 5.18% of Povidone for the development of GRFT of propranolol HCl.

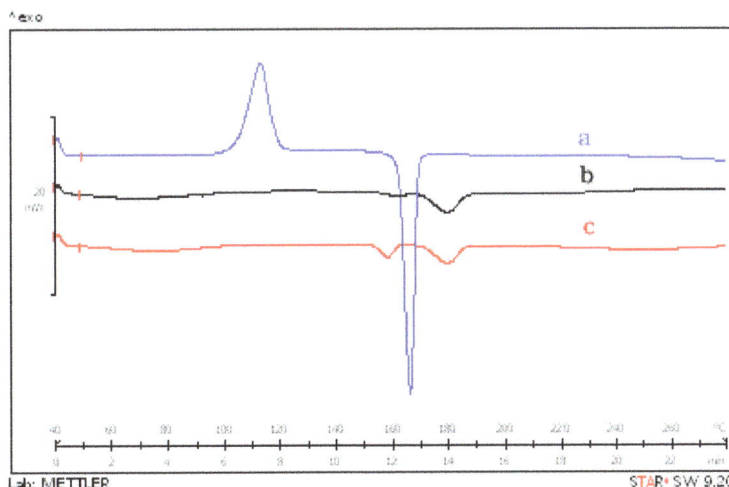

Figure 6 DSC thermogram of a) propranolol HCl, b) CMEC and c) PCMECRso.

Table 6 *In vivo* **residence time of the optimized GRFT of propranolol HCl containing barium sulfate (PCMECRsoB)**

Time (hrs)	Position of the tablet in GIT	
	Fed state	Fasted state
0.5	Stomach	Stomach
2	Stomach	Stomach
4	Stomach	Small intestine
6	Stomach	Disappeared from gastric region
8	Disappeared from gastric region	

Evaluation and validation of optimized formulations

The optimized formulation fulfilled all the criteria of physicochemical properties. *In vitro* buoyancy and dissolution studies were carried out on the prepared optimized formulations for verification of the theoretical prediction. Observed responses and predicted values for D_{1hr} and t_{90} was found to be 17.21%, 10.3 hrs and 18.43%, 10 hrs respectively. The % relative error between the predicted values and experimental values of each response was calculated and the values were found to be 2.55% and 3.0% for D_{1hr} and t_{90} respectively. From the results, it was concluded that these experimental findings are in close agreement with the model predictions which confirmed the predictability and validity of the model.

Drug interaction studies

Fourier transformation-infrared spectroscopy (FTIR)

The FTIR spectrum of propranolol HCl, CMEC and Optimized formulation are shown in Figure 5. Propranolol HCl showed characteristic secondary amine –N–H stretch at 3280 cm^{-1}, C-H stretch at 2964 cm^{-1}, Aryl C = C stretch at 1579 cm^{-1}, Aryl 0-CH$_2$ asymmetric stretch at 1240 cm^{-1}, Aryl 0-CH$_2$ symmetric stretch at 1030 cm^{-1} and the peak at 798 cm^{-1} due to alpha- substituted naphthalene [22].

The FTIR spectrum of CMEC showed the characteristic alcoholic –OH stretch at 3476 cm^{-1}, C-H stretch at

2976 cm^{-1}, -C = O stretch at 1761 cm^{-1} and -C-O-C asymmetric stretch at 1378 cm^{-1}.

Statistically optimized CMEC based formulation (PCMECRso) showed all the characteristic peaks of propranolol HCl with minor shifts in its FTIR spectrum. This spectrum showed secondary amine –N–H stretch at 3280 cm^{-1}, C-H stretch at 2974 cm^{-1}, Aryl C = C stretch at 1579 cm^{-1}, Aryl 0-CH$_2$ asymmetric stretch at 1241 cm^{-1}, Aryl 0-CH$_2$ symmetric stretch at 1031 cm^{-1} and the peak at 797 cm^{-1} due to alpha- substituted naphthalene.

Differential scanning calorimetry

DSC thermogram of propranolol HCl, CMEC and PCMECRso are shown in the Figure 6. The DSC thermogram of CMEC showed a sharp endothermic peak at 183.5 °C that corresponds its melting point. From the results, it was observed that the thermogram of statistical optimized formulation PCMECRso showed sharp endothermic peaks at 163.2 °C and 183.1 °C represents drug and polymer respectively, which indicated that slight decrease in the energy change of melting endotherm, which confirms minor extent of reduction in the crystallinity of the drug but not a significant reduction.

The absence of any changes in the FTIR spectra and DSC thermogram for the selected formulation indicated no chemical interaction between the CMEC and drug.

In vivo buoyancy studies

This study was aimed to examine whether the floating tablet system could buoyant and retain in the stomach. A radiological method was adopted to monitor the developed gastro retentive floating tablets in the gastric region of humans in different feeding conditions. The GRFT remained buoyant on gastric content under both fasted and fed states in volunteers participated in the present study. However, a difference in floating and gastric retention time was obeyed according to the feeding conditions given in Table 6.

In the fasted state, the floating tablets were observed to be buoyant on the gastric fluid up to at 2 hr as shown

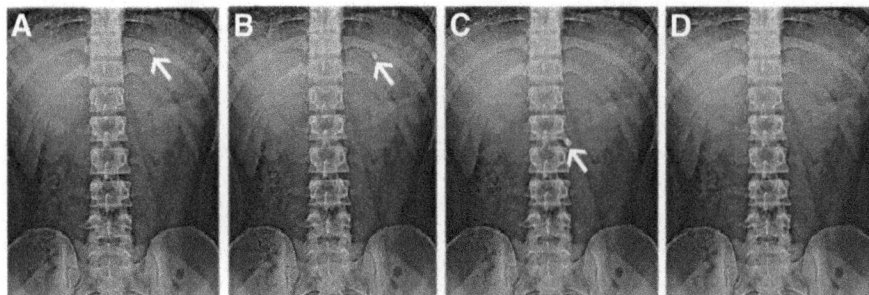

Figure 7 X- ray photographs of gastric floating tablets of PCMECRsoB containing propranolol HCl under fasted state after (a) 0.5 hrs (b) 2 hrs (c) 4 hrs (d) 6 hrs.

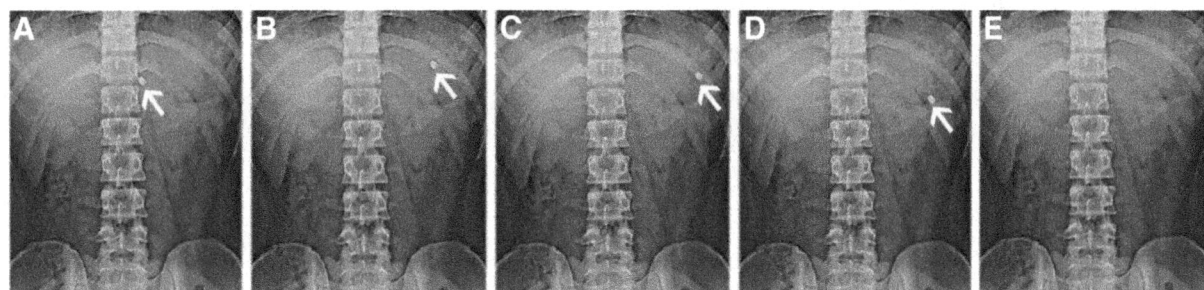

Figure 8 X- ray photographs of gastric floating tablets of PCMECRsoB containing propranolol HCl under fed state after (a) 0.5 hrs (b) 2 hrs (c) 4 hrs (d) 6 hrs (e) 8 hrs.

in Figure 7 (a&b) and were observed in the small intestine after 4 hrs as shown in Figure 7 (c) and was disappeared at 6th hr as shown in Figure 7 (d). Therefore, in such condition, the floating property did not enhance gastric retention time (GRT). The rapid emptying was attributed to periods of strong contractile activity, which occur under fasting conditions every 1.5 to 2 hrs, and effectively sweep undigested material from the stomach [20,23]. As a result of this activity, dosage form administered to fasted subjects could be emptied as rapidly as within an hour or two, depending on the presence of the strong motor induced contractile activity.

In the fed state after the high calorie high fat breakfast, the GRFT was observed to be buoyant on the gastric contents up to 6 hrs after administration as shown in Figure 8 (a) at 0.5 hrs, 8 (b) at 2 hrs, 8 (c) at 4 hrs, 8 (d) at 6 hrs and disappeared at 8th hr shown in Figure 8 (e).

Therefore, in the fed condition, the floating system showed a GRT prolonged by about 5 to 6 hrs over the fasted state.

The evaluation of the GRFT of propranolol HCl intragastric behavior in humans, showed the actual floatability of the tablet on the gastric content.

This study has demonstrated that in the fasted state under the influence of strong motor activity (the migrating myoelectric complex), there was no enhancement of GRT of gastro retentive floating tablet, where as there was a prolonged GRT of approximately 6 hrs in a fed state.

Conclusion

Thus the present study clearly indicated the applicability of the statistical optimization techniques for the prediction of the optimized concentrations of the excipients that influence the product parameters. These theoretical predictions can be verified for their experimental success as in the present case. The statistical optimization reduces the number of experiments to be carried for obtaining formulation with desired properties. Moreover the optimization is also useful in reducing the concentrations of the excipients to their optimum levels

avoiding unnecessary wastage of excipients and thereby reducing the cost of the final product. The intragastric behavior of statistically optimized GRFT of propranolol HCl in humans, showed the floatability of the tablet on the gastric content. *In vivo* evaluation demonstrated no enhancement of GRT of gastro retentive floating tablet in fasted state, where as there was a prolonged GRT of approximately 6 hrs in the fed state. From the results, it is concluded that CMEC is novel semi synthetic polymer suitable for the development of GRFT of propranolol HCl.

Competing interests
The author(s) declare that they have no competing interests.

Authors' contributions
MVS: The corresponding author involved in the literature survey, procurement of excipients, plan of research, statistical design, carrying out the bench work, statistical interpretation and drafting of the final manuscript. NSR: Co- research scholar who was involved in conducting dissolution studies and physicochemical characterization of the formulations. SAS: Co- research scholar involved in the analytical method development and interpretation of the FTIR & DSC studies. BJR: Senior research scholar involved in the *in vivo* buoyancy characterization of the formulations and he gave valuable suggestions for drafting the manuscript. KVRM: Research guide, who gave valuable suggestions in the design of experimental formulas, interpretation of the statistical data, critical review of the manuscript for intellectual content, vital and crucial review and approval of the final manuscript to be published. He also granted me permission to carry out research activities along with use of the equipment in the laboratory. All the above authors read and approved the final manuscript.

Acknowledgement
The author is thankful to UGC (University Grants Commission, India) for awarding Senior Research Fellowship for carrying out this project. One of the authors, M.V.Srikanth, is thankful to K Praveen Kumar and C Vasu for providing valuable information to carry out the research work.

Author details
[1]School of Pharmacy, International Medical University, Kuala Lumpur 57000, Malaysia. [2]A.U. College of Pharmaceutical Sciences, Andhra University, Visakhapatnam 530003, India.

References
1. Shivkumar HG, Gwda DV, Pramod Kumar TM: **Floating Controlled Drug Delivery Systems For Prolong Gastric Residence.** *Ind J Pharm Educ* 2001, 38(4):172–179.

2.   Moes AJ: **Gastroretentive dosage forms.** *Crit Rev Ther Drug Carrier Syst* 1993, **10**:143.

3.   Fell JT, Whitehead L, Collet H: **Prolonged gastric retention using floating dosage forms.** *Pharm Technol* 2000, **24**(3):82–90.

4.   Mathura RS, Sanghvi NM: **Novel drug delivery systems for captopril.** *Drug Dev Ind Pharm* 1992, **18**:1567–1574.

5.   Tripathi KD: *Antihypertensive drugs, Essentials of medical pharmacology.* 5th edition. New Delhi: Jaypee Brothers; 2003:235–236.

6.   Williams DA, Temke TL, Foyes: *Principles of medicinal chemistry, International student edition.* Philadelphia: Lippincott Williams and Wilkins; 2002:489–493.

7.   Davis SS: **Formulation strategies for absorption windows.** *Drug Discov Today* 2005, **10**(4):249–257.

8.   Singh BN, Kim KH: *Encyclopedia of pharmaceutical technology, drug delivery: oral route.* New York: Marcel Dekker; 2001:1253.

9.   Box GPE, Wilson KB: **On the experimental attainment of optimum conditions.** *J Royal Stat Soc Ser B* 1951, **13**:1.

10. Srikanth MV, Sreenivasa R, Sunil SA, Sharma GS, Uhumwangho MU, KV Rm: **Formulation and evaluation of Gastro retentive floating drug delivery system of Ofloxacin.** *Drug Inv Today* 2011, **3**(3):7–9.

11. USP 24 NF 19: *United states pharmacopoeial convention.* Philadelphia, PA: Inc.,National Publishing; 2000:1429.

12. Lazarus J, Cooper J: **Absorption, Testing, and Clinical Evaluation of Oral Prolonged-Action Drugs.** *J Pharm Sci* 1961, **50**:715.

13. Wagner JG: **Interpretation of percent dissolved-time plots derived from invitro testing of conventional tablets and capsules.** *J Pharm Sci* 1969, **58**:1253.

14. Higuchi T: **Mechanism of sustained action medication: Theoretical analysis of rate release of solid drugs dispersed in solid matrices.** *J Pharm Sci* 1963, **52**:1145–1149.

15. Korsmeyer R, Gurny R, Peppas N: **Mechanisms of solute release from porous hydrophilic polymers.** *Int J Pharm* 1983, **15**:25–35.

16. Hixson AW, Crowell JH: **Dependence of reaction velocity upon surface and agitation (I) theoretical consideration.** *Ind Eng Chem* 1931, **23**:923–931.

17. Singh BN, Kim KH: **Floating drug delivery systems: an approach to oral controlled drug delivery via gastric retention.** *J Control Release* 2000, **63**:235–259.

18. Arora S, Ali J, Ahuja A, Khar RK, Baboota S: **Floating drug delivery systems: a review.** *AAPS PharmSciTech* 2005, **6**(3):372–390.

19. Baumgartner S: **Optimisation of floating matrix tablets and evaluation of their gastric residence time.** *Int J Pharm* 2000, **195**:125–135.

20. Srikanth MV, Janaki Ram B, Sunil SA, Sreenivasa Rao N, KV Rm: **Gastroretentive drug delivery systems: novel approaches and its evaluation - a review.** *Int J Pharm Sci Rev Res* 2011, **10**(1):203–216.

21. Uhumwangho MU, Latha K, Sunil SA, Srikanth MV, Ramana Murthy KV: **Formulation of gastro-retentive floating tablets of Diltiazem hydrochloride with carnauba wax by melt Granulation technique.** *J Pharm Allied Sci* 2010, **7**(2):979–986.

22. Srikanth MV, Uhumwangho MU, Sreenivasa Rao N, Sunil SA, Janaki Ram B, Ramana Murthy KV: **Formulation and evaluation of gastro retentive floating drug delivery system for propranolol HCl.** *J Pharm Allied Sci* 2011, **8**(2):1339–1348.

23. Timmermans J, Moes AJ: **Factors controlling the buoyancy and gastric retention capabilities of floating matrix capsules: New data for reconsidering the controversy.** *J Pharm Sci* 1994, **83**:18–24.

A system dynamics model for national drug policy

Akbar Abdollahiasl[1*], Abbas Kebriaeezadeh[1,2*], Rassoul Dinarvand[3], Mohammad Abdollahi[2], Abdol Majid Cheraghali[4,5], Mona Jaberidoost[1] and Shekoufeh Nikfar[1]

Abstract

Background: Data modeling techniques can create a virtual world to analyze decision systems. National drug authorities can use such techniques to take care of their deficiencies in decision making processes. This study was designed to build a system dynamics model to simulate the effects of market mix variables (5 P's) on the national drug policy (NDP) indicators including availability, affordability, quality, and rationality. This was aimed to investigate how to increase the rationality of decision making, evaluate different alternatives, reduce the costs and identify the system obstacles. System dynamics is a computer-based approach for analyzing and designing complex systems over time. In this study the cognitive casualty map was developed to make a concept about the system then the stock-flow model was set up based on the market demand and supply concept.

Results: The model demonstrates the interdependencies between the NDP variables through four cognitive maps. Some issues in availability, willingness to pay, rational use and quality of medicines are pointed in the model. The stock-flow diagram shows how the demand for a medicine is formed and how it is responded through NDP objectives. The effects of changing variables on the other NDP variables can be studied after running the stock-flow model.

Conclusion: The model can initiate a fundamental structure for analyzing NDP. The conceptual model made a cognitive map to show many causes' and effects' trees and reveals some relations between NDP variables that are usually forgotten in the medicines affairs. The model also provides an opportunity to be expanded with more details on a specific disease for better policy making about medication.

Keywords: National drug policy, System dynamics, Modeling

Background

Everyone has the inevitable right to achieve the high standard health services, thus this is the duty of health policy makers to promote national drug policies (NDP) in line with national health objectives [1,2]. The NDP objectives are defined as making essential quality medicines available in affordable price for rational use. The NDP as a framework of integrated activities is influenced by various factors especially those arisen from inside the government and the decision making systems. The market-mix variables including product, price, promotion, place and people are also added to other complexities and issues that should be taken into account by national drug authorities (NDAs) [3].

The NDP key indicators should be compatible with health system objectives in terms of effectiveness, financial fairness and responsiveness. Monitoring the processes and their results is so essential, however lack of the live key indicators make it difficult to have a clear picture of the consequences of decisions made by NDAs [4,5].

The NDA and different parties in the ministry of health (MOH) have problems in making unified decisions that would result in amelioration or deterioration of NDP indicators. Surely, the drug systems and decision makers have limited resources and technologies to predict and evaluate the consequences of their decisions. Exploring the previous studies shows a retrospective nature of appraising evidences and key performance indicators that influence the decision making processes in the health systems [6]. In fact the consequences of some NDAs' decisions are appeared when it cannot be compensated. To overcome such a deficit in decision making, the role of simulation systems for solving the problems is reasonable [7,8].

* Correspondence: abdollahiasl@gmail.com; kebriaee@sina.tums.ac.ir
[1]Department of Pharmacoeconomics and Pharmaceutical administration, Pharmaceutical policy research center and Faculty of Pharmacy, Tehran University of Medical Sciences (TUMS), Tehran, Iran
[2]Department of Toxicology and Pharmacology, Faculty of Pharmacy and Pharmaceutical Sciences Research Center, TUMS, Tehran, Iran
Full list of author information is available at the end of the article

The NDP is a complex system involving many variables; therefore, a system thinking approach is needed to analyze the roles of influencing factors [9]. To enhance the system efficiency and integrating activities, analysis of processes and evaluation the negative/positive effects of key variables must be addressed.

Qualitative and quantitative improvement in health system necessitates NDAs to provide higher quality services but considering government downsizing and budget constraints, there is no opportunity to increase human and capital resources. Therefore, simulation-based systems can facilitate and accelerate the decision process in order to help policy makers.

System dynamic (SD) is a modeling concept that supports decision systems by breaking them into simpler and smaller subsystems. It helps:

- Shortening the decision process
- Increasing the rationality of actions
- Evaluating the different alternatives
- Reducing the costs
- Decreasing the human-derived mistakes
- Increasing reliability and validity
- Providing potentials for sensitivity analysis and repeatability.

SD founded by Jay Forrester is used to analyze the performance of complex systems [10]. It is typically used for models that represent relationships between system variables, rates of change over time and unequivocal feedbacks [11].

A rational relationship between the functions of the NDP core components and market-mixed variables as the main variables of decision making would enhance the outcomes and effectiveness of decisions. To use SD method, it is essential to add some other constant variables and relations to the model.

Although modeling technique is not a new approach in policy making, it is new in pharmaceutical affairs [12,13]. Nowadays there is no such systematic decision module in Iran while NDAs need such a tool to take care of deficiencies in decision making process. There are some negative and positive variables which affect the NDP. Therefore, building a systemic model can identify, analyze and monitor the negative/positive effects of influential factors and at the end reduces the negative effects and improves positive effects which causes the NDP to promote.

Taking the case of Iran pharmaceutical sector into account, we designed this study to analyze the effects of market mix on the NDP indicators. This study was aimed to investigate the NDP components, helps to rationalize activities and decision making, evaluates different alternatives and increases the cost-effectiveness of interventions.

Method

In fact SD models are crucial and effective tools for focusing on stock variables and the flows between them. Therefore, it seems using SD as a well-adjusted modeling technique is authentic to respond to the requirements of this study [14,15].

The model should dynamically and quantitatively simulate the core components of NDP (availability, affordability, quality and rational use). Furthermore, it should reflect the interactions between the components and the market-mix variables (price, product, place, people, and promotion). The model should also address the key influencing factors for improvement of health policies.

The NDP is composed of four subsystems: availability, affordability, quality, and rationality. The related variables were listed (Table 1) and the model was developed in a deductive basis in three phases:

- Conceptualization: in this phase, the purpose of the model, the main structure, the boundaries of system and subsystems were developed and the results were demonstrated through a casual network or a cognitive map [16-19]. In addition to the articles and documents, an expert panel (including three decision maker in IR FDA, one expert of SD and two pharmacoeconomists) formed to justify the model.
- Stock-flow modeling: the variables are categorized to level, auxiliary and constant. Then the adjusted model and mathematical equations between the variable were developed. For running the model Vensim PLE software were used. This software makes an opportunity to develop and run system dynamics models in educational or proffesional level [10,20].
- Testing and sensitivity analysis; the model was verified and validated to increase the realty of the simulation. There are some testing methods in SD that would explain in result part [21-23].

Results
Study area
The NDA in Iran -under supervision of MOH- oversees and regulates the provision and utilization of medicines through pharmaceutical division of Food and Drug Administration (IR FDA). The demand of medicines is mainly responded through registered products that are supplied by the public and private manufacturers and importers. IR FDA follows the generic approach and tries to protect domestically produced generic medicines in the market. Two-third of the Iran's 3.5 billion USD market has been supplied by local manufacturers. A half of manufacturers are presented in the stock market and their main stocks holders are the Social Security Investment Company, Melli Bank Investing Company and Alborz

Table 1 The list of variables those used in the models' subsystems (A: Auxiliary, C: Constant variable)

	Variable	Description	Availability	Affordability	Quality	Rationality
1	Affordability	Affordability	C	A		
2	Availability of domestic products	Availability of domestic products	A	C		
3	Availability of imported products	Availability of imported products	A	C		C
4	Brand Strength Dom.	Brand Strength domestic products				A
5	Brand Strength Imp.	Brand Strength imported products				A
6	Community promotion	Community promotion				A
7	Competition Dom.	Competition domestic products	A		A	
8	Consumption Dom	Consumption domestic products	A	A		
9	Consumption Imp.	Consumption imported products	A	A		
10	Cost of production	Cost of production			A	
11	Demand Dom.	Demand domestic products	A		A	
12	Demand dom/imp	Share of domestic products' demand	A		A	
13	Demand Imp	Demand imported products	A		A	
14	Diagnosis accouracy	Diagnosis accouracy				A
15	Distributors stock dom.	Distributors stock domestic products	A			
16	Distributors stock Imp	Distributors stock imported products	A			
17	Drug costs Dom.	Average costs of domestic products	A	A		
18	Drug costs Imp.	Average costs of imported products	A	A		
19	Drug Price Dom.	Average price domestic products	C	C	A	A
20	Drug price Imp.	Average price imported products	C	C	A	A
21	Efficacy	Efficacy				A
22	GDP/Capita	GDP per Capita		C		
23	Global density of pharmacies	Average density of pharmacies in the country	A			
24	Good dispensing practice	Good dispensing practice				C
25	Good lableing	Good lableing				C
26	HouseHold costs	HouseHold costs		C		
27	Import	Volume of imported products	A			
28	Importers	Number of importers	A			
29	Income	Gross national income per capita		C		
30	Induced demand	Induced demand	A			A
31	Informed consumer	Informed consumer				A
32	Intractions	Medicinal intractions				A
33	Market saturation	Market saturation	C			
34	No. distributors	Number of distributors	A			
35	No. Known Patients	Number of known patients				A
36	No. pharmacies	Number of pharmacies	A			
37	No. pharmacists	Number of pharmacists	A			
38	No. physicians	Number of physicians				C
39	No. producers	Number of producers	A			
40	OoP/Household cost	OoP/Household cost		A		
41	OoP/Income	OoP/Income		A		
42	OoP/GDP	OoP/GDP		A		
43	Out of pocket	Out of pocket	A	A		
44	Packaging quality	Packaging quality			A	

Table 1 The list of variables those used in the models' subsystems (A: Auxiliary, C: Constant variable) *(Continued)*

45	Patients purchase domestic	Patients purchase domestic products	A	A		
46	Patients purchase Imp.	Patients purchase imported products	A	A		
47	Pharmacies purchase dom.	Pharmacies purchase domestic products	A			
48	Pharmacies purchase Imp	Pharmacies purchase imported products	A			
49	Pharmacies stock domestic	Pharmacies stock domestic products	A			
50	Pharmacies stock Imp	Pharmacies stock imported products	A			
51	Physicians' K.A.P.	Physicians' Knoledge/Attitude/practice about rationality				A
52	Polypharmacy	Polypharmacy				A
53	Population	Population	C			
54	Prescriber acceptance	Prescriber acceptance				A
55	Prescription	Prescription				A
56	Prescription with injectables	Prescription with injections				A
57	Prescriptions with Ab	Prescriptions with antibiotic				A
58	Producer profit	Producer profit			A	
59	Producers' stock	Producers' stock	A			
60	Production	Production	A		A	
61	Promotion Dom.	Promotion on domestic products	A		A	A
62	Promotion Imp.	Promotion on imported products	A		A	A
63	Quality budget Dom.	Budget for quality improvement of domestic products			A	
64	Quality budget Imp.	Budget for quality improvement of imported products			A	
65	Quality Dom.	Quality index of domestic products	C		A	C
66	Quality Imp.	Quality index of imported products	C		A	C
67	R&D budget	R&D budget			A	
68	Rational prescribing	Rational prescribing				A
69	Rational use	Rational use				A
70	Rationality	Rationality	A			A
71	Real demand	Real demand				A
72	Regional density of medical centers	Regional density of medical centers	A			
73	Regional density of pharmacies	Regional density of pharmacies	A			
74	Regulatory power	Regualatory power			C	
75	RX as OTC	dispensing RX products without prescription				A
76	Safety stock	Safety stock	C			
77	Sales costs	Sales costs			A	
78	Sales value Dom.	Sales value of domestic products	A		A	A
79	Sales value Imp.	Sales value Imported of products	A		A	A
80	Saving/OOP	Saving/OOP		A		
81	Self-treatment	Self-treatment				A
82	Side effects	Side effects				A
83	Social information	Social information				A
84	Stock imported	Stock of imported products	A			
85	Total demand	Total demand	A	A		A
86	Treatment	Treatment		A	A	A
87	User stock Dom.	Stock of domestic products in homes	A			
88	User stock Imp.	Stock of imported products in homes	A			
89	Waste & Exp. Dom.	Waste & expired domestic products	A			

Table 1 The list of variables those used in the models' subsystems (A: Auxiliary, C: Constant variable) *(Continued)*

90	Waste & Exp. Imp.	Waste & expired imported products	A		
91	Willing to use	Willing to use			A
92	WTP	Willingness to pay	A	A	

Investing Company; the other half of manufacturing companies and the most importers are owned by private sectors. There are tens of distributors that distribute medicines around the country but the top five covers about 80 percent of the market. The price of all medicines is set by the government through the commission of pricing in IR FDA. The official method of pricing is cost-plus for generic medicines and external reference pricing for branded products; although some country-specific factors such as market size, anti-inflation policies, national economics and some political issues are determinants. Clinical services are provided by both public and private sectors but patients pay the same price for medicines in both sectors. The majority of the people are covered for their treatment costs by three main basic health insurers; they cover about 45 percent of health costs. The medication costs for certain illness including AIDS, TB, Malaria, Hemophilia, Thalasemia, transplantation and vaccination are covered totally by the MOH [24]. The survey on access to medicines found that most general medicines are available and affordable for all - the lowest paid workers as indicator- in both public and private sectors [25,26].

Logical framework of the model

Our suggested SD conceptual model is composed of two subsystems: NDP objectives and market mix variables. NDP is aimed to improve quality of human life mainly by equitable providing affordable quality drugs for patients who rationally need them. Market mix (5 P's) are components of a market that are aimed by marketing strategies. The interaction between NDP objectives and market mix components shaped the framework of the model.

Health system is too wide and complicated to be modeled completely in a detailed study; the framework of the model determines how deep the model is supposed to study interactions between NDP and market mix. For exploring the interactions among the variables a SD model is proposed which mainly was structured on the demand of medicines.

Firstly, a summarized cognitive map of causal loops was described (Figure 1). As mentioned before, the NDP objectives play an important role in helping the policy makers to determine the demand of patients' medicines. Therefore, the twelve main variables -Affordability, Availability, Consumption, Demand, Distribution-Points, Price, Product Supply, Promotion, Quality, Rationality, Treatment, Willingness to pay (WTP)- formed an overview on the system through the sixteen causal loops. But it was

totally obvious that many other variables should be defined to justify the model. All relations in primary structure expanded to a network of variables; to justify the subsystems some other constant or auxiliary variables were added to the model (Figure 2). The expanded model is a casual network that shows the relationships between all variables in NDP. This vast model is for demonstrating the complexity of the system and is essential to break it to smaller parts for detailed analysis.

In Iran, there are two different governmental approaches against imported medicines and domestically produced ones, therefore it was tried to consider these two approaches in studying the main NDP variables. The nature of the model leads to study it in two parts; the conceptual cognitive map was explored in part 1 and quantifying the variables and running their relationships are explained in part 2 in a stock-flow model.

Part 1–1: Availability

According to the logical framework of NDP, the causal diagram of the availability was designed based on two approaches; domestically produced products and imported ones (Figure 3). Availability has been defined as having the essential stock of the product in determined distribution points [1]. Then the number of pharmacies who distribute the product, the distance between them and the level of

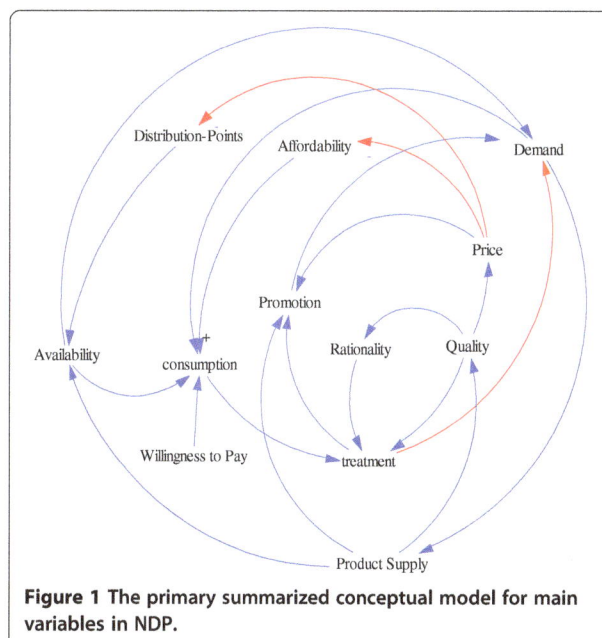

Figure 1 The primary summarized conceptual model for main variables in NDP.

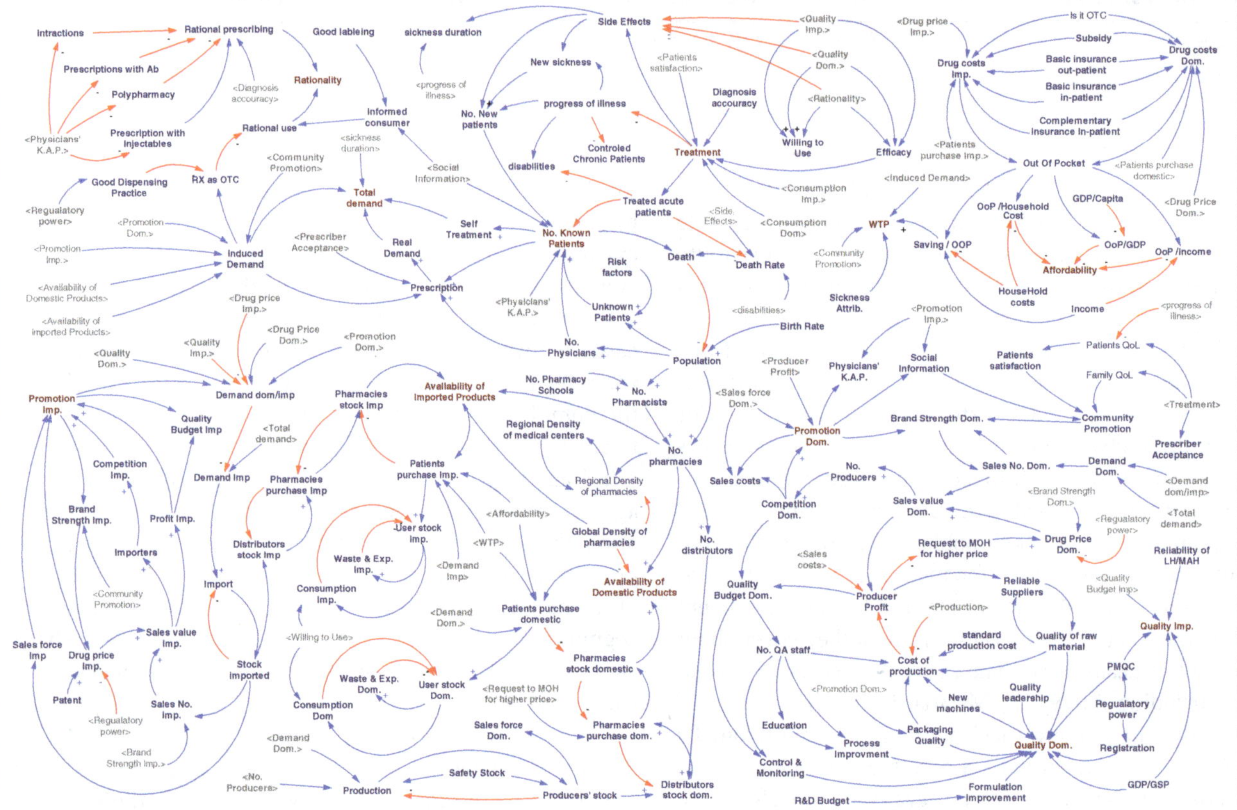

Figure 2 The expanded conceptual model for NDP.

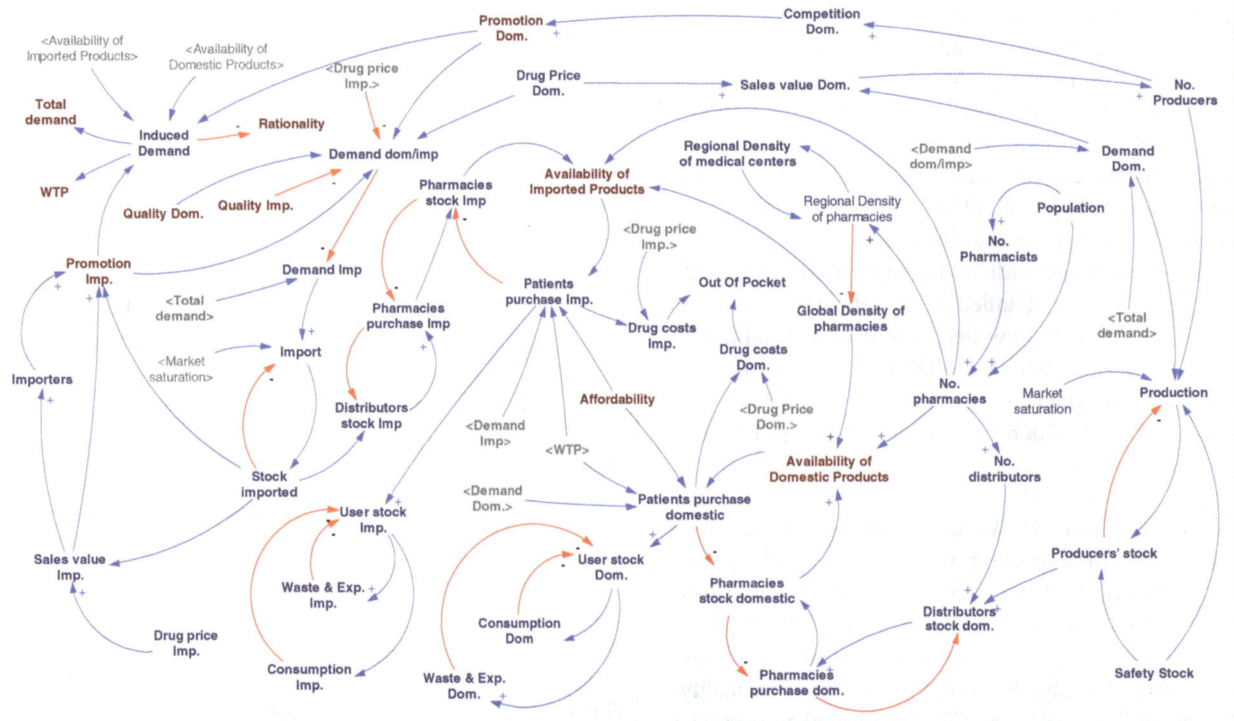

Figure 3 The conceptual model for availability.

stock for domestic and imported products determine the level of availability. In the model, both availability variables are placed in two loops that are balanced with patient purchase and pharmacy stock. Pharmacy stock for both domestic and imported product is a part of medicines supply chain which is affected by distributors' stock and purchase, production, and importation. Patients purchase is influenced by medicines consumption cycles while affordability and WTP are two main variables in these cycles. There is a variable named "demand dom/ imp" that shows the ratio of domestically produced product in the market from demand side. This item would balance the availability level of domestically produced medicines versus imported ones.

The other variables which affect the availability loops through the patients purchase are medicines' stock in patient's homes and in hospital wards; also the waste and expired medicines are effective.

The other issue in availability is "medical malls" that are places that all medical facilities and physicians' offices have been concentrated in; based on the current regulations, the number of pharmacies as the dispensing places of medicines is a function of population, distance to other pharmacies and density of medical centers. Medical malls are ideal locations for founding pharmacies but they are against the physical availability of medicines. The IR FDA as the authorized organization for regulating pharmacies allows increasing the number of pharmacies in these regions regardless to the distance to promote the fair income of pharmacies. It makes a reinforced loop to gather more medical firms in such areas and decrease the uniform distribution of pharmacies around the cities; then the level of availability declines.

Availability is not only an essential factor for access to medicines but it can induce the demand in the market. High level of stock which is in favor of availability would increase the financial costs of suppliers then they increase their sales forces whenever they are overstocked; this is one of the causes of the induced demand. Although in the market the data of demand direct the supply, the role of potential market could not be ignored. Potential market that we showed it in the model as "market saturation ratio" is the extra stock of a medicine that should be supplied in addition to real demand for market confidence. "Market saturation" variable that directly related to the safety stock of a medicine in the country, is affecting significantly on other main variable in the model.

Part 1–2: affordability

Affordability as having enough money to pay for the medicines has involved many contributors in health system. Out of pocket (OOP) /household costs, OOP/income and OOP/gross domestic products (GDP) per capita are three indicators used to show the affordability of medicines

in the model. The coverage of basic and complementary insurances for in-patients and out-patients, the government subsidy on some products such as antihemophilic factors and Iron chelators for Thalassemia, and different pricing approach for over the counter (OTC) medicines are affecting affordability through "out of pocket" (Figure 4).

Although affordability is an important factor to purchase medicines, the role of willingness to pay (WTP) should take into account. Family and social knowledge, promotional activities by suppliers, country and family economical situation, severity of illness and the opportunity costs for medication (the alternative treatments that may exist) tend patients to pay more/less for medicines (Figure 5).

Despite of different policies against domestic and imported medicines, there are more balanced (negative) than reinforced (positive) loops in this part of the model; all variables that could increase patients' OOP, would be balanced through reduction of affordability (Figure 6). Prices of domestic and imported drugs that are the most important inputs of affordability loops are the output of suppliers' requests and negotiation power of the NDA against price increase. The price variables in addition to increase of OOP, can be input of the quality system through sales increase.

Part 1–3: quality

The quality of medicines not only initiates their safety, efficacy, WTP and patient acceptance but also affects on their share in the market. A wide range of variables influence the quality of domestically produced medicines but a few factors could affect the quality of imported ones (Figure 7). Because NDA has no complete control on the quality of imported medicines in production level in the country of origin, completing registration process and enforcing post marketing quality controls are two main tools for assuring the quality.

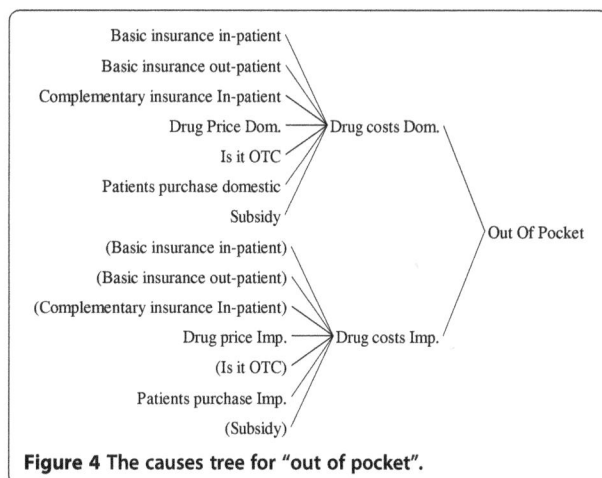

Figure 4 The causes tree for "out of pocket".

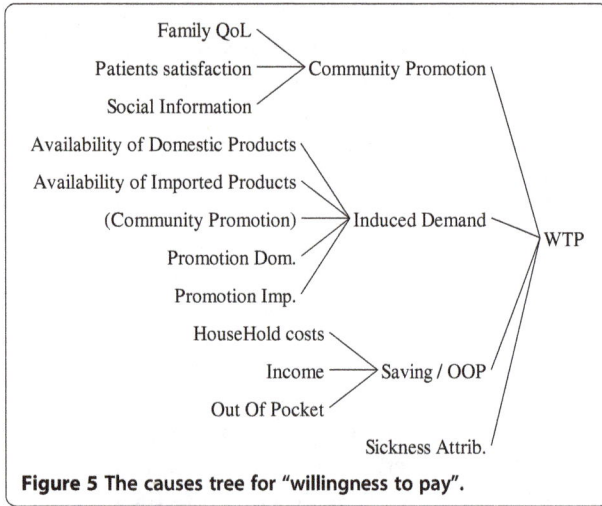

Figure 5 The causes tree for "willingness to pay".

The quality of domestic products placed in two feedback loops: the main balanced loop comes from the cost of quality which increases the cost of production and leads to decrease the quality budget due to the profit reduction. The second loop is a reinforced one coming from the

increase of demand, sales and market share due to the quality. For imported medicines, there is an only reinforced loop coming from investing on the post manufacturing quality controls and quality promotion (Figure 8).

The role of NDA is crucial in improving quality; NDA can promote the concept of quality management in local pharmaceutical companies, create the opportunity for investing on the quality with rationalizing the prices, regulating and auditing good manufacturing/distributing/storage/laboratory practices in drug supply chain, empowering registration process and post marketing quality control practices.

Part 1–4: rational use

Rational drug use as an important pillar of NDP could clinically, socially, and economically help the health system. In this model rational prescribing, good dispensing practice and giving information to patients are the main determinants of rationality. All promotional and advertising activities not only affect on the public health but also change the demand and subsequently modify activities of supply chains. Sales and promotion reinforce each other in two

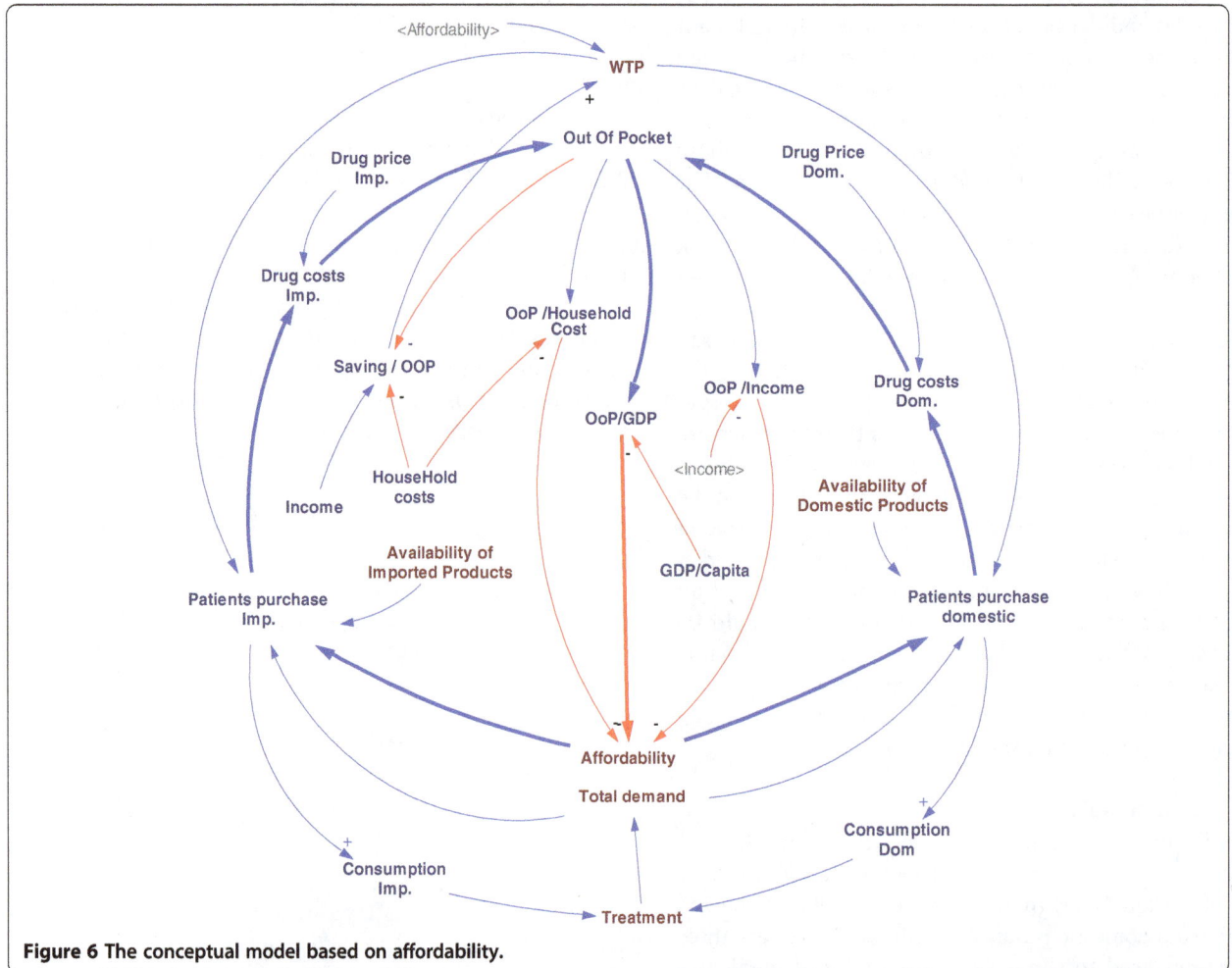

Figure 6 The conceptual model based on affordability.

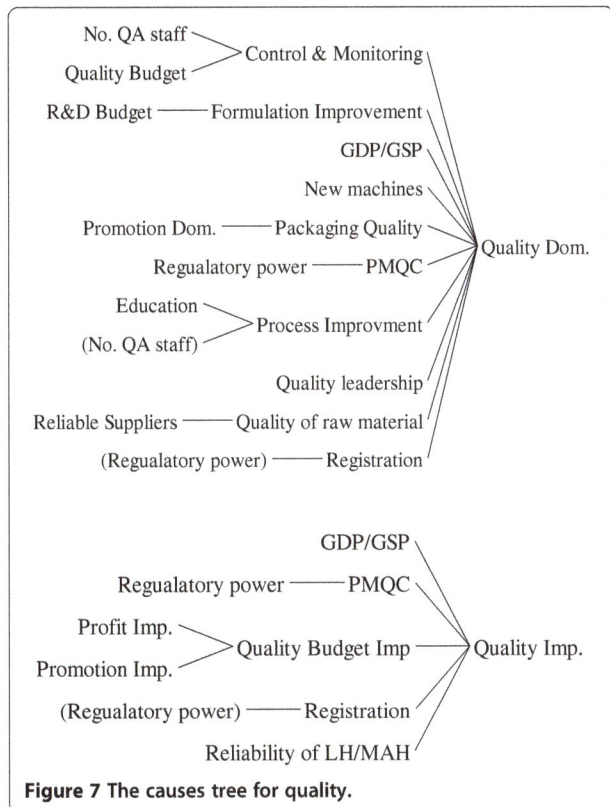

Figure 7 The causes tree for quality.

Part 1–5: Other important variables

There are some other variables in the model including population, birth and death rate, total demand, responded demand, epidemiological indices, number of physicians and pharmacists and diagnosis accuracy that help to complete system for simulation. Although treatment of patients is the main objective of medication, right diagnose, patient compliance, efficacy and side effects can change the treatment progress. Consuming the medicine is not the end of the treatment chain, many chronic diseases are never cured and patients should consume their medicine forever to control the progress of the disease or improve their quality of lives; thus they always stay on the medicine demand cycle. In spite of the demand for main illness treatment, treating the side effects and new sicknesses have some other negative forces on the treatment cycle and leads to new demands. The patients' death in chronic diseases and healing in acute ones removes the patients from the treatment cycle and reduce the demand.

Part 2–1: The stock-flow model

Figure 10 shows the stock flow diagram developed based on the mentioned conceptual casualty network. Population, demand and stock are three bunches of stock variables in the model. Population has divided into four stock variables due to age structure of the country. The incidence rates for each age group, the diagnosis rate and the standard dose of medicine would project the number of susceptible people for treatment that makes the demand. The unit used for demand variables was defined daily dose [27]. Every demand –"susceptible to

positive loops (Figure 9). Because there is an information asymmetry in health system, all activities that improve social information about the medicines and change knowledge, attitude and practice of practitioners can positively affect the rational use and prescribing behavior of the medicines.

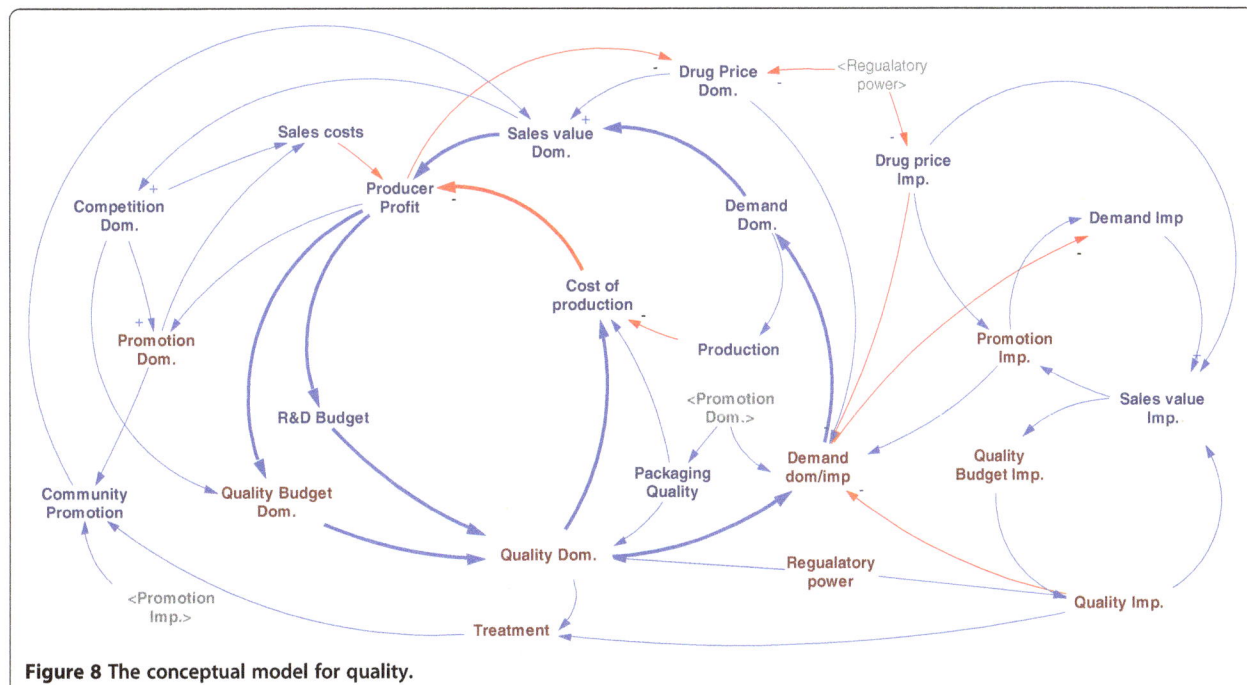

Figure 8 The conceptual model for quality.

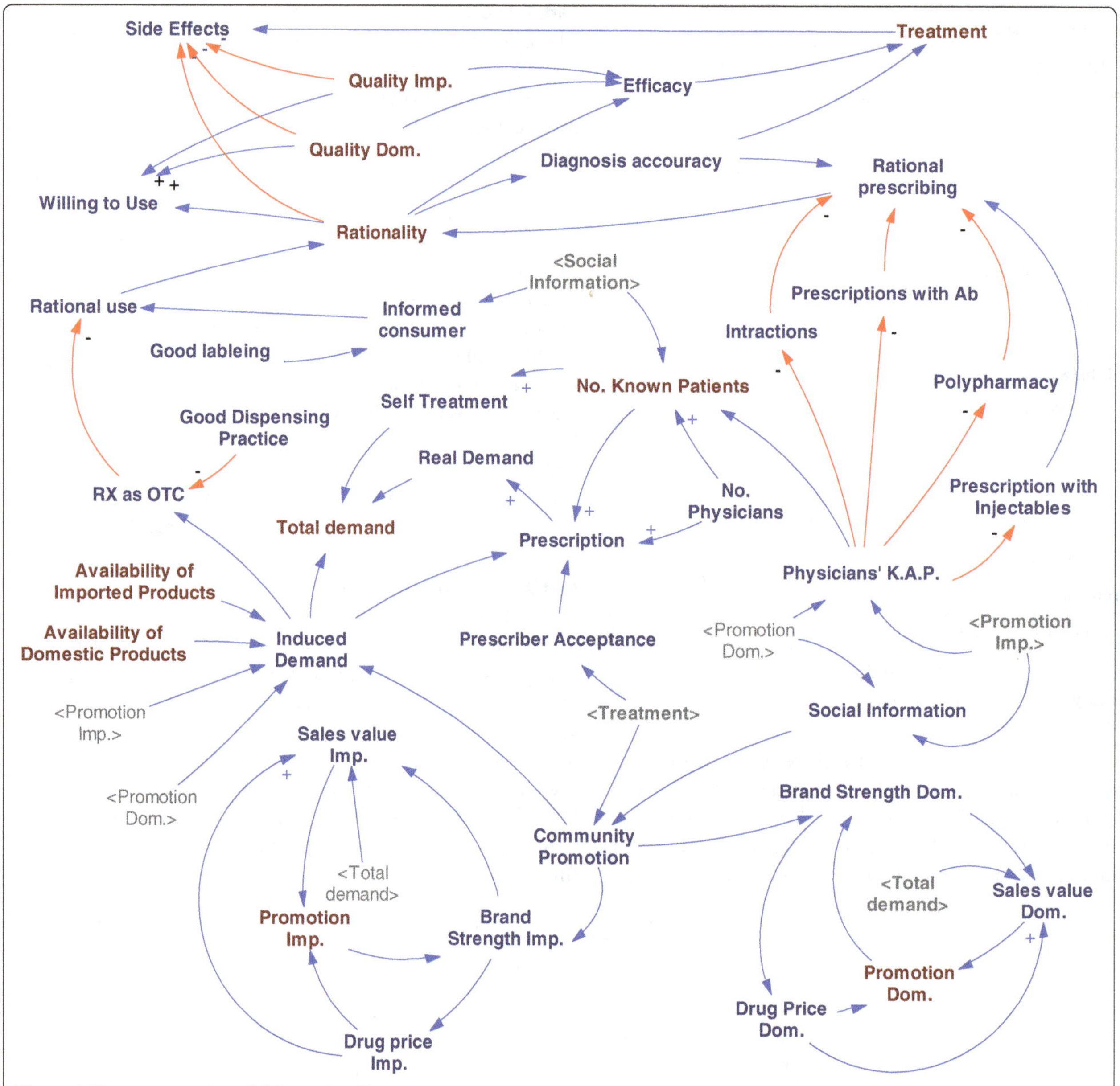

Figure 9 The conceptual model for rationality.

treat"- that is responded - diagnosed, afforded, provided, purchased and consumed -will move to the variable named "responded demand" (Figure 10). Death and stopping treatment are the exit ways of this stock variable for chronic patients; treating rate is the other exit way for acute ones.

All domestic producers and importers collect their supplied medicine in a stock variable called medicine stock. The level of medicine stock variable is higher than the demand based on market saturation rate. The variable "Medicine stock" has two existence way; all demands that can be responded including new demands and current chronic consumers would reduce the medicine

stock through these existence ways called "purchase rates" channels. The purchase rate has made by affordability, availability and WTP.

The quality and rationality related variables put their effects on auxiliary variables called "stop rate" that reduce the number of current consumers.

The variables, their units and the equations were defined on Vensim PLE (academic version) and the model was executed for a 120 months period.

The model was run without any mistakes and the influence of any changes on any variables could be explored on the time trend graphs on other variables that were made by the software.

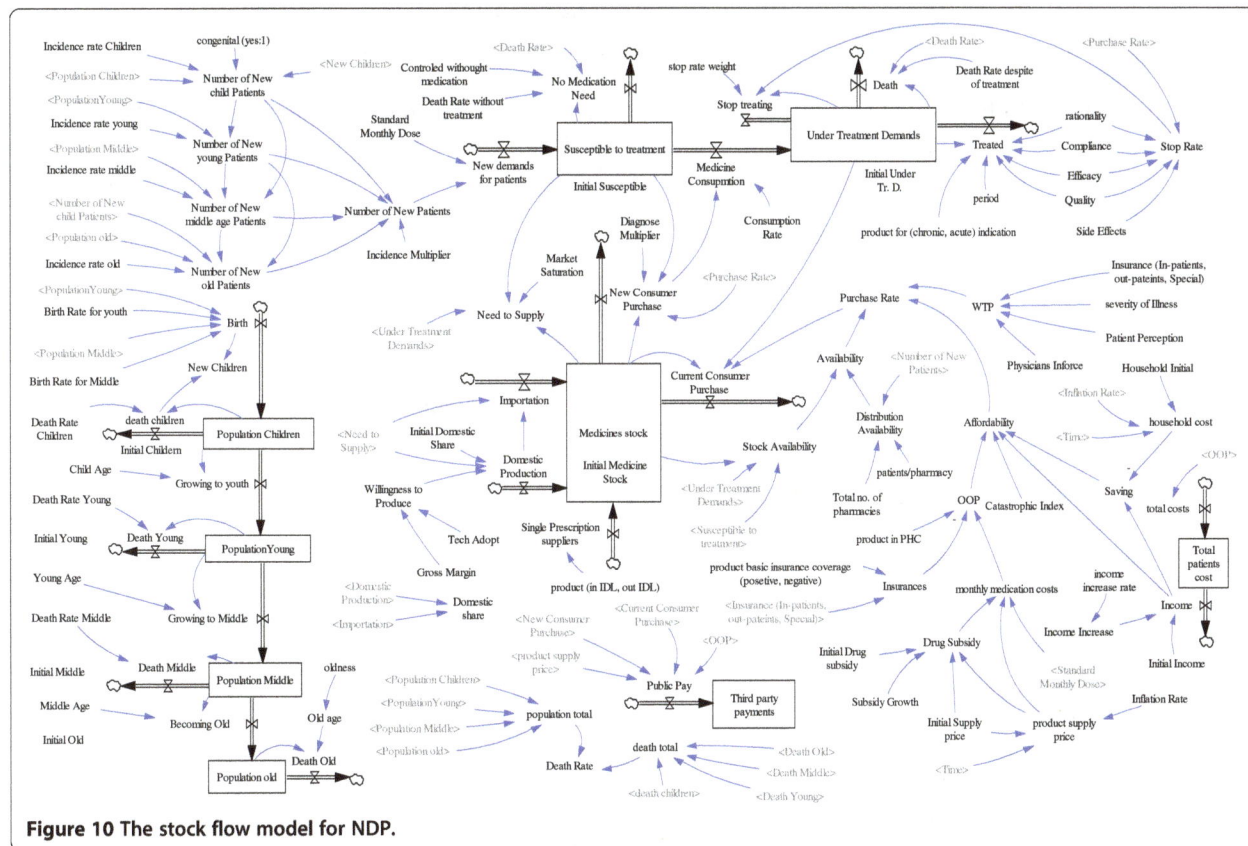

Figure 10 The stock flow model for NDP.

Part 3–1: Validity Tests and sensitivity analysis

There are a wide variety of tests for verification and validation of SD models. To assess the structure, dimensional consistency, extreme conditions and robustness of equations under stress situations are used. For testing behavior reproduction the pattern of outputs are compared with real data. Then the model was tested not only for outputs but also for internal structure [23]. Direct structure tests including extreme-conditions and dimensional consistency was done on all major variables by the software (Vensim). Also the expert panel of the study was revising the structure and casualty relations for many times to reach to the optimum situation.

For testing the structure behavior, some major variables including population groups were compared to real data but for some variables we had no real data for comparing and the expert panel tried to justify them.

Because the concept of modeling in NDP is new in Iran and there are a few written documents about it, reaching to a consensus in the expert panel on the result of the model was difficult; it is challengeable for other experts yet. Some extreme and different conditions that the model tested on them were acute versus chronic, high prevalence versus rare disease, cheap versus expensive treatment and rational high quality drugs versus irrational low quality.

Although for testing the validity, a kind of sensitivity analysis was done but for performing sensitivity analysis all rate variables and initial values are changed in a wide range (even wider than real situation) and the behavior of the model and the value of other major variables were studied. Because there are a lot of variables in the model that should be adjusted with a specific disease and its major treatments, the range of the variables' value significantly depend on the value of other variables. For example if we adjust the model with a rare congenital disease with a full subsidized medicines, availability, affordability and quality variables in the model is no sensitive to the ex-work price or death rate of adults; but it is hugely sensitive to the birth rate.

Discussion

The model is targeted to help policy makers as a decision support system (DSS) with analyzing interrelationships between availability, affordability, quality and rational use of medicines. The casual network was formed by about 140 selected variables made a crowded cognitive map in the conceptual phase that was too complex to interpret so it forced the model to break into four main subsystems. The challenges developed in defining the borders of the subsystems, caused some intersectional variables to be repeated in more than one subsystem.

The stock-flow model has been set based on the demand and supply concept. This demand was made by the population structure and incidence rates. We had to break the population to four stock variables due to the population structure of Iran. Because of the lack of disease epidemiology data in Iran we used any data from any country for covering incidence rates. It was thought this lack of data could be covered by the ability that is in SD to do a wide range of sensitivity analysis. The supply side was summarized to a few level and auxiliary variables that comes to the model as input variables, then it can be expanded to more detailed models in supplementary studies.

Availability subsystem consists of the supply side of the stock-flow model and number of pharmacies as the constant variable; although increasing the number of pharmacies can improve the availability, it cannot overwhelm the total stock situation; the total stock of the modeled medicine comes from the total demand through domestically production and imports. The number of pharmacies under the control of the government has a slow growth due to low population growth rate.

The insurance system and subsidization that play the main role in affordability subsystem present themselves as two constant variables in the stock-flow diagram. The role of insurance organizations can be explained based on the other variables in health financial system. There is a stock variable in the model that shows the cumulative medication costs of the illness and demonstrates the time when patients could fall in catastrophic expenses. The model shows only cancer and autoimmune patients can fall in the catastrophic expenses; medication for normal high burden diseases including cardiovascular, diabetes, central nervous disorders and gastro intestinal are too cheap to send patients to financial failure.

Quality and rationality in the stock-flow diagram are not in the core of the model; they can just affect the model as a foreign control knob.

It was attempted to use mathematical equations between variables than regression equations. Thus, we had to select some variables that can be adopted with it.

Conclusion

The model can initiate a fundamental structure for analyzing NDP. The conceptual model made a cognitive map for NDP that not only shows many causes and effects trees but also reveals some relations between NDP variables that are usually forgotten or ignored in the medicines affairs:

- The role of centralized medical centers in reducing the availability of medicines; although the model is silent on the effects of reducing profit of pharmacies on availability [28].

- It had already been demonstrated the increasing share of imported medicines in the market [29] but this study demonstrates the influence of importers' promotional activities on expanding the market and quality of domestically produced medicines.
- The effects of the patients' WTP on purchasing their medicines and the demand for the medicine.
- The bigger role of prescriber than consumer in rational use of medicines.
- The mutual effects of overstocking in domestic or imported products on supplying and promotion activities.
- The influence of quality and rational use on the patients' willingness to use.

There are also some special points in the model that play significant roles in the NDP that should be more notified:

- The amount of medicines that stocked in patients' homes. It can be the reason that the sales of pharmaceutical usually have no direct relation to health indices [30].
- The effects of medication on the population groups.
- The effect of brand names on the quality.
- The influence of regulatory power on the quality and the supply of medicines that was also explained in other studies [31,32].

Overall this model provides 52 control knobs for the modeler to adjust the model with a selected medicine in a specific disease. Then 121 level and auxiliary variable trends can clarify the consequences of any changes before making any decisions in the NDA.

Linking this model to some real live epidemiological and disease surveillance databases in the country could create a decision support system to help decision making.

The stock-flow model not only shows some relations between NDP variables but provide a framework for other more detailed studies.

Competing interests
The authors declare that they have no competing interests.

Authors' contributions
AA plan the project, set up the panels, developed the primary models, data analysis and drafted the paper, AK and RD conceived and revised the model and supervised the project, MA gave consultation on the study design and edited the draft, AC gave consultation on the conceptual model, SN revised the conceptual model and gave consultation on the medication procedures, MJ revised the stock-flow model and data analysis. All authors read and approved the final manuscript.

Acknowledgements
We thank Dr M. Fazeli, Dr H. Rasekh, Dr M. Cheraghali, the former managing directors of Pharmaceutical division in Iran FDA for their supports in developing the model especially in conceptualization and testing stages.

We would have a special thanks to Mr. M. Alaedini for his guidance in developing the system dynamics model.

Author details
¹Department of Pharmacoeconomics and Pharmaceutical administration, Pharmaceutical policy research center and Faculty of Pharmacy, Tehran University of Medical Sciences (TUMS), Tehran, Iran. ²Department of Toxicology and Pharmacology, Faculty of Pharmacy and Pharmaceutical Sciences Research Center, TUMS, Tehran, Iran. ³Department of Pharmaceutics, Faculty of Pharmacy, TUMS, Tehran, Iran. ⁴Food and Drug Organization, Ministry of Health and Medical Education, Tehran, Iran. ⁵Department of Pharmacology, University of Baqiyatallah Medical Sciences, Tehran, Iran.

References

1. World Health Organization: *How to develop and implement a national drug policy*. Geneva: World Health Organization; 2002.
2. World Health Organization: *WHO medicines strategy: framework for action in essential drugs and medicines policy 2000–2003*. Geneva: WHO; 2000.
3. Kaplan A: **Using the components of the marketing mix to market emergency services.** *Health Mark Q* 1984, **2**:53–62.
4. Nikfar S, Kebriaeezadeh A, Majdzadeh R, Abdollahi M: **Monitoring of National Drug Policy (NDP) and its standardized indicators; conformity to decisions of the national drug selecting committee in Iran.** *BMC Int Health Hum Rights* 2005, **5**:5.
5. Kruk ME, Freedman LP: **Assessing health system performance in developing countries: a review of the literature.** *Health Policy* 2008, **85**:263–276.
6. Paniz VM, Fassa AG, Maia MF, Domingues MR, Bertoldi AD: **Measuring access to medicines: a review of quantitative methods used in household surveys.** *BMC Health Serv Res* 2010, **10**:146.
7. Abdollahiasl A, Nikfar S, Kebriaeezadeh A, Dinarvand R, Abdollahi M: **A model for developing a decision support system to simulate national drug policy indicators.** *Arch Med Sci* 2011, **7**:744–746.
8. Lane DC, Husemann E: **Steering without Circe: attending to reinforcing loops in social systems.** *System dynamics review* 2008, **24**:37–61.
9. Homer J, Milstein B: *Optimal decision making in a dynamic model of community health*, System Sciences, 2004 Proceedings of the 37th Annual Hawaii International Conference on. IEEE; 2004:11.
10. Sterman JD: **System dynamics modeling.** *California management review* 2001, **43**:8–25.
11. Forrester JW: *System dynamics and the lessons of 35 years*, A systems-based approach to policymaking. Springer; 1993:199–240.
12. Homer JB, Hirsch GB: **System dynamics modeling for public health: background and opportunities.** *Am J Public Health* 2006, **96**:452–458.
13. Koelling P, Schwandt MJ: **Health systems: A dynamic system-benefits from system dynamics.** *Proceedings of the 2005 Winter Simulation Conference* 2005, **1–4**:1321–1327.
14. Pfaffenbichler P: **Modelling with Systems Dynamics as a Method to Bridge the Gap between Politics, Planning and Science? Lessons Learnt from the Development of the Land Use and Transport Model MARS.** *Transport Reviews* 2011, **31**:267–289.
15. Forrester JW: *Learning through system dynamics as preparation for the 21st century*. Keynote Address for Systems Thinking and Dynamic Modelling Conference for K-12 Education; 1994.
16. Albin S, Forrester JW, Breierova L: *Building a System Dynamics Model: Part 1: Conceptualization*. MIT; 2001.
17. Eden C: **Cognitive mapping and problem structuring for system dynamics model building.** *System dynamics review* 1994, **10**:257–276.
18. Größler A, Milling P: *Inductive and deductive system dynamics modeling*. The 2007 International Conference of the System Dynamics Society; 2007.
19. Grösser SN, Schaffernicht M: **Mental models of dynamic systems: taking stock and looking ahead.** *System dynamics review* 2012, **28**:46–68.
20. Brailsford S, Hilton N: In *A comparison of discrete event simulation and system dynamics for modelling health care systems*. Edited by Riley J. Glasgow, Scotland: Proceedings from ORAHS 2000; 2001:18–39.
21. Forrester JW, Senge PM: *Tests for building confidence in system dynamics models*. Cambridge: System Dynamics Group, Sloan School of Management, Massachusetts Institute of Technology; 1978.
22. Merrill JA, Deegan M, Wilson RV, Kaushal R, Fredericks K: **A system dynamics evaluation model: implementation of health information exchange for public health reporting.** *J Am Med Inform Assoc* 2013, **20**:e131–138.
23. Barlas Y: **Formal aspects of model validity and validation in system dynamics.** *System dynamics review* 1996, **12**:183–210.
24. Iran FDA: *Iran Annual Pharmaceutical Statistics*. Iran Annual Pharmaceutical Statistics; 2012.
25. HAI/WHO: *IR. Iran, Medicine prices, availability, affordability and price components*. Geneva: Essential Medicines and Pharmaceutical Policies Unit, World Health Organization, Regional Office for the Eastern Mediterranean; 2010.
26. UNFPA: *State of World Population 2012*. Washington, D.C.: UNFPA; 2012.
27. WHO: *Guidelines for ATC classification and DDD assignment*. Oslo: Norsk Medisinal depot; 1996.
28. Keshavarz K, Kebriaeezadeh A, Meshkini AH, Nikfar S, Mirian I, Khoonsari H: **Financial perspective of private pharmacies in Tehran (Iran); is it a lucrative business?** *DARU J of Pharm Sci* 2012, **20**:62.
29. Kebriaeezadeh A, Koopaei NN, Abdollahiasl A, Nikfar S, Mohamadi N: **Trend analysis of the pharmaceutical market in Iran; 1997–2010; policy implications for developing countries.** *DARU J Pharm Sci* 2013, **21**:52.
30. Abdollahiasl A, Nikfar S, Abdollahi M: **Pharmaceutical market and health system in the Middle Eastern and Central Asian countries: Time for innovations and changes in policies and actions.** *Arch Med Sci* 2011, **7**:365–367.
31. Jaberidoost M, Nikfar S, Abdollahiasl A, Dinarvand R: **Pharmaceutical supply chain risks: a systematic review.** *DARU J Pharm Sci* 2013, **12**.
32. Nassiri-Koopaei N, Majdzadeh R, Kebriaeezadeh A, Rashidian A, Yazdi MT, Nedjat S, Nikfar S: **Commercialization of biopharmaceutical knowledge in Iran; challenges and solutions.** *DARU J Pharm Sci* 2014, **22**:29.

Permissions

All chapters in this book were first published in DARU-JPS, by BioMed Central; hereby published with permission under the Creative Commons Attribution License or equivalent. Every chapter published in this book has been scrutinized by our experts. Their significance has been extensively debated. The topics covered herein carry significant findings which will fuel the growth of the discipline. They may even be implemented as practical applications or may be referred to as a beginning point for another development.

The contributors of this book come from diverse backgrounds, making this book a truly international effort. This book will bring forth new frontiers with its revolutionizing research information and detailed analysis of the nascent developments around the world.

We would like to thank all the contributing authors for lending their expertise to make the book truly unique. They have played a crucial role in the development of this book. Without their invaluable contributions this book wouldn't have been possible. They have made vital efforts to compile up to date information on the varied aspects of this subject to make this book a valuable addition to the collection of many professionals and students.

This book was conceptualized with the vision of imparting up-to-date information and advanced data in this field. To ensure the same, a matchless editorial board was set up. Every individual on the board went through rigorous rounds of assessment to prove their worth. After which they invested a large part of their time researching and compiling the most relevant data for our readers.

The editorial board has been involved in producing this book since its inception. They have spent rigorous hours researching and exploring the diverse topics which have resulted in the successful publishing of this book. They have passed on their knowledge of decades through this book. To expedite this challenging task, the publisher supported the team at every step. A small team of assistant editors was also appointed to further simplify the editing procedure and attain best results for the readers.

Apart from the editorial board, the designing team has also invested a significant amount of their time in understanding the subject and creating the most relevant covers. They scrutinized every image to scout for the most suitable representation of the subject and create an appropriate cover for the book.

The publishing team has been an ardent support to the editorial, designing and production team. Their endless efforts to recruit the best for this project, has resulted in the accomplishment of this book. They are a veteran in the field of academics and their pool of knowledge is as vast as their experience in printing. Their expertise and guidance has proved useful at every step. Their uncompromising quality standards have made this book an exceptional effort. Their encouragement from time to time has been an inspiration for everyone.

The publisher and the editorial board hope that this book will prove to be a valuable piece of knowledge for researchers, students, practitioners and scholars across the globe.

List of Contributors

Songa Ambedkar Sunil
A.U. College of Pharmaceutical Sciences, Andhra University, Visakhapatnam, 530003 India

Meka Venkata Srikanth
A.U. College of Pharmaceutical Sciences, Andhra University, Visakhapatnam, 530003 India

Nali Sreenivasa Rao
A.U. College of Pharmaceutical Sciences, Andhra University, Visakhapatnam, 530003 India

Vengaladasu Raju
A.U. College of Pharmaceutical Sciences, Andhra University, Visakhapatnam, 530003 India

Kolapalli Venkata Ramana Murthy
A.U. College of Pharmaceutical Sciences, Andhra University, Visakhapatnam, 530003 India

Mohamed S Pendekal
Department of Pharmaceutics, JSS College of Pharmacy, JSS University, SS Nagar, Mysore-15, Karnataka, India

Pramod K Tegginamat
Department of Pharmaceutics, JSS College of Pharmacy, JSS University, SS Nagar, Mysore-15, Karnataka, India

Farhad Etezadi
Sina Hospital, Tehran University of Medical Sciences, Hassan Abad sq, Tehran, Iran

Pejman Pourfakhr
Sina Hospital, Tehran University of Medical Sciences, Hassan Abad sq, Tehran, Iran

Mojtaba Mojtahedzade
Sina Hospital, Tehran University of Medical Sciences, Hassan Abad sq, Tehran, Iran

Atabak Najafi
Sina Hospital, Tehran University of Medical Sciences, Hassan Abad sq, Tehran, Iran

Reza Shariat Moharari
Sina Hospital, Tehran University of Medical Sciences, Hassan Abad sq, Tehran, Iran

Kourosh Karimi Yarandi
Sina Hospital, Tehran University of Medical Sciences, Hassan Abad sq, Tehran, Iran

Mohammad Reza Khajavi
Sina Hospital, Tehran University of Medical Sciences, Hassan Abad sq, Tehran, Iran

Taskina Ali
Department of Physiology, Bangabandhu Sheikh Mujib Medical University, Dhaka, Bangladesh
Department of Physiology, Faculty of Medical Sciences, Tarbiat Modares University, Tehran, Iran

Mohammad Javan
Department of Physiology, Faculty of Medical Sciences, Tarbiat Modares University, Tehran, Iran

Ali Sonboli
Department of Biology, Medicinal Plants and Drugs Research Institute, Shahid Beheshti University, Tehran, Iran

Saeed Semnanian
Department of Physiology, Faculty of Medical Sciences, Tarbiat Modares University, Tehran, Iran

AJ Rajamma
Department of Pharmacognosy, KLE University's College of Pharmacy, Bangalore 560010, India

HN Yogesha
Department of Pharmaceutics, Acharya & BM Reddy College of Pharmacy, Soladevanahally Hesaraghatta road, Bangalore 560090, India

SB Sateesha
Department of Pharmaceutics, Acharya & BM Reddy College of Pharmacy, Soladevanahally Hesaraghatta road, Bangalore 560090, India

Zahra Gharibnaseri
Department of Pharmacoeconomics and Pharmaceutical Administration, Faculty of Pharmacy, Tehran University of Medical Sciences, Tehran, Iran

Abbas Kebriaeezadeh
Department of Pharmacoeconomics and Pharmaceutical Administration, Faculty of Pharmacy, Tehran University of Medical Sciences, Tehran, Iran
Department of Toxicology and Pharmacology Faculty of Pharmacy, Tehran University of Medical Sciences, Tehran, Iran

Shekoufeh Nikfar
Department of Pharmacoeconomics and Pharmaceutical Administration, Faculty of Pharmacy, Tehran University of Medical Sciences, Tehran, Iran
Food and Drug Laboratory Research Center, Ministry of Health and Medical Education, Tehran, Iran

Gholamreza Zamani
Department of Pediatrics, Faculty of Medicine, Tehran University of Medical Sciences, Tehran, Iran

Akbar Abdollahiasl
Department of Pharmacoeconomics and Pharmaceutical Administration, Faculty of Pharmacy, Tehran University of Medical Sciences, Tehran, Iran

Farzaneh Nabati
Department of Medicinal Chemistry, Faculty of Pharmacy, Tehran University of Medical Sciences, Tehran, Iran

Faraz Mojab
Department of Pharmacognosy, School of Pharmacy, Shahid Beheshti University of Medical Sciences, Tehran, Iran

Mehran Habibi-Rezaei
School of Biology, College of Science, University of Tehran, Tehran, Iran

Kowsar Bagherzadeh
Department of Medicinal Chemistry, Faculty of Pharmacy, Tehran University of Medical Sciences, Tehran, Iran

Massoud Amanlou
Department of Medicinal Chemistry, Faculty of Pharmacy, Tehran University of Medical Sciences, Tehran, Iran
Medicinal Plants Research Center, Tehran University of Medical Sciences, Tehran, Iran

Behnam Yousefi
School of Advanced Medical Technologies, Tehran University of Medical Sciences, Tehran, Iran

Rezvan Zabihollahi
Hepatitis and AIDS department, Pasteur institute of Iran, Tehran, Iran

Elahe Motevaseli
School of Medicine, Tehran University of Medical Sciences (TUMS), Tehran, Iran

Seyed Mehdi Sadat
Hepatitis and AIDS department, Pasteur institute of Iran, Tehran, Iran

Ali Reza Azizi-Saraji
Hepatitis and AIDS department, Pasteur institute of Iran, Tehran, Iran

Sogol Asaadi-Dalaie
Hepatitis and AIDS department, Pasteur institute of Iran, Tehran, Iran

Mohammad Hossein Modarressi
School of Medicine, Tehran University of Medical Sciences (TUMS), Tehran, Iran

Puji Astuti
Pharmaceutical Biology Department, Faculty of Pharmacy, Universitas Gadjah Mada, Yogyakarta, Indonesia

Esti D Utami
Pharmacy Department, Faculty of Medicinal and Health Sciences, Universitas Jenderal Soedirman, Purwokerto, Indonesia

Arsa W Nugrahani
Sekolah Tinggi Ilmu Farmasi (STIFAR), Pharmacy Foundation, Semarang, Indonesia

Sismindari Sudjadi
Pharmaceutical Chemistry Department, Faculty of Pharmacy, Universitas Gadjah Mada, Yogyakarta, Indonesia

Fahimeh Moradi-Afrapoli
Department of Pharmacognosy, Faculty of Pharmacy, Tehran University of Medical Sciences, Tehran, Iran
Department of Pharmacognosy, Faculty of Pharmacy, Mazandaran University of Medical Sciences, Sari, Iran

Behavar Asghari
Department of Phytochemistry, Medicinal Plants and Drugs Research Institute, Shahid Beheshti University, Tehran, Iran

Soodabeh Saeidnia
Medicinal Plants Research Centre, Faculty of Pharmacy, Tehran University of Medical Sciences, Tehran, Iran

Yusef Ajani
Institute of Medicinal Plants, ACECR, Tehran, Iran

Mobina Mirjani
Department of Pharmacognosy, Faculty of Pharmacy, Tehran University of Medical Sciences, Tehran, Iran

Maryam Malmir
Medicinal Plants Research Centre, Faculty of Pharmacy, Tehran University of Medical Sciences, Tehran, Iran

Reza Dolatabadi Bazaz
Department of Medicinal Chemistry, Faculty of Pharmacy, Tehran University of Medical Sciences, Tehran, Iran

Abbas Hadjiakhoondi
Department of Pharmacognosy, Faculty of Pharmacy, Tehran University of Medical Sciences, Tehran, Iran
Medicinal Plants Research Centre, Faculty of Pharmacy, Tehran University of Medical Sciences, Tehran, Iran

Peyman Salehi
Department of Phytochemistry, Medicinal Plants and Drugs Research Institute, Shahid Beheshti University, Tehran, Iran

Mattias Hamburger
Department of Pharmaceutical Sciences, University of Basel, Basel, Switzerland

Narguess Yassa
Department of Pharmacognosy, Faculty of Pharmacy, Tehran University of Medical Sciences, Tehran, Iran
Medicinal Plants Research Centre, Faculty of Pharmacy, Tehran University of Medical Sciences, Tehran, Iran

Sha Sha Chu
Department of Entomology, China Agricultural University, Haidian District, Beijing 100193, China

Guo Hua Jiang
Analytic and Testing Center, Beijing Normal University, Haidian District, Beijing 100875, China

Zhi Long Liu
Department of Entomology, China Agricultural University, Haidian District, Beijing 100193, China

Mohammad Bayat
Department of Anatomy, School of Medicine, Tehran University of Medical Sciences, Tehran, Iran

Abolfazl Azami Tameh
Anatomical Sciences Research Center, Kashan University of Medical Sciences, Kashan, Iran

Mohammad Hossein Ghahremani
Department of Toxicology - Pharmacology, School of Pharmacy, Tehran University of Medical Sciences, Tehran, Iran

Mohammad Akbari
Department of Anatomy, School of Medicine, Tehran University of Medical Sciences, Tehran, Iran

Shahram Ejtemaei Mehr
Department of Pharmacology, School of Medicine, Tehran University of Medical Sciences, Tehran, Iran

Mahnaz Khanavi
Department of Pharmacognosy, School of Pharmacy, Tehran University of Medical Sciences, Tehran, Iran

Gholamreza Hassanzadeh
Department of Anatomy, School of Medicine, Tehran University of Medical Sciences, Tehran, Iran
Department of Neuroscience, School of Advanced Medical Technology, Tehran University of Medical Sciences, Tehran, Iran

Esmaeil Moazeni
Aerosol Research Laboratory, Department of Pharmaceutics, School of Pharmacy, Tehran University of Medical Sciences, Tehran, Iran

Kambiz Gilani
Aerosol Research Laboratory, Department of Pharmaceutics, School of Pharmacy, Tehran University of Medical Sciences, Tehran, Iran

Abdolhossein Rouholamini Najafabadi
Aerosol Research Laboratory, Department of Pharmaceutics, School of Pharmacy, Tehran University of Medical Sciences, Tehran, Iran

Mohamad reza Rouini
Department of Pharmaceutics, School of Pharmacy, Tehran University of Medical Sciences, Tehran, Iran

Nasir Mohajel
Aerosol Research Laboratory, Department of Pharmaceutics, School of Pharmacy, Tehran University of Medical Sciences, Tehran, Iran

Mohsen Amini
Department of Medicinal Chemistry, School of Pharmacy and Drug Design & Development Research Center, Tehran University of Medical Sciences, Tehran, Iran

Mohammad Ali Barghi
XRD Research Laboratory, School of Sciences, Tehran University, Tehran, Iran

Tamires Cardoso Lima
Department of Physiology, Federal University of Sergipe, CEP 49100-000, São Cristóvão, Sergipe, Brazil

Marcelo Mendonça Mota
Department of Physiology, Federal University of Sergipe, CEP 49100-000, São Cristóvão, Sergipe, Brazil

José Maria Barbosa-Filho
Laboratório de Tecnologia Farmacêutica, Federal University of Paraíba, Caixa Postal 5009, CEP 58051-970, João Pessoa, Paraíba, Brazil

Márcio Roberto Viana Dos Santos
Department of Physiology, Federal University of Sergipe, CEP 49100-000, São Cristóvão, Sergipe, Brazil

Damião Pergentino De Sousa
Department of Physiology, Federal University of Sergipe, CEP 49100-000, São Cristóvão, Sergipe, Brazil

Soodabeh Saeidnia
Medicinal Plants Research Center, Tehran University of Medical Sciences, P. O. Box 14155–6451, Tehran, Iran

Mitra Ghamarinia
Department of Chemistry, Faculty of Science, Golestan University, Gorgan, Iran

Ahmad R Gohari
Medicinal Plants Research Center, Tehran University of Medical Sciences, P. O. Box 14155–6451, Tehran, Iran
Medicinal Plants Research Center, Faculty of Pharmacy, Tehran University of Medical Sciences, PO Box 14155–6451, Tehran, Iran

Alireza Shakeri
Department of Chemistry, Faculty of Science, Golestan University, Gorgan, Iran

Sanjay Shah
Delhi Institute of Pharmaceutical Sciences & Research (Formerly College of Pharmacy), University of Delhi, Pushp Vihar, Sector III, New Delhi 110017, India

Sarika Madan
Delhi Institute of Pharmaceutical Sciences & Research (Formerly College of Pharmacy), University of Delhi, Pushp Vihar, Sector III, New Delhi 110017, India

SS Agrawal
Delhi Institute of Pharmaceutical Sciences & Research (Formerly College of Pharmacy), University of Delhi, Pushp Vihar, Sector III, New Delhi 110017, India

Alvala Ravi
G.Pulla Reddy College of Pharmacy, Mehdipatnam, Hyderabad 500 028, AP, India

Mallika Alvala
Birla Institute of Technology and Science, Pilani-Hyderabad Campus, Hyderabad 500 078, AP, India

Venkatesh Sama
G.Pulla Reddy College of Pharmacy, Mehdipatnam, Hyderabad 500 028, AP, India

Arunasree M Kalle
Department of Animal Sciences, School of Life Sciences, University of Hyderabad, Hyderabad 500046, India

Vamshi K Irlapati
Institute of Life Sciences, University of Hyderabad Campus, Hyderabad, AP 500 046, India

B Madhava Reddy
G.Pulla Reddy College of Pharmacy, Mehdipatnam, Hyderabad 500 028, AP, India

Rouzbeh Jahanbakhsh
Department of Pharmaceutics, Faculty of Pharmacy, Tehran University of Medical Sciences, Tehran 14174, Iran

Fatemeh Atyabi
Department of Pharmaceutics, Faculty of Pharmacy, Tehran University of Medical Sciences, Tehran 14174, Iran
Nanotechnology Research Centre, Faculty of Pharmacy, Tehran University of Medical Sciences, Tehran 14174, Iran

Saeed Shanehsazzadeh
Department of Biomedical Physics and Engineering, School of Medicine, Tehran University of Medical Sciences, Tehran, Iran

Zahra Sobhani
Department of Pharmaceutics, Faculty of Pharmacy, Tehran University of Medical Sciences, Tehran 14174, Iran

Mohsen Adeli
Department of Chemistry, Sharif University of Technology, Tehran, Iran
Department of Chemistry, Faculty of Science, Lorestan University, Khoramabad, Iran

Rassoul Dinarvand
Department of Pharmaceutics, Faculty of Pharmacy, Tehran University of Medical Sciences, Tehran 14174, Iran
Nanotechnology Research Centre, Faculty of Pharmacy, Tehran University of Medical Sciences, Tehran 14174, Iran

Dandigi M Panchaxari
Department of Pharmaceutics, KLEU's college of Pharmacy, Nehru Nagar, Belgaum, Karnataka 590010, India

Sowjanya Pampana
Department of Pharmaceutics, KLEU's college of Pharmacy, Nehru Nagar, Belgaum, Karnataka 590010, India

Tapas Pal
Research Scientist, R&D divison, Sparsha Pharma International Pvt. Ltd., Hyderabad, India

Bhavana Devabhaktuni
Research Scientist, R&D divison, Sparsha Pharma International Pvt. Ltd., Hyderabad, India

Anil Kumar Aravapalli
Department of Pharmaceutics, KLEU's college of Pharmacy, Nehru Nagar, Belgaum, Karnataka 590010, India

Anchal Sankhyan
Chitkara College of Pharmacy, Chitkara University, Chandigarh-Patiala Highway, Rajpura, Patiala, Punjab 140401, India

Pravin K Pawar
Chitkara College of Pharmacy, Chitkara University, Chandigarh-Patiala Highway, Rajpura, Patiala, Punjab 140401, India

Ketan Patel
Center for Novel Drug Delivery Systems, Department of Pharmaceutical Sciences and Technology, Institute of Chemical Technology, University under Section 3 of UGC Act – 1956, Elite Status and Center of Excellence – Govt. of Maharashtra, TEQIP Phase II Funded, N. P. Marg, Matunga (E), Mumbai 400 019, India

Vidur Sarma
Center for Novel Drug Delivery Systems, Department of Pharmaceutical Sciences and Technology, Institute of Chemical Technology, University under Section 3 of UGC Act – 1956, Elite Status and Center of Excellence – Govt. of Maharashtra, TEQIP Phase II Funded, N. P. Marg, Matunga (E), Mumbai 400 019, India

Pradeep Vavia
Center for Novel Drug Delivery Systems, Department of Pharmaceutical Sciences and Technology, Institute of Chemical Technology, University under Section 3 of UGC Act – 1956, Elite Status and Center of Excellence – Govt. of Maharashtra, TEQIP Phase II Funded, N. P. Marg, Matunga (E), Mumbai 400 019, India

Chao-an Su
Lishui Agricultural Academy of Sciences, Lishui, Zhejiang 32300, China

Xiao-yan Xu
Laboratory of Cellular and Molecular Biology, Sichuan Academy of Chinese Medicine Science, Chengdu 610041, China

De-yun Liu
Lishui Agricultural Academy of Sciences, Lishui, Zhejiang 32300, China

Ming Wu
Laboratory of Cellular and Molecular Biology, Sichuan Academy of Chinese Medicine Science, Chengdu 610041, China

Fan-qing Zeng
Lishui Agricultural Academy of Sciences, Lishui, Zhejiang 32300, China

Meng-yao Zeng
Laboratory of Cellular and Molecular Biology, Sichuan Academy of Chinese Medicine Science, Chengdu 610041, China

Wei Wei
Laboratory of Cellular and Molecular Biology, Sichuan Academy of Chinese Medicine Science, Chengdu 610041, China

Nan Jiang
Laboratory of Cellular and Molecular Biology, Sichuan Academy of Chinese Medicine Science, Chengdu 610041, China

Xia Luo
Laboratory of Cellular and Molecular Biology, Sichuan Academy of Chinese Medicine Science, Chengdu 610041, China

Azadeh Manayi
Department of Pharmacognosy, Faculty of Pharmacy, Tehran University of Medical Sciences, Tehran, Iran

Mahnaz Khanavi
Department of Pharmacognosy, Faculty of Pharmacy, Tehran University of Medical Sciences, Tehran, Iran Traditional Iranian Medicine and PharmacyResearch Center, Tehran University of Medical Sciences, Tehran, Iran

Soodabeh Saiednia
Medicinal Plants Research Center, Faculty of Pharmacy, Tehran University of Medical Sciences, Tehran, Iran

Ebrahim Azizi
Department of Pharmacology and Toxicology, Faculty of Pharmacy, Tehran University of Medical Sciences, Tehran, Iran

Mohammad Reza Mahmoodpour
Department of Pharmacognosy, Faculty of Pharmacy, Tehran University of Medical Sciences, Tehran, Iran

Fatemeh Vafi
Department of Pharmacognosy, Faculty of Pharmacy, Tehran University of Medical Sciences, Tehran, Iran

Maryam Malmir
Med.UL, Faculty of Pharmacy, University of Lisbon, Lisbon, Portugal

Farideh Siavashi
Microbiology Department, Faculty of Sciences, University of Tehran, Tehran, Iran

Abbas Hadjiakhoondi
Department of Pharmacognosy, Faculty of Pharmacy, Tehran University of Medical Sciences, Tehran, Iran
Medicinal Plants Research Center, Faculty of Pharmacy, Tehran University of Medical Sciences, Tehran, Iran

Maryam Hamzeloo Moghadam
Traditional Medicine and Materia Medica Research Center and Department of Traditional Pharmacy, School of Traditional Medicine, Shahid Beheshti University of Medical Sciences, Tehran, Iran

Jamileh Firouzi
Department of Marine Science and Technology, Science and Research Branch, Isalmic Azad University, Tehran, Iran

Soodabeh Saeidnia
Medicinal Plants Research Center, Faculty of Pharmacy, Tehran University of Medical Sciences, Tehran, Iran

Homa Hajimehdipoor
Traditional Medicine and Materia Medica Research Center and Department of Traditional Pharmacy, School of Traditional Medicine, Shahid Beheshti University of Medical Sciences, Tehran, Iran

Shahla Jamili
Department of Marine Biology, Science and Research Branch, Isalmic Azad University, Tehran, Iran

Abdolhossein Rustaiyan
Department of Chemistry, Science and Research Branch, Isalmic Azad University, Tehran, Iran

Ahmad R Gohari
Medicinal Plants Research Center, Faculty of Pharmacy, Tehran University of Medical Sciences, Tehran, Iran

Eun-Jin Yang
Jeju Biodiversity Research Institute (JBRI), Jeju Technopark, Jeju 699-943, Korea
Department of Chemistry, Cosmetic Science Center, Jeju National University, Jeju 690-756, Korea

Young Min Ham
Jeju Biodiversity Research Institute (JBRI), Jeju Technopark, Jeju 699-943, Korea

Wook Jae Lee
Jeju Biodiversity Research Institute (JBRI), Jeju Technopark, Jeju 699-943, Korea

Nam Ho Lee
Department of Chemistry, Cosmetic Science Center, Jeju National University, Jeju 690-756, Korea

Chang-Gu Hyun
Department of Chemistry, Cosmetic Science Center, Jeju National University, Jeju 690-756, Korea
LINC Agency, Jeju National University, Ara-1-dong, Jeju 690-756, Korea